PEDIATRIC EMERGENCY NURSING

PEDIATRIC EMERGENCY NURSING

Susan J. Kelley, R.N., M.S.
Assistant Professor
Maternal Child Health Graduate Program
School of Nursing
Boston College
Chestnut Hill, Massachusetts

APPLETON & LANGE
Norwalk, Connecticut/San Mateo, California

0-8385-7790-3

Notice: Our knowledge in clinical sciences is constantly changing. As new information becomes available, changes in treatment and in the use of drugs become necessary. The author(s) and the publisher of this volume have taken care to make certain that the doses of drugs and schedules of treatment are correct and compatible with the standards generally accepted at the time of publication. The reader is advised to consult carefully the instruction and information material included in the package insert of each drug or therapeutic agent before administration. This advice is especially important when using new or infrequently used drugs.

88 89 90 91 92 / 10 9 8 7 6 5 4 3 2 1

Prentice-Hall of Australia, Pty. Ltd., Sydney
Prentice-Hall Canada, Inc.
Prentice-Hall Hispanoamericana, S.A., Mexico
Prentice-Hall of India Private Limited, New Delhi
Prentice-Hall International (UK) Limited, London
Prentice-Hall of Japan, Inc., Tokyo
Prentice-Hall of Southeast Asia (Pte.) Ltd., Singapore
Whitehall Books Ltd., Wellington, New Zealand
Editora Prentice-Hall do Brasil Ltda., Rio de Janeiro

Kelley, Susan J.
    Pediatric emergency nursing / Susan J. Kelley.
        p.   cm.
    Includes bibliographies.
    ISBN 0-8385-7790-3
    1. Pediatric emergencies. 2. Emergency nursing. I. Title.
    [DNLM: 1. Emergencies—in infancy & childhood—nurses'
instruction. 2. Pediatric Nursing.   WY 159 K29p]
RJ370.K45   1988
618.92'0025—dc19

Production Editor: John Williams
Designer: Kathleen Peters Ceconi

PRINTED IN THE UNITED STATES OF AMERICA

To my husband Ron,
for your love and support

To my mother and father,
for your love, guidance, and
generosity throughout the years

Contributors

Martha A.Q. Curley, R.N., M.S.N., C.C.R.N.
Critical Care Clinical Nurse Specialist
Staff Development and Research
　Department
The Children's Hospital
Boston, Massachusetts

Sandra Dandrinos-Smith, R.N., M.Ed.
Staff Educator
Department of Nursing
New England Medical Center Hospitals
Boston, Massachusetts

Ruth A. Fisk, R.N., M.S., C.P.N.P.
Clinical Services Manager
New England Health Resources
Boston, Massachusetts

Nancy Sullivan Flint, R.N., M.S.
Practitioner–Teacher
Department of Pediatric Nursing
Rush–Presbyterian–St. Luke's
　Medical Center
Chicago, Illinois

Linda S. Goodale, R.N.C., M.S.
Assistant Director of Nursing
Pediatrics
Boston City Hospital
Boston, Massachusetts

Elena Hopkins-Lotz, R.N., M.S., P.N.P.
Clinic Nurse Manager
Pediatrics, Martha Elliot Clinic
The Children's Hospital
Boston, Massachusetts

Susan J. Kelley, R.N., M.S.
Assistant Professor
Maternal Child Health Graduate Program
School of Nursing
Boston College
Chestnut Hill, Massachusetts

Catherine Kneut, R.N., M.S.
Clinical Nurse Specialist–Pediatrics
Nursing Education and Research
Rhode Island Hospital
Providence, Rhode Island

Wendy J. Liston, R.N., M.S.
Former Instructor
School of Nursing
Boston College
Chestnut Hill, Massachusetts

Martha C. Miller, R.N.
Manager, Clinical Programs
Clinical Research Department
Richards Medical Company
Memphis, Tennessee

Sarah B. Pasternack, R.N., M.A.
Nurse Manager
The Children's Hospital
Boston, Massachusetts

Anne Phelan, R.N., M.S.
Staff Nurse Level II and
　Trauma Coordinator
Emergency Department
The Children's Hospital
Boston, Massachusetts

Carole T. Roberts, R.N., M.S.
Adjunct Instructor
School of Nursing
Boston College
Chestnut Hill, Massachusetts

Kathleen Rourke, R.N.C., B.S.N.
Nurse Practitioner
Department of Orthopaedics
Harvard Community Health Plan
Boston, Massachusetts

**Maureen Ellis Schnider, R.N.,
    M.S., C.S.**
Psychiatric Nursing Clinical Specialist
Department of Psychiatric Nursing
Boston City Hospital
Boston, Massachusetts

Arlene M. Sperhac, R.N., Ph.D.
Former Associate Professor
School of Nursing
Boston College
Chestnut Hill, Massachusetts

Contents

Preface

As emergency nursing practice has advanced in the 1980s, the need for increased knowledge related to pediatric emergencies has become evident. Existing emergency nursing texts tend to relegate pediatric emergencies to a single chapter or to several brief sections, while pediatric nursing texts are primarily concerned with the care of hospitalized children and rarely address initial emergency care. As a result, the specialized knowledge needed by emergency nurses caring for pediatric patients has not been readily available in a single source. In an attempt to meet this need, *Pediatric Emergency Nursing* focuses on the initial phase of emergency nursing management of the critically ill or injured child. It provides comprehensive information on the nursing management of emergent and urgent pediatric conditions as well as some common nonemergent problems.

Pediatric Emergency Nursing was written for emergency nurses practicing within a variety of settings including emergency departments that treat both children and adults, pediatric emergency departments, and the prehospital setting. It also serves as a reference for nurses practicing in any situation in which an acutely ill or injured child may be encountered, such as the ambulatory care, school health, or community setting.

Pediatric Emergency Nursing has been written from the perspective that nursing expertise is essential to the successful management of the acutely ill or injured child in the emergency department. Each chapter provides a comprehensive approach to the nursing care of the child and family. Topics are organized within a nursing process framework that includes the assessment, intervention, and evaluation of the pediatric emergency client. Nursing Care Guides are provided in each chapter to summarize nursing care and to assist in the formulation of nursing diagnoses. The nursing diagnoses used were selected from the 72 nursing diagnoses approved to date by the North American Nursing Diagnosis Association.

Principles of child development are integrated throughout the text. The emotional and educational needs of the child and family are emphasized, with the viewpoint that the client includes not only the child but also family members.

Topics are organized into three major areas: psychosocial emergencies, multisystem emergencies, and emergencies that primarily involve individual systems. Psychosocial emergencies such as child abuse, sexual assault, depression, suicide, psychosis, acute grief reactions, and sudden infant death syndrome are discussed in the first four chapters. Emergencies that are life-threatening and that involve multiple systems are presented in the next five chapters. These include in-depth discussions of resuscitation of the newborn, cardiopulmonary resuscitation of infants and children, multiple trauma, burns, and poisonings. The remaining 13 chapters are organized according to the system most affected by the illness or injury.

Because of space limitations, every pediatric problem that could be encountered in the emergency setting was not included; that amount of information would fill several volumes. Instead, topics were selected according to their significance and prevalence in the emergency setting. Some topics, because of their importance, are intentionally covered in more depth than others.

Extensive use of tables throughout the text facilitates access to vital information. The numerous illustrations enhance the reader's understanding of pediatric disease processes, injuries, and nursing interventions. In addition to reference citations, bibliographies are provided in each chapter for readers who may choose to research a topic further. The appendices include discharge instructions for parents for a variety of pediatric illnesses and injuries. Normal pediatric laboratory values, growth charts, and recommended immunization schedules are also included in the appendices.

Pediatric Emergency Nursing is designed to help nurses combine their clinical experience with a current reference source. Most importantly, it is hoped that *Pediatric Emergency Nursing* will contribute to the improved emergency nursing care of infants, children, and their families.

Acknowledgments

The completion of this book was made possible by the support and work of many dedicated individuals. I am especially grateful to the contributing authors who were willing to share their clinical expertise and to give so generously of their time, despite their busy schedules.

I would like to express my appreciation to the following individuals who helped make this book possible: Lorna Bernhard Grazio, R.N., B.S., for providing several of the drawings by sexually abused children; Mary McClain, R.N., M.S., for her willingness to share the SIDS checklist and form; Barton B. Schmitt, M.D., for permission to reproduce the photographs found in Chapter 1; and Richard DeNise, M.D., for the radiographs used in the respiratory and gastrointestinal chapters.

I would also like to acknowledge Yoshio Saito, Director of the Boston College Audiovisual Department, and his staff for their assistance in the preparation of art work. I am especially grateful to Judy Sweeney and Ann DuPuis for their excellent word processing skills and patience with multiple manuscript revisions.

My sincere gratitude goes to the staff of Appleton & Lange, especially Stuart Horton, Nursing Editor, and John Williams, Production Editor, for their cooperation, guidance, and dedication throughout this lengthy project.

Most importantly, I would like to extend my warmest appreciation to my husband Ronald Verni, who provided the love, support, and computer assistance that allowed me to complete this book.

1 | Child Abuse and Neglect

Susan J. Kelley

Child abuse and neglect are significant social and health problems in the United States. The emergency department nurse must keep an open mind to the fact that child abuse occurs frequently. Although child abuse has existed for centuries, its comprehensive identification and treatment is a relatively recent development. In 1962 Dr. C. Henry Kempe introduced the concept of "battered child syndrome." Not until 1967, however, had all states passed child abuse laws.

Estimates of the actual scope of the problem have been difficult to ascertain for several reasons. First, definitions of child maltreatment vary greatly across jurisdictions and among various professional disciplines. Second, cases of child maltreatment that are reported to child protective services may represent only the "tip of the iceberg." It is difficult to estimate how many cases remain unidentified and therefore unreported to officials.

The National Incidence study conducted by the National Center on Child Abuse and Neglect was the first national study of child abuse and neglect to use common and consistent definitions in their data collection. Data were collected from 26 sample counties in ten states to project national estimates of the incidence and severity of child abuse and neglect. The National Incidence study is considered to be a milestone in research on child abuse and neglect.[1]

The National Incidence study projects that at least 652,000 children are abused or neglected annually in the United States. The incidence rate is 10.5 children per 1000, or 1.5 percent of children under the age of 18 years. The National Incidence study acknowledges that these figures are conservative. The report states that very likely the actual number of children abused and neglected annually in the United States is at least 1 million.

The National Incidence study's estimates of the age distribution of maltreated children has important implications for emergency department nursing. Although substantial numbers of children of all ages are involved, the maltreatment incidence rate of adolescents is more than twice the rate for preschool children. The maltreatment incidence rate for elementary school-aged children was also found to be nearly twice the rate of preschool children. When the severity of the injury or impairment related to abuse is examined, however, preschool children sustain a disproportionately high rate of 74 percent of the fatalities. These statistics indicate that although the incidence rate for maltreatment increases with age, the younger age groups appear to be at a greater risk for severe injury and impairment.

Important factors were identified in relationship to sex distribution. Although the incidence rates for males and females were virtually identical when all forms of maltreatment were considered, several differences between the groups were identi-

1

fied. The incidence rate for physical abuse of males decreases with age above the 3- to 5-year age group. Adolescent females are more likely to experience all forms of abuse compared to their male counterparts. The incidence rate of sexual abuse is highest among adolescent females, but half of the female victims are in the younger age groups.

THEORETICAL FRAMEWORKS

Various theoretical frameworks have been attempted to explain the complex phenomena of child abuse. While the majority of models have focused on parental and family dysfunction, other models incorporate environmental influences.

The mental illness, or psychiatric model, was one of the first frameworks from which child abuse was viewed. The basic premise of this model is that factors within the individual abuser are responsible for the abuse. The psychiatric model theorizes that parents who abuse their children are psychiatrically disturbed.[2] According to this model, the alleviation of the problem therefore lies with treating the abusive parent rather than changing social conditions or the victim's behavior. This model is rather limited in scope. Although some parents who abuse their children may be psychiatrically disturbed, the majority are not. Helfer and Kempe estimate that less than 10 percent of parents who abuse their children are psychiatrically disturbed.[3]

When a psychologic disturbance is observed in the abuser, it is often what is referred to as role reversal. Role reversal is characterized by a distorted perception of child development on the part of the abusive parent.[4] In these situations the abusive parents have many unmet emotional needs. Such parents often expect to be cared for and nurtured by the child rather than to view the child as the dependent member of the family.

The theoretical model offered by Helfer and Kempe combines both social and psychologic variables in explaining the etiology of child maltreatment. According to this psychosocial model, three factors must be present for child maltreatment to occur: (1) a special parent, (2) a special child, and (3) stress. Characteristics that make a parent special are low self-esteem, unrealistic expectations of the child, inadequate parenting skills, and unmet emotional needs. Attributes that are thought to make the child special include prematurity, chronic illness, or a physical handicap. Stress, the third variable necessary, may be present either acutely or chronically. The quantity and quality of the stress can vary.[5]

This framework is more comprehensive than the psychiatric model because it incorporates two additional components: the child's attributes and parental or environmental stress. Certain characteristics in the child, such as prematurity, mental retardation, physical handicaps, and congenital malformations, have been identified as overrepresented in cases of child abuse.[6] The relationship between child abuse and stress is clearly supported when examining the influence of poverty upon child abuse. Although child abuse can be found in all income groups, children from low income families are much more likely to suffer maltreatment than are children from other income groups.[7]

The environmental stress model or sociologic model attributes child maltreatment to forces within society. This model focuses on the high level of violence in our society and the belief that when families are prone to stress, violence is likely to result. Our society is viewed as violent and one in which corporal punishment and physical violence against children is generally condoned. Straus et al[8] report that 70 percent of Americans view spanking and slapping children as normal and necessary. Stress is viewed as a factor necessary for abuse to occur. The stress may be acute or chronic and can include poverty, social isolation, and family or marital discord.

Social learning theory has also been used to explain the violence and aggression involved in child abuse. Social learning theory hypothesizes that aggression and violence are learned rather than instinctive.[9] According to social learning theory, violent behavior is learned within the family and is transmitted from generation to generation. Aggression can be learned through both direct and vicarious experiences. According to Straus, each generation learns to be violent by being a participant in a violent family.[10]

Child maltreatment has also been viewed within the model of the ecology of human development. According to this model, child abuse and neglect are created by a confluence of forces that lead to a pathologic adaptation by caregivers and, to a lesser extent, the child. Parents, children, and their environment are seen as complementing each other in cases of child abuse.[11,12]

The human ecology model incorporates concepts from some of the various models previously described. Child maltreatment is conceptualized as a social-psychologic phenomenon that is determined by multiple forces at work in the individual (otogenic development), family (microsystem), community (exosystem), and the culture (macrosystem). Cultural support for the use of physical force against children and the inadequate use of family support systems are identified as necessary conditions for child maltreatment. The ecologic model is the most encompassing of the various theoretical frameworks currently available.

PARENTAL CHARACTERISTICS

It is important to keep in mind that all parents possess the potential to abuse their children. Only approximately 10 percent of child abusers have a past history of psychiatric disorders. Many factors contribute to the reason a parent abuses a child, including a combination of individual, familial, and societal factors. Stress factors, such as economic difficulty, crowded or inadequate housing, and unemployment, often contribute to the parent's abusive potential. Parenting factors that often contribute include unrealistic expectations of the child, lack of preparation in parenting, and poor role models. Psychologic factors may include poor impulse control, substance abuse, and depression. Abusive parents are often socially isolated without adequate social support from extended family members or friends.

Another major factor is the type of parenting one received as a child. Many abusive parents were abused as children, and these parents relate to their child as their parents related to them—through physical or emotional abuse. Since everyone to some degree internalizes the way they were raised, it is important to keep in mind that abusive parents have unmet emotional needs. They are therefore unable to meet their child's basic emotional needs. To make matters worse, they look to the child to meet their own emotional needs and are often disappointed. Table 1–1 summarizes the characteristics of abusive parents.

IMPACT OF CHILD ABUSE AND NEGLECT

Many studies have attempted to identify the impact of abuse. Research on the developmental sequelae of child maltreat-

TABLE 1-1. CHARACTERISTICS OF ABUSIVE PARENTS

Low self-esteem
Social isolation
Unrealistic expectations of their child
Unmet emotional needs
Role reversal
Substance abuse
Multiple stressors

ment indicates that various areas of a child's development are adversely affected. Research findings indicate that abuse and neglect effects the intellectual, emotional, and social development of the child.

Studies that have examined intelligence performance of abused children indicate that mental retardation is more prevalent in this population.[13-17] It is difficult to determine, however, whether mental retardation antedates child abuse and therefore places the child at risk or is one of its effects. To answer this question several related factors must be further examined. First, the intelligence of the parents and siblings of mentally deficient abused children must be considered. Second, the intrauterine environment of the mentally deficient abused child must be carefully evaluated as a possible cause of mental retardation. Abuse prior to the birth of the child, in the form of drug and alcohol abuse or inflicted physical injury due to battering, must be considered. Various types of neglect, such as poor nutrition and lack of prenatal care during pregnancy, are other possible contributors to developmental delays. Child maltreatment often precedes the birth of the child.

In addition to effecting intelligence performance, research findings have indicated that abuse and neglect also effect the emotional and social development of the child.[18-20] The association between child maltreatment and adverse developmental outcomes has therefore been established. Longitudinal studies must be conducted, however, to prospectively examine parent-child relationships and subsequent developmental sequelae over longer periods of time, beginning in the first trimester of pregnancy.

Nurses must be knowledgeable about all possible indicators of abuse and neglect, especially those that are manifested before a child suffers a serious injury, emotional impairment, or developmental delay. Early recognition and intervention are the key to prevention of subsequent abuse.

TYPES OF CHILD MALTREATMENT

When at any time in a child's life his physical or emotional needs are not met or trauma is inflicted, the child is a victim of maltreatment.

The four basic categories of child maltreatment are (1) physical abuse, (2) neglect, (3) emotional abuse, and (4) sexual abuse. (Sexual abuse of children will be discussed separately in the chapter to follow.)

Physical Abuse

The physical abuse of children is defined as any inflicted injury by the parent or caretaker. This includes injuries that are intentional as well as those that are the result of a parent losing control. Physical abuse may be the result of corporal punishment. Parents who ''overdiscipline'' their children often have good intentions, and the abuse may take place while they are attempting to ''teach the child a lesson'' and to change what they perceive as unacceptable or ''bad'' behavior.

Parents' unrealistic expectations of their children is one problem that can lead to abuse. This is the direct result of parents' lack of knowledge and understanding of normal or age-appropriate behavior. For instance, some parents actually believe that their infant cries only for attention or to annoy them.

History. Identification of inflicted injuries is often difficult, since children possess an amazing ability to injure themselves in limitless ways. To distinguish between accidental and nonaccidental injuries, the nurse must first elicit a careful history from the parent (and child when possible) and then compare the explanation to the existing injury. If a discrepancy exists between the parents' account of the mechanism of injury and the physical findings, abuse should be suspected. Another important factor to determine is the distance of the home from the hospital where they seek care. If the parents travel great distances to the treatment facility, bypassing closer hospitals, they may be trying to avoid detection. Abusive parents also seek care at many different treatment facilities to prevent being identified as abusers.

Knowledge of normal growth and development is important in assessing possible cases of abuse. For instance, if the mother of a 1-month-old infant with a skull fracture states that the baby rolled over in the crib and fell out onto the floor, abuse should be suspected because infants are not capable of rolling over until 3 to 5 months of age. Likewise, nonaccidental fractures of the limbs are unusual in infants who have not yet learned to walk. Table 1-2 summarizes the characteristics of histories that should alert the nurse to the possibility of child abuse.

Assessment

Physical Indicators. A complete physical assessment should be conducted on all children in whom child abuse or neglect is suspected. Table 1-3 summarizes the indicators of physical abuse.

TABLE 1-2. CHARACTERISTICS IN THE HISTORY OF CHILD ABUSE

History given by parent is inconsistent with existing injury
Absence of any history or explanation for injury
Parent reluctant to give information
Child is developmentally incapable of specified self-injury
Delay in seeking medical care
Inconsistencies or changes in the history
History of repeated injuries or hospitalizations
Inappropriate response to severity of injury

BRUISES. Bruises are the most common manifestation of physical abuse. Normal active children may have bruises and a few traumatic scars, especially on their chin, knees, elbows, and forehead. Bruises on the buttocks (Fig. 1-1), perineum, trunk, back of legs, head (Fig. 1-2), neck (Fig. 1-3), or genitals (Figs. 1-4, and 1-5) may indicate abuse, however.[21]

Bruises or welts in the configuration of objects frequently used to strike chil-

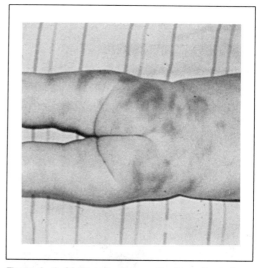

Figure 1-1. Multiple bruises on the lower back, buttocks, and thighs of a young child beaten with a paddle. Bruises in these locations indicate physical punishment. *(Figures 1-1 through 1-19 are courtesy of Barton D. Schmitt, M.D., The Children's Hospital, Denver.)*

TABLE 1–3. CLINICAL INDICATORS OF PHYSICAL ABUSE

Bruises
  In various states of healing
  In configuration of object used to strike child
  Located on face, thighs, genitals, back
Burns
  Submersion burns
  Cigarette burns
  In configuration of heating object
  Circumferential rope burns to wrist, ankles, torso
  Scald burns
Human bite marks
Head trauma
  Skull fractures
  Subdural hematomas
  Separation of sutures due to chronic subdural
    hematoma
  Subgaleal hematoma
	Ocular manifestations
	  Hyphema
	  Retinal detachment
	  Intraocular hemorrhage
	  Subconjunctival bleeding
	Neck trauma
	  Subluxation or dislocation due to shaking
	Fractures
	  Multiple fractures in various stages of healing
	  Spiral fractures (forcible twisting)
	  Transverse fractures (blunt trauma)
	  Rib fractures
	  Fragmentation at the epiphysis
	Blunt abdominal trauma
	  Often leaves little external evidence
	  Peritoneal or mesenteric bleeding
	  Persistent vomiting or abdominal pain
	  Hypovolemic shock
	  Injury to liver, spleen, pancreas, duodenum,
	    jejunum, kidneys

dren indicate abuse. These configurations include the characteristic "loop" mark from an extension cord (Fig. 1–6), linear mark from a belt or strap (Fig. 1–7), and wooden spoon, buckle, or hand print (Fig. 1–8).

Bruises in various stages of healing should be considered suspicious (Fig. 1–9). It is important to compare the reported date of injury to the age of the existing bruise(s) and to be alert for discrepancies. Table 1–4 provides a general guide for esti-

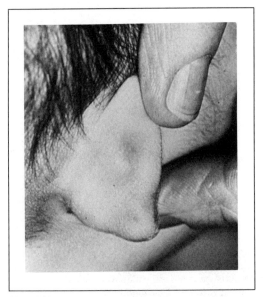

Figure 1–2. Inflicted bruise mark behind the ear that was the result of the child being pulled by the ear.

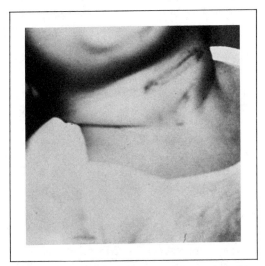

Figure 1–3. Fourteen-month-old who was choked by his stepfather. Bruises or cuts on the neck such as these are usually from a choking or strangling attempt.

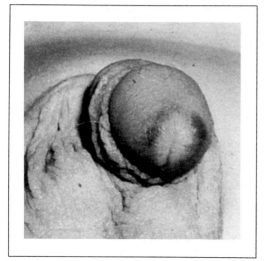

Figure 1–4. A pinch-mark bruise on the end of the penis caused by fingernails. Note the two small crescent-shaped bruises that face each other. This injury was inflicted when the child was punished for touching his penis.

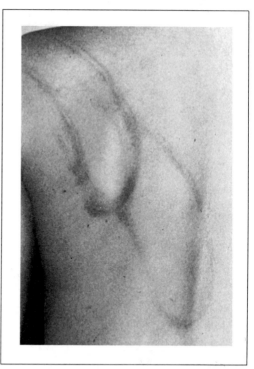

Figure 1–6. Bruises in this configuration are referred to as loop marks and are the result of being struck with a doubled-over extension cord, lamp cord, or rope.

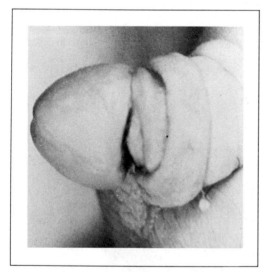

Figure 1–5. Fifteen-month-old male with deep groove to the penis from having it repeatedly tied off with a string. The child's father claimed he was using this method to keep his son's diapers dry.

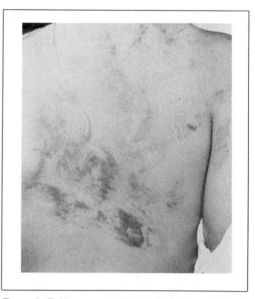

Figure 1–7. Numerous belt-mark bruises on the back and upper arm of an abused school-aged female.

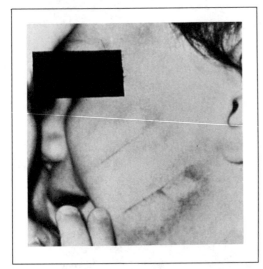

Figure 1-8. Fresh bruising on the cheek from a slap across the child's face. The configuration of the bruise indicates the child was struck from the front.

TABLE 1-4. GENERAL GUIDE TO ESTIMATION OF AGE OF BRUISES

Color	Age
Reddish purple	14 to 48 hr
Dark purple	1 to 4 days
Greenish yellow	5 to 7 days
Brownish yellow	7 to 10 days

mating the age of bruises. If a history of easy bruising is given, a prothrombin time (PT), partial thromboplastin time (PTT), and platelet count should be obtained.

BURNS. Inflicted burns are involved in 5 to 10 percent of substantiated cases of child abuse. In two thirds of these cases the child is under 3 years of age.[22] Children who repeatedly come to the emergency department with burns should be carefully evaluated for abuse.

Burns intentionally inflicted often leave identifiable patterns on the skin.

Figure 1-9. Multiple inflicted bruises on the child's lower abdomen, groin, and genitals in various stages of healing.

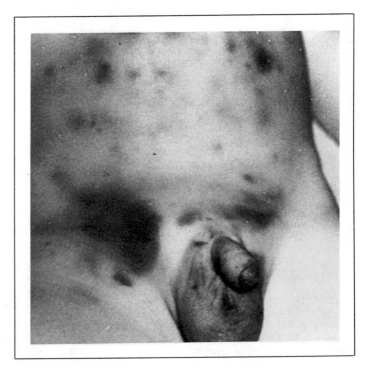

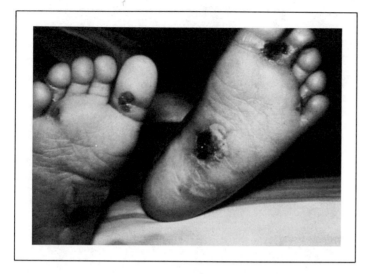

Figure 1-10. Inflicted cigarette burns on the soles of a child's feet.

Round cigarette or cigar burns are often found on the soles of the feet, palms of the hands, buttocks, torso, or other locations where the lesions would normally be concealed. When a cigarette burn is inflicted, the burn is usually 8 to 10 mm in diameter and is indurated at the margins (Fig. 1-10).

Tap water scald burns often have non-accidental injury as their etiology. Scald burns can be the result of the child being submerged in very hot water. Inflicted immersion burns often appear ''sock-like'' on the feet (Fig. 1-11), ''glove-like'' on the hands, and ''donut-like'' on the buttocks (Fig. 1-12) or genitalia. The extent of the submersion burn will depend on the temperature of the water, duration of exposure, and presence of clothing. Water tem-

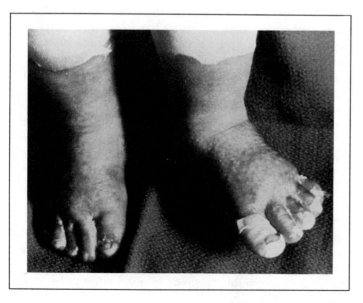

Figure 1-11. Forced immersion burns of both legs in a toddler.

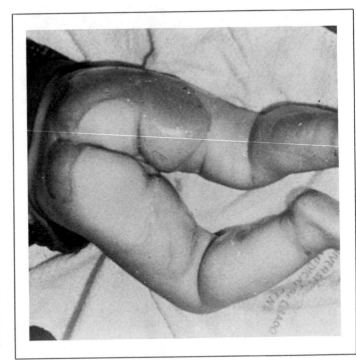

Figure 1–12. Child forced to sit in scalding hot water, resulting in a donut-shaped burn to the buttocks and legs. The unburned skin is the result of the child being forcibly held down against the bottom of the tub and spared prolonged contact in that area by the hot water.

peratures of 130F (54C) or higher can cause a full thickness burn in less than 30 seconds. The presence of clothing tends to cause more severe burns because there is longer contact with the skin. Accidental hot water burns are usually not as clearly demarcated on the edges as inflicted immersion burns. Inflicted immersion burns are often symmetrical, whereas accidental burns are usually asymmetrical. Inflicted burns tend to be full thickness, whereas the accidental burns are often partial thickness.[23,24]

A dry burn in the pattern of a heating object such as an iron, electric stove burner, hot plate, curling iron, or radiator is often inflicted (Fig. 1–13). Toddlers in the process of being toilet trained have been known to be placed on radiators to dry their wet diapers, with resultant burns to the buttocks. Suspicions should be raised when treatment of a child's burns

are delayed over 24 hours or the parent who was not home at the time of the "accident" brings the child to the emergency department.

Children who have been bound or "tied up" may have circumferential rope burns or tissue necrosis at the wrists, ankles (Fig. 1–14), knees, neck, and torso. Suspicious marks may also be observed at the corners of the mouth or sides of the face as the result of a child being gagged. A gag leaves down-turned lesions at the corner of the mouth. Abused infants and young children are often gagged or have clothes or objects stuffed in their mouths to stop their crying.

OTHER CUTANEOUS LESIONS. Human bites should always be considered suspicious. Human bite marks should be measured to determine if they were inflicted by an adult or child. Human bite marks appear

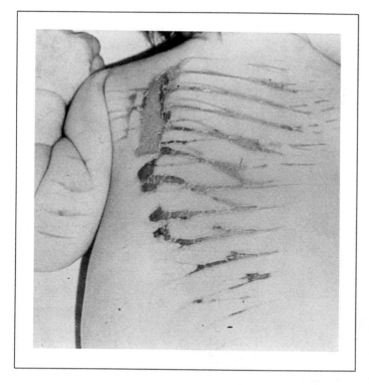

Figure 1-13. This 2-month-old has dry burns to his back and arms that were the result of being forcibly held against a hot grate.

as circular lesions 1½ to 2 inches in diameter. Adult-sized human bite marks indicate abuse (Fig. 1-15). A torn frenulum may be the result of an infant having a bottle forced into the mouth (Fig. 1-16).

Areas of baldness or swelling of the scalp may be the result of pulling the child by the hair. This is often referred to as traction or traumatic alopecia. In this type of alopecia the scalp is clear, unlike the scalp

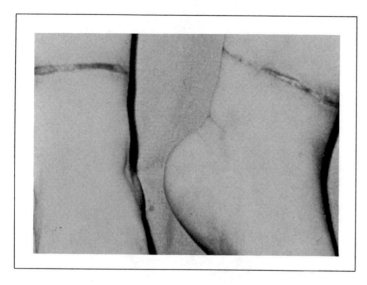

Figure 1-14. Rope marks on the ankles of a child who was tied to a bed with narrow rope on several occasions while his mother went out for the evening.

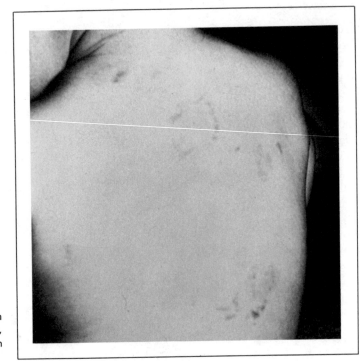

Figure 1–15. Human bite marks on this boy's back have the distinctive, paired, crescent-shaped bruises from teeth marks.

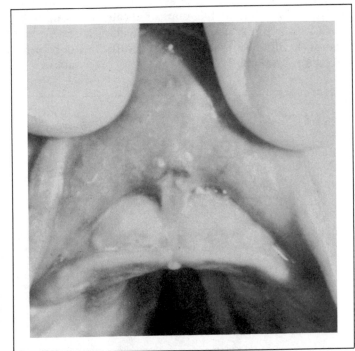

Figure 1–16. Five-month-old infant with torn upper frenulum of 1 to 2 days duration. This type of injury is caused by forced feeding with a bottle, often in an effort to quiet a crying infant. Bruises and tears to the upper lip may remain hidden unless the lip is everted and carefully examined.

in scalp infection or eczema. Broken hair often remains in cases of traction alopecia.[25]

FRACTURES. The skeletal system is commonly traumatized when children are maltreated. Fractures and dislocations that are inconsistent with the history of the mechanism injury are highly suspect, especially in children under the age of 2. Dislocations of the shoulder and elbow are often the result of pulling the child roughly by the arm. Resultant dislocations of the elbow are often referred to as "handmaiden's elbow." Spiral fractures of the long bones are often the result of an intentional twisting of the extremity by a caretaker. Spiral fractures are always considered suspicious. Multiple fractures in various stages of healing, especially involving the epiphyses and metaphyses, indicate repetitive abuse. Multiple fractures are often seen in the ribs, skull, and extremities. Fragmentation at the epiphysis may be the result of vigorous shaking of a young child. Fractures of the humerus, skull, nose, or facial structures are frequently the result of abuse. The possibility that multiple fractures are related to an underlying disease process such as osteogenesis imperfecta, scurvy, syphilis, rickets, neoplasm, or osteomyelitis should be considered. The presence of these rare disorders can be ruled out by the appropriate diagnostic procedures.

HEAD INJURIES. Inflicted head injury is a major cause of death and disability in abused children. Inflicted head injuries may be the result of direct trauma or vigorous shaking. Subdural hematomas in children may be the result of abusive treatment, such as direct trauma to the head from being struck, thrown, dropped, or even shaken severely. Shaking a child can result in the tearing of fragile cerebral veins resulting in lethal intracranial bleeding. Most children

showing evidence of cerebral injury have soft tissue swelling or a skull fracture. Some children with acute brain damage, however, have negative skull films and no cutaneous evidence of a blow to the head. In these cases a computerized axial tomography scan (CAT scan) may show evidence of brain hemorrhage.[26]

Repeated minor injuries due to shaking an infant or child may result in cumulative brain damage manifested as mental retardation or seizure disorders.[27] The infant's weak neck muscles and disproportionately large head predispose them to whiplash.[28] Additional evidence of a shaking injury may be provided by the evidence of intraocular hemorrhage and grip marks on the upper arms or shoulders (Fig. 1–17).

EYE INJURIES. Eye or orbital injuries are common in child abuse. There may or may not be external evidence of trauma. Pathology may include periorbital hematomas, fractures of the orbital or facial bones, subconjunctival hemorrhage, dislocated lens, retinal detachment, retinal hemorrhage,

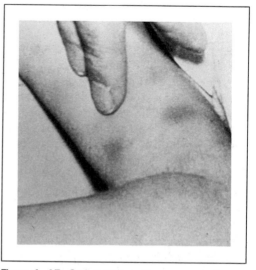

Figure 1–17. Grab marks on the upper arm from a child being forcibly held during a violent shaking.

hyphema, corneal abrasion, and optic atrophy. Funduscopic examination is therefore essential in suspected cases of child abuse.[29]

EAR INJURIES. The external ear may show evidence of contusions. Ecchymosis on the internal surface of the pinna may be the result of "boxing" the ear and crushing it against the skull. A direct blow to the ear may also cause hemotympanum and perforation of the tympanic membrane. The presence of discoloration behind the ear (Battle's sign) may be a further indication of a basilar skull fracture.[30]

ABDOMINAL TRAUMA. Abdominal injuries in childhood rank second only to head trauma as the leading cause of death in child abuse.[31] Blunt abdominal trauma, the result of punching or kicking a child in the abdomen, may lead to intra-abdominal hemorrhage with little external sign of trauma. Generally the blow is to the mid-abdomen. The child may have persistent vomiting, abdominal pain, or even hypovolemic shock. Internal organs that may be injured by blunt trauma include the pancreas, duodenum, jejunum, mesentery, liver, spleen, and kidneys.

The high mortality rate resulting from these injuries may be due to exsanguinating intra-abdominal hemorrhage, a delay in seeking medical attention, or failure of emergency personnel to make the correct diagnosis when life-threatening surgery is still possible.[32] Severe internal injuries may not be immediately detected due to the parent's failure to give an accurate history of trauma and little or no external evidence of abdominal trauma being present at the time of examination.

Munchausen's Syndrome by Proxy. Munchausen's syndrome by proxy is a form of child abuse in which a parent or caregiver fabricates an illness or injury in a child.

The syndrome was named after Baron Von Munchausen, an eighteenth century storyteller who entertained people with fabricated stories. The term Munchausen's syndrome was first given to adults who fabricated illness with false medical histories and altered laboratory and physical findings. Later the term Munchausen's syndrome by proxy was used to describe cases in which parents fabricate a medical disorder in their child.[33]

The child victims of Munchausen's syndrome by proxy usually range in age from infancy to 10 years. The older child may aid in his or her parents' deceptions to protect them or because of intense fear of retribution by the abusive parents. False histories given by parents often include seizures, apnea, cardiopulmonary arrest, hematuria, and hematemesis. Parents may induce physical findings in their children by suffocation, administration of drugs or toxic substances, or placing their own blood in the child's urine, vomitus, or stool specimens.

Most reported cases of Munchausen's syndrome by proxy involve the child's mother. Often the mother has Munchausen's syndrome with the same physical complaints as her child. In many reported cases the mother has had some nursing or medical training and is adept at making falsified information appear credible. The mother often appears genuinely concerned over her child's illness.

Clinical indicators of Munchausen's syndrome by proxy are summarized in Table 1–5.

Behavioral Indicators of Physical Abuse. A wide range of behavior is exhibited by physically abused children. These behaviors may include (1) extreme withdrawal, (2) indiscriminate friendliness and display of affection, (3) appearance of being frightened of parents and of going home, (4) inappropriate reactions to hospital proce-

TABLE 1–5. CLINICAL INDICATORS OF MUNCHAUSEN'S SYNDROME BY PROXY

Recurrent illnesses for which no cause is identified	Discrepancies between the history and physical findings
Unusual symptoms that do not make clinical sense	
Symptoms that are only observed by the parent(s)	Numerous hospitalizations at many different hospitals
Frequent visits to various emergency departments with negative physical findings	The mother has some form of allied health or nursing education
Presence of drugs in a toxic screen that induced the symptom in the child	

dures, such as failure to cry after an injection or other painful procedure, or (5) a look of apprehension when hearing other children cry.

Neglect

Neglect is the most prevalent form of child maltreatment. Child neglect usually involves acts of omission, or failure to meet the basic needs of a child. These basic needs include food, shelter, clothing, medical care, and a safe environment. Neglect is often unintentional due to lack of money, education, parenting skills, motivation, or appropriate judgment. Physical neglect, as opposed to physical abuse, is more often chronic than episodic. In addition to physical neglect, a child may be subjected to emotional, medical, or educational neglect.

Neglect is often not obvious, and many cases go undetected for long periods of time. Identification of neglect often calls for value judgments because neglect is difficult to distinguish from poverty. It is important to consider what the family should be doing versus what they are economically capable of doing.[34]

Assessment

Physical Indicators. Physical indicators of neglect include malnourishment, poor hygiene, and inappropriate dress, such as light clothing in the winter or very soiled clothing. Bald patches on the scalp of an infant may be the result of the infant lying

in the crib in one position for extended periods of time. The child may have evidence of inadequate medical care, including unattended medical problems or lack of proper immunization. It is sometimes difficult to differentiate between medical neglect and noncompliancy. When harm to the child is the result, it is medical neglect. Neglected children often have numerous, untreated dental caries and other dental problems. Neglected children may have a history of numerous accidental injuries due to inadequate supervision. There may be a history of truancy and school avoidance. Infants and young children may be brought to the emergency department because of abandonment.

Behavioral Indicators. Behavioral indicators of neglect include developmental delays, particularly in the area of language development. Malnourished children generally do poorly in school due to a low energy level and inability to concentrate. Neglected children often fall asleep during class due to inadequate sleep at night. Neglected infants and toddlers may appear dull, inactive, and excessively passive.

Table 1–6 provides a summary of clinical indicators in child neglect.

Failure to Thrive Syndrome. Nonorganic failure to thrive (FTT) is a term used to describe infants whose poor weight gain is without apparent physical cause and is therefore believed to be related to environmental factors (Figs. 1–18 and 1–19). Or-

TABLE 1-6. CLINICAL INDICATORS OF NEGLECT

Malnutrition	Numerous unattended dental caries
Failure to thrive syndrome	Developmental delays
Poor housing, such as unsanitary or unsafe conditions	Appears dull, inactive, and excessively passive and fatigued
Unattended medical problems	Abandonment
Lack of proper immunizations	Lack of supervision
Poor hygiene	Educational neglect, such as truancy
Inappropriate dress or clothing	
Bald patches on scalp of infant who is allowed to lie in crib in one position for extended periods of time	

ganic FTT refers to infants and children who fail to grow adequately as the result of an identified medical condition, which may include a cardiac, metabolic, endocrine, or neurologic disorder.

FTT usually becomes apparent in the first year of life. The criteria for FTT diagnosis is usually based on the infant or child falling below the third percentile for weight on an anthropometric chart. Appendix D contains anthropometric charts for height and weight that can be used by emergency department nurses to identify cases of FTT.

The condition of nonorganic FTT is assumed to arise from disturbed parenting, which may range from outright maternal neglect, hostility, and food deprivation to indifference and incompetence.[35] The term ''maternal deprivation'' has often been used to describe the mothers of FTT infants. This term connotes an unloving and withdrawn mother who intentionally neglects her child, which is not always the case. Other maternal characteristics, including stress factors and lack of social support systems, may also contribute to a woman's inability to function successfully in her role as a mother. Although adequate income does not exclude children from FTT, poverty appears to increase the risk.

A significant finding reported in the literature is that the mothers of FTT infants and children recall their own childhood family problems.[36-39] Recollections of unhappy childhood experiences include physical, sexual, and emotional abuse; inadequate nurturance; alcoholic parents; divorce; and psychiatrically disturbed mothers. These findings are very impor-

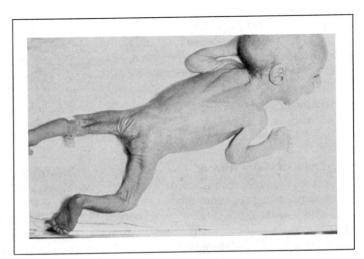

Figure 1-18. Failure to thrive in a 3-month-old who had gained only 1 ounce since birth.

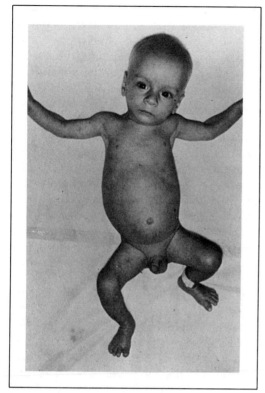

Figure 1–19. Same infant as in Figure 1–18 after significant weight gain during hospitalization.

tant and support the belief in intergenerational parenting behaviors and difficulties. The transmission of attachment behavior across generations has been reported.[40] Mothers of securely attached infants were found to have higher self-esteem scores and more positive recollections of childhood relationships with their mothers, fathers, and peers than mothers of anxiously attached infants. Intergenerational patterns of parenting styles are a common theme reported in the child abuse literature. Many abusive and neglectful parents were themselves maltreated as children. In turn, they relate to their own children in the way that they themselves were treated as children.[41]

Perceived lack of social support

among FTT mothers is another important finding reported in the literature.[42-44] FTT mothers in one study reported significantly less social support from neighbors and family members alike. Although these mothers reported having relatives nearby, they were less likely to see these relatives on a regular basis than the control group. The FTT mothers were also less likely to have telephones in their homes. These findings indicate that lack of an adequate social support system could be an important contributing factor to the emotional status and coping abilities of FTT mothers.[45]

MATERNAL-CHILD RELATIONSHIPS. Maternal perceptions of their FTT infants are often reported to be different. In one study mothers of FTT infants were significantly more likely than the control group to report perceptions of their child as "sickly" and as having feeding, sleep, and discipline problems. The FTT mothers often perceive their infants as vulnerable to illness or death. A mother's perception of her infant as defective or different is likely to influence her feelings and interactions with the child.[46]

Mothers of FTT infants are often found to be less responsive to their infants than mothers of non-FTT children. Some FTT mothers are hostile and neglectful with their infants. Mothers of FTT infants are often less affectionate toward their infants than other mothers.

A typology of family environments that can lead to FTT in an infant has been developed. Three basic patterns of family difficulty were identified. The first pattern involves a recent loss to the mother. Mothers in this group were able to restore adequate nurturance as their depression lifted. The second pattern of difficulty involved families living in impoverished physical circumstances. Maternal depression was again a factor in the disruption of the mother-child interaction. The prognosis for these children was less favorable than in the first group. The third pattern involved neglect of the child and a hostile mother-child interaction. Mothers in this group perceived their children as "bad" instead of "ill." These children had the least favorable prognosis and in some instances warranted foster placement.[47]

FTT infants and young children who arrive at the emergency department and are found to be below the third percentile in weight and height should be admitted to the hospital for a comprehensive evaluation. Infants and children with nonorganic FTT usually gain weight while in the hospital.

Emotional Abuse
Emotional abuse is the result of parents failing to provide a nurturing environment in which a child can fully develop emotionally and intellectually. While physical and sexual abuse is always accompanied by emotional abuse, emotional maltreatment can be inflicted independently. Emotional abuse can be just as devastating to a child's well-being as other forms of abuse. Emotional abuse includes constant criticism, beratement, belittlement, verbal abuse, and threats and exposure to spousal abuse or other forms of domestic violence.

Assessment

Physical Indicators. Emotional maltreatment is more difficult to identify and document than physical maltreatment. There is rarely enough objective data to prove cases of emotional abuse. Physical indicators of emotional abuse may include persistent vomiting, sleep disorders, enuresis, speech disorders, hyperactivity, or FTT syndrome. Like neglect, emotional abuse is a chronic impediment to normal development.

Behavioral Indicators. The emotionally abused child may demonstrate behavior that is disruptive, excessively passive or aggressive, overly compliant, unreasonably demanding, or underdemanding. Neurotic traits associated with emotional abuse include sleep disorders, inhibition, and fearfulness. Psychoneurotic reactions include hysteria, obsession, compulsion, phobias, and hypochondria. Emotional abuse in adolescents may be manifested by alcohol or drug abuse and runaway behavior. Table 1–7 summarizes the clinical indicators of emotional abuse.

Management
It is common for health care professionals when encountered with an abused or neglected child to have sympathy for the child and feelings of anger toward the abuser. When encountering an abusive parent it is important to be understanding and empathetic. It is always counterproductive to display anger. Likewise, one should never act disapprovingly of the parent in front of the abused child. Every effort must be made not to overidentify with the child. The abused child can only be helped through services for the entire family. It is unrealistic to think that every child who comes from a suboptimal home environment should be removed from the parents. In many cases this would be a great disservice to the child, who usually loves the parent despite the maltreatment.

A multidisciplinary approach to child

TABLE 1–7. CLINICAL INDICATORS OF EMOTIONAL ABUSE

Failure to thrive syndrome
Feeding disorders
Sleep disorders
Developmental delays
Speech disorders
Hyperactivity
Excessive passive or aggressive behavior
Depressed or suicidal behavior

abuse in the emergency department, including nurses, physicians, and social workers, is advantageous for several reasons. First, consultation with other health care professionals in the emergency department is helpful in validating suspicions of child abuse and neglect. Because accidental and nonaccidental injuries are often difficult to differentiate, several clinical opinions are useful in collecting and interpreting objective data. It is important to have more than one professional interview with the child and parents so that each history obtained can be carefully compared for any inconsistencies. A child protection multidisciplinary team approach is also useful so that members can share their thoughts and feelings and provide support to each other. It is important to establish an emergency department protocol that clearly outlines the management of child abuse cases and the responsibilities of each member of the child protection team. Sharing the demands of managing child abuse cases is lessened when the responsibilities are shared with other health care professionals. Case conferences, including all members of the emergency department staff who treated a child, should be held after difficult child abuse cases. This will serve as an opportunity for staff to ventilate their feelings of anger and disbelief.

Documentation. Careful documentation in all cases of suspected abuse and neglect is of the utmost importance. It is not enough to write "multiple bruises in various stages of healing noted." Rather, each bruise, lesion, or burn needs to be described in detail according to size, location, color, and shape. Color photographs should be taken whenever possible. In some jurisdictions parental permission to take the child's photograph is needed, while other jurisdictions allow photographs to be taken without parental con-

sent. Even the most severely abused children are often physically healed at the time of a court hearing. The photographs will help the judge or jury to understand the extent of injury. All significant statements by both parent(s) and child should be carefully recorded using as many direct quotes as possible. The behavior of the child and parents should be carefully described. Medical records, including the nurse's notes, are often subpoenaed and introduced as medical evidence. The nurse therefore has a great responsibility in carefully reporting all of the facts and never providing subjective opinion.

Disposition. The disposition of the child from the emergency department will depend on many variables. One must look at how serious the presenting injury is and under what circumstances it occurred. The most important single factor to assess is whether this child is at immediate risk for further abuse if returned home from the emergency department. If it is perceived that the child is at risk upon returning home, the child may be temporarily removed from the home through (1) admission to the hospital, (2) placement in the home of a relative such as a grandparent or aunt, or (3) placement in an emergency foster home.

Often a temporary removal from the home allows time for the parent to receive necessary support services. In extreme cases if the parent refuses to allow the child to be admitted to the hospital or to be temporarily placed, an emergency "care and protection" order can be obtained from a judge over the telephone in most jurisdictions. This gives the hospital authority to temporarily remove the child from the home pending a further investigation into the child's safety, and it allows time for arrangement of support services for the family.

TABLE 1–8. RESPONSIBILITIES OF THE EMERGENCY DEPARTMENT NURSE IN CHILD ABUSE

Thorough knowledge of physical and behavioral indicators of child abuse and neglect	Reporting of all suspected cases of abuse and neglect to the appropriate child protection agency
Case identification	Assessment of the extent of immediate risk to child if returned home
Obtaining careful history and comparing it to existing injury	Consideration of crisis hospitalization or foster placement if child is unsafe returning home
Observation of interactions between parent and child	
Collaboration with other members of the health care team	Arrangement for support services and interventions for family prior to returning the child home
Careful documentation of all objective data	Emotional support to child and parents

Reporting Suspected Child Abuse and Neglect. Child abuse legislation in each of the 50 states mandates the reporting of suspected child abuse and neglect. The conditions for reporting, who are mandated reporters, to which agency one reports, and protection for those who report "in good faith" are all defined by individual state statutes. It is important to be knowledgeable in child abuse laws in the jurisdiction in which one practices. In most states nurses are identified as mandated reporters. Statutes of many states include penalties for those who fail to report suspected cases of abuse and neglect. Those who report in "good faith" are generally immune from criminal and civil liability. It is important to understand that only a suspicion of abuse or neglect is necessary for reporting a case. Actual proof or evidence is not required by law to report a suspected case.

Reporting a suspected case should never be viewed as an accusation or punitive action but rather as a (1) referral for further investigation into the child's environment and well-being and (2) referral for social services for the entire family. Reporting should never be used as a threat to force cooperation nor should parents ever be told they will be given a "second chance" and that no report will be filed. If a report is not made immediately after a suspicion has been raised, there may be subsequent injury to the child and a delay in services for the family. Also, if a health care professional had reason to suspect child abuse and failed to report it and the child was reinjured, the health care provider could be held liable for those injuries.[48]

Nurses should always inform the parents that a report is being made and should explain the purpose of the report. Parents need to know that the report is not a criminal complaint but rather a referral for services. They should also be told to expect a telephone call or home visit from a caseworker from the child protective services agency as a follow-up to the report. Once the parents have been informed of the nurse's suspicions, their behavior should be carefully observed for signs of elopement. Table 1–8 summarizes the emergency department nurse's responsibilities in cases of child abuse.

NOTES

1. National Center on Child Abuse and Neglect. *National Study of the Incidence and Severity of Child Abuse and Neglect: Executive Summary.* Washington, D.C.: U.S. Department of Health and Human Services, U.S. Government Printing Office, 1982.
2. J.J. Spinetta, & D. Riglu. The child abusing parent: A psychological review. *Psychological Bulletin* 77(1972):296–304.
3. R.E. Helfer, & C.H. Kempe. *Child Abuse and Neglect.* Cambridge, Mass.: Harper & Row, 1976.
4. M. Morris, & R. Gould. Role reversal: A

necessary concept in dealing with the battered child syndrome. In *Neglected/Battered Child Syndrome,* New York: Child Welfare League of America, 1963.

5. Helfer & Kempe, *Child Abuse and Neglect,* pp. 777–779.
6. W.N. Friedrick, & J.A. Boriskin. The role of the child in abuse: A review of the literature. *American Journal of Orthopsychiatry 46,* no. 2(1976):580–590.
7. National Incidence Study, p. 9.
8. M. Straus, R. Gilles, & S. Steinmetz. *Behind Closed Doors: Violence in the American Family.* New York: Doubleday, Anchor Press, 1980, p. 55.
9. A. Bandura. *Aggression: A Social Learning Analysis.* Englewood Cliffs, N.J.: Prentice Hall, 1973.
10. Straus, *Behind Closed Doors,* p. 122.
11. J. Garbarino. The human ecology of child maltreatment: A conceptual model for research. *Journal of Marriage and the Family 39,* no. 11(1977):721–736.
12. J. Belsky. Child maltreatment: An ecological integration. *American Psychologist 35,* no. 4(1980):320–335.
13. E. Elmer, & G.S. Gregg. Developmental characteristics of abused children. *Pediatrics 35,* no. 4(1967):596–602.
14. C.M. Morse, O.J. Sahler, & S.B. Friedman. A three-year follow-up study of abused and neglected children. *American Journal of Diseases in Children 120,* no. 11(1970):439–446.
15. A. Sandgrund, R.W. Gaines, & A.H. Green. Child abuse and mental retardation: A problem of cause and effect. *American Journal of Mental Deficiency 79(1974):327–330.
16. B. Egeland, & A. Sroufe. Developmental sequelae of maltreatment in infancy. *New Directions for Child Development 11(1981):77–92.
17. E. Goldenstein, M.J. Fitch, F.A. Wendell, & G. Knapp. Child abuse, its relationship to birthweight, apgar score and developmental testing. *American Journal of Diseases in Children 132(1978):790–793.
18. A. Green. Self-destructive behavior in battered children. *American Journal of Psychiatry 135,* no. 5(1978):579–582.
19. C. George, & M. Main. Social interactions

of young abused children: Approach, avoidance, and aggression. *Child Development 50(1979):306–318.
20. E.M. Kinard. Emotional development in physically abused children. *American Journal of Orthopsychiatry 50,* no. 4(1980):686–696.
21. A. Shaw. Child abuse. *Topics in Emergency Medicine,* October 1982, 75–79.
22. U.S. Department of Health, Education and Welfare. *National Analysis of Official Child Abuse and Neglect Reporting—1977.* Washington, D.C.: National Center on Child Abuse and Neglect, 1979, pp. 49–53.
23. S. Ludwig. Child abuse. In G. Fleisher, & S. Ludwig (Eds.), *Textbook of Pediatric Emergency Medicine,* Baltimore: Williams & Wilkins, 1983, pp. 1030–1031.
24. R.M. Reece, & M. Grodin. Recognition of nonaccidental injury. *Pediatric Clinics of North America 32,* no. 1(February 1985):48.
25. Ludwig, Child abuse, p. 1031.
26. Shaw, Child abuse, pp. 75–79.
27. J. Caffey. The whiplash shaken infant syndrome. *Pediatrics 54(1974):396–403.
28. Ludwig, Child abuse, p. 1035.
29. Shaw, Child abuse, pp. 77–78.
30. Ludwig, Child abuse, p. 1036.
31. C.E. Cooper. Child abuse and neglect: Medical aspects. In S.M. Smith (Ed.), *The Maltreatment of Children.* Baltimore: University Park Press, 1978, pp. 17–21.
32. Shaw, Child abuse, p. 78.
33. J.G. Jones, H.L. Butler, B. Hamilton, et al. Munchausen syndrome by proxy. *Child Abuse and Neglect 10(1986):33–40.
34. Ludwig, Child abuse, p. 1054.
35. M. Field. Follow-up developmental status of infants hospitalized for nonorganic failure to thrive. *Journal of Pediatric Psychology 9,* no. 2(1984):241–256.
36. M. Kotelchuck, & E.H. Newberger. Failure to thrive: A controlled study of familial characteristics. *Journal of the American Academy of Child Psychiatry 22,* no. 4(1983):322–328.
37. J. Fischhoff, C.F. Whitten, & M.G. Pettit. A psychiatric study of mothers of infants with growth failure secondary to maternal deprivation. *Journal of Pediatrics 79,* no. 2 (1971):209–215.

38. C.F. Haynes, C. Cutler, J. Gray, & R.S. Kempe. Hospitalized cases of nonorganic failure to thrive: The scope of the problem and short term lay health visitor intervention. *Child Abuse and Neglect: The International Journal* 8, no. 2(1984):229–242.

39. E. Pollitt, A.W. Eichler, & C.K. Chan. Psychosocial development and behavior of mothers of failure to thrive children. *American Journal of Orthopsychiatry* 45, no. 4(1975):525–537.

40. M.H. Ricks. The social transmission of parental behavior: Attachment across generations. In I. Bretherton, & E. Waters (Eds.), *Growing Points of Attachment Theory and Research*. Monograph of the Society for Research in Child Development. 50, nos. 1–2(1984):211–279.

41. R.S. Kempe, & C.H. Kempe. *Child Abuse*. Cambridge, Mass.: Harvard University Press, 1978.

42. Kotelchuck, & Newberger, Failure to thrive, pp. 322–328.

43. R.J. Gagan, J.M. Cupoli, & A.H. Watkins. The families of children who fail to thrive: Preliminary investigations of parental deprivation among organic and nonorganic cases. *Child Abuse and Neglect: The International Journal* 8, no. 1(1984):93–103.

44. Pollitt, Eichler, & Chan. Mothers of failure to thrive infants, pp. 525–537.

45. Kotelchuck, & Newberger. Failure to thrive, pp. 322–328.

46. Gagan, Cupoli, & Watkins. Families of children who fail to thrive, pp. 93–103.

47. S.L. Evans. Failure to thrive: A study of forty-five children and their families. *Journal of the American Academy of Child Psychiatry* no. 2(1972):111–119.

48. C.A. McKittrick. Child abuse: Recognition and reporting by health professionals. *Nursing Clinics of North America* 16(March 1981):109.

BIBLIOGRAPHY

Ainsworth, M. Patterns of infant-mother attachment: Antecedents and effects on development. *Bulletin of the New York Academy of Medicine* 61, no. 9(1985):771–791.

Ayoub, C., & Pfeifer, D. Burns as a manifestation of child abuse and neglect. *American Journal of Diseases in Children* 433(September 1979):910–914.

Bandura, A. *Aggression: A Social Learning Analysis*. Englewood Cliffs, N.J.: Prentice Hall, 1973.

Belsky, J. Child maltreatment: An ecological integration. *American Psychologist* 35, no. 4 (1980):320–335.

Berger, D. Child abuse simulating near-miss sudden infant death syndrome. *Journal of Pediatrics* 95(1979):554–556.

Bittner, S., & Newberger, E. Pediatric understanding of child abuse and neglect. *Pediatric Review* 2(1981):197–207.

Campbell, J., & Humphrey, S.J. *Nursing Care of Victims of Family Violence*. Reston, Va.: Reston, 1984.

Dine, M.S., & McGovern, M.E. Intentional poisoning of children—An overlooked category of child abuse. *Pediatrics* July 1982, 32–35.

Egeland, B., & Sroufe, A. Developmental sequelae of maltreatment in infancy. *New Directions for Child Development* 11(1981):77–92.

Elmer, E. A follow-up study of traumatized children. *Pediatrics* 59, no. 2(1977):273–279.

Elmer, E., & Gregg, G.S. Developmental characteristics of abused children. *Pediatrics* 40, no. 4(1967):596–602.

Evans, S.L. Failure to thrive: A study of forty-five children and their families. *Journal of the American Academy of Child Psychiatry* 11, no. 2(1972):111–119.

Field, M. Follow-up developmental status of infants hospitalized for nonorganic failure to thrive. *Journal of Pediatric Psychology* 9, no. 2(1984):241–256.

Fischhoff, J., Whitten, C.F., & Pettit, M.G. A psychiatric study of mothers of infants with growth failure secondary to maternal deprivation. *Journal of Pediatrics* 79, no. 2 (1971):209–215.

Friedrick, W.N., & Boriskin, J.A. The role of the child in abuse: A review of the literature. *American Journal of Orthopsychiatry*, 46, no. 4(1976):580–590.

Gagan, R.J., Cupoli, J.M., & Watkins, A.H. The families of children who fail to thrive: Preliminary investigations of parental deprivation among organic and nonorganic cases.

Child Abuse and Neglect: The International Journal 8, no. 1(1984):93–103.

Garbarino, J. The Human ecology of child maltreatment: A conceptual model for research. *Journal of Marriage and the Family* 39, no. 11(1977):721–736.

George, C., & Main, M. Social interactions of young abused children: Approach, avoidance, and aggression. *Child Development* 50(1979):306–318.

Goldenstein, E., Fitch, M.J., Wendell, F.A., & Knapp, G. Child abuse, its relationship to birthweight, Apgar score, and developmental testing. *American Journal of Diseases in Children* 132(1978):790–793.

Green, A. Self-destructive behavior in battered children. *American Journal of Psychiatry* 135, no. 5(1978):579–582.

Groothuis, J., Altemeier, W., Robarge, J., et al. Increased child abuse in families with twins. *Pediatrics* November 1982, 769–773.

Gully, K.J., Dengerink, H.A., Pepping, M., & Bergstrom, D. Sibling contribution to violent behavior. *Journal of Marriage and the Family* 5(1981):333–337.

Haynes, C.F., Cutler, C., Gray, J., & Kempe, R.S. Hospitalized cases of nonorganic failure to thrive: The scope of the problem and short term lay health visitor intervention. *Child Abuse and Neglect: The International Journal* 8, no. 2(1984):229–242.

Helfer, R.E., & Kempe, C.H. *The Battered Child* (3rd ed.). Chicago: University of Chicago Press, 1980.

Helfer, R.E. Preventing the abuse and neglect of children. *Pediatric Basics* 23(April 1979): 4–7.

Helfer, R.E., & Kempe, C.H. *Child Abuse and Neglect.* Cambridge, Mass.: Harper & Row, 1976.

Holter, J.C. Child abuse. *Nursing Clinics of North America* 14(1979):417–427.

Johnson, S.H. *Nursing Assessment and Strategies for the Family at Risk: High Risk Parenting* (2nd ed.). Philadelphia: Lippincott, 1986.

Jones, J.G. Munchausen's syndrome by proxy. *Child Abuse and Neglect* 10(1986):33–40.

Josten, L. Prenatal assessment guide for illuminating possible problems with parenting. *American Journal of Maternal Child Nursing* 6 (1981):113–117.

Kempe, C.H. Cross-cultural perspectives in child abuse. *Pediatrics* April 1982, 497–498.

Kempe, R.S., & Kempe, C.H. *Child Abuse.* Cambridge, Mass.: Harvard University Press, 1978.

Kinard, E.M. Emotional development in physically abused children. *American Journal of Orthopsychiatry* 50, no. 4(1980):686–696.

Kotelchuck, M., & Newberger, E.H. Failure to thrive: A controlled study of familial characteristics. *Journal of the American Academy of Child Psychiatry* 22, no. 4(1983):322–328.

Kreitzer, M. Legal aspects of child abuse: Guidelines for the nurse. *Nursing Clinics of North America* 16(March 1981):149–160.

Maurer, J.A. Clues for early detection of child abuse in the emergency department. *Point of View* July 1980, 18–19.

McCraken, J. Be suspicious . . . recognize child abuse. *Point of View* July 1980, 19.

McDonald, A.E., & Reece, R. Child abuse: Problems of reporting. *Pediatric Clinics of North America* November 1979, 785–791.

McKittrick, C.A. Child abuse: Recognition and reporting by health professionals. *Nursing Clinics of North America* 16(March 1981):103–115.

Morris, M., & Gould, R. Role reversal: A necessary concept in dealing with the battered child syndrome. In *Neglected/Battered Child Syndrome.* New York: Child Welfare League of America, 1963.

Morse, C.M., Sahler, O.J., & Friedman, S.B. A three-year follow-up study of abused and neglected children. *American Journal of Diseases in Children* 120, no. 11(1970):439–446.

National Center of Child Abuse and Neglect. *National Study of the Incidence and Severity of Child Abuse and Neglect: Executive Summary.* Washington, D.C.: U.S. Department of Health and Human Services. U.S. Government Printing Office, 1982.

Ortman, E. Attachment behaviors in abused children. *Pediatric Nursing* 5(1979):25–29.

Pollitt, E., Eichler, A.W., & Chan, C.K. Psychosocial development and behavior of mothers of failure to thrive children. *American Journal of Orthopsychiatry* 45, no. 4(1975):525–537.

Reece, R.M. Child abuse and neglect. *Emergency Medicine Clinics of North America* 1(April 1983):207–216.

Reece, R.M., & Grodin, M.A. Recognition of nonaccidental trauma. *Pediatric Clinics of North America* 132(1985):41–60.

Ricks, M.H. The social transmission of parental behavior: Attachment across generations. In Bretherton, I., & Waters, E. (Eds.), *Growing Points of Attachment Theory and Research.* Monograph of the Society for Research in Child Development, 50, no. 1–2(1984):211–279.

Rosenberg, N., & Bottenfield, G. Fractures in infants: A sign of child abuse. *Annals of Emergency Medicine* April 1982, 178–180.

Sandgrund, A., Gaines, R.W., & Green, A.H. Child abuse and mental retardation: A problem of cause and effect. *American Journal of Mental Deficiency* 79(1974):327–330.

Shaw, A. Child abuse. *Topics in Emergency Medicine* October 1982, 75–79.

Shnaps, Y., Frand, M., & Rotem, Y. The chemically abused child. *Pediatrics* 68(1981):119–121.

Solomons, G. Trauma and child abuse. *American Journal of Diseases in Children* 134(May 1980):503–505.

Spinetta, J.J., & Riglu, D. The child abusing parent: A psychological review. *Psychological Bulletin* 77(1972):296–304.

Straker, B., & Jacobson, R.I. Aggression, emotional maladjustment and empathy in the abused child. *Developmental Psychology* 17, no. 6(1981):762–765.

Straus, M.A. Measuring intra-family conflict and violence: the conflict tactics scales. *Journal of Marriage and the Family* no. 2(1979):75–88.

Straus, M., Gilles, R., & Steinmetz, S. Behind closed doors: Violence in the American family. New York: Doubleday, Anchor Press, 1980.

U.S. Department of Health, Education, and Welfare. *Federal Standards for Child Abuse and Neglect, Prevention and Treatment Programs and Projects.* Publication no. 105-76-1190. Washington, D.C.: Office of Human Development Services, March 1978.

EMERGENCY DEPARTMENT CARE GUIDE FOR CHILD ABUSE AND NEGLECT

Nursing Diagnosis	Interventions	Evaluation
Alteration in parenting related to inflicted injury	Provide emotional support to parent and child	Acknowledge parents' frustrations
	Refer family for social services	Family is referred for social services
	Assess child for evidence of inflicted injuries or neglect	Parents agree to participate in service plan
	Arrange for visiting nurse or homemaker services	Parents demonstrate positive parent-child interactions
	Assess whether abuse is episodic or chronic behavior	
	Assess child's response toward parent	
	Observe parent-child behavior	
Potential for further injury related to subsequent abuse or neglect	Assess parent(s) approach to discipline	Parents describe their approach to discipline
	Encourage nonphysical approach to discipline	Child protective service agency is notified and becomes involved in case
	Assess parents' ability to control violent behavior	Child is protected from subsequent abuse
	Report all suspected cases of abuse or neglect to child protective agency	Multidisciplinary approach is used

Nursing Diagnosis	Interventions	Evaluation
	If child is at immediate risk, admit to hospital or consider emergency foster placement	
	Use multidisciplinary approach	
	Identify community resources for family	
Knowledge deficit related to normal child growth and development	Discuss goals for attainment of parenting skills	Parents increase knowledge of normal child growth and development
	Teach parents normal age-appropriate expectations	Parents acknowledge need to change style of discipline
	Identify style of discipline and effectiveness	Parents have realistic expectations of child
	Provide anticipatory guidance	
Altered growth and development related to chronic abuse and neglect	Refer parents for counseling	Parents enroll child in early intervention program or preschool program
	Refer child to early intervention program	Parents provide appropriate stimulation in the home
	Discuss ways to promote development	
	Provide nutrition education	
Fear related to possibility child will be removed from home	Never threaten parents with removal of child from the home	Parents demonstrate an understanding of all procedures
	Prepare parents for emergency removal of child by explaining that it is in the best interest of the child and parents	
	Inform parents that a report of suspected child abuse has been made	
	Inform parents to expect a visit from the child protective agency	
Anxiety related to feelings of guilt, embarassment	Use a nonjudgmental approach	Parents demonstrate a decrease in anxiety
	Acknowledge positive aspects of parents' behavior	
	Assure parents of confidentiality	
Ineffective individual coping related to lack of support system, history of abuse as child, stress	Discuss with parents the difficulty and demands of being a parent	Parent establishes and uses a positive social support system
	Discuss the parents' needs	Parent copes effectively with stress
	Discuss alternate forms of discipline that are non-physical	Parents demonstrate appropriate use of community resources

(Continued)

Nursing Diagnosis	Interventions	Evaluation
	Assist with identification of strengths, weaknesses, resources	
	Encourage participation in a self-help group such as Parent's Anonymous	
	Assist parents in identification of social support systems	

2
Sexual Abuse of Children

Susan J. Kelley

Few clinical encounters for emergency department nurses carry the intense moral, legal, social, and professional implications as contact with a sexually abused child. The physical, emotional, and behavioral stress placed upon the child as the result of sexual misuse can be overwhelming. Despite the growing awareness that sexual abuse is a significant problem in the United States, the majority of health care professionals feel inadequately prepared to respond comfortably and effectively when confronted with a case of sexual abuse. It is important for the emergency department nurse to be adequately prepared in this area. The psychologic trauma the child suffers can be alleviated by informed, sensitive, and appropriate intervention on the part of the nurse involved. The sexually abused child or adolescent should be given priority in the emergency department.

Sexual abuse refers to any sexual activity or contact between a child and adult, whether by force or consent. It is important to keep in mind that children are incapable of informed consent when it comes to sexual activity with an adult. Children are unaware of the moral, legal, and physical implications of the sexual activity. Sexual abuse includes a wide range of behaviors, including exhibitionism, fondling or manipulation of the genitals, oral-genital contact, vaginal or rectal intercourse, the insertion of foreign objects into the geni-

tals or rectum, and the use of children in pornography or prostitution.

Sexual abuse is one of the most common and least reported crimes against children. Reliable estimates of the magnitude of the problem of childhood sexual abuse are difficult to obtain. One reason is the lack of precise working definitions of child sexual abuse. There is also a lack of standardized data collection methods. There is no way to estimate the number of cases that go undetected and therefore unreported.

One of the first studies to determine the extent of sexual abuse among children in the United States was published in 1969 by Vincent DeFrancis. DeFrancis estimated the number of sexually abused children in the United States to be between 50,000 and 100,000 a year.[1] In 1983 the National Center on Child Abuse and Neglect reported 71,961 cases of child sexual abuse.[2]

There is considerable variation in the prevalence rates for child sexual abuse reported in the literature. Reported prevalence rates range from 6 percent to 62 percent of all females and from 3 percent to 31 percent for all males.[3] Even the lowest rates reported indicate that child sexual abuse is a significant problem in our society. Many cases of child sexual abuse are detected in the emergency department.

Child sexual abuse involves victims and offenders from all socioeconomic, racial, and cultural backgrounds. Although female victims are reported more often than males, there are probably more male victims than previously realized. Male victims may go unreported for a variety of reasons. First, the offender is usually male. Some may therefore view the relationship as homosexual and consensual, even though there may be a significant difference in age between the offender and victim. Another reason why male victims and their parents do not report the victimization is that the abuse may be perceived as a threat to the child's masculinity. In such cases the parents do not want others to know of the abuse to keep their child from being labeled as homosexual or as unable to defend himself.

Clinical data are increasingly suggesting that boys may be at equal risk for sexual victimization because they are the target of habitual pedophiles and child pornography collectors. Males also appear to be more at risk for victimization through child prostitution rings. Male victims who seek treatment in emergency departments are often younger and report a higher incidence of violence than do female victims. Abuse by relatives is more common with female victims, while male victims report more acquaintance assaults by nonrelatives.[4]

LEARNED HELPLESSNESS THEORY

Child sexual abuse is an example of human helplessness and can be viewed through the learned helplessness theory.[5] Sexually abused children often experience a sense of loss of control or helplessness when victimized by an adult. Most children are taught to respect and obey all adults, including not only their own parents but all caretakers, teachers, relatives, and others in authority positions. In general children are taught blind obedience to

adults. Therefore when the adult introduces inappropriate sexual behavior, the child feels incapable of escaping.[6] As stated by Sgroi, "The ability to lure a child into a sexual relationship is based upon the all-powerful and dominant position of the adult or older adolescent perpetrator, which is in sharp contrast to the child's age, dependency, and subordinate position. Authority and power enable the perpetrator, implicitly, or directly to coerce the child into sexual compliance."[7] The child learns early on in the relationship with the offender that he or she is incapable of avoiding the sexual advances of the offender. Often the child attempts to end the behavior but is usually unsuccessful. As Summit[8] describes, the sexually abused child is just as powerless within the intimidating or ingratiating relationship as the adult rape victim would be at the point of a knife.

Most sexually abused children blame themselves for the abuse. This attribution of self-blame leads to feelings of low self-esteem, guilt, and vulnerability.

IMMEDIATE AND LONG-TERM EFFECTS OF CHILD SEXUAL ABUSE

There is insufficient documentation of the specific effects of sexual abuse. Existing studies have produced conflicting opinions on the seriousness of such experiences. Initial reactions of child victims reported in the literature include fear, anxiety and depression, anger, hostility, guilt, shame, and low self-esteem.[9]

The long-term effects reported most often include depression, self-destructive behavior, poor self-esteem, difficulties in interpersonal relationships, and a tendency toward revictimization and substance abuse.[10]

Many variables determine the child's reaction to sexual abuse. These variables include the child's relationship to the offender, the amount of force used, the nature of the sexual activity, and the reaction of family members.

THE RELATIONSHIP OF THE OFFENDER TO THE VICTIM

In the majority of cases of child sexual abuse the perpetrator is well known to the victim and the victim's family, and therefore has legitimate access to the child. The child victim's reaction varies according to the relationship of the offender to the victim. The greater the emotional distance between the victim and the perpetrator, the less emotional trauma is experienced. An outside offender who is a total stranger will usually have less of an impact than an offender who is well known to the child.

Intrafamilial sexual abuse, or incest, occurs when the perpetrator is a family member. The terms intrafamilial sexual abuse and incest refer to sexual activity between a child and parent, step-parent, surrogate parent figure (i.e., common law spouse or foster parent), siblings, or an extended family member such as a grandparent, cousin, aunt, or uncle. The degree of emotional impact will vary with the closeness of the relationship. When the offender is a stranger, the sexual encounter is more likely to be a one-time offense. When the perpetrator is known to the victim, the child is more likely to be the subject of repeated exposure to sexual activity. When a child is sexually abused by an adult who is a parent or other close, respected, authority figure, there is likely to be a great deal of psychologic confusion. In general the most acute problems occur when the offender is the victim's parent. Likewise the child's guilt will be more pronounced if the offender is a family member. If disclosing the abuse results in punishment of the offender or breaking up of the family, the parents and siblings may blame the child.[11] In these cases the victim will feel rejected, unsupported, unprotected, guilty, and abandoned.

USE OF FORCE VERSUS PERSUASION

The degree of force or violence used by the perpetrator is another determinant of the child's reaction. When violence or physical force is used, the experience will be frightening to the child. The child often fears loss of his or her life or serious bodily harm. Physical force is rarely used or needed, however, to engage the child in sexual activity. Most often the child is engaged in the sexual activity through persuasion, misrepresentation of norms and morals, threats, bribes, and rewards. The offender misuses his or her position as a trusted adult authority figure to gain emotional and physical control over the child. The number of incidents and the length of time over which incidents of sexual assault occur are extremely important. The longer the sexual abuse has been occurring the longer the child has been pressured to keep the activity a secret. Generally a single incident, although disruptive, may be easier for a child to integrate than a series of incidents occurring over time.[12]

OFFENDERS

To understand the type and extent of trauma experienced by the child, it is necessary to understand the offender and the nature of the offense. Professionals and laypersons alike have many misconceptions about the type of person who would molest an innocent young child. Often the image of the "dirty old man" comes to mind. The abuser is often thought to be someone who is a stranger to the child or someone who is sexually frustrated, single, homosexual, or mentally incompetent. Many offenders, however, are married, are successful in their careers, and appear to lead normal lives. Although reported less often, females have also been known to sexually abuse children.

One whose sexual desires and responses are directed either partially or exclusively toward children is often referred to as a pedophile. According to Groth,[13] pedophiles are classified according to whether their behavior is a chronic condition or fixation, or an acute situation and regression in their sexual life-style. The fixated pedophile has little or no meaningful involvement in peer relationships. From adolescence on he has been sexually attracted to significantly younger people. He feels compelled to interact sexually with children and creates opportunities to be in their company. This person appears to be sexually "addicted" to children.[14]

The regressed pedophile differs in that he has had positive adult relationships. He turns to children for sexual gratification when the adult relationships become conflictive. Typically this offender is married, and a situation develops that threatens this relationship. Feeling overwhelmed by the resulting stresses, he becomes involved sexually with one or more children. His pedophilic behavior appears to be an effort to cope with specific life issues.[15]

The nature of the interaction between the offender and the victim reveals the motivational intent of the offender. Offenses fall into two basic categories: pressured sex contacts and forced sex contacts. In sex-pressure offenses the pedophile uses enticement, persuasion, cajolement, or entrapment, whereby he takes advantage of the child by placing the child in a situation in which he or she feels indebted or obligated. Bribes or rewards of affection, attention, money, gifts, and good

times are used to persuade the victim to cooperate. The aim is to gain sexual control over the child by developing a willing or consenting sexual relationship. At some level the offender cares for the child, is emotionally involved, and is usually nonviolent. In the majority of sex-pressure offenses the offender is well known to the child.

The second category, the sex-force offense, is characterized by the threat of harm or the actual use of physical force to overpower the child. The sexual act constitutes the extent and duration of the relationship and therefore is usually only a temporary involvement. In this category the sadistic offense is the extreme. In such offenses the offender actually derives pleasure from hurting the child. The physical and psychologic abuse as well as degradation of the child is necessary for the experience of sexual excitement and gratification in the offender.[16]

TYPES OF SEXUAL ABUSE

The type of sexual contact involved between the child and adult is one of the least understood aspects of the problem. Most people imagine that the sexual assault of a child by an adult will be a brutal and violent act with forcible penetration. While such violent attacks do occur occasionally, most often the sexual abuse will be nonviolent and without vaginal intercourse. The sexual activity may include exhibitionism, fondling of the genitals, participation in pornography or prostitution, masturbatory activities, oral-genital contact, and vaginal or rectal intercourse. Refer to Table 2-1 for a summary of types of child sexual abuse.

The sexual activity usually involves a steady progression or escalation in the type of abuse performed. The abuse is often presented to the child as a "game"

TABLE 2–1. TYPES OF SEXUAL ABUSE OF CHILDREN

Exhibitionism
Fondling of breasts, vagina, buttocks, penis
Digital penetration of vagina or rectum
Oral-genital contact
Vaginal-penile contact
Vaginal-penile penetration
Penile-rectal penetration
Insertion of foreign objects into vagina, rectum, or urethra
Pornography
Prostitution

or a "secret." It often begins with exhibitionism by the offender or with the offender viewing the child naked. The activity may then involve masturbation by the offender in front of the child, after which the offender may encourage the child to imitate this behavior. Later the activity typically progresses to fondling, digital penetration of the vagina or rectum, and oral-genital contact. Finally the activity may involve vaginal or rectal intercourse. In some cases the offender will not attempt vaginal intercourse but instead will rub his penis against the genitorectal region of the female child. This is often referred to as "dry intercourse." In many cases the sexually naive female will confuse this with vaginal penetration and will state during an interview that the offender placed his penis inside her vagina. Later, during the physical examination, the hymenal ring may be found to be intact, and it may appear that the child is lying when in fact she is trying to describe dry intercourse.

Often in the course of repeated digital penetration and partial penile penetration of the vagina, the introitus, or vaginal opening, is gradually stretched in diameter. When the child is later subjected to full penile penetration there is not always the extent of trauma that would be expected. Likewise the rectal opening can be dilated gradually over a period of time and may

not appear as traumatized as one would expect when sodomy is reported.

PRESENTATION TO THE EMERGENCY DEPARTMENT

There are generally three ways in which the sexually abused child may come to the emergency department. First, the child may present with a chief complaint of sexual abuse or assault. In this case the child has disclosed the sexual abuse and is believed by the parent or caretaker. The parents seek medical and legal advice as well as counseling services. Second, the child may have a nonspecific or a somatic complaint, such as headache or abdominal pain, or a behavioral change for which no cause can be identified. Further questioning of the child and family in regard to social problems or reasons why the child may be experiencing unusual stress may reveal a recent or past history of sexual abuse. In these cases the child and family are reaching for professional help. In the third and most common type of presentation to the emergency department, physical indicators of sexual abuse are evident, such as trauma to the genitals or signs of a sexually transmitted disease. The child may initially deny sexual abuse when questioned but after an in-depth interview may disclose the abuse. The parents may also deny any prior knowledge of abuse and are often shocked to learn the child has been abused.

History. There are a variety of physical and behavioral indicators of child sexual abuse that may be elicited in the history given by the parent or detected in the physical assessment. Recognition of sexual abuse is dependent on the emergency department nurse's knowledge of the dynamics and clinical indicators of sexual abuse. Physical indicators in the history of

TABLE 2-2. PHYSICAL INDICATORS OF CHILD SEXUAL ABUSE

Trauma to the genitals or rectum	Pregnancy, especially in young adolescents
Vaginal or rectal bleeding	Complaint of vaginal or rectal pain
Vaginal, penile, or rectal lacerations	Gait disturbance
Vaginal or penile discharge	Sexually transmitted disease
Unusual dilatation of vaginal or rectal opening	Gonorrhea
Increased pigmentation at rectum	Chlamydia
Dysuria or frequency	Syphilis
Foreign bodies in the urethra, vagina, or rectum	Herpes genitalis
Vaginal or penile discharge	Venereal warts

the female child include vaginal discharge or bleeding, vaginal trauma or irritation, presence of a sexually transmitted disease (STD), rectal lacerations or bleeding, foreign bodies in the vagina or rectum, and dysuria. Pregnancy in a young adolescent (10 to 14 years of age) should also be considered suspicious, especially if the adolescent attempts to conceal the pregnancy for a long period of time. The possibility of a forced sexual experience should be pursued in such cases.

The physical indicators of sexual abuse in a male child that should be elicited in the history include dysuria, penile discharge, foreign bodies in the urethra or rectum, rectal bleeding or laceration, or trauma to the penis or testicles. Table 2–2 summarizes the physical indicators of sexual abuse.

A careful history of any of the behavioral indicators of sexual abuse should be elicited. Behavioral indicators are more prevalent than physical indicators and include an infant or child who appears un-usually frightened when having diapers or undergarments removed, a child who refuses to sleep alone, or one who barricades or locks the bedroom door to prevent the offender from entering the bedroom. The sexually abused child may become obsessed with cleanliness, demonstrated by taking excessive numbers of baths to conceal blood or secretions. Sexually abused children often become preoccupied with sexual matters. They may make precocious remarks or ask questions indicating their increased awareness of sexual matters. There may be a history of frequent and compulsive masturbation. Sexually abused children often act out sexually with peers, siblings, and sometimes adults. A history of any regressed behavior should be elicited. Table 2–3 summarizes the behavioral indicators of sexual abuse in children.

Interviewing the Parents. Whenever possible the child and parents should be interviewed separately. Ideally one staff member should interview the child while

TABLE 2-3. BEHAVIORAL INDICATORS OF CHILD SEXUAL ABUSE

Sexual acting out with siblings, peers, or adults	Excessive fears
Preoccupation with sexual matters	Refusal to sleep alone at night
Precocious knowledge of adult sexual behavior	Eating disorders, such as overeating or loss
Excessive masturbation	of appetite
Aggressive or hostile behavior	Depression
Regressive behavior	Suicidal or self-destructive behavior
Enuresis	Substance abuse
Encopresis	Runaway behavior
Sleep disorders, such as night terrors or nightmares	Unusual behavior during examination of genitalia

another staff member interviews the parents. If the parents remain present during the interview, the child may be reluctant to identify the offender, especially if it is a relative or friend of the family. Children are often threatened by their parents not to disclose the abuse. Parents may be hesitant to reveal their suspicions or to identify the offender, especially if it is a family member or friend. It is not uncommon for all involved to attempt to protect the identity of the offender.

Most parents react with alarm when they discover that their child has been sexually abused or is even suspected of having been abused. Often the child does not understand the significance of the incidence at the time it occurs. The intense emotional reactions of parents at the time of disclosure can therefore be frightening to the child. Often the child misinterprets parental display of anger and thinks that the anger is directed toward him or her. This only serves to compound any fear and guilt the child is already experiencing. Even when the child and parents are not trying to protect the offender, the child is often very embarrassed to describe the details of the sexual activity with the parents present. Unfortunately children often view themselves as willing participants in the sexual abuse and fear that their parents will be angry with them and hold them responsible.

The information needed from the parents includes why they feel their child has been abused and who they suspect abused their child. If the parents claim they do not know who has abused their child they should be asked who has access to the child (i.e., baby sitter, day-care teacher, relatives). Parents should be carefully questioned regarding any family history of sexual victimization. It is not unusual for more than one child in a nuclear or extended family to be victimized by the same offender.

Parents need an opportunity to express their shock, disbelief, concerns, anger, and any other feelings they are experiencing without the child present. Parents of female victims are often concerned with what they perceive as "loss of virginity." Parents of male victims are usually concerned with what they perceive to be a threat to the child's masculinity and often fear the child may become homosexual as a result of victimization by a male offender. Parents need reassurance that their child should be able to adjust and integrate the experience over time with appropriate counseling and support.

Parents often need as much support as the child victim. They should be forewarned that their child may demonstrate regressive behavior, become very clingy, refuse to be left alone, experience eating and sleeping disorders, and develop school phobias. Child victims may also engage in regressive or sexual acting-out behaviors. Parents will cope more effectively if they know in advance that these types of behaviors are typical reactions to the sexual abuse. Parents should be informed that these behavioral problems should resolve in time with support from the parents and therapy. Regardless of how well the child and family appear to be coping, they should be strongly encouraged to seek therapy for their child and for themselves. The referral for therapy should be made directly from the emergency department. This will increase the likelihood that the parents will follow through for therapy. Otherwise the parents may feel the best approach is to attempt to "forget" the experience and to deny the need to seek therapy.

Interviewing the Child. The child should be interviewed prior to the physical examination whenever sexual abuse is suspected. Children are often upset or embarrassed after the physical examination and as a result are reluctant to discuss the abuse.

There are several important objectives of the interview with the sexually abused child. First, it is important to determine if the child has been sexually abused to prevent further abuse and to offer the appropriate medical, legal, and psychologic interventions. The second objective is to assess the child's emotional status and the extent of psychologic trauma. The third objective is to identify the offender(s) to determine whether the child is at subsequent risk of abuse or retaliation if returned home upon discharge from the emergency department.[17]

Child victims can be further traumatized by repeated interviews. It is important to keep the number of staff who interview the child to a minimum. It is crucial to prevent numerous and repetitive interviews with a succession of emergency department staff, such as the triage nurse, primary clinical nurse, physician, psychiatric nurse, and social worker. It is traumatic for the child to repeatedly relate the history of abuse. The staff member with the most skill and experience should be chosen to interview the child. That individual can then share the information obtained from the interview with other emergency department staff. If the child has previously reported the abuse to a child protective worker or law enforcement official and is at the emergency department for medical treatment, it may be unnecessary for a staff member to interview the child. In such cases the necessary information can be obtained from the parent, child protective worker, or police officer.

Once a rapport with the child has been established, the child should be separated from the parent and interviewed alone in a quiet, private room. Initially the child may be reluctant to separate from the parents and will need reassurance that

they approve of the separation and will be nearby if needed.

The first step in the interview is to establish a trusting relationship with the child by conveying interest, sincerity, and respect for the child. Explain your role as a nurse and that you want to help the child. Initially discuss topics that are nonthreatening to the child, such as school, friends, sports, favorite television programs. Next, determine the child's understanding of why he or she is in the emergency department. This may give insight into the child's perception of the situation. Sometimes the child does not realize that he or she is at the hospital because of the abuse. Also determine if the child has any fears. The child may describe fear of retribution by the offender or other family members for disclosing the abuse. Many times the child is afraid that he or she has done something wrong and will now be punished. Determining the child's fears and concerns early on in the interview provides the nurse an opportunity to reassure the child that he or she has done nothing wrong and will be safe. Attempt to establish credibility with the child by telling the child that you have talked to many children who have had similar experiences. Child victims often act surprised to hear this. Children, like adults, often feel alone in their situations and need reassurance that they are not the only ones who have experienced this traumatic event.

Ask the child if he or she has any requests. The child may ask you to promise not to share the information obtained during the interview with parents and others. Such promises should never be made. Rather, explain to the child that to help the child you need to share information from the interview with others.

Once the child appears comfortable, slowly move into the purpose of the interview. Initially try to obtain general information regarding the abuse or assault and then elicit the specific details. Avoid asking the child too many questions. Let the child tell the story at his or her own pace. The child's limited vocabulary may interfere with the interviewer's ability to communicate and gather important information. Determine what terms the child uses to describe the genitals and other private parts of the body, such as breasts, penis, rectum, and vagina. Children often have "pet" names such as "pee-pee", "bum," "hot cakes," and "couchie" for their genitals. Often parents can provide you with this information prior to the interview. If not, have the child point to various body parts on anatomic drawings or dolls to obtain this information. (Anatomically correct dolls and anatomic drawings will be discussed in further detail in the section to follow on age-appropriate media). Once you have determined the child's terms for the various body parts, the interviewer must also use the child's terms. The time of crisis is not the appropriate time to teach the child the proper terms of anatomy. The interviewer's vocabulary should be kept simple and concise.

Information obtained from the child should include the name of the offender(s), types of sexual acts committed, the number of incidents, the time and location of the abuse, as well as the use of any violence, force, threats, or bribes. Children should be asked if they have any "secrets" or play any "special games." Often the sexual abuse has been presented to the child as something "fun" or "special." The use of threats should be elicited. Typical threats made to child victims include, "if you tell anyone, I won't love you any more" or "I'll kill your parents if you tell anyone about our secret." Such threats are very real to the child and serve as a tremendous source of fear and pressure not to disclose the abuse. Threats and other

pressures to keep the activity a secret are often as emotionally traumatizing as the sexual acts themselves.

Because of the prevalent exploitation of children in pornography and sex rings, each child victim should be asked if any photographs or movies were ever taken of the sexual activity. The child should also be asked if they were ever shown any adult or child pornography by the perpetrator. Often adults will show the child victim sexually explicit material in an attempt to desensitize the child and normalize the sexual behavior. The involvement of multiple victims or multiple offenders should always be explored. Often in cases of intrafamilial abuse the child knows of other siblings involved. In cases of extrafamilial abuse the child may also know of other children or perpetrators involved in the sexual activity.

Careful documentation of the content of the interview is crucial, using as many direct quotes from the child as possible. Be certain to clarify all information with the child.

Sexual abuse cases are extremely stressful for all professionals involved. Although it is difficult, the interviewer must avoid indicating his or her own negative feelings during the interview. Children integrate the negative reactions of adults into their own thoughts and feelings. Often the details of the sexual activity that are elicited from the child are disturbing to the interviewer. The interviewer must therefore be aware of any negative facial expressions, body language, and particularly, verbal responses that indicate he or she is upset. Remarks such as "you poor thing" or "what he did to you was terrible" will only intensify the child's own anxiety. At the same time, however, the interviewer can make very clear to the child that the sexual abuse is not acceptable through such statements as, "what he did to you was wrong'' or ''adults are not supposed to do that with children.'' Most importantly, children need constant reassurance that they have done nothing wrong and that the offender is totally responsible for the abuse.

Age-Appropriate Media. Because of fear, embarrassment, and lack of a sophisticated adult vocabulary, sexually abused children often have great difficulty describing their thoughts and feelings about the abuse. For sexually abused children, questions can stimulate many emotions and can trigger an inability to respond verbally, which can cause additional assessment and treatment problems. Sexually abused children need age-appropriate ways to ventilate their fear, anger, aggression, hostility, and feelings surrounding

the issues of sexual abuse.[18] Communication can be facilitated through the use of anatomically correct dolls, anatomic drawings, picture drawing, and puppets. Each of these materials should be available in the emergency department.

Anatomically Correct Dolls. Anatomically correct dolls, such as those in Figure 2–1, are valuable clinical tools for interviewing the sexually abused child in the emergency department. Anatomically correct dolls include the genitals, rectal opening, and breasts. A complete set that includes an adult male, adult female, male child, and female child should be available. Before the dolls are introduced to the child, it should be explained that ''these are special dolls that have all of the body parts, just like real people.'' Suggest to the child that

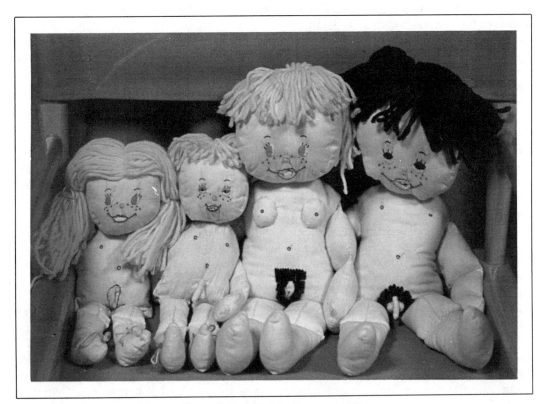

Figure 2–1. Anatomically correct dolls.

you both undress the dolls. Next, have the child describe all of the body parts on a male and a female doll. As stated earlier, this will help identify which terms the child uses for the genitalia. Observe how the child reacts to the presence of genitals on the dolls.

The child should then be asked to point to anyplace on the child doll where he or she was touched. With the adult doll the child can be asked to identify anywhere that he or she saw the offender without clothes or was made to touch the offender. The child can then be asked to demonstrate "what happened" between the child and offender. Sexually abused children are often quite graphic in demonstrating with the dolls the sexual acts performed. Children will often demonstrate intercourse, digital penetration, and oral-genital activity with the dolls. All behaviors should be carefully observed and described with detail in the nurse's notes.

Anatomic Drawings. Anatomic drawings are another means of facilitating communication with the sexually abused child. Anatomic drawings are simple line illustrations of male and female preschool, school age, adolescent, and adult figures.[19] After they are explained to the child the child is asked to either circle or place an "X" on the area of the figure where the child was touched by the offender. The adult illustrations can be used in a similar fashion to indicate where the child may have touched the perpetrator or viewed him without clothing. Each anatomic drawing should then be carefully labeled with the child's name, patient number, and interviewer and entered into the medical record.

Picture Drawings. Encouraging the sexually abused child to draw pictures is an effective way to communicate thoughts and feelings related to the abuse. Communicating through picture drawings is a non-

threatening mode of communication for the sexually abused child.[20] Most children enjoy drawing pictures. The materials needed are easily accessible and inexpensive.

In addition to whatever pictures are drawn spontaneously, the child should be encouraged to draw a self-portrait, a portrait of the offender, a family portrait, and a picture of "what happened" in relation to the abuse. The impact of the sexual abuse is highly individualized and is reflected in the child's drawings.

Self-portraits drawn by sexually abused children often contain the genitalia, reflecting their increased awareness, concern, and anxiety with those body parts. Sexually abused children often draw themselves with hands missing, reflecting their feelings of helplessness as a result of the victimization. Self-portraits may also reflect other characteristics, such as low self-esteem, poor body image, and gender identity confusion.[21] Figures 2–2 to 2–5 are

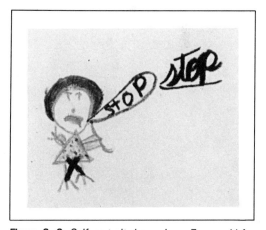

Figure 2–2. Self-portrait drawn by a 7-year-old female who was being sexually abused by her stepfather. Of special significance is the sign she is holding that says "STOP" and the large "X" she has placed over her genital region. *(Reproduced with permission from S.J. Kelley. Interviewing the sexually abused child: Principles and techniques. Journal of Emergency Nursing 11, no. 5(1985):234–241.)*

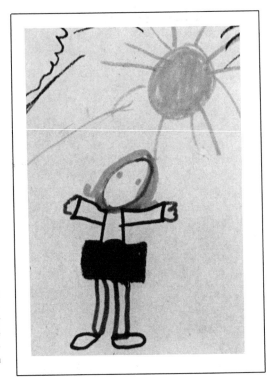

Figure 2-3. Self-portrait drawn by 7-year-old female sexual assault victim treated in the emergency department for the assault and for gonorrhea. The rectangular figure at her pelvic region is an example of how some sexually abused children will compartmentalize the genital region in their drawings in an effort to protect an area that has been traumatized.

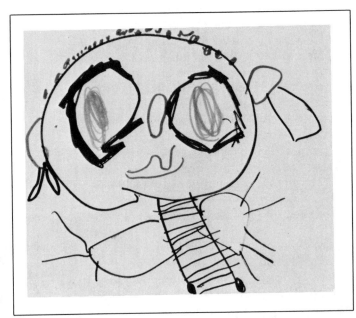

Figure 2-4. Self-portrait drawn by 5-year-old female who was sexually abused by her 15-year-old stepbrother. The prominent eyes are suggestive of a child who is fearful and unable to trust.

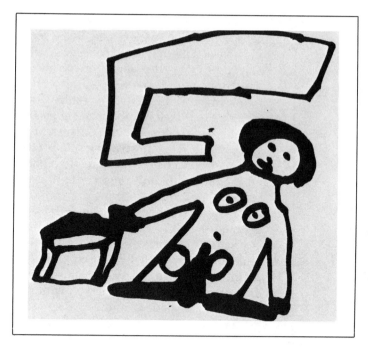

Figure 2–5. Self-portrait drawn by a 9-year-old male who was sexually abused at overnight camp by his camp counselor. The prominent genitals indicate his increased awareness of the genitals after sexual victimization. The inclusion of breasts on a male figure is unusual and reflects his gender identity confusion after a sexual experience with another male. In his right hand is a suitcase. *(Reproduced with permission from S.J. Kelley. Interviewing the sexually abused child: Principles and techniques. Journal of Emergency Nursing 11, no. 5(1985): 234–241.)*

examples of self-portraits drawn by sexually abused children.

Children should be encouraged to draw a portrait of the offender. This often helps the child to verbalize thoughts and feelings related to the abuse. Often both positive and negative feelings toward the offender are elicited from the child while drawing these pictures.[22] Figures 2–6 and 2–7 are examples of pictures of offenders drawn by sexually abused children.

Sexually abused children should also

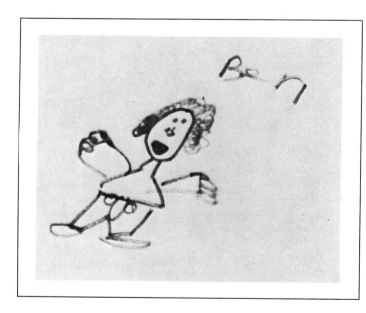

Figure 2–6. This portrait of the offender was drawn by the 9-year-old male victim whose self-portrait was shown in Figure 2–5. The prominent genitals and increased emphasis on the mouth are significant and related to the type of abuse that occurred. *(Reproduced with permission from S.J. Kelley. Interviewing the sexually abused child: Principles and techniques. Journal of Emergency Nursing 11, no. 5(1985):234–241.)*

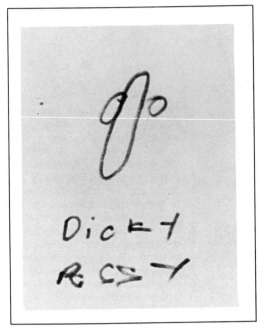

Figure 2–7. Drawing of offender's genitals by 9-year-old male victim who was sexually assaulted by a male social worker. After being sexually abused, child victims often become preoccupied with the genitals and sexual matters.

be asked to draw pictures of what happened in relation to the abuse. Some sexually abused children are capable of graphically portraying the abuse or assault in their drawings. Drawing pictures of the event enables children to organize their thoughts and feelings about the abuse on paper prior to verbalization. Such pictures also assist the child in recalling some of the details of the abuse, which are often helpful in identifying and prosecuting the offender. Often these pictures are convincing to adults who may have originally doubted the child's accusations.[23] Figures 2–8 to 2–10 are pictures of the sexual assault drawn by sexually abused children. All pictures drawn by sexually abused children should be carefully marked with the child's name, patient number, date, and the name of the interviewer and should be entered into the medical record.

Assessment. The physical examination of the child is reserved for last. Children un-

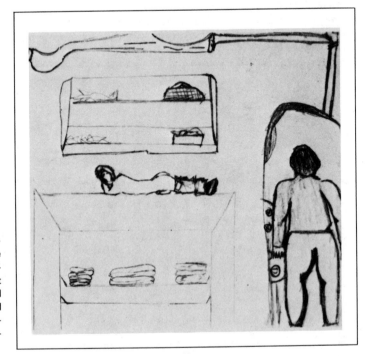

Figure 2–8. Drawing of "what happened" to a 9-year-old male rape victim. The victim (lying on the table) was tricked into believing that he was going to have a physical examination by an 18-year-old neighbor (standing on right) but instead was sodomized by the offender.

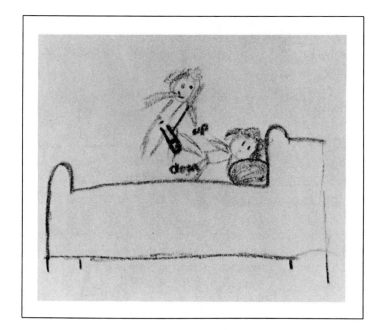

Figure 2–9. Drawing depicting rape scene of an 8-year-old female incest victim. Drawings such as this illustrate how the child forms a clear mental image of the abuse. *(Reproduced with permission of Anthony J. Jannetti, Inc., Publisher, from S.J. Kelley. Drawings: Critical communications for sexually abused children. Pediatric Nursing 11(1985):421–426.)*

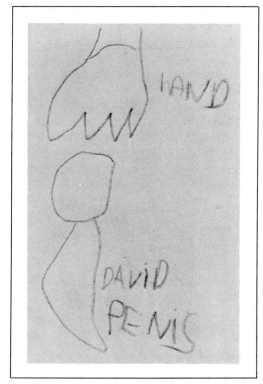

Figure 2–10. Picture drawn by 6-six-year-old female showing how she was forced to touch the penis of an adult male.

der the age of 12 years should be examined by a pediatrician. Female sexual assault victims over the age of 12 should be examined by a gynecologist. All procedures should be carefully explained to the child and parents. The physician and nurse should examine the child together to prevent the child from being subjected to this often frightening experience more than once. If the child desires, one or both parents should remain in the examination room. An uncooperative child should never be restrained during the examination, as this will cause further emotional trauma. If necessary the child should be sedated and then examined. If lacerations need to be sutured or foreign objects removed from the vagina, rectum, or urethra, the child should be examined and treated under general anesthesia in the operating room by a surgeon or gynecologist.

The age and emotional state of the child will determine what type of examination and position will be used. In the prepubertal female child, only the external

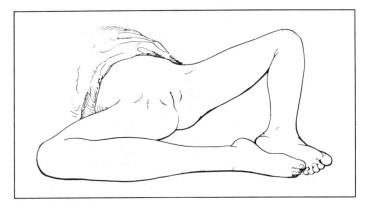

Figure 2-11. Girl in the frog-leg position for examination of the external genitalia. *(From G.R. Fleisher, & S. Ludwig (Eds.). Textbook of Pediatric Emergency Medicine. Baltimore: Williams & Wilkins, 1983, p. 604.)*

genitalia needs to be examined, unless there is an indication of an internal laceration or hematoma. The very young female will be most comfortable being examined while sitting on a parent's lap in a frog-leg position (Fig. 2-11). The cooperative child should be allowed to hold her labia majora apart during the examination of the genitalia. This will give the child a sense of control during the examination. With the older, prepubescent female the knee-chest position (Fig. 2-12) is usually well tolerated. The child is placed on the examination table and lies prone, with her knees tucked under her chest. This allows easy visualization of the perineum, labia majora and minora, introitus, and hymenal ring. As the child takes deep breaths, allowing her abdomen to sag forward, the vaginal orifice will fall open. The prepubertal vagina is quite short, and vaginal lacerations or foreign bodies are easily observed.

If an internal examination of the vaginal canal is necessary, a small pediatric vaginal speculum, nasal speculum, or pediatric laryngoscope may be used. The standard lithotomy position is used for older and pubescent females. It is always important to determine if this is the patient's first gynecologic examination. Reassurance from the nurse present may alleviate some of the child's anxiety.

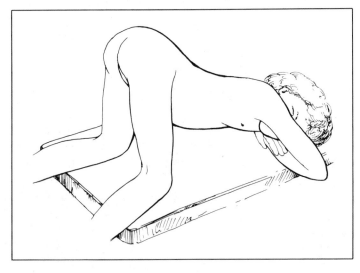

Figure 2-12. Girl in the knee-chest position with exaggerated lordosis and relaxed abdominal muscles. The examiner can inspect the interior wall of her vagina by gently separating her buttocks and labia using an otoscope without an attached speculum for illumination. *(From G.R. Fleisher, & S. Ludwig (Eds.). Textbook of Pediatric Emergency Medicine. Baltimore: Williams & Wilkins, 1983, p. 604.)*

Any signs of trauma, including lacerations, ecchymosis, hematomas, abrasions, erythema, dried blood or secretions, or foreign bodies, should be noted. A description of the condition of the hymenal ring is recorded. The rectal area should also be observed for signs of trauma. Common sites for nongenital trauma include the upper thighs, buttocks, and upper arms.

Male victims should be carefully examined for any trauma to the penis, testicles, or urethra. The rectal area should be carefully examined for bleeding, lacera-

tions, or hematomas. Increased pigmentation of the rectal area or unusual dilatation may indicate repeated rectal penetration.

If there is a history of a recent assault, the female and male victim should be examined with a Wood's lamp to detect the presence of dried semen in the perineum, rectum, abdomen, or thighs and their surrounding regions. Seminal fluid will fluoresce on clothing for up to six months.

Collection of Evidence. A child sexual abuse/assault form, such as in Figure 2–13, will assist emergency department staff in

---

CHILD AND ADOLESCENT SEXUAL ASSAULT VICTIM ASSESSMENT TOOL

Demographic Data

1. Name: _____ Hospital Number: _____

2. Address: _____ Telephone No.: _____

   _____

3. Date of Birth: _____ Sex: _____ Male _____ Female

4. School: _____

5. Parents: Mother _____

   Father _____

6. Address: _____

7. Brought to ED by: _____ Relationship: _____

8. Address: _____ Telephone No.: _____
   (If different
   than above) _____

Emergency Department Visit

9. Date: _____ Time: _____

10. Chief Complaint: _____
    (State in patient's
    or parent's terms) _____

(*Continued*)

Figure 2–13. A victim assessment form for sexual abuse or assault of a child or adolescent.

11. Date(s) of sexual assault: _____

   Time: _____

History

12. Name of offender *(if known):* _____

13. Address *(if known):* _____

14. Age: _____   Sex: _____   Race: _____

15. Relationship *(if any)* to offender: _____

16. Type(s) of sexual abuse; describe:

   Penetration: _____   Ejaculation: _____

17. Use of violence or threats; describe:

   Weapons used: _____

   Bribes used: _____

18. Since incident, has victim:

   Urinated   _____ Yes   _____ No

   Defecated   _____ Yes   _____ No

   Showered/washed perineum   _____ Yes   _____ No

   Changed clothes   _____ Yes   _____ No

   If yes, describe:

19. Is victim sexually active: _____ Yes   _____ No

20. LMP began: _____

   Normal: _____ Yes   _____ No

21. Emotional status of child/adolescent in ED:

Figure 2–13. *(Continued)*

Physical Examination

22. *Female:* Describe condition or abnormalities *(ecchymosis, lacerations, secretions, blood)* of:

Vulva: _____

Vaginal introitus: _____

Vaginal canal: _____

Cervix: _____

Hymen: _____

Perineum: _____

Anus: _____

23. *Male:* Describe condition or abnormalities *(ecchymosis, lacerations, secretions, blood)* of:

Penis: _____

Urethra: _____

Rectum: _____

Testicles/Scrotum: _____

Laboratory Data

24. Two fixed slides *(air dried)* from each site of contact: _____ Yes _____ No

25. Wetmount *(NS with cover slip):* _____ Yes _____ No

26. Presence of sperm: _____ Yes _____ No

If yes, was it: _____ Motile _____ Nonmotile

27. Acid phosphatase:

Site(s)	Positive	Negative
Vaginal	_____	_____
Rectal	_____	_____
Perineum	_____	_____
Thighs	_____	_____
Abdomen	_____	_____

28. Urinalysis: _____

29. Serology *(Hinton or VDRL)* obtained: _____

30. Pregnancy test: _____

Figure 2–13. *(Continued)*

31. GC cultures of: *(obtain all, regardless of history)*

    Throat   _____
    Vagina (female)   _____
    Urethra (male)   _____
    Rectum   _____

Medications

32. STD prophylaxis: _____ Yes _____ No

    Drug: _____ Dosage: _____

33. Contraceptive currently in use: _____ Yes _____ No

    If yes, describe:

34. Postcoital contraceptive prescribed: _____ Yes _____ No

    Drug: _____ Dosage: _____

Case Information

35. Police notified: _____ Yes _____ No

    If yes, detective's/officer's name: _____

    Precinct: _____ Telephone No.: _____

36. Chain of evidence:

37. Specimens transferred by: _____

    to: _____

    Date/Time: _____

38. Examining physician: _____

39. Examining nurse/victim's counsellor: _____

Follow-Up Care

40. Medical follow-up appointment: _____ Yes _____ No

    Doctor: _____ Location: _____

    Date/Time: _____

Figure 2-13. *(Continued)*

41. Crisis intervention follow-up services: _____ Yes   _____ No

     Name: _____ Location: _____

     Date/Time: _____

42. Child protective service report filed: _____ Yes   _____ No

     Date: _____

Figure 2-13. *(Continued)*

gathering and organizing the necessary data. Each emergency department should have a protocol for the collection of evidence in cases of child sexual abuse or assault. The protocol should also specify careful labeling of all specimens and documentation of chain of evidence. There must be documentation each time evidence is transferred from one person to another. Some emergency departments have "rape kits" available for collection of evidence. The following specimens should be collected as indicated by history.

Clothing. If the abuse reported has been a recent assault, the child's clothing should be examined for any sign of struggle, blood, or semen stains. Clothing worn during the assault should be preserved in a paper bag. A plastic bag should never be used, since the presence of warm, damp air can cause a chemical change. Disposition of the clothing should be noted in the patient's chart.

Gonococcal Cultures. Gonorrhea cultures should be obtained from the pharynx, rectum, vagina, and urethra (in male victims). Because children tend to minimize the types of sexual activity that took place, each of these areas should be cultured regardless of history. For instance, a child who denies a history of oral intercourse should have a pharyngeal culture obtained anyway because of the possibility that the child may be denying the oral intercourse due to embarrassment or fear. While children rarely fabricate allegations of sexual abuse, they often initially minimize the extent of the abuse. If there is no penile discharge, a urethral culture may be obtained from the male victim by having him place the first few drops of urine, without prior cleansing, in a sterile urine culture container and then immediately plating the urine on the Thayer-Martin medium.

Serologic Test for Syphilis. A serologic test for syphilis (Hinton or Venereal Disease Research Laboratory [VDRL] test) should be obtained on all children. If the abuse was a recent assault this will serve as a baseline, and the test should be repeated in 6 to 8 weeks.

Seminal Fluid or Sperm. If there has been a recent assault (within 72 hours) involving vaginal or rectal penile penetration, secretions should be examined at high power under a microscope for the presence of motile or nonmotile sperm. The secretions can be aspirated from the vagina or rectum with a plastic eyedropper and placed on a slide prepared with normal saline and a coverslip. Two slides from each site of contact should also be obtained for legal use. These slides are air dried and remain without slip covers. All slides should be carefully labeled with the patient's name, hospital number, site, and date. The secretions should also be tested for the presence of semen, using an acid phosphatase test. Commercial products are available to facilitate rapid, accurate, test results. Areas where the perpetrator may have ejaculated, such as the buttocks, perineum, thighs, and abdomen, should also be tested with acid phosphatase.[24]

Pregnancy. A pregnancy test should be performed on all females who are postmenarchal. If negative the pregnancy test should be repeated in 6 weeks.

Pubic Hair and Nail Clippings. Foreign pubic hairs should be gently combed from the victim's pubic hair. A pubic hair from the victim must be plucked, using a tweezer, to serve as a control. The pubic hairs from the assailant and victim should be placed in separate envelopes and carefully labeled.

If the victim scratched the offender during a struggle, then the fingernails should be clipped or scraped underneath, placed in an envelope, and carefully labeled.

Management. Table 2–4 provides a summary of the nurse's responsibilities in cases of child sexual abuse or assault.

Prophylaxis for gonorrhea in child sexual assault victims remains controversial. If the sexual activity occurred more than 48 hours prior to seeking medical attention in the emergency department, prophylaxis is not necessary if the appropriate cultures are obtained and the patient is likely to return for treatment and repeat culturing. If the sexual assault has occurred within 48 hours of the visit, prophylaxis may be given.

For children less than 40 kg, amoxicillin, 50 mg/kg orally, may be given in a single dose. If the child is over 40 kg, amoxicillin, 3 g orally, is given in a single dose. Probenecid, 25 mg/kg to a maximum of

TABLE 2–4. EMERGENCY DEPARTMENT NURSE'S RESPONSIBILITIES IN CHILD SEXUAL ABUSE

Case identification
Rapid triage of case as a priority
Conduct-sensitive interview using age-appropriate media
Physical assessment
Evidence collection
Prevention of pregnancy, sexually transmitted disease, and subsequent abuse
Reporting of all suspected cases to child-protective agency
Referral of child and family for therapy and follow-up medical care

1 g, is given orally with the amoxicillin. Using oral amoxicillin instead of an intramuscular (IM) injection of penicillin spares the child from another source of trauma and is as effective.[25]

Children who are allergic to pencillin and who are under 8 years of age may be treated with spectinomycin, 40 mg/kg IM. Children over 8 years who are allergic to pencillin may be treated with tetracycline. If the child is less than 40 kg, the dose of tetracycline is 40 mg/kg/day orally in 4 divided doses for 5 days; children greater than 40 kg are treated with 500 mg orally 4 times a day for 5 days.[26]

The need for pregnancy prevention will depend on the victim's age, menstrual history, and type of sexual activity reported. If the victim is postmenarchal and in the second half of her menstrual cycle, and the rape has occurred within 12 hours, a postcoital contraceptive may be offered. Lo-Ovral, 4 tablets at once, and 3 tablets 12 hours later is often prescribed since it has few side effects (nausea and vomiting).

As in all cases of child abuse, the emergency department staff must determine if the child victim is safe from further abuse or retribution if he or she returns home. If the child appears to be at immediate risk for subsequent harm, an alternative disposition such as hospital admission or foster placement must be considered. All child and adolescent victims should be referred for counseling and medical follow-up. If possible the referral for follow-up services should be made within the same institution. This not only provides continuity of care but also prevents the child and family from going to a second agency where they must again share the sensitive information regarding the abuse or assault.

Reporting Cases of Suspected Sexual Abuse. The sexual abuse of children is a crime in every state in the United States. The specific laws pertaining to child sexual assault vary from one jurisdiction to another. Emergency department nurses need to be knowledgeable about their own jurisdiction's laws pertaining to child sexual abuse. Nurses need to work cooperatively with law enforcement without violating patient confidentiality.

The reporting of child sexual abuse is mandated in each of the 50 United States. The official agency to which one reports varies, however, with each jurisdiction. Nurses are mandated reporters of child abuse in almost every state and should take this obligation seriously. In most cases the reporting is made to the child protection agency or the local police department.

NOTES

1. V. DeFrancis. *Protecting the Child Victim of Sex Crimes.* Denver: American Humane Association, 1969, p. 50.
2. U.S. Department of Health and Human Services, National Center on Child Abuse and Neglect. *National Study on Child Abuse and Neglect.* Denver: American Humane Association, 1984.
3. D. Finkelhor. *A Sourcebook on Child Sexual Abuse.* Beverly Hills, Calif.: Sage Publications, 1986, p. 19.
4. A.R. DeJong. Sexual abuse of children: Sex, race, and age dependent variations. *American Journal of Diseases of Children* 136, no. 2(1982):129–134.
5. S.J. Kelley. Learned helplessness in the sexually abused child. *Issues in Comprehensive Pediatric Nursing* 9, no. 3(1986):193.
6. Kelley, Learned helplessness, p. 195.
7. S.M. Sgroi. *Handbook of Clinical Intervention in Child Sexual Abuse.* Lexington, Mass.: Lexington Books, 1982, p. 9.
8. R.C. Summit. Beyond belief: The reluctant discovery of incest. In M. Kirkpatrick (Ed.), *Women in Context.* New York: Plenum, 1981.
9. Finkelhor, *A Source Book on Child Sexual Abuse,* p. 152.
10. Ibid., p. 162.
11. S.M. Sgroi. Child sexual assault: Some guidelines for intervention and assessment. In A.W. Burgess (Ed.), *Sexual Assault of Children and Adolescents.* Lexington, Mass.: Lexington Books, 1978, pp. 135–137.
12. Ibid.
13. A.N. Groth. Patterns of sexual assault against children and adolescents. In A.W. Burgess (Ed.), *Sexual Assault of Children and Adolescents.* Lexington, Mass.: Lexington Books, 1978, pp. 3–9.
14. Ibid.
15. Ibid.
16. Ibid., pp. 10–14.
17. S.J. Kelley. Interviewing the sexually abused child: Principles and techniques. *Journal of Emergency Nursing* 11, no. 5(1985):234–235.
18. S.J. Kelley. The use of art therapy with sexually abused children. *Journal of Psychosocial Nursing* 22, no. 12(1984):12.
19. A.N. Groth. *Anatomic Drawings.* Newton, Mass.: Forensic Mental Health Associates, 1984.
20. S.J. Kelley. Drawings: Critical communications for sexually abused children. *Pediatric Nursing* 11, no. 6(1985):421–426.
21. Ibid.
22. Ibid.
23. Ibid.
24. G.P. Lenehan, S. Bowie, & N. Ruksnaitis. Rape victim protocol and chart use in the emergency department. *Journal of Emergency Nursing* 9, no. 2(1983):84.

25. S. Ludwig. Sexual abuse. In G. Fleisher, & S. Ludwig (Eds.), *Textbook of Pediatric Emergency Medicine.* Baltimore: Williams & Wilkins, 1983, p. 1053.
26. Ibid.

BIBLIOGRAPHY

Burgess, A.W., ed. *Sexual Assault of Children and Adolescents.* Lexington, Mass.: Lexington Books, 1978.
Burgess, A.W., Hartman, C., McCausland, M., & Powers, P. Response patterns in children and adolescents exploited through sex rings and pornography. *American Journal of Psychiatry* 141(1984):656–662.
DeFrancis, V. *Protecting the Child Victim of Sex Crimes,* Denver: American Humane Association, 1969.
DeJong, A.R. Sexual abuse of children: Sex, race, and age dependent variations. *American Journal of Diseases of Children* 136(1982):129–134.
DeYoung, M. *The Sexual Victimization of Children.* Jefferson, N.C.: McFarland, 1982.
Finkelhor, D. *A Sourcebook on Child Sexual Abuse.* Beverly Hills, Calif.: Sage Publications, 1986.
Finkelhor, D. *Child Sexual Abuse.* New York: Free Press, 1984.
Friedrich, W.N. Behavior problems in the sexually abused young child. *Journal of Pediatric Psychology* 11(1986):47–57.
Fromuth, M.E. The relationship of childhood sexual abuse with later psychological and sexual adjustment in a sample of college women. *Child Abuse and Neglect* 10(1986):5–15.
Groth, A.N. *Anatomic Drawings.* Newton,

Mass.: Forensic Mental Health Associates, 1984.
Groth, A.N. *Men Who Rape.* New York: Plenum, 1979.
Herman, J., & Hirschman, L. Families at risk for father-daughter incest. *American Journal of Psychiatry* 138(1981):967–970.
Kelley, S.J. The use of art therapy with sexually abused children. *Journal of Psychosocial Nursing* 22(1984):12–18.
Kelley, S.J. Interviewing the sexually abused child: Principles and techniques. *Journal of Emergency Nursing* 11(1985):234–241.
Kelley, S.J. Drawings: Critical communications for the sexually abused child. *Pediatric Nursing* 11(1985):421–426.
Kelley, S.J. Learned helplessness in the sexually abused child. *Issues in Comprehensive Pediatric Nursing* 9(1986):193–207.
Khan, M., & Sexton, M. Sexual abuse of young children. *Clinical Pediatrics* 22(1983):369–372.
Lenehan, G.P., Bowie, S., & Ruksnaitis, N. Rape victim protocol and chart for use in the emergency department. *Journal of Emergency Nursing* 9(1983):83–90.
Mannarino, A.P., & Cohen, J.A. A clinical-demographic study of sexually abused children. *Child Abuse and Neglect* 10(1986):17–23.
Miller, E.L. Interviewing the sexually abused child. *Maternal Child Nursing* 10(1985):103–105.
Summit, R. Beyond belief: The reluctant discovery of incest. In Kirkpatrick, M. (Ed.), *Women in Context.* New York: Plenum, 1981.
Summit, R. The child abuse accommodation syndrome. *Child Abuse and Neglect* 7(1983):177–193.
U.S. Department of Health and Human Services. *National Study on Child Abuse and Neglect.* Denver: American Humane Association, 1984.

EMERGENCY DEPARTMENT CARE GUIDE FOR THE SEXUALLY ABUSED CHILD

Nursing Diagnosis	Interventions	Evaluation
Rape trauma syndrome related to sexual assault or abuse	Provide emotional support to child or adolescent during history and physical examination Assess child for behavioral	Child and family members are able to disclose abusive experience Child is able to tolerate physical examination and

Nursing Diagnosis	Interventions	Evaluation
	and physical indicators of sexual assault Collect necessary evidence Alleviate any feelings of self-blame Advocate for victim through complex legal system Contact victim in 24 to 48 hours to assess emotional status	evidence collection without further emotional trauma Child and family members agree to participate in counseling services
Alteration in parenting related to intrafamilial sexual abuse	Protect child from further sexual abuse by removing offender or child Report suspected cases of child sexual abuse to child protective agency or legal authorities Assess other children in home for risk Assess for use of alcohol or drugs by offender Assess mother's ability to support and protect child	Child is protected from repeat abuse by removal of offender from home Child protective services are notified and become involved Other children in home are protected from abuse Child's mother demonstrates supportive and protective behaviors
Potential for infection	Administer appropriate antibiotic for prophylaxis of sexually transmitted disease (STD)	Child is treated prophylactically for STD
Ineffective family coping related to incest	Assess whether other children are at risk of sexual abuse Refer entire family for evaluation and therapy Assess nonabusing parent's reaction to child's disclosure Assess for other types of family violence, such as child physical abuse or spouse abuse	Family members agree to participate in therapy Other children in family are protected from sexual abuse Child's mother exhibits protective behaviors
Anxiety related to disclosure of victimization	Identify and alleviate any of child's feelings of guilt or self-blame Reassure child that he or she has done nothing wrong and that the abuser is entirely responsible Use age-appropriate media to communicate with child Refer child victim for therapy	Child verbalizes thoughts and feelings related to sexual abuse Child's feelings of guilt and self-blame are alleviated Child communicates through age-appropriate media

3 | Sudden Infant Death Syndrome

Linda S. Goodale
Susan J. Kelley

Sudden infant death syndrome (SIDS) is the sudden and unexpected death of an apparently healthy infant, for which no medical cause is found, despite the performance of a post-mortem examination. SIDS, formerly called ''crib death'' or ''cot death'' is the most common cause of death in children greater than 1 month of age and less than 1 year. It affects approximately 7000 children annually in the United States, with an incidence rate of 2 deaths per 1000 live births. The peak incidence of SIDS is between 2 and 4 months of age, although it can occur anytime in the first year of life. SIDS seems to occur more frequently in the winter months. It affects males disproportionately.[1] Table 3–1 summarizes some of the currently hypothesized causes of SIDS.

Although SIDS occurs more frequently in low socioeconomic groups and in high-density population areas, it can and does occur in all socioeconomic groups and cultures. It has been documented as having been present since biblical times, and despite continued research and medical intervention, the incidence of SIDS has not lessened in recent years.

Most SIDS deaths occur during sleep, at home, with the highest occurrence between midnight and 8 AM. The infant usually dies quietly. Crib linens and blankets may show a sign of increased motor activity prior to death.

SIDS RISK FACTORS

As research results are gathered and examined, it appears that infants who succumb to SIDS may not have been as healthy as previously thought. They may have subtle physiologic defects of neurologic, cardiac, respiratory, or metabolic nature, indicating that SIDS is probably not caused by a single mechanism but may result from a variety of complex factors.[2]

Several factors have been identified that may predispose infants to an increased risk of SIDS. These infant risk factors are summarized in Table 3–2. Maternal risk factors associated with SIDS are summarized in Table 3–3.

History. While resuscitation efforts are attempted, a careful history regarding the circumstances surrounding the death should be obtained in a sensitive manner by the nurse. The information needed is summarized in Figure 3–1. An emergency department form such as seen in Figure 3–1 is helpful in obtaining the necessary information in cases of suspected SIDS.

Children can suffer SIDS at any time

TABLE 3–1. CURRENTLY HYPOTHESIZED CAUSES OF SIDS

Proposed Causes	Description of Findings
Cardiac imbalance (Schwartz, 1976)	Ventricular fibrillation led to unbalanced cardiac innervation; elevated Q-T intervals were thought to cause death, but this was refuted in some recent studies
Infection (Scott, Gardner, McQuillin, et al., 1978)	In a study of 104 infant autopsies, 31 died of SIDS, with only 7 showing viral infections. Of the 73 children dying of causes other than SIDS, 2 showed evidence of infections. Researchers concluded that infection probably does not cause SIDS but may trigger SIDS in infants at risk
Electrolyte imbalance (Blumenfeld, Mantell, Catherman, et al., 1979)	Sodium, potassium, chloride, calcium, magnesium, urea nitrogen, creatinine, and protein levels for control and SIDS victims were tested in postmortem vitreous humors with no significant differences found
Hypoglycemia (Cox, Geulpa, & Terragon, 1976; Polak & Wigglesworth, 1976)	In 1970, hypoglycemia was thought to result from pancreatic islet-cell hyperplasia. Although this is possible, most recent studies refute the earlier hypothesis connecting hypoglycemia to SIDS
Allergic reaction (Clark, Yunginger, Bonnes, et al., 1979)	Since 1972, it has been widely accepted that hypersensitivity to house dust can effect the respiratory system by causing an overwhelming anaphylactic reaction and death. Studies have not shown an elevated antibody level in SIDS victims, however
Diphtheria, pertussis, and tetanus (DPT) immunization (Valdes-Dapena, 1980)	This was considered to cause death in 1979 when four babies died in Tennessee after receiving these immunizations. The Food and Drug Administration, the National Institute of Child Health and Human Development, and the Center for Disease Control found, however, that the deaths did not exceed the number that might have been expected in the general population. Furthermore, the vaccine is usually administered at 4 months of age, precisely when infants are most at risk for SIDS
Thymic petechiae (Krous, 1984)	Pathologically increased regulatory intrathoracic pressure from sudden complete occlusion of the upper airway at or near the end of expiration was thought to cause SIDS; however, this has been generally disputed in current literature
Abnormal maternal placentas (Naeye, 1977)	A number of researchers have suggested that abnormalities of the placenta can cause damage during gestation and later risk for SIDS
Morphologic abnormalities (Merritt & Valdes-Dapena, 1984; Naeye, 1974)	Postmortem examinations of infants between 1973 and 1976 have indicated signs of hypoxia and hypoxemia. These findings have been confirmed by numerous researchers

Reproduced with permission from S. Swoiskin. SIDS: Nursing care for survivors. Journal of Pediatric Nursing 1(1986):35.

of day and in any location. Although most deaths occur at home during nighttime hours, SIDS victims have died in car seats, with babysitters, and even in doctors' offices and hospitals. Typically children are found to have died during a sleeping period and are discovered in the early morning or after a nap.

The child's condition preceding the death may include a slight upper respiratory infection, and many children have been seen by their primary healthcare provider shortly prior to their death.

The person finding the child may describe in great detail the child's clenched fists, blood-tinged froth in the nose and mouth, and the child lying in a face-down position or cramped into a corner of the

TABLE 3-2. INFANT RISK FACTORS IN SIDS

Prematurity
Low birth weight
Resuscitation at birth or in the newborn period
Low Apgar score
Product of multiple birth
Apnea
Low socioeconomic status
Progressive growth lags
Feeding problems
Black infants
Males

Adapted from R.M. Reece. SIDS. In R.M. Reece (Ed.), Manual of Emergency Pediatrics (3rd ed.). Philadelphia: W. B. Saunders, 1984, p. 315, and from S. Swoiskin, SIDS: Nursing care for survivors. Journal of Pediatric Nursing 1(1986):33–39.

TABLE 3-3. MATERNAL RISK FACTORS IN SIDS

Maternal youth (less than 20 years old)
Multiparity
Poor prenatal care
Home delivery
Narcotic use
Cigarette smoking
Prior fetal losses
Low socioeconomic status

Adapted from R.M. Reece. SIDS. In R.M. Reece (Ed.), Manual of Emergency Pediatrics (3rd ed.). Philadelphia: W.B. Saunders, 1984, p. 316, and from S. Swoiskin. SIDS: Nursing care for survivors. Journal of Pediatric Nursing 1(1986):33–39.

EMERGENCY DEPARTMENT INFORMATION FORM

Patient Information

Name _____ Age _____   Sex: M _____ F _____

Birthdate: _____

Last seen alive: Date _____   Time _____

Found dead: Date _____   Time _____

By whom: _____

Place: crib, parents' bed, other _____

Position _____

Appearance of infant: Body temperature _____

Color of skin _____

Nasopharyngeal discharge: Yes _____   No _____

Resuscitative Efforts

CPR: Yes _____   No _____

Intracardiac medication: Yes _____   No _____

Other medication *(please specify)* _____

Figure 3-1. An emergency department information form. *(M. McClain, project coordinator. SIDS: A Guide for Emergency Department Personnel. Boston: Massachusetts Center for Sudden Infant Death Syndrome, 1984.)*

Birth and Medical History

Birth weight _____ Gestational age _____ Birthplace _____

Source of medical care _____

Well-baby visits: Yes _____ No _____ Unknown _____

                   Most recent visit _____

                   Most recent weight _____

                   Immunizations: Yes _____ No _____ Date _____

Type of feeding: Breast _____ Bottle _____ Both _____

Illness in last 2 weeks: Yes _____ No _____

                   Cold, sniffles, stuffy nose _____

                   GI symptoms _____

                   Other minor/major _____

                   Describe _____

Medical Examiner _____

Autopsy: Yes _____ No _____ By whom _____

Parental Data

Mother _____ Age _____ Father _____ Age _____

Address _____

Telephone _____ Emergency phone _____

Pregnancy complications _____

Type of delivery _____ Anesthesia _____

Complications during labor, delivery, or neonatal period _____

_____

_____

Figure 3–1. *(Continued)*

Previous infant deaths: Yes _____ No _____ Cause _____

Numbers of siblings _____

Report filed by _____

Date _____

CPR = Cardiopulmonary resuscitation; GI = gastrointestinal

Figure 3–1. *(Continued)*

crib or cradle. The nurse should explain to the family that these findings are typical in cases of SIDS.

Management. Families may arrive in the emergency department by police, ambulance, or private transportation. Upon arrival at least one nurse or other staff member should be assigned to remain with family members while other staff members participate in resuscitation efforts. Resuscitation procedures should be no different than with any other infant in cardiac arrest. (Refer to Chapter 6) Figure 3–2 provides a summary of interventions in the form of a checklist that can be used by emergency department personnel to assure that each of the appropriate interventions is completed in cases of SIDS.

The family should be taken to a private area of the emergency department. It is crucial for the emergency nurse to recognize the unusually devastating effect that a SIDS death has on the surviving family. While the death of an older family member is traumatic, death of an infant is different because the natural expectations of the family are completely shattered. Furthermore, when the death is sudden and unexpected, as in the case of SIDS, additional stress is placed upon the family.[3]

The first contacts at the time of the infant's death are extremely important, and parent's long remember what was said to them.[4] Generally families are in a state of

shock and will need to express a variety of emotions, including shock, disbelief, guilt, and anger. Many parents think they may have caused their child's death. Emergency department personnel need to approach family members in a supportive, nonthreatening manner. Unfortunately some parents who lose infants to SIDS are wrongly accused of child abuse or murder by health care providers or legal authorities. Such accusations only serve to increase existing feelings of extreme guilt and despair.

It is important to assist in notifying other significant family members, the primary health care provider, and clergy that the family is present in the emergency department.

The time during attempted resuscitation provides an opportunity for the family to begin to grasp the gravity of the situation. Parents of infants who die of SIDS should be continually reassured that everything possible is being done for their child in the emergency department.

Parents should be told directly and openly of their child's death using the child's name. They should be told that it appears the child died of SIDS and that an autopsy must be performed to confirm the diagnosis. It should be stressed that SIDS is not the fault of parents either through something they did or did not do. Parents should be informed that SIDS is not contagious or hereditary, that it is not predict-

CHECKLIST FOR SUDDEN INFANT DEATH

_____ Resuscitation

_____ Staff person assigned to family members

_____ Primary care physician notified

_____ Medical examiner notified

_____ Clergy called (hospital chaplain and/or family clergy) if parents desire

_____ Family notification of death and tentative cause (essential family members present in emergency department)

_____ Family permitted to see baby

_____ Family allowed to express grief; respond to individual needs

_____ Family members understand how they may receive autopsy report

_____ If tentative SIDS diagnosis, SIDS facts pamphlet given to family

_____ Family informed of follow-up services by Massachusetts SIDS Center

_____ ED chart completed (including ED form)

_____ ED staff conference

Patient's name _____

Staff member _____

Date _____

Figure 3–2. An emergency department (ED) checklist for SIDS. _(M. McClain, project coordinator. SIDS: A Guide for Emergency Department Personnel. Boston: Massachusetts Center for Sudden Infant Death Syndrome, 1984.)_

able or preventable, and that it is not caused by suffocation or pneumonia. Parents may not remember all that is told them during this time but will eventually recall this important and reassuring information.[5]

Family members should be strongly encouraged to see and hold their infant after they have been informed of the death. The baby should be bathed and wrapped in a blanket. All tubes, including intravenous (IV) tubes and catheters, should either be removed or, if legally required to be left in place, clipped short and covered to make them as unobtrusive as possible. A nurse should be prepared to accompany the family during this time. The opportunity to hold or view the infant allows families to focus on the death of the infant as a reality and may serve to reassure the family that their baby's body has not been damaged or mutilated during the resuscitation.

Permission for a postmortem examination should be obtained at an appropriate opportunity. Whether or not required by law, a postmortem examination is important to the management of SIDS families. It may assist in dealing with normal parental guilt and eventually with the issue of having subsequent children. Many parents will have misconceptions about postmortem examinations. Any myths or misinterpretations should be identified and corrected, and the benefits and risks of the examination should be discussed.

It is helpful to explain to the parents that an autopsy is a medical procedure similar to an operation and is performed in a respectful manner. Second, in addition to ruling out injury, an autopsy will eliminate or confirm any unsuspected illness or congenital anomaly as the cause of death. Third, in cases in which an autopsy is not performed, the family may later come to regret the decision because of lingering doubts about the cause of death.[6]

These difficult tasks should be undertaken with patience and sensitivity and can be shared by various members of the health care team. When a postmortem examination is obtained, parents should be notified of the preliminary findings within 48 hours of the death.

The tragic, unexpected death of a child causes considerable and sometimes permanent distress in families. This difficult time may be exacerbated when parents are young or have had no previous experience with death. Immediate professional intervention can make a positive impact on the course of the family's life.

SIDS programs exist in most states across the United States to provide a variety of services to families whose infants have died from SIDS. These services usually include crisis intervention for families, educational endeavors, and liaison services between the local medical examiner and the families of SIDS victims. The appropriate SIDS program should be notified by emergency department personnel of an infant's death as soon as possible. Table 3–4 provides a listing of SIDS programs throughout the country.

Ideally, families should be visited at home by a nurse, social worker, or other health care provider shortly following the infant's death. The reporting of preliminary postmortem findings may offer an appropriate time for an extensive counseling session. This type of counseling session may greatly benefit the family and offer an opportunity to explore issues and concerns around the death. Many state and regional programs may provide this service without charge to bereaved families.

Volunteer programs may offer help as well. The National Sudden Infant Death Syndrome Foundation, a group composed of bereaved parents, has numerous chapters across the country. Local chapters may provide written information for parents and health care providers as well as beneficial peer support for parents.

It must be stressed that families bereaved by SIDS are often unable to reach out for services and that initial referrals and follow-ups made from the emergency department can be critical to the long-term mental health and recovery of the entire family. Many emergency departments take an active role establishing follow-up care for families. Nurses in this capacity may be instrumental in coordinating state

TABLE 3-4. SIDS CENTERS AND PROGRAMS

National Organizations		

National SIDS Clearinghouse
1555 Wilson Blvd., Suite 600
Rosslyn, VA 22209
	National Sudden Infant Death
	  Syndrome Foundation
	Two Metro Plaza, Suite 205
	8240 Professional Place
	Landover, MD 20785
		Council of Guilds for Infant
		  Survival
		P.O. Box 3841
		Davenport, IA 52808

State Programs		

Alabama
Fern Shinbaum, R.N., M.S.N.
SIDS Information Counseling
  Program
Family Health Administration
434 Monroe St.
Montgomery, AL 36130-1701
	Connecticut
	Verdel Bolden
	SIDS Program
	State Department of Health
	  Services
	79 Elm St.
	Hartford, CT 06115
		Illinois
		Lori Bennett
		SIDS Information & Counseling
		  Program
		Illinois Department of Public
		  Health
		Division of Family Health
		535 West Jefferson St.
		Springfield, IL 62761

Alaska
Almeda Amoureux, R.N.
Alaska SIDS Information
  & Counseling Program
Family Health Section
State Department of Health and
  Social Services
Pouch H-06B
Juneau, AK 99811
	Colorado
	Sheila Marquez, R.N.
	Colorado SIDS Program, Inc.
	1330 Leyden St., Suite 134
	Denver, CO 80220
		Indiana
		Diane Oliver, R.N.
		SIDS Information & Counseling
		  Program
		Statewide SIDS Case Manage-
		  ment System
		Indiana State Board of Health
		1330 West Michigan St.
		Indianapolis, IN 46206

Arizona
Virginia B. Harris, R.N., B.S.N.
Office of Maternal & Child
  Health
Child Development Section
1740 W. Adams St.
Phoenix, AZ 85007
	Delaware
	Richard Vehslage, A.C.S.W.
	SIDS Information & Counseling
	  Program
	Division of Public Health
	Cooper Building
	Dover, DE 19901
		Kentucky
		Ida Lyons, R.N.
		SIDS Information & Counseling
		  Program
		Kentucky Department for Hu-
		  man Resources
		Bureau for Health Services
		Division for Maternal & Child
		  Health
		275 East Main St.
		Frankfort, KY 40621

Arkansas
Pat Braswell, R.N., C.P.N.P.
SIDS Information & Counseling
  Program
Arkansas Department of Health
4815 West Markham
Little Rock, AR 72201
	Florida
	Betsy Jones, R.N.
	Florida SIDS Program
	Florida State Department
	  of Health & Rehabilitative
	  Services
	Children's Medical Services
	1417 Winewood Blvd.
	Bldg. 5, Suite 127
	Tallahassee, FL 32301	

California
Lyn Headley, M.D.
SIDS Information & Counseling
  Program
California Department of Health
  Services
Maternal & Child Health Branch
2151 Berkeley Way, Annex 4
Berkeley, CA 94704
	Georgia
	Susan Williamson, R.N.
	Georgia SIDS Progam
	Child Health Program
	Division of Public Health
	878 Peachtree St. N.E., Suite
	  212
	Atlanta, GA 30306
		Maine
		Kathleen Jewett, R.N., M.S.
		Maine SIDS Program
		Maine Department of Human
		  Services
		Division of Public Health Nurs-
		  ing
		Statehouse, Station 11
		Augusta, ME 04333

	Hawaii
	Sharon Morton, R.N.
	Hawaii SIDS Information &
	  Counseling Program
	Kapiolani Children's Medical
	  Center
	1319 Punabou St., 7th Floor
	Honolulu, HI 96826	

(Continued)

TABLE 3–4. *(Continued)*

State Programs

Maryland
Stanford B. Friedman, M.D.
Maryland SIDS Information &
    Counseling Program
University of Maryland School
    of Medicine
Medical School Teaching Facil-
    ity
10 South Pine St., Suite 400
Baltimore, MD 21201

Massachusetts
Mary McClain, R.N., M.S.
Massachusetts Center for SIDS
Boston City Hospital
Ambulatory Care Center
4th Floor, South
818 Harrison Ave.
Boston, MA 02118

Michigan
Bonnie Haun, R.N., M.S.
SIDS Information & Counseling
    Program
Genessee County Health
    Department
310 West Oakley
Flint, MI 48503

Karen Braniff, R.N., M.S.N.
Wayne County SIDS Center
c/o Childrens Hospital of
    Michigan
5310 St. Antoine
Detroit, MI 49502

Pamela Walsh
Macomb County Health
    Department
43525 Elizabeth
Mount Clemens, MI 48043

Minnesota
Kathleen Fernbach, P.H.N.
Minnesota Sudden Infant Death
    Center
Minneapolis Children's Medical
    Center
2525 Chicago Ave., S.
Minneapolis, MN 55404

Mississippi
Fran Baker, M.S.W.
SIDS Information & Counseling
    Program
Mississippi State Board of
    Health
P.O. Box 1700
Jackson, MS 39215

Nebraska
Jane Jensen, R.N., M.S.N.
Nebraska SIDS Program
VNA of Omaha
10840 Harvey Circle
Omaha, NE 68154

Nevada
Ann Malone, R.N.
505 East King St., Room 205
Carson City, NV 89710

New Mexico
Beverly White, R.N.
SIDS Information & Counseling
    Program
University of New Mexico
School of Medicine
Office of Medical Investigator
Albuquerque, NM 87131

New York
Christine Blenninger, R.N., M.A.
New York City Information
    & Counseling Program
    for Sudden Infant Death
Office of the Medical Examiner
520 First Ave., Room 506
New York, NY 10016

E. Jean Scully, M.S.W.
New York State Eastern Region
Sudden Infant Death Syndrome
    Center
School of Social Welfare
Health Sciences Center
Level 2, Room 099
State University of New York
Stony Brook, NY 11794

Fe A. Cardona, M.D., M.P.H.
New York State SIDS Informa-
    tion & Counseling Program
Division of Children's Services
State Department of Health
Tower Building, Empire State
    Plaza
Room 821
Albany, NY 12237

M. Gabrielle Weiss, B.P.S.
Western New York SIDS Center
University of Rochester
601 Elmwood Ave.
Box 777
Rochester, NY 14642

North Carolina
Reid Tatum-Merritt, B.S.N.
North Carolina SIDS Information
    & Counseling Program
Department of Human Re-
    sources
Division of Health Services
MCH Branch
P.O. Box 2091
Raleigh, NC 27602

Oklahoma
Wallace Johnson, M.S.W.
SIDS Information & Counseling
    Program
Oklahoma State Department of
    Health
1000 Northeast 10 St.
Room 709
P.O. Box 53551
Oklahoma City, OK 73152

Oregon
Marianne Reny, P.N.P., M.P.H.
SIDS Information & Counseling
    Program
Maternal & Child Health Pro-
    gram
Oregon State Health Division
P.O. Box 231
Portland, OR 97207

Janice Cramm, B.A.
Counseling Division, America
SIDS Institute
1425 S.W. 20th. St.
Portland, OR 97201

Pennsylvania
David Gordon
Pennsylvania SIDS Center
Hershey Medical Center
Pennsylvania State University
P.O. Box 850
Hershey, PA 17033

Rhode Island
Linda Hanley, R.N.
SIDS Information & Counseling
    Program
Rhode Island Department of
    Health
Division of Family Health
75 Davis St., Room 302
Cannon Building
Providence, RI 02908

TABLE 3–4. *(Continued)*

State Programs		
South Carolina	*Tennessee*	*Vermont*
Betty Johnson	Millicent Stuntz, R.N., M.P.H.	Claire LeFrancois, R.N., M.P.H.
SIDS Information & Counseling	Tennessee SIDS Program	Vermont Health SIDS Program
Program	100 9th Ave. N, 3rd Floor	Medical Services
South Carolina Department of	Department of Health	P.O. Box 70
Health & Environmental	& Environment	1193 North Ave.
Control	Division of Maternal & Child	Burlington, VT 05402
Division of Children's Health	Health	
2600 Bull St.	Nashville, TN 37216	
Columbia, SC 29201		
South Dakota		
Mary Jaeger, R.N.		
SIDS Information & Counseling		
Program		
Division of Health Services		
Joe Foss Building		
523 E. Capitol		
Pierre, SD 57501		

and regional services and care involving other members of the health care team, such as the primary provider. Such involvement can strengthen the effectiveness of the health care team in crisis events.

It may be beneficial for emergency department staff and prehospital personnel to meet following cases of SIDS to discuss feelings and concerns regarding unsuccessful resuscitation efforts and the family's tragic loss. The emotional drain on the emergency department staff must be taken into account and addressed. A case conference may also serve as an opportunity to evaluate the staff's intervention with the family to continually improve upon the manner in which families are assisted in dealing with such devastating losses.[7]

NOTES

1. R.M. Reece, Sudden infant death syndrome. In R.M. Reece, (Ed.), *Manual of Emergency Pediatrics* (3rd ed.). Philadelphia: W.B. Saunders, 1984, p. 315.

2. Ibid.
3. S. Swoiskin. "Sudden infant death: Nursing care for the survivors. *Journal of Pediatric Nursing* 1(1986):35.
4. M. McClain. Sudden infant death syndrome: An update. *Journal of Emergency Nursing* 11(1985):230.
5. Reece, Sudden infant death syndrome, p. 318.
6. McClain, Sudden infant death syndrome, p. 232.
7. Ibid., pp. 232–233.

BIBLIOGRAPHY

Defrain, J. *Coping with Sudden Infant Death.* Lexington, Mass.: D.C. Heath, 1982.

Mandell, F., McAnulty, E, & Reece, R.M. Unexpected death of an infant sibling. *Pediatrics* 72(1983):652–657.

McClain, M. Sudden infant death syndrome: An update. *Journal of Emergency Nursing* 11(1985):227–233.

Merritt, T.A., Valdes-Dapena, M. SIDS research update. *Pediatric Annals* 13(1984):193–205.

R.M. Reece, Sudden infant death syndrome. In Reece, R.M., (Ed.), *Manual of Emergency Pedi-*

atrics (3rd ed.). Philadelphia: W.B. Saunders, 1984, pp. 314–319.

Sperhac, A. Sudden infant death syndrome. *Nurse Practitioner* 7(1982):38–41.

Swoiskin, S. Sudden infant death: Nursing care for the survivors. *Journal of Pediatric Nursing* 1(1986):33–39.

EMERGENCY DEPARTMENT CARE GUIDE FOR SURVIVING FAMILY MEMBERS OF SUDDEN INFANT DEATH SYNDROME

Nursing Diagnosis	Interventions	Evaluation
Grieving, related to the death of infant by SIDS	Remain with parents during resuscitation procedures	Parents express grieving behavior
	Inform parents of the infant's death in as sensitive a manner as possible	Family members verbalize feelings of denial, anger, and loss
	Reassure parents that all that was possible was done to resuscitate their baby	
	Allow parents to grieve in their own, individual manner	
	Allow the parents the opportunity to hold their baby's body	
	Provide crisis intervention	
Alterations in family processes related to death of infant by SIDS	Notify other family members or clergy of family's presence in the emergency department	Family members and clergy are available for support in the emergency department
	Notify SIDS center of infant's death so that follow-up services can be arranged	
	Assist families in identification of social supports	
	Provide crisis intervention to family members	
Post-trauma response related to death of infant	Alleviate any feelings of guilt the parents are experiencing	Parents experience a decrease in guilt and re-experiencing of event
	Encourage the parents to talk about the baby	Parents experience a decrease in sleep and eating disturbances
	Inform parents that it is normal to have dreams about their baby and to experience eating and sleep disturbances	
	Encourage parents to join SIDS support groups through local SIDS Center	

Nursing Diagnosis	**Interventions**	**Evaluation**
Knowledge deficit related to SIDS	Educate the parents about SIDS	Parents are able to understand basic facts about SIDS in the emergency department
	Inform them that the baby's death was not their fault; the death was not caused by anything they did or did not do; their baby did not suffocate; and autopsy will confirm the cause of death	Parents will participate in services of SIDS center
	Provide the parents literature on SIDS	Parents will receive an autopsy report confirming the cause of death as SIDS within 48 hours
	Refer family to local SIDS center	

4

Psychiatric Emergencies in Children and Adolescents

Maureen Ellis Schnider

Little has been written for nurses on the management of children and adolescents with psychiatric emergencies. This chapter will focus on nursing care of these patients. Guidelines and Suggestions for assessment and intervention will give the nurse a greater understanding of these clinical situations for more confidence when managing such problems in the emergency department. Etiologic descriptions and management strategies for specific clinical problems, including depression and suicide, psychosis, and other psychiatric problems, will be presented. Techniques for conducting interviews with children and adolescents will be discussed, and suggestions will be provided on how emergency department nurses can use themselves therapeutically.

People of all ages come to an emergency setting in crisis. Simply put, a crisis occurs because the individual's usual coping mechanisms are not functioning effectively or at all.[1] The individual or family needs help to strengthen or to restore those mechanisms that enable them to deal with stresses imposed by internal and external forces.

When a young child experiences a psychiatric emergency, usually the family is no longer able to cope with the child's behavior and the effect it has on the family.[2] The adolescent's emergency may occur with family members or privately, but the crisis situation within the family is still present.

The goal of crisis intervention is to help the individual and family return to their previous level of functioning or, if possible, to an even more optimal level.[3] Depending on the nature of the problem and the individuals involved, children and their families may exhibit varying levels of understanding and insight into their problems. It is not uncommon to find denial of the problem by both children and parents. It is therefore imperative to obtain careful histories from the children and their families. It is best to interview the identified patient and the parents separately when at all possible. (More about this will be discussed in the section covering the interview process.)

The nurse dealing with the patient in crisis must be calm, reassuring, and able to assess and intervene fairly quickly. Emergency department nurses must convey to the patient that they are in control and will help the child and his family regain some of the control they feel they have lost. This will decrease the anxiety and enable the patient and family to deal more effectively with the crisis.[4]

When working with patients whose

problems are psychiatric, it is important that the nurse take a look at oneself and one's own feelings. Many professionals are made anxious by psychiatric problems and are often highly ambivalent about having to deal with them. The constellation of feelings engendered may include anger, fear, disdain, sympathy, empathy, and acceptance. These are usually generated by the nature of the nurse's understanding of psychiatric problems, his or her past experience with them, prejudices, and how stable the emotional life of the nurse is at present. It is necessary for the nurse to look at himself or herself and to deal with the feelings he or she is experiencing so that the nurse may interact with the patient in a way that is therapeutic and causes no further discomfort to either the patient or the nurse. To do this the nurse must be honest with himself or herself and must explore the nature of any problem areas that may exist.

There have been many references made to the "therapeutic relationship" in nursing.[5-7] Establishing a rapport with a patient of any age and with any problem so that the patient can feel trusting enough to disclose his or her feelings is paramount.[8,9] There should be mutual, goal-oriented communication to help the patient feel comfortable so that both the patient and nurse can approach the problem and find a solution.

This bond will not occur immediately but can develop over the course of an interview, when the person who is trying to provide assistance is objective, honest, accepting, and empathetic to and tolerant of what the patient is experiencing.

When these situations are difficult for nurses, nurses should seek support from other professionals so that through recognizing and dealing with the problem they may go on to manage other such situations effectively.

Conducting the Interview

Assessing the problem and why the patient or family has sought care should be the first priority in managing the psychiatric emergency.[10-12]

Much valuable information can be collected during the interview. It is the task of the interviewer to establish an atmosphere conducive to the sharing of this information, incorporating the ingredients of comfort, respect, a nonjudgmental attitude, privacy, and an approach geared to the developmental level of the patient.[13,14]

A developmental approach, which is least threatening, is most successful. The use of toys, art, and puppets are often very fruitful in obtaining information from children as well as in assisting them in feeling more comfortable in their interactions with the nurse.[15,16] Asking children to draw or act out with puppets what they are thinking or feeling or an event that took place is often helpful. This can also be done with dolls and other illustrative toys and play things. It is imperative to use language that is easy for the child to understand and to allow the child to use phrases or special labels for objects, for which the nurse should request an explanation (e.g., children often have a variety of names for body parts).

The adolescent may pose special problems that a younger child may not. Frequently the adolescent may test the interviewer through actions or affect (i.e., acting distant or difficult to engage).[17] The nurse should convey to the adolescent that he or she is sincerely interested, cares, and is willing to listen and try to help. It is important that the nurse respond to what the adolescent is feeling rather than react to his or her behavior, which can often be annoying or difficult.

Children should be interviewed separately from their parents whenever possible. Preferably the adolescent should be interviewed first, before his parents. This helps to reassure the adolescent that the interviewer respects what he or she has to share and that the interviewer is not already biased by what the parents may have previously reported had they been interviewed first.

If all efforts to assist the child to feel comfortable while alone with the interviewer are unsuccessful, the child should not be forced to leave his or her parents, as this would further stress the child. Parents who do not wish their child to be interviewed alone, however, should be assured (matter of factly) that this is a standard procedure and that it is important for all involved to have a chance to share their thoughts and feelings with the examiner. Often much pertinent information is obtained from the child or parents outside the presence of the others in situations where the presence of others may inhibit disclosure.

Major areas to explore during the assessment are the child's significant relationships, cognitive and behavioral functioning, sense of identity and body image, and the integrated development of body functions.[18,19] Specific assessment data will be addressed in the discussion of clinical problems.

Depression

Depression in children and adolescents is frequently manifested. Depression is defined as a reaction to a loss, real or imagined, originating from an internal or external source.[20] It is characterized by feelings of dejection, unhappiness, and low spirits. Depression can be helped by removing the external source, when possible. A neurotic depression occurs when tension and anxiety are expressed in feelings of poor self-esteem, inferiority, hopelessness, and somatic disturbances.[21]

Depression can be looked at as a symptom of dysfunction within the family system and society.[22] The family is involved, whether it be in contributing to the development of the problem or in the effect the problem has on how the rest of the family unit functions.

Particular external sources currently contributing to the development of depression in children are changes in the family structure and function, for example, divorce; more parents employed outside the home; isolation from extended family (e.g., grandparents); death of a loved one; role confusion and discrepancy in societal expectations; demands upon children (e.g., exposure to confusing behavior, drugs, promiscuous sexual behavior); and school disturbances or difficulties. Sources of internal stress can arise from difficulty in managing the developmental tasks of a particular stage, resulting in feelings of inferiority, worthlessness, and poor self-esteem.

History and Assessment. A young child who is depressed may not exhibit the same signs and symptoms that are associated with adolescent and adult depression; therefore proper identification and treatment of the problem does not always occur. It is therefore important to be aware of the symptomatology (as well as the etiology) of depression in children and adolescents.

Depression in children and adolescents cuts across boundaries of ethnicity, socioeconomics, and religion. It is easy to see that the family system as well as the personality of the child can contribute to its occurrence. Deciphering the exact nature of the problem may take some time and will necessitate looking at a variety of factors influencing the child. Examining the problem in terms of a family context is important, since the problem is affected by, and in turn affects, the family.

Manifestations of childhood depression include the following: sadness, acting-out behavior, boredom, restlessness, lethargy, low self-esteem, self-deprecation, ambivalence toward loved ones, and feelings of guilt. Changes in behavior may include increased aggressiveness, promiscuity, changes in school performance, school failure, accident proneness, disturbances in sleep, and changes in appetite.[23-26]

These same indicators as well as others may be present in adolescents. For example, changes in appearance (not caring as much about appearance), disturbances in peer relationships (particularly increased isolation), slowed speech and body movements, increased somatic complaints, and delinquency may be manifested.[27-29]

Emergency management of the depressed child and adolescent includes obtaining a pertinent history, ensuring safety, identifying the problem, and providing support through the crisis. This includes assessment of the parent-child relationship for both data collection and disposition planning.

General assessment considerations were mentioned earlier as well as the importance of approaching the child and family in a therapeutic and nonjudgmental manner. Other areas to explore in the assessment of the depressed child or adolescent include the parents' specific concerns, how parents perceive the child's behavior has changed at home or at school, and how the child's relationships have changed. It is also important to obtain pertinent developmental and school histories as well as a family history, including changes in relationships or recent losses. Identification of significant stressors and precipitants is extremely important, although the family may not always be able to pinpoint these as such. The child and family should be questioned regarding the use of drugs and alcohol (including toxic screening when indicated) and significant

medical, psychiatric, and pharmaceutic history. The area of suicidal ideation needs also to be explored by asking whether the child has ever felt like killing himself or herself and whether he or she has ever acted on these feelings. The nurse should also ask how the child is feeling about this at present.[30-34]

Finally, it is important to assess through the history how the child has coped with stress in the past and to identify those coping mechanisms that have already been employed to deal with the current problem. This includes ascertaining how parents, school personnel, and other agencies have tried to help the child and who is currently involved in trying to manage the problem.

Management. Intervention is geared toward the goal of assisting the family in dealing with the crisis. It is necessary to first identify what is best for the child, particularly in terms of safety. It will be important to work with the family to assess what they can manage and what resources and supports they can draw upon for help once they leave the emergency setting. This may include family members, friends, or other agencies. It is helpful when making these plans to outline the problem for the family so that they may make informed decisions.[35]

Support is often the key factor in helping the family make decisions while in crisis, and the use of a supportive, professional attitude cannot be emphasized enough. This support extends to incorporating the family into the planning as much as possible to bolster the family's existing strengths and assist them to regain faltering ones.

Disposition will be based on assessment of the child's needs and the resources of the family. The disposition may range from sending the child home with a referral to an appropriate outpatient

agency to arranging for alternative placement of the child in a medical or psychiatric facility or other appropriate setting,
such as foster care, group home, or shelter. The professional should be aware of
appropriate resources within the geographic area or have access to people who
can assist in locating resources for children
and families in need.

Suicide

Suicidal behavior can take many forms, including suicidal ideation, gesture/attempt,
and completed suicide. Suicidal ideation
describes the individual having thoughts
about hurting or killing himself, while a
gesture or attempt means acting on these
thoughts. These actions range from minor
self-inflicted lacerations or ingestions, for
example, to more severe self-destructive
acts. It is imperative that any or all of these
actions be taken seriously. Whether it is a
cry for help or attention-seeking behavior,
the impulse is serious and the ramifications potentially fatal. All incidents should
be treated by the health provider as extremely serious and should be assessed
and managed as such.

History and Assessment. The following
variables, which have been found to be
risk factors in the etiology of suicidal behavior, should be elicited in the history:

- Age. (Suicide is particularly high among
  persons aged 15 to 24 years, although it
  appears that young children are attempting suicide with increasing frequency.)
- Sex. (Males have more completed sui-
  cides and tend to use more potentially
  lethal methods, such as guns and hanging, while females have a higher number of suicide attempts, usually through
  ingestions.)
- History of previous attempts. (With
  each attempt the potential for success increases.)

- History of loss. (E.g., death, loss of self-
  esteem, which can be recent or past, real
  or threatened.)
- Preoccupation with death. (Especially if
  the preoccupation is recent.)
- Lack of plans for the future.
- Atypical attitudes toward death. (E.g,
  viewing death as romantic, which can be
  frequently found in adolescents.)

There may be a sudden lifting of
symptoms of depression at this time. This
relief may have resulted from making the
decision to die, and with that relief comes
the energy to attempt suicide. The suicidal
individual may demonstrate impulsive-
ness and poor judgment and may feel that
there are no available supports. The suicidal child or adolescent may report delu-
sions and command hallucinations (hearing voices telling him or her to kill himself
or herself), which are always extremely serious.[36-42]

Management. Emergency management of
the suicidal child or adolescent includes
initial medical assessment and stabilization, the first goal in any emergency situation; assessment and initiation of safety
factors; the psychologic assessment, covering pertinent history and risk factors;
and disposition.

Children who have made suicide attempts and who express suicidal ideation
or feelings should never be left alone and
should be watched extremely closely (including removal of potentially dangerous
objects) until it is determined that the suicidal impulse has diminished and the patient's judgment has improved.

Disposition of the child who has made
a suicide attempt is often difficult, usually
due to the lack of readily available resources. In those cases in which the child
requires medical as well as psychiatric
treatment, an admission to an inpatient
medical or combined medical/psychiatric
unit is usually appropriate, as long as psy-

chiatric treatment is also available. Children who require only psychiatric intervention, however, have more limited options. In the case of the child who continues to be actively suicidal, admission to a unit on which he can be managed safely is the number one priority.[43-45] Due to the scarcity of inpatient psychiatric units for children in some areas, this necessitates admission to an inpatient pediatric medical unit where the staff will need to provide safety as a minimum and, optimally, a psychologically therapeutic environment. There are also times when an adult psychiatric unit is the only available placement option. This is often frightening for the child and is a strain on the staff, since they may not be well versed in the special needs of the child. When this is the only choice, however, support should be given to the child and family to make the transition as smooth as possible.

In some cases the child or adolescent may be considered able to safely return home with family or to alternative housing (relatives, foster care) if proper support is provided. This usually occurs when the child who has attempted to harm himself or herself feels, either through the response received from others or through changes in the perception of the situation and its precipitants, that he or she no longer wants to die. This disposition should be made only after careful assessment of the client and family and when it is felt that the child and significant others are comfortable about their ability to keep the child safe. This option should be coupled with a great deal of support, assurance that they can return to the emergency department at any time, and a follow-up phone call or visit, the next day (or whenever deemed appropriate).

Referrals for psychiatric treatment for the child and family should also be made from the emergency department. When this is done it is often advantageous to follow up fairly soon. This gives the client and family the message that you care and further encourages them to seek treatment. Such encouragement is often needed.

It is helpful to have a list of appropriate referral sources readily available in the emergency department. Often people in crisis find a great deal of comfort in having the name of a person or agency whom they can call. This may be the extra support they need to see them through until they make contact and receive more extensive help. Emergency departments that have psychiatric crisis teams available at all times have the advantage of being able to provide clients with the referral source on site, which enables the patient and family to establish contact immediately with the individual or representative of an agency with whom they may become involved.

Legal policies vary from state to state, so it is prudent for emergency department nurses and crisis team members to familiarize themselves with the laws in their area regarding children's and families' rights, especially in the areas of mental health and psychiatric commitment. At times it may be necessary to act in a way which is against the wishes of the parents if it is in the best interests of the child, but this can only be done in states where the laws support this action.

Psychosis

Psychosis in children is a severe disorder characterized by behavior that deviates markedly from age-appropriate norms.[46] The incidence of this disorder is not known, and the etiologic theories vary, being primarily divided between psychogenic and biological schools of thought.

The psychogenic theory views psychosis as the mechanism by which the child blocks out the real world in response to stress and anxiety in his environment. This theory places responsibility on the parents for having some role as causative agents. The biological theory looks at psychosis as reflecting disturbances in physiologic arousal or in cognition or perception.[47]

The psychosis is seen as a disturbance in the development of ego functioning, so that the resulting impairment of important ego functions along the developmental continuum are displayed through inappropriate behaviors for a given age. For example, in very young children alterations are seen in their ability to individuate and to relate to others. In later years one may see more impairment in reality testing and personality integration. Psychosis in adolescence will often be demonstrated by impaired thought processes, an impaired sense of identity, and difficulty in relating to others.[48]

Descriptive factors that can be attributed to psychoses of childhood and adolescence include the following: pervasive and ongoing disturbances in relatedness; lack of sense of personal identity; disturbances in intellectual development (blunted, fragmented); problems in speech development or lack of any speech; sensory perception problems; a tendency to be preoccupied with inanimate objects; bizarre or stereotyped movements and behaviors; panic outbursts; and resistance to change in the environment.[49]

Some of the common characteristics and behaviors found in children with these disorders are disturbances in affect; an inability to communicate (including mutism and echolalia); temper tantrums (including rages directed against self and others and self-mutilating behavior); perseveration, or compulsiveness aimed at maintaining sameness in the environment; apparent sensory deficits (although none may actually be present); lack of demonstrated awareness of an understanding of common dangers; and a lack of self-care skills development.[50]

The area of psychosis in children is broad, and there are several areas of diagnoses in which these patients may be grouped. Some of these categories may overlap, and specific classification may not be the appropriate goal in the emergency setting. So that the nurse will have some understanding of these diagnostic categories, however, they will be discussed briefly here.

The following descriptions have been taken from the works of the Group for the Advancement of Psychiatry's Committee for Child Psychiatry.[51]

The psychoses of infancy and early childhood have been divided into early infantile autism, interactional psychotic disorders, and other psychoses of infancy and early childhood.

Early infantile autism appears to develop during the first few months or years of life, at which time the infant fails to develop an attachment to the mother figure. Characteristics and behaviors displayed by these children include aloofness, lack of awareness of human contact, preoccupation with inanimate objects, problems in speech development, resistance to change, stereotyped and bizarre movements, disturbances in eating and sleeping, and the possibility of impaired intellectual development.

The interactional psychotic disorder describes children who may develop normally the first year of life but who in the following year(s) may develop an overattachment to the mother figure with resultant inability to master the developmental tasks of separation and individuation.

The psychotic process may have its onset in the second to fourth year, often in response to a threat (real or imagined) to the mother-child relationship. The child exhibits regressive behaviors, displays increased anxiety over separation, and may begin to show much of the symptomatology previously discussed under infantile autism, thus possibly resembling this other disorder.

Children who do not fall into either of these diagnostic categories but who may exhibit features of each and who show some deviation in development, including emotional aloofness and autistic behaviors, may be classified under the group of other psychosis of infancy and early childhood. These children differ from those previously mentioned in that they may show some positive adaptive behaviors and strengths in personality development. They must be differentiated from those children who are markedly depressed, who imitate a psychotic parent, who are extremely anxious and inhibited, or who display problems secondary to cognitive difficulties.

The later childhood years may be divided into the category of schizophreniform psychotic disorder and other psychosis of later childhood. The schizophreniform disorder usually has its onset between the ages of 6 and 13 years, with gradual development of symptoms followed by severe phobic reactions, profound anxiety, and withdrawal resulting in autistic behaviors and distorted reality testing. Some characteristics also displayed by adults may be present in this disorder, including paranoid thinking, catatonic behavior, and other disturbances in thought processes.

Children with this disorder do not necessarily develop schizophrenia, and children in this age group have a fairly good prognosis for recovery from the initial episode.

Types of psychosis other than schizophreniform may be classified under other psychosis, such as psychotic reactions of a bipolar illness (manic-depressive episodes), which are rarely seen, and schizoaffective type disorder.

The psychoses of adolescence include the acute confusional state, which is characterized by an acute onset with extreme anxiety, depression, and confusion. There is usually the absence of a true thought disorder, and these individuals are often able to form and maintain relationships with others, despite problems with identity formation. They also usually do possess some ability to adapt.

Differential diagnoses with this state include schizophrenia, dissociative reactions, and other emotional problems common in adolescents, such as depression, anxiety, and feelings of depersonalization.

The other psychosis of adolescence category includes disorders such as regression (severe) with associated thought disorder and other psychotic manifestations, differentiated from schizophrenia; some transient dissociative states; and dissociative states with hysterical features.

Prognosis in this age group for recovery from psychotic episodes may be good, although these episodes may indicate an underlying personality disorder.

Some adolescents will also present with schizophrenia, adult type, and although episodes may be acute and may resolve quickly, some pictures of more chronic and recurring illness will be seen.

Management. Intervention strategies for the psychotic child or adolescent in the emergency setting include maintaining safety for both the child and others, decreasing the anxiety of the child and family, and assisting the family to identify what measures must be taken to best meet the needs of the child. This will entail providing the family with a great deal of support and encouragement to look at the situation and to make decisions that will benefit not only the child but, optimally, the entire family.

Health care providers interacting with the family will need to help the parents to feel less guilt, to identify and begin to resolve some of their ambivalence and confused feelings to be able to participate in decision making, and to observe and assess the dynamics between the child and parents[52] while staying particularly attuned to those behaviors that may be inappropriate or dysfunctional.

It may be necessary in some cases for the nurse to act as a buffer between the child and parents in situations that are potentially explosive and that could endanger someone, either physically or emotionally. Assisting people to remain calm and to feel as unthreatened as possible is most optimal, both during the crisis period and when decisions are being made. All members of the family need to feel that they are being listened to and that their feelings are being respected. Allowing both child and parents (and other family members when appropriate) to express themselves and responding to these expressions will enable everyone to feel that they are being treated fairly and that their concerns are being acknowledged and addressed.

Parents are often confused and frightened about their child's behavior, whether it is an acute problem or one that has been going on for a longer period of time. Explaining as simply as possible what may be going on with the child psychiatrically usually enables parents to better help their child.

The child may also be extremely frightened, whether it be due to an awareness of what is happening to him or to the function of the psychotic process (i.e., paranoid thinking, confusion). He or she will need a great deal of reassurance and support that people are there to help, not to hurt, and that he or she will be kept safe. The child will often need constant observation, either to maintain safety (for himself or herself or others) or to decrease anxiety and fear. If keeping the parents and child together results in a situation that is too stressful or potentially explosive, it will be in the best interests of everyone to separate them either until the situation is defused or until the disposition plans can be made.

Mechanical restraint should be used only as a last resort, for example, when it is the only way to keep the patient from harming himself or herself, either through intent or confusion; or when he or she is unable to be controlled and is of danger to others or is in danger of running away. Chemical restraint may be necessary through the use of psychotropic medication and should be prescribed by a physician who is experienced in its use only after careful assessment. Commonly used medication groups include the minor and major tranquilizers, antianxiety agents, sedatives, and, at times, antidepressants or mood elevators. These latter two groups are less likely to be used in an emergency situation, since they are more suited to treating disorders over a longer time period.

Disposition will again depend on the condition of the child, the family situation, and the available resources. Obviously children who are in danger of hurting themselves or others or who are out of control in general require admission to a safe facility. For those children who are suffering from either an acute episode or a disorder of longer standing but who are not in acute danger, it may be feasible for them to be managed at home until a more thorough assessment can be made and a program located to most appropriately meet their needs. Depending on the resources available, it might be possible to arrange for admission to an appropriate inpatient unit or treatment program directly from the emergency setting. Should this occur, as when the child requires admission for maintenance of a safe environment, both the child and the family need support and reassurance that these measures are being taken in the best interests of the child. Admission to a psychiatric treatment program is a difficult decision for any family to make regardless of the circumstances, and understanding this is important to be able to support and help the family in this process.

Some children suffering from psychotic disorders do not require admission to an inpatient program but need referral for further evaluation and treatment. Emergency settings should have the mechanism to either directly provide appropriate referrals or to refer the family to someone who can make the referral. Staff in the emergency setting should also include available members who can provide support to those families who are in need of crisis intervention, even if they are already involved in treatment but for some reason are unable to reach their own therapist at a given time.

Sleep Terror Disorder

Children will occasionally be brought to the emergency setting in the midst of or following an episode of "night terror," or sleep terror disorder. This syndrome has been described as a disorder of arousal in which the child repeatedly experiences abrupt awakening, usually accompanied by a panicked scream. Episodes commonly occur shortly after the onset of sleep (non-REM sleep; approximately one-half hour to 3 hours following entrance into sleep) and last for 1 to 10 minutes. The child will be found sitting up in bed, displaying severe anxiety and agitation. This may be accompanied by perseverative movements (such as plucking at the blanket), sweating, dilated pupils, and increased heart and respiratory rate. Those in attendance are unable to calm or comfort the child until the confusion and anxiety lessen. The child has no recall of a dream following the event (as in the experience of a nightmare) but may remember a feeling of extreme fear and parts of a dream just prior to waking. Usually there is no memory of the episode the following morning.[53]

Predisposing factors include fatigue, stress, and nighttime doses of tricyclic antidepressants or neuroleptic medications. These episodes must be differentiated from REM nightmares, hallucinations oc-

curring just prior to sleep, and epileptic seizures.[54]

Sleep terror disorder occurs in about one to four percent of the population, with an estimated greater number having an isolated episode. It is more prevalent in male children, with an age of onset between 4 and 12 years. Extremely variable courses are reported, with frequency of episodes ranging from daily intervals to numbers of weeks between events. There is no consistently accompanying psychopathology seen in these children, and the disorder usually disappears over time in early adolescence.[55]

Families need reassurance and support to cope with these episodes, as they can be frightening to witness as well as experience. The parents need to be educated as to the characteristics, predisposing factors, and theory behind the disorder so that their anxiety can be diminished and they can help their child avoid situations (as much as possible) that may serve to trigger these attacks.

Acute Grief Reaction

Children may be brought to the emergency setting in acute crisis at some point following the death of or sudden separation from a loved one. This process of acute grieving can be extremely distressing to both child and family, and there are measures that health professionals can employ to assist the clients during these times. These may also favorably influence prognostic outcomes for the child and family.

Lindemann,[56] in his classic work on acute grief, described symptomatology common to persons experiencing grief over a loss, regardless of its origin (i.e., type of death or separation). This syndrome has some universal characteristics and predictable behaviors, which, if understood by the person experiencing the loss and by those involved in helping to support the person, can make the experience more manageable.

Lindemann described the somatic and psychologic symptomatology of acute grief as follows: sighing respirations, especially when the individual is talking about his grief; feeling exhausted; a hollow feeling in the stomach; lack of appetite; feeling of things being unreal; feeling emotionally distant from others; a tendency to be intensely preoccupied with the image of the lost person; a preoccupation with feelings of guilt; feelings of irritability and anger/ hostility toward others; and a fear that these symptoms indicate that the individual is "going crazy." Conduct patterns may also change, especially those somehow reminiscent of the deceased.[57]

Apparently the duration of the reaction depends on how well the individual deals with the grief and begins to resolve the loss. This resolution entails the individual releasing his preoccupation with the dependency on the lost one, adjusting to life and the environment without the loved one, and establishing new emotional relationships.[58]

People surrounding the grieving person can help in this process by allowing the person to share his or her sorrow. This can be done through encouraging and sometimes even pushing the person to talk about the loss (especially when the person consistently avoids thinking or talking about the lost individual), acknowledging the person's fears and reassuring him or her that what he or she is experiencing is part of the normal grieving process, and encouraging and supporting the person in his or her attempts to carry on with his or her life and to form new relationships.

Parents will often be confused and frightened by the behavioral changes in their child and will often be at a loss as to how to manage the changes and to help the child. This helplessness may be compounded if the other family members are also grieving, as when someone close to the whole family is lost (i.e., death of parent, sibling, grandparent). In this case everyone needs support to understand the grief process and how teaching can help others resolve it. Parents will require education on how to talk with their children about death (in a manner appropriate to the developmental level of the child) and on how it is permissible for both parents and children to share the grief, not hide it, and come to some resolution together. Sometimes it will be helpful to refer parents or families to support groups dealing with specific losses, as many people find it helpful to share what they are experiencing with others who have had similar trials.

There are cases in which grieving does take on abnormal features. These "morbid"[59] reactions are described by Lindemann as:

1. Delayed reaction. This can happen even years later and can be triggered by something in connection with the lost loved one or by a spontaneous event in the life of the individual.
2. Distorted reactions. These reactions are characterized by overactivity, with feelings of happiness rather than loss, or acquisition of symptomatology of the last disease or cause of death of the loved one; exacerbation of medical diseases with some possible psychogenic origins, such as asthma, rheumatoid arthritis and ulcerative colitis; changes in close relationships; hostility directed at specific persons (i.e., the treating doctor); and affectual changes (i.e., "wooden features," flat affect) as a result of the individual's attempts to deal with his or her feelings, which he or she thinks are abnormal.

Other characteristics include an inability to generate activity spontaneously without the aid of others; maladaptive behaviors (self-punitive acts, physical and emotional); and agitated depression with a high potential for suicide risk. These individuals require referral for more in-depth psychotherapeutic treatment. The outcome will depend on how well the individual deals with his or her grief in terms of resolving it most appropriately. The outcome can also be influenced by premorbid personality integration and functioning.

VIOLENCE

Occasionally a child or adolescent will be brought to the emergency setting who is violently out of control or on the verge of being so. These situations are anxiety provoking for everyone, including the patient, and thus should be managed as quickly and safely as possible. Emergency staff can use certain techniques and procedures to resolve the crisis expediently and with minimal threat.

Tupin identifies three categories of strategies that can be employed in the management of violent patients to establish control on an immediate, short-term basis. These include psychotherapeutic techniques, environmental-physical controls, and pharmacologic measures.[60] Psychotherapeutic measures involve interventions geared to calming the patient and to decreasing the anxiety and potential explosiveness of the situation. These measures involve reassuring the patient that he or she is being listened to, is respected, and that action will be taken to address his or her problem. It is necessary to convey to the patient that he or she will be kept safe and that others will be kept safe also. The measures also include helping the patient control himself or herself, if necessary. It is imperative that these actions be undertaken in a nonthreatening manner and that the patient be assured that no one

will try to hurt him or her. Specific techniques include the following:

- Introduce yourself (even if the patient appears confused or unaware, as they often understand more than is apparent), and calmly explain what you are going to do.
- After assessing the patient's sensorium, orient him or her, speaking simply, to the surroundings; assure him or her that you are going to try to help; decrease stimuli as much as possible (particularly if behavior is drug induced)[61] and use simple explanations before initiating any procedures.
- Avoid all unnecessary procedures, particularly intrusive ones.[62]
- Try to keep one person with the patient to provide consistency.
- Do not express fear to the patient, either verbally or through body language, as the individual's threatening behavior is often a defense against his or her own anxiety and fear, which may be increased if he or she feels that those around him or her are feeling as much lack of control as he or she is[63] (this is especially true with children, who, because of their developmental level, need to know and feel that the adults around them are in control).
- State to the patient calmly that he or she must stop his or her verbal abuse so that you can better listen to him or her and understand the problem.
- Remember that verbal abuse can indicate the possibility of physically threatening behavior and be careful not to antagonize the patient.
- Set consistent limits and do not allow yourself to be manipulated.
- Reinforce the positive by encouraging the patient to talk to you about what is bothering him or her.
- Do not crowd the patient, as this will also serve to increase his or her anxiety

and may provoke him or her to more aggressive behavior.

- Allow the person to have some control and to make some choices (within appropriate limits), as this will serve to make him or her feel less threatened and will provide him or her with some self-esteem.
- Take threats seriously; do not try to manage a potentially serious and dangerous situation alone.

Should the patient lose control and require physical restraint, apply the restraints as quickly and smoothly as possible to decrease the possibility of harm to the patient and others. Reassure the patient that his or her behavior can be contained. Have personnel standing by (when possible) who are trained to deal with this situation (i.e., security guards, mental health workers). Explain beforehand, if possible, what is going to happen and how it will be done. Again, reinforce that no one wants to hurt him or her, and that you are trying to help. Keep someone with the patient at all times when he or she is restrained, both for safety and to decrease the patient's fear and anxiety. If conversation seems to agitate the individual, then remain silent; stay within the area to visualize the patient clearly. If speaking with the patient is not contraindicated, then help him or her to verbalize rather than to act out his feelings.[68] Should an injection of medication be necessary, explain that it is being done to calm him or her, not as a punishment. Release the patient from restraints as soon as it is possible to do so but only after careful assessment indicates that he or she can control his or her behavior.

The patient may also be managed psychopharmaceutically when acute agitation exists despite attempts at other measures. Commonly used agents include barbiturates, antianxiety medications, and antipsychotics. Any of these medications may be useful, and each group may also have its drawbacks.[69] The person prescribing the medication as well as the nurse who is administering it should be familiar with those agents commonly used in their emergency setting to manage these problems.

Disposition will depend on underlying causes of the behavior, and the reader should refer to other sections in which disposition alternatives for specific clinical syndromes are discussed.

NOTES

1. D. Aguilera, & J. Messick. *Crisis Intervention Therapy for Psychological Emergencies.* St. Louis: Mosby, 1982, p. 1.
2. H.J. Brad, & G. Caplan. A framework for studying families in crisis. *Social Work* 5, no. 3(1960):57.
3. Aguilera, & Messick, *Crisis Intervention Therapy,* p. 14.
4. R. McKinnon, & R. Michels. *The Psychiatric Interview in Clinical Practice.* Philadelphia: W.B. Saunders, 1971, p. 402.
5. A.W. Burgess. *Psychiatric Nursing in the Hospital and Community* (4th ed.). Englewood Cliffs, N.J.: Prentice Hall, 1985, pp. 84–111.
6. F.M. Carter. *Psychosocial Nursing Theory and Practice in Hospital and Community Mental Health* (3rd ed.). New York: Macmillan, 1981, pp. 98–128.
7. J. Haber, A. Leach, S. Scheedy, & B.F. Sideleau. *Comprehensive Psychiatric Nursing* (2nd ed.). New York: McGraw-Hill, 1982, pp. 76–77.
8. J.G. Gorton, & R. Partridge (Eds.). *Practice and Management of Psychiatric Emergency Care.* St. Louis: Mosby, 1982, p. 191.
9. J. Bumbalo. Nursing assessment and diagnosis: Mental health problems of children. *Topics In Clinical Nursing* 5, no. 1(April 1983):41–51.
10. Gorton, & Partridge, *Practice and Management of Psychiatric Emergency Care,* p. 189.

11. A.C. Slaby, L.R. Tancredi, & J. Lieb. *Clinical Psychiatric Medicine*. Philadelphia: Harper, 1981, pp. 552–556.
12. S. Talley, & M.C. King. *Psychiatric Emergencies. Nursing Assessment and Intervention*. New York: Macmillan, 1981, p. 17.
13. Gorton, & Partridge, *Practice and Management of Psychiatric Emergency Care*, p. 191.
14. Talley, & King, *Psychiatric Emergencies*, p. 17.
15. Bumbalo, Mental health problems of children, pp. 41–51.
16. James E. Simmons. *Psychiatric Examination of Children* (3rd ed.). Philadelphia: Lea & Febiger, 1981, pp. 1–26, 60.
17. Gorton, & Partridge, *Practice and Management of Psychiatric Emergency Care*, p. 191.
18. Bumbalo, Mental health problems of children, pp. 41–51.
19. Simmons, *Psychiatric Examination of Children*, pp. 1–26, 60.
20. A. Child, C. Murphy, & M. Rhyne. Depression in children: Reasons and risks. *Pediatric Nursing* 6, no. 4(July/August 1980): 9–10.
21. Ibid., pp. 9–10.
22. A. Mellencamp. Adolescent depression: A review of the literature with implications for nursing care. *Journal of Psychosocial Nursing* 19, no. 9(September 1981):15.
23. Child, Murphy, & Rhyne, Depression in children, pp. 12–13.
24. C. Deuber. Depression in the school aged child. Implications for primary care. *The Nurse Practitioner* 7, no. 8(September 1982): 26–30.
25. B. Curran. Suicide. *Pediatric Clinics of North America* 26, no. 4(November 1979):740.
26. B. Nelms, & M. Brady. The depressed school aged child. *Pediatric Nursing* 6, no. 4(July/August 1980):15–19.
27. Curran, Suicide, p. 740.
28. S. Inamdar. G. Siomopoulos, M. Osborn, & E. Bianchi. Phenomenology associated with depressed moods in adolescents. *American Journal of Psychiatry* 136, no. 2(February 1979):158.
29. American Academy of Pediatrics, Committee on Adolescence. Teenage suicide. *Pediatrics* 66, no. 1(July 1980):144.
30. J.M. Finigan. Assessment of childhood and adolescent depression and suicide potential. *Journal of Emergency Nursing* 12, no. 1(January/February 1986):35–40.
31. Nelms, & Brady, The depressed school aged child, pp. 15–19.
32. Bumbalo, Mental health problems of children, pp. 41–51.
33. Child, Murphy, & Rhyne, Depression in children, pp. 10–12.
34. American Academy of Pediatrics, Teenage suicide, pp. 145–146.
35. Curran, Suicide, p. 745.
36. Ibid., pp. 737–745.
37. S. Friedman, P. Friedman, & H. Juseman. Judging the degree of risk through the clinical interview. *The Mount Sinai Journal of Medicine* 45, no. 4(July/August 1978):463–468.
38. L. Eisenberg. Adolescent suicide: On taking arms against a sea of trouble. *Pediatrics* (1980):318–319.
39. American Academy of Pediatrics, Teenage suicide, pp. 144–145.
40. Finigan, Assessment of childhood and adolescent depression and suicide potential, pp. 35–40.
41. Slaby, Tancredi, & Lieb, *Clinical Psychiatric Nursing*, pp. 556–561.
42. C. Smith, & E. Bope. The suicide patient. The primary care physician's role in evaluation and treatment. *Postgraduate Medicine* 79, no. 8(June 1986):196–197.
43. Curran, Suicide, p. 745.
44. Eisenberg, Adolescent suicide: On taking arms against a sea of trouble, p. 319.
45. Smith, The suicide patient, p. 198.
46. Group for the Advancement of Psychiatry. The Committee on Child Psychiatry. *Psychopathological Disorders in Childhood: Theoretical Considerations and a Proposed Classification, Volume VI*. Report No. 62(June 1966):251.
47. R.B. Murray, & M. Wilson. *Psychiatric Mental Health Nursing: Giving Emotional Care*. Englewood Cliffs, N.J.: Prentice Hall, 1983, p. 657.
48. The Committee on Child Psychiatry, *Psychopathological Disorders*, pp. 251–252.
49. Murray, & Wilson, *Psychiatric Mental Health Nursing*, p. 657.
50. Ibid., pp. 657–658.

51. The Committee on Child Psychiatry, *Psychopathological Disorder*, pp. 253–258.
52. Murray, & Wilson, *Psychiatric Mental Health Nursing*, p. 661.
53. American Psychiatric Association. *Diagnostic and Statistical Manual of Mental Disorders* (3rd ed.). Washington, D.C.: American Psychiatric Association, 1980, pp. 84–85.
54. Ibid., pp. 84–85.
55. Ibid., p. 85.
56. E. Lindemann. *Symptomatology and Management of Acute Grief*. Paper read at the Centenary Meeting of the American Psychiatric Association, Philadelphia, May 15–18, 1944, pp. 1–9.
57. Ibid., pp. 1–4.
58. Ibid., p. 3.
59. Ibid., pp. 4–8.
60. J. Tupin. The violent patient: A strategy for management and diagnosis. *Hospital and Community Psychiatry* 34, no. 1(January 1983):37.
61. Ibid., pp. 37–38.
62. Ibid.
63. Ibid., p. 38.
64. R.L. Anders. Management of violent patients, *Critical Care Update* 10, no. 1(January 1983):41–48, 53.
65. P.M. Fahrney. The secure emergency department.*Emergency Medicine* 15, no. 9(May 15, 1983):41–45, 48–49.
66. M.A. Teszle. Management of behavioral emergencies in the hospital emergency department. *Topics in Emergency Department* 4, no. 4(January 1983):8–16.
67. E.G. Boettcher. Preventing violent behavior. An integrated theoretical model for nursing. *Perspectives in Psychiatric Care* 21, no. 2(April–June 1983):54–58.
68. Tupin, The violent patient, p. 38.
69. Ibid.

BIBLIOGRAPHY

Aguilera, D., & Messick, J. *Crisis Intervention. Therapy for Psychological Emergencies*. St. Louis: Mosby, 1982.

American Academy of Pediatrics, Committee on Adolescence. Teenage suicide. *Pediatrics* 66(1980):144.

American Psychiatric Association. *Diagnostic and Statistical Manual of Mental Disorders* (3rd ed.). Washington, D.C.: American Psychiatric Association, 1980.

Bumbalo, J. Nursing assessment and diagnosis: Mental health problems of children. *Topics in Clinical Nursing* 1(1983):41–51.

Burgess, A.W. *Psychiatric Nursing in the Hospital and Community* (4th ed.). Englewood Cliffs, N.J.: Prentice Hall, 1985.

Carter, F.M. *Psychosocial Nursing. Theory and Practice in Hospital and Community Mental Health* (3rd ed.). New York: Macmillan, 1981.

Child, A., Murphy, C., & Rhyne, M. Depression in children: Reasons and risks. *Pediatric Nursing* 6(1980):9–10.

Curran, B. Suicide. *Pediatric Clinics of North America* 26(1979):740.

Deuber, C. Depression in the school aged child. Implications for primary care. *The Nurse Practitioner* 7(1982):26–30.

Eisenberg, L. Adolescent suicide on taking arms against a sea of trouble. *Pediatrics* (1980):318–319.

Finigan, J.M. Assessment of childhood and adolescent depression and suicide potential. *Journal of Emergency Nursing* 12(1986):35–40.

Friedman, S., Friedman, P., & Juseman, H. Judging the degree of risk through the clinical interview. *The Mount Sinai Journal of Medicine* 45(1978):463–468.

Gorton, J.G., & Partridge, R., eds. *Practice and Management of Psychiatric Emergency Care*. St. Louis: Mosby, 1982.

Group for the Advancement of Psychiatry, The Committee on Child Psychiatry. *Psychopathological Disorders in Childhood Theoretical Considerations and A Proposed Classification: Volume VI*. Report No. 62(1966):251.

Haber, J., Leach, A., Scheedy, S. & Sideleau, B.F. *Comprehensive Psychiatric Nursing* (2nd ed.). New York: McGraw-Hill, 1982.

Inamdar, S., Siomopoulos, G., Osborn, M., & Bianchi, E. Phenomenology associated with depressed moods in adolescents. *American Journal of Psychiatry* 136(1979):58.

Lindemann, E. *Symptomatology and Management of Acute Grief*. Paper read at the Centenary meeting of the American Psychiatry Association. Philadelphia, May 15–18, 1944, pp. 1–9.

McKinnon, R., & Michels, R. *The Psychiatric Interview in Clinical Practice.* Philadelphia: W.B. Saunders, 1971.

Mellencamp, A. Adolescent depression: A review of the literature with implications for nursing care. *Journal of Psychosocial Nursing* 19(1981):15.

Nelms, B., & Brady, M. The depressed school aged child. *Pediatric Nursing* 6(1980):15–19.

Murray, R.B., & Wilson, M. *Psychiatric Mental Health Nursing: Giving Emotional Care.* Englewood Cliffs, N.J.: Prentice Hall, 1983.

Simmons, J.E. *Psychiatric Examination of Children* (3rd ed.). Philadelphia: Lea & Febiger, 1981.

Slaby, A.E., Tancredi, L.R., & Lieb, J. *Clinical Psychiatric Medicine.* Philadelphia: Harper, 1981.

Smith, C., & Bope, E. The suicide patient. The primary care physician's role in evaluation and treatment. *Postgraduate Medicine* 79(1986): 196–97.

Talley, S., & King, M.C. *Psychiatric Emergencies. Nursing Assessment and Intervention.* New York: Macmillan, 1981.

Tupin, J. The violent patient: A strategy for management and diagnosis. *Hospital and Community Psychiatry* 34(1983):37.

EMERGENCY DEPARTMENT CARE GUIDE FOR PSYCHIATRIC EMERGENCIES

Nursing Diagnosis	Interventions	Evaluation
Alterations in thought processes related to extreme anxiety, psychosis, or drug intoxication	Use nonthreatening approach; Speak to patient in simple terms that are easily comprehended; Administer medications as indicated and monitor for side effects; Establish trusting, nonthreatening relationship	Patient communicates more coherently; Patient begins to share thoughts and feelings; Patient feels calmer and safer
Potential for violence to self, related to depression	Assess patient for suicide risk; Implement suicide precautions; provide safe environment; Assess for ingestion of toxic substances (i.e., obtain toxic screen specimens); Prepare patient for admission to hospital or psychiatric treatment facility, when appropriate	Patient is prevented from harming self or others in the emergency department
Ineffective family coping related to presence of multiple stressors	Assess family's coping abilities; Identify social supports; Encourage family to seek therapy	Family members identify social supports; Family members agree to seek therapy

(Continued)

Nursing Diagnosis	Interventions	Evaluation
Ineffective individual coping related to internal conflicts	Convey trust and sincerity Identify patient's social supports Assist patient in identification and verbal expression of thoughts and feelings Accept patient's feelings Provide for appropriate disposition or referral	Patient expresses thoughts and feelings Patient is able to identify social supports Patient cooperates with disposition
Impaired social interactions related to individual or personal stressors	Assess patient's social supports Speak in simple terms Use patient's name when addressing him or her	Patient is able to access social supports Patient is able to communicate with emergency department staff
Disturbance in self-concept related to low self-esteem	Use a nonjudgemental approach Assist patient to identify individuals in his or her life who care for him or her	Patient is able to acknowledge personal strengths as well as weaknesses

5

Resuscitation of the Newborn

Sarah B. Pasternack

The imminent birth of an infant coupled with the potential need to resuscitate the infant presents some unique challenges for emergency department personnel. Often the mother's prenatal and general medical history is unknown. Any pre-existing maternal or fetal complications may not be immediately evident to staff members. If the birth was unattended, there may be no information about the infant's condition at birth or at delivery. The infant may not be responsive upon arrival in the emergency department, and the parents are likely to be distraught.

Delivery and resuscitation of a newborn are not frequent occurrences in most emergency departments, and staff members are often not as familiar with the management of perinatal and neonatal emergencies as they are with other urgent situations. It is understandable that the urgency of the situation, compounded by the simultaneous needs of the infant and parents, can present a tense situation for staff members.

It is essential that every emergency department staff develop a plan for the eventuality of emergency delivery and neonatal resuscitation. This is especially true if the emergency facility is freestanding, that is, not located in a hospital, or if the emergency department is in a hospital with no obstetric or pediatric department. Each member of the team should be prepared to assume an appropriate role in the management of a neonatal emergency.

The American Heart Association recommends that personnel who provide emergency services demonstrate expertise in Basic and Advanced Life-Support techniques for neonates and children.[1] In many emergency departments both nurses and physicians are required to obtain American Heart Association certification in Advanced Life-Support. Educational in-service programs on emergency delivery and newborn resuscitation should be provided at periodic intervals to update knowledge and skills of staff members. A list of equipment for care of the newborn at the time of delivery and during resuscitation can be found in Table 5–1.

HIGH-RISK CONDITIONS FOR THE NEWBORN

Most births that occur outside a health facility, enroute to a hospital, or in an emergency department are precipitous or result from a delay in reaching assistance. These factors in and of themselves often place an

TABLE 5–1. EQUIPMENT FOR INFANT DELIVERY AND RESUSCITATION IN THE EMERGENCY DEPARTMENT

Essential Items		

Emergency delivery kits
  Sterile scissors
  Sterile umbilicae tape or plastic cord clamps
Suction catheters, sizes 6 F, 8 F, 10 F
Infant bulb suction syringes
Infant blankets (warmed if possible)
Stockinette (3 to 5 inches wide)
Warming source (radiant heater, warming lights, plastic wrap, hot packs, etc.)
ECG monitor (capable of setting alarms at lower limit of 60 and upper limit of 180)
Neonatal-sized ECG electrode pads
Infant-sized face masks
Resuscitation bags, 750 ml capacity, with reservoir
Anesthesia bag, 750 ml capacity, with in-line pressure manometer
Miller laryngoscope blades, sizes 0 and 1
Magill forceps
Endotracheal tubes, uniform diameter and tapered, sizes 2.5 to 4.0, at least two of each size
Extra batteries and bulbs for laryngoscope
Endotracheal tube stylets
Laryngoscope
	Wall suction
	Wall oxygen, with warmer
	Portable oxygen
	Cutdown trays
	Umbilical catheterization trays 3.5 F, to 5.0 F umbilical catheters
	Dextrose solutions (10%, 20%, 25%, 50%)
	Pediatric IV solutions, such as $D_5/0.25$ NS
	Normal saline for injection, USP
	Sterile water for injection, USP
	Lactated Ringer's injection, USP
	Albumin 5% and 25% solutions
	Drugs
	  Sodium bicarbonate, neonatal, 0.5 mEq/ml (4.2%), 10-ml amps
	  Epinephrine, 1:10,000 solution
	  Heparin 10 µg/ml solution
	  Calcium chloride
	  Naloxone (Narcan), neonatal solution, 0.02 mg/ml, 2-ml amps
	  Isoproterenol (Isuprel), 0.2 mg/ml
	  Atropine, 0.4 mg/0.5 ml solution
	  Dopamine, 40 mg/ml solution
	  Defibrillator, with neonatal size paddles
	  Conductive paste
	Doppler blood pressure device or sphygmomanometer
		Premature- and infant-sized disposable blood pressure cuffs
		Stethoscopes
		Volumetric infusion pumps (capable of delivering at least 1 ml/hr; battery powered)
		Infant scale
		Nasogastric tubes and feeding tubes, sizes 5 F and 6 F
		Sterile towels, gowns, gloves
		Surgical masks, hats
		Povidine iodine preps
		Alcohol preps
		Needles, IV catheters (various sizes)
		Syringes (various sizes)
		Microtainers, heparinized and plain
		Capillary blood tubes, heparinized and plain
		Blood gas syringes (heparinized)
		Lancets
		Glass slides
		Culture tubes
		No. 11 surgical blades
		Sutures, needles
		Blood glucose reagent strips
		Suture sets
		Sterile 2 × 2 and 4 × 4 sponges
		Thermometer (rectal)
		Neonatal-sized arm boards
		Tincture of benzoin
		Identification bands
		Adhesive tape

Desirable Items (But Not Essential)		
Electronic blood pressure/vital signs monitor	Transcutaneous O_2 monitor	Prewarmed isolette, with portable oxygen supply

infant at high risk. There are, however, numerous other factors that are associated with high risk for the newborn. They may originate during the prenatal, perinatal, or neonatal period. Factors most frequently implicated in producing high risk for infants are listed in Table 5–2.

ASSESSMENT AND MANAGEMENT OF THE NEWBORN

Imminent Delivery
When a laboring pregnant female is brought to the emergency department, the nurse quickly and systematically assesses

TABLE 5-2. FACTORS ASSOCIATED WITH HIGH RISK FOR THE NEWBORN

I. Prenatal	II. Perinatal	III. Neonatal

A. *Maternal conditions*
Maternal age <16 or
   >35 years
Drug, alcohol abuse
Diabetes, thyroid, renal,
   heart, or lung disease
Hypertension, chronic or
   pregnancy induced
Bleeding, especially in early
   pregnancy or in third trimester
Premature rupture of
   membranes
Fever
Infection
Inadequate or no prenatal
   care
	Premature labor
	Meconium-stained amniotic
	   fluid
	Prolapsed cord
	Maternal hypotension, sei-
	   zures, respiratory arrest
	Rapid labor
	Placenta previa
	Abruptio placenta
		Traumatic delivery
		Premature birth
		Infection
		Acidosis
		Hypoxia
		Respiratory distress
		Hypothermia
		Hypovolemia
		Congenital anomalies,
		   especially cardiac
		Intracranial hemorrhage

B. *Fetal conditions* Multiple gestation Abnormal fetal size or position Abnormality of fetal heart rate or rhythm Acidosis		

Adapted from J.W. Graef, & T.E. Cone, Jr. (Eds.). *Manual of Pediatric Therapeutics* (3rd Ed.). Boston: Little, Brown, 1985, pp. 120–121; and from J.P. Cloherty, & A.R. Stark (Eds.). *Manual of Neonatal Care.* Boston: Little, Brown, 1980, p. 56.

the mother's vital signs, contractions, and fetal heart tones. The nurse should also attempt to ascertain whether the membranes have ruptured and how long ago the membranes ruptured. While the mother is being examined to determine the progress of her labor, the nurse should take note of the woman's general physical status and behavior. This is undoubtedly a stressful time for the mother. Therefore it is essential that staff members proceed in a calm but deliberate manner.

If the infant's father or a "significant other" is present, this person should be instructed briefly and allowed to remain with the mother. This individual can provide valuable emotional support while emergency department personnel attend

to the mother's needs and prepare for the delivery and possible resuscitation of the infant. Long-standing emergency department practices of automatically excluding family or significant others from treatment areas should be re-evaluated and individualized. Unless the family or significant other is disruptive to the care of the mother or infant, more harm than benefit may result from exclusion.

It is essential that all emergency department nurses be able to recognize the signs of imminent delivery (Table 5-3) and act accordingly. Management of emergency delivery and care of the mother in the immediate postpartum period is beyond the scope of this chapter and will not be addressed here.

TABLE 5-3. PHYSICAL AND BEHAVIORAL SIGNS OF IMMINENT DELIVERY

Involuntary catching of breath and pushing, even subtly, during a contraction
Thrashing about in bed; absorption in self; change in breathing patterns; expressing the feeling, "I can't go on any longer." (These behaviors often indicate the transition phase of labor, which may be immediately followed by delivery.)
Increasing bloody show
Increased facial flushing and diaphoresis
Increased sensation of pressure in pelvis
Beginning of "blossoming" of the anus
Appearance of fullness at perineum
"Crowning"—appearance of head at introitus. (In multipara, birth is very imminent. In primipara, birth may be up to 30 minutes later. When head stays visible between contractions, birth is nearing.)

Copyright 1979, American Journal of Nursing Company with permission from B. Jennings. Emergency delivery: How to attend to one safely. MCN: American Journal Maternal-Child Nursing 4(May-June 1979):153.

Assessment

Airway. One of the most important physiologic changes occurring at birth is transition from fetal respiration through placental gas exchange to extrauterine breathing through the nose and respiratory tract. It is believed that this change is effected by two processes: (1) activation of certain chemoreceptors in the aorta and carotid arteries, and (2) cutaneous receptors that are sensitive to extrauterine temperature and tactile stimuli.[2] A clear, patent airway is a necessary prerequisite for the infant's ability to take a breath.

During a vaginal delivery pressure on the infant's thorax in the birth canal aids in expelling a good amount of fetal lung fluids. Since it may not be possible to ascertain the infant's condition prior to delivery, it is advisable to bulb suction the mouth, and then the nose, when the head is delivered.

The infant should be dried and wrapped in a towel or blanket immediately after delivery, prior to cutting the cord. The friction of drying helps to stimulate the infant's breathing and crying. Wrapping the infant helps conserve body heat. (See section on thermoregulation later in this chapter.)

Except in situations in which the infant is endangered (i.e., pale, cyanotic, flaccid), the cord should not be clamped and cut until pulsation ceases. This usually takes 30 to 40 seconds. Early clamping should be avoided because doing so may deprive the infant of as much as 30 ml/kg of blood.[3] During this time it is important that the infant be held at the level of the mother's introitus. Holding the infant higher than the introitus or placing him or her on the mother's abdomen (a common practice) before the cord is cut may cause hypovolemia in the infant.[4] Conversely, holding the infant below the introitus or "milking" the cord should be avoided, as these practices may result in hypervolemia, polycythemia, or impaired respiratory status for the infant.[5]

Bulb suctioning the mouth and nares may be repeated, as necessary, before and after the cord is cut. For most healthy infants bulb suctioning will sufficiently clear the airway. Prolonged catheter suctioning of vigorous infants during the first 5 to 10 minutes of life is contraindicated because it may result in vomiting, hypoxia, apnea, or bradycardia.[6-8] When bulb suctioning is insufficient, an 8- or 10-F suction catheter using pressures no greater than −100 mm Hg (−136 cm of water) or a DeLee mucus trap may be used.[9] Suction periods should be no greater than 10 seconds, and 100 percent oxygen should be administered between suctionings.[10] The oxygen can be blown over the infant's face or administered by mask and bag as necessary.

If the infant is born with thick meconium (not merely meconium-stained fluid), different procedures should be used to suction the infant. A DeLee mucus trap suction catheter should be used as soon as the head is delivered.[11] It is essential that meconium be cleared from the infant's airway prior to the onset of breathing. This will prevent, or minimize at least, meconium aspiration and complications such as pneumonia, respiratory distress, and pneumothorax. The infant born with thick meconium should therefore be immediately intubated, and tracheal suctioning should be performed.

Suction should be directly applied to the endotracheal tube, as it is slowly withdrawn from the trachea.[12-14] One should not attempt to pass catheters through the endotracheal tube because their diameter is too small for clearing thick tenacious mucus. The laryngoscope blade is left in place to permit reintubation and suctioning.[15,16] Since deep tracheal suctioning can result in bradycardia, it is essential that the infant's heart rate be monitored continuously during this procedure.

After tracheal suctioning has been performed a second time, the infant should be gently ventilated with oxygen. It is desirable to also suction the stomach at this time to reduce the likelihood that regurgitated meconium will be aspirated.[17] This tracheal suctioning procedure is also indicated when there has been severe vaginal bleeding during birth.[18]

Apgar Evaluation. The Apgar score is a rapid method of evaluating the newborn against five objective criteria: heart rate, respiratory effort, color, muscle tone, and response to stimulation (Table 5-4). The Apgar scoring method is highly useful in the emergency department because it is reliable, is quickly performed, and is the most useful method of assessing a newborn's well-being or need for resuscitation. A wall chart or other suitable convenient means should be used to make the Apgar scoring system visible to emergency department personnel.

Based on the infant's condition, he or she is given a score of 0, 1, or 2 for each of the five signs at 1 minute and again at 5 minutes of age. The sum of these scores each time this evaluation method is used is the infant's Apgar score. It is important for emergency department personnel to remember that few infants achieve a score of 9 or 10. Table 5-5 summarizes interpretation of Apgar scores and the indicated interventions.

Initial Assessment. It is not necessary that a thorough newborn assessment be performed in the emergency department. The infant should be observed for any obvious abnormalities and skin lesions. In addi-

TABLE 5-4. APGAR EVALUATION OF THE NEWBORN

Sign	Score		
	0	1	2
Heart Rate	Absent	Less than 100/min	Over 100/min
Respiratory effort	Absent	Slow, irregular, or weak	Vigorous cry
Color	Blue, pale	Pink body, blue extremities	Completely pink
Muscle tone	Limp, flaccid	Some flexion of extremities	Active motion; good extremity flexion
Reflex irritability[a]	Absent	Grimace	Cough, sneeze, or cry

[a]Elicited by insertion of nasal catheter or cutaneous stimulation of soles of the feet.

TABLE 5-5. APGAR SCORE INTERPRETATION AND INTERVENTIONS

Apgar Score	Interpretation	Interventions
8-10	Vigorous infant	Oral and nasal bulb suction Keep infant warm and dry
5-7	Mild asphyxia just prior to birth	Vigorous stimulation by slapping soles of feet or rubbing back Blow 100% O_2 by face If response sluggish, ventilate with 80-100% O_2 via bag and mask
3-4	Moderate depression	Ventilate with bag and mask 30 times per minute, using pressures of 20-25cm H_2O If no response, decompress stomach with NG tube, intubate and resume ventilation Administer $NaHCO_3$ if arterial blood gases indicate acidosis
0-2	Severe asphyxiation	Resuscitate immediately

Adapted from G.A. Gregory. Resuscitation of the newborn. In W.C. Shoemaker, W.L. Thompson, & P.R. Holbrook (Eds.). Textbook of Critical Care. Philadelphia: W.B. Saunders, 1984, p. 24; and from J.W. Graef, & T.E. Cone, Jr. (Eds.). Manual of Pediatric Therapeutics (3rd ed.). Boston: Little, Brown, 1985, p. 133.

tion, two specific assessment measures should be carried out after the infant has stabilized but within the first 10 to 15 minutes of life. The first measure, passage of a suction catheter through each nostril to the posterior pharynx, is done to detect choanal atresia. This should be done as soon as possible because bilateral obstruction of the posterior nares at the junction of the nasopharynx can be lethal. Since neonates are obligate nose breathers, choanal atresia forces the infant to use the mouth for breathing, and the infant will show signs of respiratory distress within a short period of time. If it is impossible to pass the catheter bilaterally, an oral airway should be inserted as an initial measure, even if the infant appears pink and vigorous. Orotracheal intubation can later be performed by a qualified professional.

The second technique, passage of a number 10-F DeLee suction catheter with a mucus trap through the mouth into the stomach and aspiration of at least 2 to 3 ml gastric contents should also be done in the emergency department. This measure is performed for several reasons. The first is to rule out esophageal atresia. If the cathe-

ter meets with obstruction or if gastric contents cannot be obtained (the catheter may advance but merely coil upon itself when it meets obstruction), esophageal atresia should be suspected. If the tube advances but it is possible to aspirate more than 25 ml of fluid from the stomach, it is possible that the infant may have a small bowel obstruction.[19]

Some forms of esophageal atresia or bowel anomalies may occur concomitantly with tracheal anomalies. All infants with these suspected disorders should therefore be observed closely and not allowed to feed until they can be more thoroughly evaluated and the anomalies ruled out or confirmed. Infants with esophageal atresia or small bowel obstruction are likely to have copious secretions that may need to be removed frequently by suction.

After gastric contents are obtained, the tube may be withdrawn. The gastric contents should be labeled with the time the specimen was obtained and other pertinent identifying data and reserved. A smear can be prepared from the gastric fluid for gram strain to determine the risk of infection. The remaining amount of fluid should accompany the infant to the nursery where the neonatologist may elect to use the fluid to perform the "shake test" to predict the likelihood of respiratory distress syndrome. This test is especially useful when an infant is premature, born with thick meconium, or if the infant experiences respiratory distress at birth. For the shake test results to be accurate, it is important that the gastric aspirate be obtained during the first hour of life.[20]

Most emergency departments have cameras that take instantly developing photographs. It is suggested that emergency department staff members take two photographs of any baby born in the emergency department or born prior to arrival in the emergency department. This practice is common in delivery rooms. Photographs should be taken regardless of whether the infant is normal, ill, or stillborn. One copy of the photograph can be given to the parents, and one should be retained in the emergency department files. (Do not insert in the medical record. Take a third photograph if one is to be placed in the record.)

Maternity nurses have found that a photograph of the baby is invaluable for parents if they must be separated from the baby for any length of time (i.e., if the baby must be transferred to a regional neonatal intensive care center), if the baby's prognosis is poor, or if the baby dies. If the baby is stillborn, the photograph should be taken and offered to parents. They may initially refuse, but later (even months later) parents may request the photo. Maternity nurses have learned that it is wise to place the second photo in a file in case the family accidentally loses the first one.

Management of the Vigorous Newborn

If the infant is responsive, vigorous, appears healthy, and has an Apgar score of 8 to 10, there is very little intervention indicated. In fact, unnecessary invasive mea-

sures are clearly contraindicated. The infant should be observed at frequent intervals (approximately every 15 minutes) to ascertain color and respiratory rate. Once the infant has been stabilized, heart rate can be obtained every 30 to 60 minutes unless the infant experiences respiratory or color changes. Acrocyanosis, a condition in which the infant's extremities remain blue, mottled, and cool to touch, is a common phenomenon during the first 24 to 48 hours of life. This condition in and of itself presents no cause for alarm. All observations of the infant made by the nurse should be documented in the infant's record. The normal range of vital signs for the newborn is given in Table 5-6.

Temperature Regulation

Heat production and temperature regulation in neonates is quite different from that of the older child and adult. In addition, thermoregulation differs between full-term and premature infants. The term newborn has fat deposits and the ability to use specialized chemical processes to aid in heat production when he or she is exposed to cold. The premature infant has little, if any, fat deposits, and heat loss generally exceeds the infant's ability to produce body heat. The large body surface area of infants in comparison to body weight makes them highly vulnerable to heat loss.

When the infant emerges from the warmth of his mother's uterus, his or her body temperature falls rapidly as he or she is exposed to room temperature (convection). Failure to keep the infant dry results in heat loss from evaporation. Placing the infant on unwarmed surfaces for purposes of examination or resuscitation causes heat loss due to conduction.

If the infant is forced to maintain body temperature in response to cold stress, his or her rate of metabolism and oxygen consumption rise. The infant rapidly progresses to acidosis and/or hypoglycemia if he or she must continue to struggle to

TABLE 5-6. AVERAGE VITAL SIGNS DURING THE FIRST FOUR HOURS OF LIFE

Age	Temperature	Apical Pulse	Respiratory Rate	Blood Pressure[a] (According to Weight)
Birth	37C–37.8C, rectally (98.6F–100F)	160–180	60–80 (irregular)	1001–2000 g: 34–58 systolic 18–36 diastolic
One-half hour	36C–37C, axillary (96.8F–98.6F)	120–160	40–60 (irregular)	2001–3000 g: 44–64 systolic 22–42 diastolic
1–4 hours	36.5C–37.5C, axillary (97.7F–99.5F)	120–140	30–60 (irregular)	>3000 g: 50–80 systolic 24–52 diastolic

[a]Proper cuff size is essential to accuracy of blood pressure measurement; cuff width for most neonates is 2.5 to 4.0 cm.

maintain body temperature. The infant's body temperature may initially be measured rectally to rule out imperforate anus. Care should be taken to insert the thermometer no more than 2 to 3 cm into the rectum. Thereafter only axillary temperatures should be taken.

Employing measures designed to maintain the infant's body temperature is an important responsibility for the nurse. It is most important that the infant be kept warm and dry at all times following delivery. All towels and blankets that become moist should be removed immediately and the infant wrapped securely with dry blankets. If possible warmed blankets should be used. Neonates lose a very large amount of heat through their heads. The nurse can fashion a hat from a length of stockinette knotted at one end. This is an effective method of conserving the neonate's body heat. If the infant is vigorous, he or she can be wrapped and placed in the mother's or father's arms. Skin-to-skin contact between the infant and the mother's body is another excellent method for keeping a healthy newborn warm following delivery. If this method is used, it is essential that both mother and baby be warmly covered, or a warming hood should be used.

If the infant cannot be held or if he or she is ill, the nurse must make sure the infant is kept warm. This is especially true if the infant must be resuscitated. If there is no incubator or warmed resuscitation bed available in the emergency department, the nurse can use measures listed in Table 5-7.

Overheating the infant during his stay in the emergency department is an unlikely but possible consequence of overzealous application of external heat. Hyperthermia in the neonate may result in apnea. The infant's temperature should therefore not be allowed to exceed the limits given in Table 5-6. If the infant has become too warm, merely uncovering him or

TABLE 5-7. SOURCES OF EXTERNAL HEAT FOR THE NEONATE BORN IN THE EMERGENCY DEPARTMENT

Radiant hood or panel
Warming lights
Infant warming pad[a] (placed under infant)
Commercially manufactured disposable neonatal thermal wraps
Rubber glove filled with warmed water[a]
Hot packs[a] (disposable type or plastic-covered moist towels heated in microwave oven)

[a]Extreme caution must be taken to prevent burning the infant. These methods all require adequate layers of cloth between the infant's skin and the heat source. Note also that warmed gloves and hot packs must be replaced, as they lose heat.

her for a short period of time should remedy the problem. Frequent axillary temperatures (every 15 to 30 minutes) should be taken and recorded until the infant's temperature remains stable for one hour.

Parent-Infant Bonding

There has been extensive research into the time period surrounding birth and practices used by clinicians in the perinatal and early postpartum periods. Better understanding has resulted in use of methods designed to enhance the period of time when parents become acquainted with their newborn for the very first time. This process is commonly referred to as ''parent-infant bonding.'' The initial 30 to 60 minutes after birth are considered critical to this process.

If the infant does not need medical care, the nurse should use some simple measures to enhance parent-infant bonding while the family is awaiting transfer from the emergency department. As soon as the mother is physically able, she should be given her baby. If the mother so desires, skin-to-skin contact with the infant should be afforded. The mother who plans to breast-feed can put the infant to breast at this time if this is not medically contraindicated for the infant. The father (or significant other) should remain by the mother's side. The father should be encouraged to participate as the mother touches and explores the baby. (The father should use good handwashing and wear a cover gown.)

If medical reasons prohibit or limit opportunities for holding the baby, visualization of the baby for as long as possible is an alternative. Separation of parents and infants should occur only if necessary (i.e., extensive resuscitation). The family should be afforded as much privacy as possible.

The value of using these practices, especially in the emergency department, for

promoting the well-being of the entire family should not be underestimated. Studies have shown that early parent-infant bonding experiences are an important factor in promoting good parent-child interaction and in preventing failure to thrive and child abuse during infancy.[21] Implementing measures to support parent-infant bonding in the emergency department restores a sense of normalcy to a somewhat unusual and untimely birth experience.

RESUSCITATION OF THE NEWBORN

If there is time to prepare, equipment for neonatal intubation, umbilical vessel catheterization, blood sampling, and neonatal emergency drugs should be placed within easy reach. The nurse should ensure that an adequate heat source is provided during resuscitative efforts. Despite the urgency of neonatal resuscitation, it is essential that this detail is not overlooked. It is known that a normal, full-term infant who is left naked and wet in a 25C (77F) room loses 2C (3.6F) of core body temperature within 20 minutes of birth.[22] An asphyxiated newborn encounters more difficulty than does a vigorous one in maintaining body temperatures.[23] Hypothermia in the newborn results in acidosis, which can further complicate resuscitation. Keeping the infant warm and dry is a major factor underlying the success of neonatal resuscitation. An overhead radiant heat source is the preferred method of providing warmth to the infant during emergency procedures.

Timing is of utmost importance in neonatal resuscitation. Apgar scores help identify the extent to which resuscitative measures are necessary, but it is important that resuscitation begin as soon as an asphyxiated or unresponsive infant is born rather than wasting precious time while waiting for 1- and 5-minute scores. The Apgar scoring system does, however, provide useful criteria for assessing the infant's response to resuscitation. The measures described in this section are presented in a sequential manner. In actual practice, however, they are usually instituted in rapid sequence.

Airway and Assisted Ventilation

If the infant does not respond to the methods normally used at delivery, methods to assist ventilation should be instituted immediately.

Oxygen by Mask

When respirations are depressed in the presence of a clear airway but the infant's heart rate is adequate (at least 100 per minute) and muscle tone is good, 100 percent oxygen may be administered. A well-fitting mask (size 0 or 1) that is small enough to maintain a tight face seal should be used. For greatest effectiveness the face mask should have less than 5 ml of dead space.[24] All oxygen delivered by mask should be warmed and humidified. The recommended temperature range is 32C (89.6F) to 36C (96.8F).[25] The infant should respond quickly (within 1 to 2 minutes) by demonstrating spontaneous respirations, adequate heart rate, and improved color. Color changes are most accurately assessed by checking the neonate's oral mucous membranes rather than the extremities.

Positive-Pressure Bag and Mask

If the infant's condition does not improve, positive-pressure ventilation should be instituted. Positive-pressure ventilation, consisting of bag and mask delivering 80 percent to 100 percent oxygen, is indicated when (1) cyanosis persists despite administration of 100 percent oxygen, (2) heart rate is less than 100 per minute, and (3)

respirations are absent.[26] Rate of ventilation should be 30 to 60 per minute,[27] with 40 per minute recommended as the optimal rate.[28] If the infant has not taken a breath on his own, pressure of 20 to 40 cm of water may be necessary initially.[29-31] Lower pressures should be adequate for succeeding breaths.

The infant's head position during bag and mask ventilation is critical. For the infant to benefit from the ventilations, his or her head should be in the "sniffing" position, that is, the neck is extended slightly, with the eyes directly facing the ceiling (Fig. 5-1.) Success of ventilation can be monitored by bilateral auscultation of breath sounds and symmetrical, bilateral chest-wall movements. If the infant does not show evidence of ventilation, he or she should be suctioned, the head and mask repositioned, and ventilation resumed.[32] It is important to remember that bag and mask ventilation often causes gastric distention. It is advisable to insert a feeding tube (size 5 F or 6 F) orally to relieve distention and prevent aspiration.

Endotracheal Intubation

If the bag and mask method is ineffective, or if heart rate and respirations remain depressed, the infant should be intubated under direct laryngoscopic vision. Intubation should be undertaken by professionals skilled in neonatal intubation. Gastric decompression generally precedes intubation. The laryngoscope blades used for neonates are straight (Miller) and come in size 0 (for premature infants weighing up to 2500 g) and in the longer size 1, which can be used for newborns of any size. Oral intubation is usually preferred over nasal intubation during neonatal resuscitation. Endotracheal tubes used for neonates may be straight or tapered at the distal tip (Fig. 5-2). Many clinicians prefer the straight tube because there is less chance of ob-

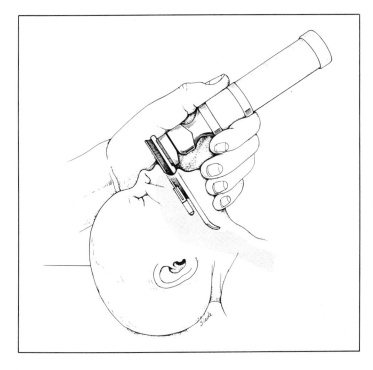

Figure 5-1. The sniffing position. The "sniffing" position (neck slightly extended, eyes directed toward ceiling) is the proper position for maximizing the neonate's airway. This position is used to administer oxygen by mask and for intubation of the neonate. *(From J.P. Goldsmith, & E.H. Karotkin. Assisted Ventilation of the Neonate. Philadelphia: Saunders, 1981.)*

struction with thick secretions. Two tubes of each size should be available. The tube selected should be the largest size possible while still permitting an air leak.[33,34] Only sterile, disposable tubes marked "IT" (implantation tested) or "Z79" should be used.[35] Table 5–8 lists various endotracheal tube sizes suitable for newborns. The infant's head should be maintained in the sniffing position during intubation (Fig. 5–1).

It is essential that the tube be properly secured to prevent displacement or accidental extubation. Correct placement may be checked by visualizing markings on the tube (through laryngoscope), by auscultation, and by observing for bilateral, symmetrical chest-wall motion. A portable chest x-ray can be used to verify tube position. Oxygen administered through an endotracheal tube should be humidified and warmed to 35C to 36C (95F to 96.8F).[36]

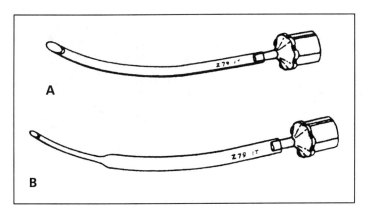

Figure 5-2. Two types of endotracheal tubes for neonates. The straight, or uniform diameter, tube (**A**) is preferred over the "Cole" type (**B**), which has a tapered distal end. *(From K.M. McIntyre, & L.A. James (Eds.). Textbook of Advanced Cardiac Life Support. Dallas: American Heart Association, 1981. Used by permission.)*

TABLE 5–8. SELECTION OF AIRWAYS, ENDOTRACHEAL TUBES, AND SUCTION CATHETER SIZES

Infant Weight	Airway Size	Endotracheal Tube Size (Internal Diameter)	Suction Catheter Size
<1000 g	000	2.5 mm	5 F
1000–1250 g	000	3.0 mm	5–6 F
1250–2000 g	00–0	3.0 mm	6 F
2500–3000 g	0	3.5 mm	8 F
>3000 g	0-1	3.5–4.0 mm	8 F

Ventilation Bags

Several types of bags are available for use in neonatal resuscitation. They may be used with masks or endotracheal tubes. Self-inflating bags are equipped with an intake valve to permit rapid reinflation (Fig. 5–3 A). Both air and oxygen mix as the bag self-inflates. Thus it is impossible to deliver high concentrations of oxygen unless an oxygen reservoir is attached (Fig. 5–3 B). One disadvantage of self-inflating bags is that it is impossible to administer oxygen passively through the mask. Another disadvantage is that the pop-off valve prevents delivery of pressure exceeding 30 to 35 cm of water. Hence a self-inflating bag is generally inadequate for initiating a neonate's first breaths. Bag volume should not exceed 750 ml because infants' tidal volumes are only 6 to 8 ml/kg.[37]

An alternative to self-inflating bags is the anesthesia bag (Fig. 5–4). The anesthesia bag is preferred for neonatal resuscitation because it is capable of delivering very high inspiratory pressures that can be monitored by way of an in-line pressure manometer. This bag is also capable of delivering various concentrations of oxygen. Because one must be able to judge accurately gas intake and gas escape from the exit port (to avoid underfilling or overfilling), this bag should be used only by a professional who has been instructed properly.

It is important that the infant not be overventilated. One should use the least amount of pressure sufficient to create chest movement, breath sounds, and pink skin color. Excessive airway pressures can cause pneumothorax and pneumomediastinum. Providing high concentrations of oxygen for unnecessarily long periods of time should also be avoided. Experts agree that an infant who is able to maintain adequate respiratory function and heart rate

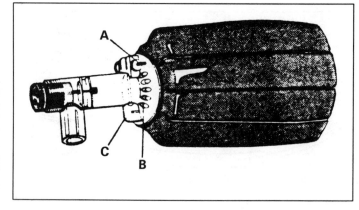

Figure 5–3A. Self-inflating resuscitation bags. Nonreservoir-type bag with gas intake (A), air intake valve (B), and pressure-limiting assembly (C). *(From K.M. McIntyre, & L.A. James (Eds.). Textbook of Advanced Cardiac Life Support. Dallas: American Heart Association, 1981. Used by permission.)*

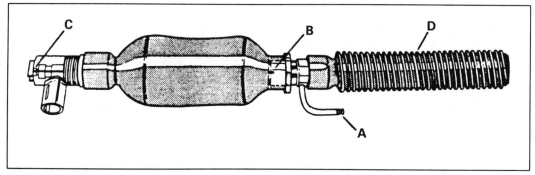

Figure 5–3B. Self-inflating resuscitation bags. Reservoir-type bag with gas intake (A), intake valve (B), pressure-limiting assembly (C), and gas reservoir (D). *(From K.M. McIntyre, & L.A. James (Eds.). Textbook of Advanced Cardiac Life Support. Dallas: American Heart Association, 1981. Used by permission.)*

should be allowed to use his own efforts. Assessment of respiratory function and heart rate should be made approximately every 30 to 60 seconds. Ventilation may be discontinued if the infant demonstrates spontaneous respirations and heart rate over 100 per minute.[38] Ventilation must be continued if there are no spontaneous respirations or if the heart rate is below 100 per minute.[39]

Circulation

Adequacy of the heart rate should be checked after the newborn has been effec-

tively ventilated for 15 to 30 seconds.[40] The American Heart Association recommends that chest compression be initiated if the neonate's heart rate is less than 60 beats per minute or if the neonate's heart rate does not rise above 80 per minute after adequate ventilation with 100 percent oxygen for 30 seconds.[41]

Chest Compressions. It is important that correct technique be used to provide chest compressions for the neonate. The American Heart Association currently advises placing the thumbs on the middle third of

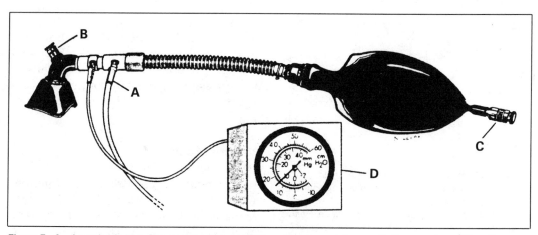

Figure 5–4. Anesthesia bag. The anesthesia bag, preferred for neonatal resuscitation, requires skill and instruction for proper use. *(From K.M. McIntyre, & L.M. James (Eds.). Textbook of Advanced Cardiac Life Support. Dallas: American Heart Association, 1981. Used by permission.)*

the sternum while using the fingers to encircle the thorax and to support the back[42] (Fig. 5–5A). The thumbs should be placed just below an imaginary horizontal line between the nipples, as shown in Figure 5–5 A.

An alternate position, shown in Figure 5–5B, may also be used. This position is used when the rescuer's hands are not large enough to encircle the infant's chest. In using this technique the rescuer first places the index finger of the hand most distant from the newborn's head just below an imaginary horizontal line between the nipples. The correct area of compression is one finger's width below this point, that is, at the location of the middle and ring fingers.[43]

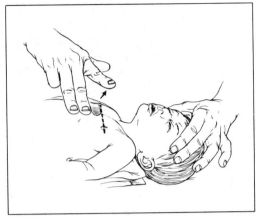

Figure 5–5B. Proper hand position for chest compressions in neonates. Two-finger compression method. Note anatomic landmarks to locate correct finger placement in both figures. *(From American Heart Association. Standards and guidelines for cardiopulmonary resuscitation and emergency cardiac care. The Journal of the American Medical Association 255:21 (June 6, 1986):2958. Used by permission.)*

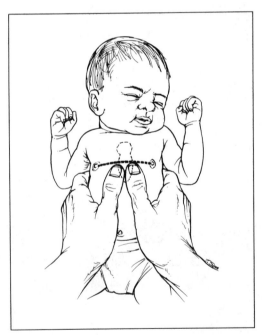

Figure 5–5A. Proper hand position for chest compressions in neonates. Side-by-side thumb placement for chest compressions in small neonates. Thumbs may also be superimposed. *(From American Heart Association. Standards and guidelines for cardiopulmonary resuscitation and emergency cardiac care. The Journal of the American Medical Association 255:21 (June 6, 1986):2958. Used by permission.)*

Compressions should be delivered smoothly at equal intervals and at a rate of 120 times per minute.[44] The fingers or thumbs should not be removed from the sternum between compressions. Positive-pressure ventilations should always accompany chest compressions. Ventilations should be interspersed between compressions at a rate of 40 to 60 per minute.[45] The neonate should be checked periodically for evidence of spontaneous heart beat and strength of brachial and femoral pulses. Compressions may be discontinued when the neonate has a heart rate of 80 beats per minute or greater.

Venous Access

Hypovolemia, which frequently accompanies neonatal asphyxia, may interfere with successful resuscitation. Hypovolemia is likely if the infant remains pale after ventilation with 100 percent oxygen or if the infant has faint pulses.[46] Partial umbilical cord occlusion in utero, maternal placenta previa, or abruptio placenta are likely antecedents of neonatal hypovolemia.[47]

The neonate's arterial blood pressure provides useful criteria for detecting hypovolemia. Table 5–6 gives average systolic and diastolic blood pressures during the first 4 hours of life that are correlated with birth weight. Use of a Doppler system or an electronic blood pressure monitor, if available, is recommended. Hypovolemia is likely if the mean arterial pressure is below the average range or if the systolic blood pressure drops more than 5 mm Hg with inspiration.[48] Table 5–9 provides simple criteria for determining hypovolemia that can be used during emergency resuscitation in the emergency department.

To provide blood or fluids to correct hypovolemia, it is necessary to have vascular access. The umbilical vein is the recommended access vessel for emergency neonatal blood transfusion or administration of other volume expanders.[49-52] The umbilical vein is easy to identify, and it is generally large enough to allow easy catheter insertion. Although catheterization of the umbilical vein is technically easier to perform than is umbilical artery catheterization, this procedure should be undertaken only by one who is experienced in neonatal procedures.

Umbilical vein catheterization is performed under sterile conditions. The nurse should prepare the cord and surrounding area carefully with an antiseptic solution and drape the infant's abdomen with sterile towels. Caps, masks, sterile gowns, and gloves should be worn. A sterile 3.5 F or 5.0 F umbilical catheter should be primed with heparinized saline (1 unit heparin: 1 ml saline) from an attached syringe.[53] The catheter is advanced until free blood flow is observed. Blood and volume expanders may then be administered through the umbilical vein. Hypertonic solutions and drugs must never be infused through this site unless an x-ray has confirmed that the catheter is in the inferior vena cava and not in the portal vein.[54-57]

Although they may be difficult to access immediately, peripheral intravenous (IV) lines should also be established. The scalp veins and foot and ankle veins are the preferred sites. A number 25 or 27 butterfly may be used for this purpose.

Volume Expanders

The volume expander of choice is O-negative blood that has been cross-matched with the mother's blood.[58-60] If cross-matched blood cannot be obtained, it is possible to obtain compatible blood by withdrawing blood from the placenta through an umbilical artery or vein.[61,62] This method does carry risks of bacterial infection and infusion of blood clots or red blood cell microaggregates.[63,64] If this method is used, a heparinized syringe

TABLE 5–9. THE RELATIONSHIP OF SKIN COLOR, CAPILLARY REFILL TIME, PULSE VOLUME, AND EXTREMITY TEMPERATURE TO HYPOVOLEMIA

Amount of Volume Depletion	Skin Color	Capillary Refill Time (Seconds)	Posterior Tibial Pulse Volume	Skin Temperature
None	Pink	<2	++++	Warm
5%	Pale	3–4	++	Cold from midcalf and midforearm out
10%	Gray	4–5	0	Cold from midthigh and upper arm out
15%	Mottled	>5	0	Entire extremity cold

From G.A. Gregory. Resuscitation of the newborn. In W.C. Shoemaker, W.L. Thompson, & P.R. Holbrook (Eds.). Textbook of Critical Care. Philadelphia: W.B. Saunders, 1984, p. 27. Used by permission.

should be used to withdraw the blood (1 to 2 units heparin per ml blood), and a blood filter should be used to administer the blood.[65,66]

Alternatives to blood include plasma, albumin, lactated Ringer's solution, or saline. It is recommended that volume expanders be administered in units of 10 to 20 ml/kg over a 5- to 10-minute period.[67,68] Additional 10-ml increments can be administered as necessary. The infant's blood pressure, hematocrit, and, if possible, arterial blood gases should be monitored during and after administration of volume expanders. It is not unusual for an infant to require more than 50 percent of his total blood volume (85 ml/kg) for correction of hypovolemia.[69,70] It is important that hypovolemia not be overcorrected. Hypertension can result in cerebral hemorrhage in the newborn infant.[71]

Drugs

Experts in neonatal resuscitation agree that adequate ventilation corrects respiratory acidosis in the asphyxiated newborn.[72-74] Drugs should be used only if the newborn infant does not adequately respond to ventilation, chest compressions, and, when indicated, volume expanders. The drugs used in acute newborn resuscitation are not as numerous as those used with older infants.

Epinephrine. Improved cardiac contractility and vasoconstriction resulting in elevated perfusion pressure are achieved by giving this drug.[75] Epinephrine is indicated if the heart rate persists below 80 per minute despite adequate ventilation with 100 percent oxygen and chest compressions.[76] The recommended dose is 0.1 to 0.3 ml/kg of 1 : 10,000 solution given every 5 minutes as necessary.[77-79] This drug may be given through a peripheral IV, umbilical vein, or by endotracheal tube.[80-82] If the endotracheal route is used, 1 to 2 ml normal

saline may be used to aid in drug delivery to tissues.[83] Intracardiac injection should be reserved as a last resort.[84,85]

Sodium Bicarbonate. If a well-ventilated infant demonstrates acidosis with a pH below 7.0, sodium bicarbonate may be administered.[86] The nurse should be aware that standard resuscitation solutions of 44 or 50 mEq sodium bicarbonate in 50 ml (7.5 percent and 8.4 percent respectively), or the "pediatric" preparation of 10 mEq/10 ml (8.4 percent), are hyperosmolar and should **never** be given to an infant without dilution. If these are the only solutions available, they may be diluted to a strength of 0.5 mEq/ml by mixing with an equal amount of 10 percent dextrose and water.[87] A 4.2 percent solution of sodium bicarbonate (0.5 mEq/ml) for administration to neonates and infants is commercially available and needs no dilution. Bicarbonate should be infused no faster than 1 mEq/kg/minute.[88] A total dose is generally 2 to 3 mEq/kg.[89,90] Blood gases and pH should be monitored carefully after administration. Raising the pH to 7.15 is generally adequate to improve cardiac output and to resolve metabolic acidosis.[91]

Dextrose. Hypoglycemia (blood glucose less than 30 mg/100 ml) can interfere with cardiac function and cause neonatal seizures. Infusion of 5 ml/kg of 20 percent dextrose solution over 3 to 5 minutes, followed by a continuous infusion of 10 percent dextrose and water should be used to raise the infant's blood glucose to 45 to 90 mg/dl.[92] The infusion rate should be 0.045 ml/kg/minute by infusion pump.[93]

Naloxone (Narcan). If it has been determined that the mother was given or took a narcotic drug within 4 hours of delivery, naloxone should be given promptly. A neonatal solution (Narcan Neonatal) supplying 0.02 mg/ml in 2-ml ampules is commercially available. The recommended dosage is 0.01 mg/kg, repeated every 2 to 5 minutes as needed.[94,95] The drug may be given IV, intramuscularly (IM), subcutaneously (SC), or by endotracheal tube.[96] If narcotic reversal occurs, the drug may need to be repeated every 1 or 2 hours because duration of narcotic action may exceed the duration of naloxone. This drug must be used with extreme caution in an infant of a narcotic-addicted mother because acute withdrawal syndrome may result.[97,98]

Other Procedures

There are several procedures that may be performed on the newborn during resuscitation and while awaiting transfer from the emergency department.

Arterial Punctures. The preferred sites for arterial punctures in newborns are the radial and temporal arteries. Use of the brachial and femoral arteries should be avoided. This procedure should be performed by a professional experienced in neonatal punctures. The site is prepared with an antiseptic, and firm pressure is applied to the site for several minutes afterward. Arterial blood samples are useful in assessing the success of resuscitative efforts through arterial blood gas and pH determinations.

Capillary Blood Samples. The nurse or physician can obtain capillary blood samples for several studies. Newborn hematocrit, blood glucose, electrolytes, and blood gases may be determined from capillary blood. The preferred sites for capillary puncture in the newborn are the lateral sides of the soles of the heels. The fingertips can also be used. Previous sites should be avoided. The extremity should be warmed prior to puncture. An antiseptic should precede puncture with either a lancet (for obtaining a few drops) or a No. 11 scalpel blade (for obtaining greater quantities).[99] The nurse may use capillary blood to determine serum glucose using commercially available reagent strips as necessary.

IV Infusions. Monitoring IV infusions (peripheral or umbilical vein) is the nurse's responsibility. Meticulous attention must be paid to the strength, volume, and rate of infusion. An infusion chart should be maintained, and infusions should be documented every 30 minutes and when medications are added and infused. Drug dosages should be double-checked for accuracy. All syringes and infusions should be clearly labeled. Infusion pumps should always be used to monitor and control infusions. Syringe pumps are most useful for newborns because infusion volumes are small, and these pumps are easily transported. Any pump capable of delivering solutions at incremental rates beginning at 0.1 ml/minute is appropriate.

The nurse should see that the umbilical venous catheter site is maintained with a sterile dressing. All peripheral IV sites are taped securely to prevent the needle from dislodging accidentally. The nurse should restrain the extremity and protect the site with a medicine cup or other available protector.

Postresuscitation Care and Preparation for Transport. After acute resuscitation has been completed, the neonate should be observed closely. It is possible that the infant may require further blood tests, x-rays, or treatment with additional drugs (i.e., vasopressors, electrolytes).

If the infant is to be transported to another facility, the parents should be informed. While awaiting transport the nurse should see that the infant is kept warm, dry, and adequately ventilated. Identification bands bearing the infant's name, time of birth, and mother's name should be applied. A copy of the infant's birth and resuscitation record should be prepared to accompany the infant to the receiving hospital. Samples of the infant's cord blood and the mother's blood should be sent to the receiving hospital with the infant.

UNSUCCESSFUL RESUSCITATION OF STILLBORN INFANT

Discontinuing Resuscitation

The decision to discontinue resuscitation is an individualized one. Factors to be weighed include the infant's response to resuscitation, length of resuscitation, presence of underlying physical problems, and the availability of adequate treatment resources. It has been demonstrated that infants unable to demonstrate spontaneous respirations within the first hour of life have a poor neurologic prognosis.[100] While it is important to give the infant any benefit of doubt, resuscitation of the newborn may not always be successful. Numerous congenital conditions (i.e., severe cardiac anomalies, diaphragmatic hernias, brain and neurologic disorders) may interfere with successful newborn resuscitation in the emergency department. Also, a woman who has had fetal demise in utero may deliver a stillborn in the emergency department or en route.

Parental Responses

Responses of parents to their newborn's death may be the result of their expectations for the child, their own life experiences, customs, values, and religious beliefs. In addition, their emotional status and perceptions of the events prior to, during, and following delivery may influence their reactions. Perinatal loss is one of the most traumatic events that can happen to parents. It brings to an abrupt end all the hopes and plans that parents envi-

sioned for their child and family. Strong attachment of both parents to an infant begins during pregnancy. Neonatal death, therefore, creates a substantial loss in the lives of the parents and family.

Support of parents by nurses is especially important at this time. Support begins in the emergency department at the time of the infant's death. Whenever possible the emergency department nurse should refer parents who have suffered a neonatal loss to maternity or pediatric nurses (or social workers) who can follow up with a home visit and provide additional support. Some communities have specialized support groups for parents who have suffered a perinatal or neonatal loss.

Viewing the Infant by Parents. Parents may ask to view the infant's body in the emergency department. This request should neither be denied nor labeled as "morbid." Rather, viewing the dead newborn helps the parents integrate the reality that a baby actually existed. This experience helps parents put the events surrounding the child's birth and death in perspective as they grieve. Seeing the infant is also important to dispel fantasies that the child was deformed.

If the newborn is actually deformed, it is still important for parents to see the child. A simple preparatory description should be given. Parents of deformed infants often formulate fantasies that are far more grotesque than the infant's actual appearance. More harm than good is done when these parents are "protected" from seeing their deformed infant. In the event they do not request it, the nurse should offer the parents time alone with their baby.

The nurse should bathe, dry, and dress the infant in a shirt and diaper and wrap him or her in a soft blanket. The room should be clear of remnants of the resuscitation (i.e., bloody instruments, tubes, needles, syringes, drug containers). The area should be as quiet and as private as possible. The nurse should explain to the parents that the infant will be cold and bluish-grey in color. The parents should be allowed to hold and unwrap the infant if they wish.

The nurse should remain with the parents long enough to assess their responses and to answer their questions. The nurse may then leave the parents alone with their child while remaining outside the room. Permitting grandparents or significant others to view the infant after death should be determined by the parents' wishes and other pertinent circumstances.

NOTES

1. American Heart Association. Standards and guidelines for cardiopulmonary resuscitation and emergency cardiac care. Reprinted from *The Journal of the American Medical Association* 255, no. 21(June 6, 1986):2983.
2. V.G. Daniels, & C.L.-H. Huang. *Companion to Neonatal Medicine.* Boston: M.T.P. Press, 1982, p. 19.
3. G.A. Gregory. Resuscitation of the newborn. In W.C. Shoemaker, W.L. Thompson, & P.R. Holbrook (Eds.). *Textbook of Critical Care.* Philadelphia: W.B. Saunders, 1984, p. 23.
4. Ibid.
5. Ibid.
6. Ibid.
7. J.W. Graef, & T.E. Cone, Jr. (Eds.). *Manual of Pediatric Therapeutics* (3rd ed.). Boston: Little, Brown, 1985, p. 133.
8. American Heart Association, Standards and guidelines, p. 2970.
9. Ibid.
10. Ibid.
11. Ibid., p. 2971.
12. Ibid.
13. Gregory, Resuscitation of the newborn, p. 25.
14. Graef, & Cone, *Manual of Pediatric Therapeutics,* p. 133.
15. Gregory, Resuscitation of the newborn, p. 25.
16. American Heart Association, Standards and guidelines, p. 2971.
17. Gregory, Resuscitation of the newborn, p. 25.
18. Ibid.
19. Ibid., p. 24.
20. J.P. Cloherty, & A.R. Stark (Eds.). *Manual of Neonatal Care.* Boston: Little, Brown, 1980, pp. 142–143.
21. M.H. Klaus, & J.H. Kennell. *Parent-Infant Bonding* (2nd ed.). St. Louis: Mosby, 1982, pp. 35–38.
22. D.E. Fisher, & J.B. Paton. Resuscitation of the newborn infant. In M.H. Klaus, & A.M. Faranoff (Eds.), *Care of the High Risk Neonate* (3rd ed.). Philadelphia: W.B. Saunders, 1986, p. 35.
23. American Heart Association, Standards and guidelines, p. 2970.
24. Ibid., p. 2971.
25. American Academy of Pediatrics/American College of Obstetricians and Gynecologists. *Guidelines for Perinatal Care.* Evanston, Ill.: American Academy of Pediatrics, 1983, p. 231.
26. American Heart Association, Standards and guidelines, p. 2971.
27. Gregory, Resuscitation of the newborn, p. 25.
28. American Heart Association, Standards and guidelines, p. 2971.
29. Ibid.
30. Gregory, Resuscitation of the newborn, p. 25.
31. American Academy of Pediatrics, *Guidelines for Perinatal Care,* p. 36.
32. American Heart Association, Standards and guidelines, p. 2971.
33. American Academy of Pediatrics, *Guidelines for Perinatal Care,* p. 36.
34. Gregory, Resuscitation of the newborn, p. 24.
35. American Heart Association, Standards and guidelines, p. 2972.
36. Fisher, & Paton, Resuscitation of the newborn infant, p. 231.
37. American Heart Association, Standards and guidelines, p. 2971.

38. Ibid.
39. Ibid.
40. Ibid.
41. Ibid., p. 2972.
42. Ibid.
43. Ibid. p., 2958.
44. Ibid., p. 2972.
45. Ibid.
46. Ibid., p. 2973.
47. Gregory, Resuscitation of the newborn, p. 26.
48. Ibid.
49. Fisher, & Paton, Resuscitation of the newborn infant, p. 36.
50. American Heart Association, Standards and guidelines, p. 2973.
51. Cloherty, & Stark, *Manual of Neonatal Care*, pp. 61, 381.
52. Graef, & Cone, *Manual of Pediatric Therapeutics*, p. 139.
53. Cloherty, & Stark, *Manual of Neonatal Care*, pp. 61, 381.
54. Ibid., p. 381.
55. Graef, & Cone, *Manual of Neonatal Care*, p. 140.
56. Fisher, & Paton, Resuscitation of the newborn infant, p. 36.
57. American Heart Association, Standards and guidelines, p. 2973.
58. Ibid.
59. Fisher, & Paton, Resuscitation of the newborn infant, p. 36.
60. Gregory, Resuscitation of the newborn, p. 27.
61. Ibid.
62. Fisher, & Paton, Resuscitation of the newborn infant, p. 36.
63. Ibid.
64. Gregory, Resuscitation of the newborn, p. 27.
65. Ibid.
66. Fisher, & Paton, Resuscitation of the newborn infant, p. 37.
67. Ibid.
68. Gregory, Resuscitation of the newborn, p. 27.
69. Ibid.
70. Fisher, & Paton, Resuscitation of the newborn infant, p. 37.
71. Gregory, Resuscitation of the newborn, p. 27.
72. Ibid., p. 25.
73. American Heart Association, Standards and guidelines, p. 2972.
74. Fisher, & Paton, Resuscitation of the newborn infant, pp. 36, 37.
75. American Heart Association, Standards and guidelines, p. 2973.
76. Ibid.
77. Ibid.
78. Fisher, & Paton, Resuscitation of the newborn infant, p. 41.
79. Gregory, Resuscitation of the newborn, p. 29.
80. Ibid., p. 28.
81. Fisher, & Paton, Resuscitation of the newborn infant, pp. 37, 41.
82. American Heart Association, Standards and guidelines, p. 2973.
83. Ibid.
84. Ibid.
85. Fisher, & Paton, Resuscitation of the newborn infant, pp. 37, 41.
86. Gregory, Resuscitation of the newborn, p. 26.
87. Cloherty, & Stark, *Manual of Neonatal Care*, p. 62.
88. Gregory, Resuscitation of the newborn, p. 25.
89. Ibid., p. 26.
90. Fisher, & Paton, Resuscitation of the newborn infant, p. 41.
91. Gregory, Resuscitation of the newborn, p. 26.
92. Ibid.
93. Graef, & Cone, *Manual of Pediatric Therapeutics*, p. 166.
94. Cloherty, & Stark, *Manual of Neonatal Care*, p. 62.
95. American Heart Association, Standards and guidelines, p. 2973.
96. Ibid.
97. Ibid.
98. Cloherty, & Stark, *Manual of Neonatal Care*, p. 62.
99. Ibid., p. 367.
100. Fisher, & Paton, Resuscitation of the newborn infant, p. 44.

BIBLIOGRAPHY

American Academy of Pediatrics/American College of Obstetricians and Gynecologists.

Guidelines for Perinatal Care. Evanston, Ill.: American Academy of Pediatrics, 1983.

American Heart Association. Standards and guidelines for cardiopulmonary resuscitation and emergency cardiac care. Reprinted from *The Journal of the American Medical Association* 255, no. 21(June 6, 1986):2983.

Cloherty, J.P., & Stark, A.R., eds. *Manual of Neonatal Care.* Boston: Little, Brown, 1980.

Daniels, V.G., Huang, C.L.-H. *Companion to Neonatal Medicine.* Boston: M.T.P. Press, 1982.

Fisher, D.E., & Paton, J.B. Resuscitation of the newborn infant. In M.H. Klaus, & A.M. Faranoff (Eds.), *Care of the High Risk Neonate* (3rd ed.). Philadelphia: W.B. Saunders, 1986, p. 35.

Graef, J.W., & Cone, T.E., Jr., eds. *Manual of Pediatric Therapeutics* (3rd ed.). Boston: Little, Brown, 1985.

Gregory, G.A. Resuscitation of the newborn. In W.C. Shoemaker, W.L. Thompson, & P.R. Holbrook (Eds.), *Textbook of Critical Care.* Philadelphia: W.B. Saunders, 1984, p. 23.

Klaus, M.H., & Kennell, J.H. *Parent-Infant Bonding* (2nd. ed.). St. Louis: Mosby, 1982.

EMERGENCY DEPARTMENT CARE GUIDE FOR RESUSCITATION OF THE NEONATE

Nursing Diagnosis	Interventions	Evaluation
Ineffective airway clearance related to amniotic fluid in airway	Immediately assess airway, breathing and circulation Position neonate on his or her back with the neck in a neutral position Place a 1-inch thick blanket under neonate's shoulder to maintain proper head position Suction the mouth and then the nose with a bulb syringe or DeLee trap	Airway becomes patent
Ineffective breathing patterns related to prematurity complicated during delivery or to asphyxia	Provide tactile stimulation to induce effective respirations Provide artificial ventilations with bag and mask if necessary Provide humidified oxygen Prepare for endotracheal intubation Continually assess vital signs	Spontaneous respirations begin Respiratory rate is adequate Vital signs are stable
Impaired gas exchange related to depressed respirations	Administer 100% humidifed oxygen Obtain arterial blood gases Assess neonate's skin color and temperature Provide artificial ventilations at 40 breaths per minute if neonate is apneic	Arterial blood gas values return to normal Neonate's skin color and warmth return to normal Spontaneous respirations occur
Alteration in cardiac output: decreased, related to asphyxia	Perform chest compressions if the heart rate is less than 60 beats per minute	Heart rate returns to normal rate and rhythm

(Continued)

Nursing Diagnosis	Interventions	Evaluation
	Administer cardiac medications as ordered	
	Administer IV fluids or blood products as ordered	
	Obtain Apgar score at 1 and 5 minutes	
Ineffective thermoregulation related to adjustment to extrauterine environment	Maintain a warm room for the delivery and neonatal resuscitation	Neonate's body temperature returns to normal
	Place the neonate under preheated radiant warmers	
	Dry the infant to remove amniotic fluid	
Alterations in family processes related to delivery of neonate in emergency department	Provide emotional support to neonate's mother and other family members	Family members demonstrate coping abilities
	Continually inform family members of infant's status	
	Allow parents to view the infant as soon as he or she is stabilized	

6

Cardiopulmonary Resuscitation of Infants and Children

Sandra Dandrinos-Smith
Susan J. Kelley

The death of an infant or child is a tragic and often preventable event. Pediatric cardiopulmonary arrest is one of the most difficult encounters the emergency nurse confronts. In the pediatric arrest situation more is required of the emergency nurse than skilled intervention. Successful resuscitation of the pediatric patient depends on a knowledge of the etiology and pathophysiology related to cardiopulmonary arrest, early identification of a prearrest situation, well-developed pediatric assessment skills, and excellent organizational skills. Although 10,000 children in the United States die each year, most individual treatment centers have limited experience with the infant or child in cardiac arrest.

Etiology and Pathophysiology

Unlike the adult population, few primary cardiac arrests occur in infancy (0 to 1 years) and childhood (1 to 16 years). Most cardiopulmonary arrests follow a prolonged hypoxic episode. Because of the prolonged episodes of hypoxia associated with cardiopulmonary arrest in children, the outcome of cardiopulmonary resuscitation (CPR) in the pediatric population is often poor, with a mortality rate in excess of 90 percent.[1]

The major events that may necessitate resuscitation in the pediatric population include:

- Major trauma
- Suffocation caused by foreign bodies
- Smoke inhalation
- Sudden infant death syndrome
- Infectious diseases
- Drowning/near drowning
- Respiratory failure
- Congestive heart failure
- Seizures
- Severe dehydration

Although most pediatric cardiac arrests are respiratory in origin, cardiac arrest as a primary event does occur in this population. Causes of primary cardiac arrest include abnormalities of the heart and its conduction system (particularly following cardiac surgery), metabolic acidosis, drug ingestion, trauma to the chest, and electrocution.[2]

Anatomic and physiologic differences in the infant's and child's respiratory system predispose them to frequent respiratory difficulties. The entire respiratory tract of the infant and child is narrower than that of an adult. One millimeter of edema at the glottic area can cause a 65 percent decrease of air exchange in infants and small children while only causing hoarseness in the adult. Infants are particularly at a disadvantage. In addition to their very narrow airway, they have large tongues, and their epiglottis is large, v-shaped, and lies cephalic, obligating them to breath through their nose. Since the infant's nasal passages are extremely narrow, they can easily be obstructed by secretions or foreign bodies. To complicate matters, during the first few months of life the infant has poor head control, which can compromise air exchange by head and neck flexion alone. Also, the larynx and trachea in both the infant and young child is very flexible; hyperextension of the neck by a well-meaning rescuer may actually cut off rather than open their airway. The first cartilage of the trachea, the cricoid cartilage, is the narrowest portion of the infant's and child's airway, whereas the larynx at the area of the vocal cords is the narrowest portion of the adult's airway. Consequently edema from a tight-fitting endotracheal tube or infection of the laryngeal tracheal area may only cause a sore throat and hoarseness in the adult while causing severe stridor and respiratory distress in infants and young children.

Preterm infants during the first weeks of life are particularly at risk for respiratory difficulties. They have poor medullary response to PCO_2 levels, resulting in apnea or periodic breathing. Preterm infants are also at high risk for respiratory infection and may have varying degrees of surfactant insufficiency, resulting in respiratory difficulties. Hypoglycemia and cold stress in this population, with or without respiratory pathology, can also lead to a respiratory arrest. (Refer to Chapter 5 on neonatal resuscitation for further information.)

In addition to the above pulmonary causes of respiratory arrests, other events that can lead to respiratory arrests include seizures, increased intracranial pressure, metabolic disturbances, suffocation, poisonings, and drug overdoses. Although sudden cardiac arrests are uncommon in children, they can occur as the result of congenital cardiac disease or cardiac infections. Cardiac arrests can also follow shock due to hypovolemia or overwhelming sepsis.

Hypoxia

Throughout infancy and childhood metabolism is high, so there is an increase in O_2 consumption contributing to the rapidity of hypoxia. The child's brain has a particularly high requirement for O_2. Even a slight decrease in the usual oxygen supply can affect neuron functioning, causing changes in behavior and a decrease in mental acuity. Infants and young children can become restless, anxious, and irritable in the beginning stages of hypoxia. This may be demonstrated by thrashing about, crying, anxious faces, and wrinkling of the forehead, followed by lethargy and unresponsiveness. Older children may demonstrate confusion and disorientation as well.

The respiratory system response to hypoxia includes an increased rate of breathing. The cardiovascular system response includes tachycardia followed by bradycardia, hypotension, and diaphoresis. Cutaneous manifestations of hypoxia include cyanosis, diaphoresis, and mottling.[3] The patient in the emergency department should therefore be observed for changes in heart and respiratory rates as well as changes in behavior (see Table 6–1 for normal pulse and respiratory rates) and skin color. It should be noted that infants may not exhibit respiratory and cardiac compensations during hypoxic episodes. Instead they may suddenly present with

TABLE 6-1. NORMAL RESTING PULSE AND RESPIRATORY RATES ON AN AFEBRILE CHILD

Age	Pulse	Respirations
Newborn	110–160	30–50
2 yr	100–140	28–32
4 yr	90–96	24–28
6 yr	80–90	24–26
10 yr	80–84	22–24
12 yr	78–80	18–20

bradycardia rapidly leading to a cardiac arrest.

When prolonged hypoxia occurs, the body shifts to anaerobic metabolism, which leads to metabolic acidosis. This is accompanied by a respiratory acidosis as the PCO_2 level rises. Hypoxia, acidosis, and hypercarbia depress the myocardium, causing dysrhythmias that can be fatal. Many young children and infants, however, can tolerate a pH as low as 7.10 for extended periods without cardiovascular dysfunction.[4]

It is vital that the emergency department nurse recognize the symptoms of hypoxia and make appropriate interventions immediately. A decrease or lack of O_2 to the heart muscle may quickly cause bradycardia followed by asystole requiring a full cardiopulmonary resuscitation.

History. A designated member of the emergency department staff should obtain a rapid but thorough history from family members who witnessed the cardiac arrest or events leading to it. Of particular importance is the length of time the child has been breathless or pulseless prior to the initiation of CPR or arrival at the hospital. A detailed account of the circumstances surrounding the child's illness or accident should be elicited as well as any significant past medical history or allergies. A history of the child's activities and behavior in the previous 24 hours should also be carefully elicited. If the child has been transported to the hospital by prehospital care providers, a careful history of treatments and procedures initiated in the field should be obtained.

Assessment. The infant or child should be immediately disrobed while assessing airway, breathing, and circulation, as discussed in the section to follow on basic life support. Immediate interventions should be made in the event of absence of respirations, respiratory difficulties, bradycardia, or asystole. Vital signs should be obtained. The child's skin should be assessed for cyanosis, mottling, temperature, diaphoresis, dependent lividity, bruising, or cutaneous lesions associated with the mechanism of injury. The head should be inspected and palpated for signs of deformity, fracture, laceration, of other sign of trauma. The pupils should be assessed for size and reactivity. Hypoxia causes dilated, fixated pupils. Extraocular movements should be assessed, which are asymmetric in structural coma. The neck should be inspected for signs of deformity, trauma, subcutaneous air, and the position of the trachea. The chest should be auscultated for breath sounds and observed for spontaneous movement and obvious chest wall trauma. Heart sounds should be auscultated. Distant heart sounds can be secondary to pericardial effusion. Displaced sounds may indicate a tension pneumothorax. The abdomen should be assessed for signs of trauma, distention, or rigidity. The extremities should be inspected for fractures and presence and strength of pulses.[5]

Basic Life Support

The steps in initiating basic life support are outlined in Table 6-2.

Establishing Unresponsiveness. Infants and children should normally respond to tactile stimulation by crying or moving. To

TABLE 6-2. THE SEQUENCE OF CPR

1. Determine unresponsiveness or respiratory difficulty
2. Call for help
3. Position the victim
4. Open the airway
5. Determine whether the patient is breathing
6. Breathe for the victim
7. Circulation: check the pulse
8. Activate the emergency medical service system
9. Perform chest compressions
10. Coordinate compressions and breathing

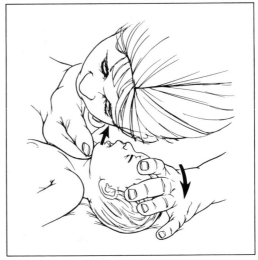

Figure 6-1. Head tilt/chin lift. *(From American Heart Association. Standards and guidelines for cardiopulmonary resuscitation and emergency cardiac care. The Journal of the American Medical Association 255:21 (June 6, 1986):2956. Used by permission.)*

establish unresponsiveness the infant or child should be called to loudly and shaken.

Call for Help. If the patient is unresponsive, limp, has absence of respirations, or has respiratory difficulties, the nurse should call for help and proceed by positioning the patient on his or her back so that he or she can be evaluated and prepared for CPR. If the nurse is alone and the child is not breathing and is pulseless, CPR should be performed for 1 minute before calling for help.

Positioning the Victim. In order for CPR to be effective, the victim must be placed on his or her back on a firm, flat surface. It should be remembered that trauma is the number one cause of death in children more than 1-year-old. Because of their large heads relative to body size, infants and children frequently receive head and spine injuries. If the patient has been involved in an accident, the nurse should make certain that the head and neck are firmly supported and are not rolled, twisted, or tilted backward or forward while positioning for CPR.

Opening the Airway. Since the majority of arrests in the pediatric population are respiratory, proper airway management is the key to a successful resuscitation. Once

it has been established that the infant or child is unconscious and has been placed in a supine position, the airway should be opened. This is accomplished by the head-tilt/chin-lift maneuver (Fig. 6-1). Because of the soft, pliable airway in infants and children up to approximately 4 to 6 years of age, this group should not have their necks hyperextended, since some believe that hyperextension may cut off rather than open their airway. Instead, infants and young children should be placed in a neutral or "sniffing" position (slight head tilt). To augment the head tilt, the rescuer lifts the chin, with its attached structures, including the tongue, from the airway. The nurse's fingers are placed under the bony part of the lower jaw at the chin, and the chin is lifted upwards. The jaw thrust maneuver is the safest technique for opening the airway when neck injury is suspected. The jaw maneuver is performed by placing two to three fingers under each side of the lower jaw at its angle and lifting the jaw upward (Fig. 6-2).[6]

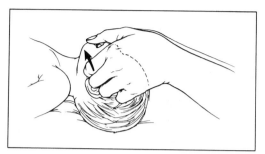

Figure 6-2. Jaw thrust. *(From American Heart Association. Standards and guidelines for cardiopulmonary resuscitation and emergency cardiac care. The Journal of the American Medical Association 255:21 (June 6, 1986):2956. Used by permission.)*

Older children may have increasing head extension if cervicle spine injury is not suspected. Once the airway is opened, breathing status is assessed.

Assessing Respirations. While maintaining an open airway, the nurse should assess whether or not the patient is breathing. The rescuer places his ear over the patient's nose and mouth to feel and to listen for air exchange while observing the patient's chest and abdomen for respiratory movement. If spontaneous or effective breathing is absent, rescue breathing should be initiated. In infants adequacy of ventilation is assessed by observing free, uniform expansion of the lower chest and upper abdomen. In older children and adolescents uniform upper chest expansion indicates adequate ventilation. Auscultation is also necessary to confirm gas exchange by first listening over the trachea to determine if gas exchange is occurring through the central airway. Next, breath sounds should be auscultated bilaterally to assess for peripheral aeration and symmetrical lung expansion.[7]

Assisted Ventilation. Positioning alone may be enough to establish spontaneous respirations in the infant or child. If spontaneous breathing does not occur, however, rescue breathing should be started in the following manner. In infants both the nose and mouth should be covered by the rescuer's mouth (Fig. 6-3). In children only the mouth is covered by the rescuer's mouth, and the nose is pinched closed. Two small breaths (1.0 to 1.5 seconds per breath) are given, with a pause between them for the rescuer to take a breath.[8] The American Heart Association (AHA) recommends that infants receive 20 breaths per minute or one breath every 3 seconds. Children should receive 15 breaths per minute or one breath every 4 seconds.

The appropriate volume to be given is the volume that will make the chest rise and fall. If breaths are given slowly, an adequate volume will be provided at the lowest possible pressure, thereby reducing the risk of gastric distention. Adjuncts for airway and ventilation will be discussed in the section on advanced cardiac life support.

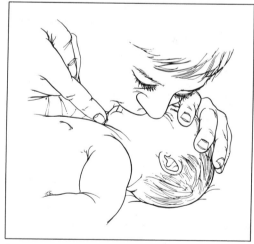

Figure 6-3. Mouth-to-mouth and nose seal. *(From American Heart Association. Standards and guidelines for cardiopulmonary resuscitation and emergency cardiac care. The Journal of the American Medical Association 255:21 (June 6, 1986):2956. Used by permission.)*

Circulation: Assessing the Pulse. Because infants have short, thick necks, the carotid pulse is difficult to assess. Also, because ineffective cardiac activity can often be palpated over the child's thin chest wall, the presence of an apical pulse may not be meaningful.[9] The palpation of a strong brachial or femoral pulse is therefore necessary to determine that cardiac output is adequate. Palpation of the brachial pulse is accomplished by palpating the inner aspect of the infant's arm halfway between the elbow and the axilla with the rescuer's thumb on the outside of the arm and the index and middle fingers pressed against the humerus until the pulse is felt (Fig. 6–4). Beyond the first year of life the carotid artery may be used. Continuous electrocardiogram monitoring should be initiated as soon as possible. Continuous blood pressure monitoring is essential to determine the effectiveness of cardiac function. An ultrasound or Doppler device may be necessary to detect low systolic blood pressures.

Cardiac Compressions. In many cases a quick response to a witnessed respiratory arrest will prevent asystole in the infant and child. If pulselessness or severe bradycardia is established, however, cardiac compressions will need to be performed immediately to establish at least a minimum blood supply to the brain. Every second the brain is without oxygenation decreases the chances of a successful outcome.

INFANTS. The AHA (1986) recommends the following for performing chest compressions on infants. Identify an imaginary line over the sternum, between the nipples (Fig. 6–5). The index finger of the hand furthest from the infant's head is placed just under the intermammary line where it intersects the sternum. The area of compression is one finger's width below this

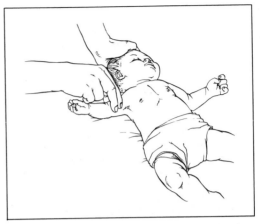

Figure 6–4. Locating and palpating brachial pulse. *(From American Heart Association. Standards and guidelines for cardiopulmonary resuscitation and emergency cardiac care. The Journal of the American Medical Association 255:21 (June 6, 1986):2958. Used by permission.)*

intersection, at the location of the middle and ring fingers. Using two or three fingers, the sternum is compressed to a depth of 0.5 to 1.0 inch at a rate of at least 100 times a minute. Chest compressions and artificial respirations should be implemented in a 5:1 ratio for both one and two rescuers.[10]

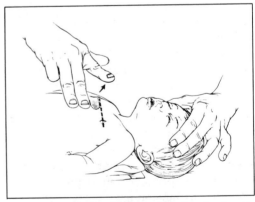

Figure 6–5. Locating finger position for chest compressions in infant. *(From American Heart Association. Standards and guidelines for cardiopulmonary resuscitation and emergency cardiac care. The Journal of the American Medical Association 255:21 (June 6, 1986):2958. Used by permission.)*

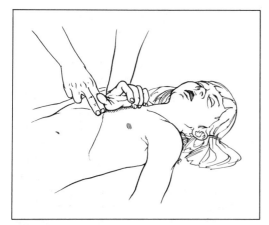

Figure 6-6. Locating hand position for chest compressions in child. *(From American Heart Association. Standards and guidelines for cardiopulmonary resuscitation and emergency cardiac care. The Journal of the American Medical Association 255:21 (June 6, 1986):2958. Used by permission.)*

CHILDREN. In children cardiac compressions are performed one finger breadth above the costal-sternal notch on the sternum (Fig. 6-6). The heel of only one hand should be used for children under 8 years of age with the heel of both hands, one over the other, for children older. The depth of compressions should be 1.0 to 1.5 inches for children under 8 years of age and 1.5 to 2 inches for children 8 years and older. The rate should be 80 to 100 compressions per minute. Infants and children of all ages should be placed in a horizontal, supine position on a hard surface while compressions are being performed. Mechanical chest compressors should not be used for infants or children.

Advanced Cardiac Life Support

Adjuncts for Airway and Ventilation

Bag-Valve-Mask Devices. In the emergency department bag-valve-mask with oxygen should replace mouth-to-mouth resuscitation as soon as possible; however, mouth-to-mouth resuscitation should never be withheld while waiting for the appropriate equipment to arrive. Resuscitation bags should be self-inflating and should have a reservoir to permit delivery of nearly 100 percent oxygen. Devices without oxygen reservoir adaptations often deliver lower concentrations of supplemental oxygen than desired. They should not contain a pressure relief valve. Ideally a manometer should be attached to monitor airway pressure.[11]

Masks should be available in a variety of pediatric sizes and shapes. A mask should be chosen that provides an airtight seal. Masks that are transparent are preferable, since vomitus can be more readily observed. The airway should be opened, as described in the section on basic life support. A secure seal is achieved with one hand securing the mask while the other hand squeezes the bag.

It may be advisable for the nurse to quickly suction the patient before beginning bag-valve-mask breathing to prevent forcing secretions or foreign matter from the upper airway into the lungs. Table 6-3 provides the appropriate sized nasal suction catheters based on the patient's age. Larger size suction catheters should be used for oral suctioning, since it is difficult to clear the oral airway with small lumen catheters.

Oropharyngeal Airways. Oropharyngeal airways can be useful during bag-valve-mask ventilation. Oropharyngeal airways assist in keeping the tongue separated from the back of the pharynx and prevent approximation of the central incisors. Oropharyngeal airways should never be inserted in the conscious patient, since vomiting and aspiration may be induced. Pediatric oropharyngeal airways come in a variety of sizes ranging from 000 for infants to adult size airways for adolescents. The proper size can be established by placing the airway along the side of the face so

TABLE 6–3. SUGGESTED SIZES
FOR ENDOTRACHEAL TUBES
AND SUCTION CATHETERS[a]

Age	Internal Diameter of Tube (mm)	Suction Catheters
Newborn	3.0	6 F
6 mo	3.5	8 F
18 mo	4.0	8 F
3 yr	4.5	8 F
5 yr	5.0	10 F
6 yr	5.5	10 F
8 yr	6.0	10 F
12 yr	6.5	10 F
16 yr	7.0	10 F
Adult (F)	7.5–8.0	12 F
Adult (M)	8.0–8.5	14 F

[a]Endotracheal tube selection for a child should be based on the child's size, not age. One size larger and one size smaller should be allowed for individual variations.
Reproduced with permission from American Medical Association. Standards and guidelines for cardiopulmonary resuscitation and emergency cardiac care. Journal of the American Medical Association 255, no. 21(June 6, 1986):2841–3044.

that the flange is at the level of the central incisors and the bite block portion is parallel to the palate. The tip of the palate should approximate the angle of the mandible.[12]

Endotracheal Intubation. In the pediatric arrest situation endotracheal intubation may be necessary for adequate ventilation or for the delivery of emergency medications. Indications for endotracheal intubation include (1) inability to ventilate the unconscious patient, (2) cardiac or respiratory arrest, (3) inability of the patient to protect his or her airway, and (4) the need for prolonged artificial ventilation.[13]

A wide variety of laryngoscopic blades are available, although personal preference may vary. Usually a No. 1 straight miller blade is used for infants and toddlers and a No. 2 straight miller or curved MacIntosh is used for children; however, No. 3 curved MacIntosh blades should be available for larger children and

adolescents. Suggested sizes for endotracheal tubes are contained in Table 6–3.

Because the cricoid cartilage is the smallest portion of the child's airway and tends to form a "natural cuff," cuffed endotracheal tubes are rarely used with children under 8 years of age. Oral intubation is performed more quickly than nasal intubation in the emergency situation; but if nasal intubation is preferred, neosynephrine nose drops may be helpful in shrinking the mucous membrane lining of the nose so that a larger diameter tube may be inserted. Magill forceps and guidewires should also be available for intubation. The nurse should make certain that appropriately sized suction catheters are ready for use. Prior to the intubation the patient should receive 100 percent oxygen by bag-mask breathing. Frequently atropine is administered to prevent bradycardia during the intubation process. The patient's pulse should be monitored by an electrocardiogram. During the intubation the heart rate should be watched closely. If the patient becomes bradycardic (heart rate less than 80 beats per minute in an infant and less than 60 beats per minute in a child) during intubation or if ventilation is interrupted for more than 30 seconds, the procedure should be terminated and the patient ventilated with a bag-valve-mask device.

After intubation is performed correct placement may be checked by careful bilateral auscultation and visualization of chest movement. If breath sounds are not equal, the tube should be withdrawn slightly and breath sounds reevaluated. A chest radiograph will confirm proper placement. On an anteroposterior (AP) film, the tip of the endotracheal tube should be at a T-2 or T-3 vertebral level or directly between the lower edges of the medial aspect of the clavicles.[14] The tube should be thoroughly secured following the intubation. One popular method of securing both nasal and oral endotracheal tubes is the "cloth tape-suture method." The skin between the nose and upper lip is dried and is painted with tincture of benzoin. A narrow strip of cloth tape with one pleat in the middle is centered between the nose and upper lip after the tincture of benzoin is dry. 00-silk on a cutting needle is then tied around the tube and is sutured to the pleat on the cloth tape (not on the skin). Two or three pieces of adhesive tape may be used to secure the tube. If respiratory distress or absence of respirations continues postintubation, bag breathing will need to be continued. In the case of airway obstruction, such as in croup or epiglottitis, spontaneous respirations may resume and only O_2 or compressed air may be needed.

Drug Therapy. The preparation and administration of emergency drugs may be the most challenging part of the pediatric resuscitation process. Although many of the drugs used for adult and pediatric patients are the same, drug dosages and, in some cases, drug concentrations are different. Pediatric medication dosages are calculated according to the patient's weight or body surface area. With the exception of multiple trauma patients, who need to be immobilized, the child's weight should be obtained immediately upon arrival. Patients already in cardiac arrest, however, should have their weights estimated. Nurses can become proficient in accurately estimating weights by practicing estimations of weights on nonacute pediatric patients. A list of commonly used arrest drugs and their dosages per kilogram or body surface area should be posted in clear sight in the resuscitation area. The drugs used in pediatric advanced life support are described in Table 6–4.

Oxygen Therapy. Oxygen, preferably 100 percent, humidified, must be adminis-

TABLE 6–4. DRUGS USED IN PEDIATRIC ADVANCED LIFE SUPPORT

Drug	Dose	How Supplied	Remarks
Atropine sulfate	0.02 mg/kg/dose	0.1 mg/ml	Minimum dose of 0.1 mg (1.0 ml)
Calcium chloride	20 mg/kg/dose	100 mg/ml (10%)	Give slowly
Dopamine hydro-chloride	2–20 µg/kg/min	40 mg/ml	Alpha-adrenergic action dominates at 15–20 µg/kg/min
Dobutamine hydro-chloride	5–20 µg/kg/min	250 mg/vial lyophilized	Titrate to desired effect
Epinephrine hydro-chloride	0.1 ml/kg (0.01 mg/kg)	1:10,000 (0.1 mg/ml)	1:1,000 must be diluted
Epinephrine infusion	Start at 0.1 µg/kg/min	1:1,000 (1 mg/ml)	Titrate to desired effect (0.1–1.0 µg/kg/min)
Isoproterenol hydro-chloride	Start at 0.1 µg/kg/min	1 mg/5 ml	Titrate to desired effect (0.1–1.0 µg/kg/min)
Lidocaine	1 mg/kg/dose	10 mg/ml (1%) 20 mg/ml (2%)	—
Lidocaine infusion	20–50 µg/kg/min	40 mg/ml (4%)	—
Norepinephrine infusion	Start at 0.1 µg/kg/min	1 mg/ml	Titrate to desired effect (0.1–1.0 µg/kg/min)
Sodium bicarbonate	1 mEq/kg/dose or 0.3 × kg × base deficit	1 mEq/ml (8.4%)	Infuse slowly and only if ventilation is adequate

Reproduced with permission from American Medical Association. Standards and guidelines for cardiopulmonary resuscitation and emergency cardiac care. Journal of the American Medical Association, 255, no. 21(June 6, 1986):2841–3044.

tered in all cases of cardiorespiratory arrest. Frequently bradycardia will be resolved by the administration of oxygen combined with bag-valve-mask breathing without any further interventions. Oxygen should improve arterial oxygen tension, which may improve oxygen content, and tissue oxygen delivery.[15]

Any patient who is suspected of being hypoxemic should be given oxygen. A variety of oxygen delivery devices are available for pediatric patients who do not require endotracheal tubes or artificial ventilation. The type of device chosen should depend on the patient's age, condition, and oxygen requirements.

Nasal cannulas deliver humidified oxygen through nasal prongs. When 100 percent oxygen is run at a flow of 4 to 6 L per minute, the final oxygen delivery to the patient is 30 to 40 percent oxygen. Oxygen hoods are used to deliver oxygen to infants. They maintain a controlled environment for oxygen, humidity, and temperature. Oxygen concentrations as high as 80 to 90 percent can be administered. Prolonged use of high concentrations of oxygen must be closely monitored because of the potential toxicity to the infant's lungs or eyes.

Oxygen tents also provide a controlled environment for oxygen, humidity, and temperature and are capable of delivering oxygen concentrations between 21 and 50 percent. Disadvantages of placing a critically ill patient in an oxygen tent is that access to the patient is impeded, and careful observation for changes in skin color or facial expression may be hindered. Also, children often become frightened and combative when placed in an oxygen tent. If a child cries for extended periods of time in the tent, he or she is not benefiting from the oxygen therapy, and an alternative device for delivering oxygen should be used.

A variety of oxygen masks are available for pediatric patients. A disadvantage of a facial mask is that if the patient were to vomit with the mask in place, the likelihood of aspiration is increased.

Simple facial masks are capable of delivering moderate amounts of oxygen. It is difficult, however, to measure exact amounts of oxygen delivered. Partial rebreathing masks have a combined face mask and reservoir mask that deliver a higher oxygen concentration than simple face masks. Nonrebreathing masks are combined face mask and reservoir bag devices with nonrebreathing valves incorporated into the face mask. Oxygen can be administered at concentrations up to 100 percent. Nonrebreathing masks are therefore preferable for oxygen therapy with patients who are hypoxic and in a prearrest state.[16]

Intravenous Therapy. Establishing a secure intravenous line for drug and fluid administration is a crucial but often difficult step in resuscitating the pediatric patient. Central venous administration of medications in resuscitation is preferable to peripheral administration. Peripheral sites are often inadequate in getting drugs into the central circulation. In addition, a peripheral line may be difficult to insert in the pediatric patient in cardiac arrest, and in some cases a venous cut down in the distal saphenous vein may be necessary. The femoral and external jugular veins are used most often for central venous access. The femoral vein, however, is preferable, since its cannulation does not necessarily interfere with other resuscitation interventions.

Intraosseous vascular access can be used in an emergency situation to administer fluids and drugs when venous access is unavailable. Intraosseous access is obtained by the placement of a rigid needle, preferably a bone marrow needle (although spinal and butterfly needles are sometimes used), into the marrow of the anterior tibia.[17] Drugs and fluids in the same dosages and amounts used intravenously may be administered. Although this method of vascular access has reportedly been used since the late 1930s,[18] there is little data on its effectiveness during cardiopulmonary resuscitation.

Ringer's lactate or 5 percent dextrose in normal saline is usually administered during cardiac arrest. The emergency department nurse should monitor and record intravenous fluid intake very carefully during the resuscitation. Burettes, volume control pumps, or microdrips should be used to administer intravenous solutions to pediatric patients. Cerebral or pulmonary edema can result from fluid overload in infants and young children, especially those with renal compromise.

When intravenous access is impossible, the endotracheal route may be used for the administration of epinephrine, atropine, or lidocaine. Usually the same doses as recommended in the intravenous route are given. Diluting the drug in 1 to 2 ml of normal saline may aid drug delivery into the peripheral airways.

When both the intravenous and endotracheal routes are inaccessible, resuscitation medications may be injected into the heart. Intracardiac injection, however, is associated with significant trauma and should therefore be reserved for cases only in which the other routes are unavailable.[19]

Drugs Used for Control of Heart Rate and Rhythm

Lidocaine. Lidocaine in a bolus of 1mg/kg is given intravenously to the child with ventricular fibrillation or ventricular tachycardia or to the symptomatic child with ventricular ectopy. Lidocaine works by reducing the automaticity of ventricular pacemakers. Thus it increases the fibrillation threshold. Lidocaine may be given prior to cardioversion to treat symptomatic ventricular tachycardia. If ventricular tachycardia or ventricular fibrillation is not corrected following defibrillation or cardioversion and bolus lidocaine therapy, a lidocaine drip should be administered. Table 6–5 describes the preparation and dose of the lidocaine drip.[20]

Adverse effects of lidocaine include nausea, vomiting, lethargy, paresthesias, tinnitus, disorientation, and seizures. Central nervous system signs usually appear first, followed by symptoms of cardiac toxicity that may include depression of myocardial contractility, ventricular irri-

TABLE 6–5. PREPARATION OF INFUSIONS

Drug	Preparation	Dose
Isoproterenol, epinephrine, norepinephrine	0.6 × body weight (kg) is mg added to diluent[a] to make 100 ml	Then 1 ml/hr delivers 0.1 µg/kg/min; titrate to effect
Dopamine, dobutamine	6 × body weight (kg) is mg added to diluent to make 100 ml	Then 1 ml/hr delivers 1.0 µg/kg/min; titrate to effect
Lidocaine	120 mg (3ml of 4% solution) into 100 ml of 5% dextrose in water, 1200 µg/ml	Then 1 ml/kg/hr delivers 20 µg/kg/min

[a] Diluent may be 5% dextrose in water, 5% dextrose in half normal saline, normal saline, or Ringer's lactate.
Reproduced with permission from American Medical Association. Standards and guidelines for cardiopulmonary resuscitation and emergency cardiac care. Journal of the American Medical Association 255, no. 21(June 6, 1986):2841–3044.

tability, heart block, and drug-induced asystole. The metabolism of lidocaine is dependent on liver metabolism. The dosage must therefore be adjusted for children with liver disease.[21]

Atropine Sulfate. Atropine sulfate is a common drug used during pediatric resuscitation. Atropine has parasympatholytic action, with both peripheral and central effects. It is used for symptomatic bradycardia in a dosage of 0.02 mg/kg intravenously, with a minimum dose of 0.1 mg and a maximum single dose of 1.0 mg. The dose may be repeated in 5 minutes to a maximum total dose of 1.0 mg in a child and 2.0 mg in an adolescent. Atropine may be given endotracheally in the same dose used intravenously. Atropine may produce tachycardia, which is generally well tolerated in infants and children. Adverse effects of atropine may include paradoxical bradycardia, atrial and ventricular tachyarrhythmia, and myocardiac ischemia.[22]

Isoproterenol. Isoproterenol is a pure beta-adrenergic receptor stimulator that produces increases in blood pressure, heart rate, conduction velocity, and cardiac contractility associated with peripheral vasodilation.[23] Isoproterenol is infused according to the dose and preparation described in Table 6–4. Isoproterenol is used for bradyarrhythmias that are not responsive to atropine. Adverse effects of isoproterenol include tachyarrhythmias and myocardial ischemia. It should be used with extreme caution in children on digitalis.[24]

Drugs Used to Improve Cardiac Output and Blood Pressure

Epinephrine. Epinephrine is most commonly used when heart action has stopped or is slow and noneffective. It is used to try to change a fine fibrillation pattern to a coarse pattern prior to defibrillation. Epinephrine causes vasoconstriction, with a resultant increase in systolic and diastolic blood pressure, increases the contractile state of the heart, stimulates spontaneous contractions, and increases heart rate. It also produces vasodilation of the coronary and cerebral vasculature. The usual dose is 0.1 ml/kg of the 1 : 10,000 solution given intravenously. It may be repeated as often as every 5 minutes if necessary. Epinephrine may be given endotracheally, although the intravenous route is preferred. Intracardiac administration should be avoided. Epinephrine may also be given by constant infusion. Table 6–5 describes the dose and preparation for constant infusion. Epinephrine should not be mixed with sodium bicarbonate, since mixing will inactivate the epinephrine.

Calcium Chloride. The actions of calcium include increased myocardial contractility, increased ventricular excitability, and increased conduction velocity through the ventricular muscles.[25] According to the 1986 AHA standards, calcium is indicated only when hypocalcemia has been documented. It may be considered in the treatment of hyperkalemia, hypermagnesemia, and calcium-channel blocker overdose.[26] When indicated calcium is given in a dose of 20 mg/kg and should be infused slowly while monitoring for bradycardia. The adverse effects include hypercalcemia, which may lead to an arrest in systole and which is an untreatable condition in which even external cardiac compression will not be beneficial.[27]

Dopamine. Dopamine is both an alpha- and beta-adrenergic stimulant that increases blood flow to the renal and mesenteric vessels. It also increases peripheral vascular resistance, which increases blood pressure. Dopamine is indicated in the treatment of hypotension or poor peripheral circulation in the postresuscitation setting or in shock failing to respond to fluid resuscitation. Dopamine is infused intravenously, preferably through a central line, beginning with 5 to 10 μg/kg/minute and may be increased to 20 μg/kg/minute in an effort to improve blood pressure, perfusion, and urine output.[28] Dopamine should not be mixed with sodium bicarbonate. Side effects of dopamine include tachycardia and tachyarrhythmias. Nausea and vomiting may also occur.

Dobutamine Hydrochloride. Dobutamine hydrochloride is an inotropic drug that increases myocardial contractility and cardiac function. It is indicated in the child with poor myocardial function. It may be used as a first line drug or in the patient who initially fails to respond to dopamine. Dobutamine is infused in a dose range of 5 to 15 μg/kg/minute.[29]

Sodium Bicarbonate. Respiratory acidosis develops at the onset of respiratory failure. Rising levels of carbon dioxide produce a fall in pH. The initial approach to an infant or child in cardiac arrest should be geared to adequate ventilation and intubation to correct the acidosis and hypoxemia. Then epinephrine should be administered. Following these procedures sodium bicarbonate may be administered in the patient with documented metabolic acidosis,[30] since metabolic acidosis further impairs cardiac and pulmonary function. The initial dose is 1 mEq/kg (1 ml/kg of 8.4 percent solution) given intravenously. A dilute solution (0.5 mEq/ml) should be used with infants, since adult strength (1 mEq/cc, 8.4 percent) sodium bicarbonate is hyperosmolar and can cause cerebral vessel rupture in infants due to a rapid shift of fluids from the tissues to the vascular space. Sodium bicarbonate can be diluted 1 : 1 with sterile H_2O (0.5 mEq/ml) before adminis-

tration to infants.[31] Also, infant sodium bicarbonate (0.5 mEq/cc, 4.2 percent) is now commercially prepared and widely available. Subsequent doses of sodium bicarbonate may be given every 10 minutes as indicated by arterial pH values.

Excessive sodium bicarbonate administration may result in metabolic alkalosis, which can cause impaired oxygen delivery, electrolyte imbalance, and decreased fibrillation threshold.

Hypoglycemia

Because glucogenesis is sluggish in the preterm and newborn infant, there is frequently an imbalance between glucose production and utilization. Hypoglycemia in this population can lead to seizures or respiratory arrest. Dextrose (25 percent solution) in an initial dose of 2 cc/kg is often given intravenously during resuscitation in infants and young children. Subsequent doses are based on serum levels.

Defibrillation and Cardioversion

Ventricular fibrillation is relatively uncommon in the pediatric population; therefore the AHA does not recommend unmonitored defibrillation in infants and children. When an infant or child without a pulse is found, efforts should be directed toward airway management, ventilation, and circulatory support of the pediatric patient. Only if ventricular fibrillation is demonstrated by electrocardiogram should defibrillation be attempted.

Defibrillation works by producing a mass polarization of myocardial cells with the intent that a spontaneous sinus rhythm returns.[32] Hypoxemia and acidosis must also be corrected. A defibrillator with appropriately sized paddles should be available at all times. A paddle of 4.5 cm in diameter is recommended for infants and a paddle 8 cm in diameter for children. Nurses should have practice changing from one size paddle to another so that this may be done quickly during an emergency. Electrode cream, saline-soaked gauze pads, or electrode paste can be used for interface between the paddle-electrode and chest wall. Alcohol pads should never be used, as they can cause serious burns. Care must be taken so that the cream, paste, or saline gauze from one paddle does not touch the other.

Emergency personnel should be cleared from contact with the patient and bed. It is recommended that 2 watt-seconds (joules)/kg be given to infants and children. The dose should be doubled if initially unsuccessful. This formula should be clearly posted on the defibrillator. One paddle should be placed to the right of the sternum at the second rib and the second in the left midclavicular line at the xyphoid level. Adverse reactions from defibrillation can include myocardial injury from excessive current or from multiple discharges delivered in rapid succession. If electrode skin interfaces are inadequate, damage to the skin and subcutaneous tissue can occur.[33]

Cardioversion is used to convert rapid symptomatic supraventricular or ventricular tachycardias to sinus rhythms in a patient who is also hypotensive, in cardiac failure, or in a patient who has poor perfusion. The synchronizer circuit must be activated on the defibrillator. The synchronizer circuit allows timed depolarization synchronized with the patient's depolarization.[34] The dose is 0.2 to 1.0 watt-seconds (joules)/kg. The dose may be increased with subsequent attempts or in the presence of acidosis, hypoxemia, hypoglycemia, or hypothermia.

Secondary Interventions

Hypothermia. Because of the infant's and young child's relatively large body surface area in comparison to weight, a large amount of heat is lost from the skin. In an emergency situation overhead radiant warmers should be used to help maintain temperature while allowing patient exposure for observation and treatment. Blood, peritoneal lavage, and intravenous fluids should be warmed before administration. Nurses should instruct emergency medical service personnel to keep the patient warm during transport.

Nasogastric Tube Insertion. During the resuscitation process the stomachs of infants and children frequently become distended with air, causing a decrease in lung expansion and sometimes a vagal response leading to bradycardia. Feedings are more frequent in infants and children, and the chance of a full stomach during an emergency situation is quite high. Nasogastric tubes should therefore be inserted immediately to reduce the risk of aspiration and to relieve pressure on the diaphragm. If severe trauma is observed, an orogastric tube may be inserted.

Volume Expansion. Volume expansion may be necessary for the pediatric trauma patient or the severely dehydrated patient. Children have a greater sympathetic response to blood loss than adults. The normal blood volume is 80 cc/kg of body weight. Blood losses of 20 to 30 percent of the total blood capacity causes hypovolemia. Unlike adults, the infant and child will maintain their blood pressure for a longer period of time, then it may suddenly drop. Pediatric patients with symptomatic hypovolemia should have their blood loss replaced with whole blood, fresh frozen plasma, crystalloid solution, such as Ringer's lactate or normal saline, or colloid solution, such as 5 percent albumin, in aliquots equal to 25 percent of their total blood volume, or 20 cc/kg. Fluid administration should be carefully controlled and recorded.

Foley Catheterization. An indwelling urinary catheter should be inserted to accurately measure urinary output. A urine collection bag may be used initially on infants and young children. Urine output should be accurately recorded.

Termination of Resuscitation in the Emergency Department

The decision to terminate resuscitation efforts in the emergency department is the responsibility of the senior physician. The decision is usually made when the heart is unresponsive to advanced cardiac life-support measures after an extended period of time. Since the heart tolerates hypoxemia better than the brain, normal heart function may return, but varying degrees of permanent brain damage can result. Decisions to terminate CPR, however, are rarely made on the basis of brain death alone in the emergency department. Although unresponsive pupils, unconsciousness, and a history of extended time lapse between arrest and resuscitation may suggest possible brain damage, the extent of damage cannot be evaluated or determined during the resuscitation in the emergency department.

Psychosocial Support

A nurse, social worker, or physician should be assigned to remain with parents and other family members during resuscitation efforts. Parents should be brought to a private location, removed from the resuscitation area, and provided continual information on their child's status. Emergency department staff should offer to contact other family members or clergy to inform them of the parents' presence in the emergency department.

Parents should be reassured that everything possible is being done for their child. When necessary parents should be prepared for the worst, and false hope should never be given. Any guilt that the parents are experiencing should be alleviated when possible by a calm, nonjudg-

mental approach from emergency department staff.

If the resuscitation efforts are unsuccessful, the parents should be informed of the child's death as soon as possible. Parents should be given an opportunity to express their anger, disbelief, and sorrow. Many parents, if given the opportunity, will choose to see, touch, or hold their deceased child while in the emergency department. This allows the parents an opportunity to begin the grieving process. An emergency nurse should offer to remain with the family during this time. Prior to the viewing of the deceased child, the child and resuscitation area should be made as presentable as possible. Parents should be prepared ahead of time for the child's appearance.

A parent who has lost a child should never be sent home unaccompanied. The emergency nurse can offer to contact the closest relative or friend to come to the emergency department. The child's primary care provider should also be contacted. If the parents so desire, a member of the clergy may be called to the emergency department to perform last rites or to comfort the grieving family.

Emergency staff should also inform the parents of where the child's body will be sent from the emergency department, such as to the hospital, city, or county morgue. An autopsy may be requested by the attending physician to determine the cause of death. In some jurisdictions an autopsy of all sudden deaths in young persons is required by law. The emergency nurse may also offer to contact an undertaker for the family. The emergency department staff should also have the opportunity to discuss the arrest event among peers and to give feedback and support to each other and to the prehospital team. A psychiatric liaison nurse or social worker should be available to listen to the staff discuss their feelings individually or as a group.

Parent Education. Since most pediatric cardiopulmonary arrests can be prevented, nursing's major responsibilities occur before the arrest stage. Preventive teaching during noncrisis visits by family members is a major role of the emergency department nurse. From the time of an infant's birth nurses have the unique opportunity to teach parents about the importance of car restraining devices, proper supervision of children, necessary precautions with potentially harmful household items, and ways to ensure adequate health care maintenance for their child and other family members.

Nurse Education. In addition to performing basic life support, many nurses have successfully completed advanced cardiac life support courses and are responsible for educating other health care professionals in both basic and advanced cardiac life support. Nurses also have an important role in teaching prehospital care providers emergency care of children.

Since pediatric resuscitations are infrequent in most emergency departments, the emergency department nurse should arrange mock pediatric resuscitation practice sessions on a regular basis. The sessions can be utilized to identify learning needs as well as to give the staff greater confidence in dealing with the pediatric arrest situation. Also, postarrest conferences involving all members of the resuscitation team should be conducted after each resuscitation effort in the emergency department. These will serve to review any problems encountered in resuscitation management.

NOTES

1. American Heart Association. Standards and guidelines for cardiopulmonary resuscitation and emergency cardiac care. *Journal of the American Medical Association* 225, no. 21(1986):2961.
2. Coffey, R.J. Cardiopulmonary resuscitation in infants and children. In E.F. Crain, & J.C. Gershel (Eds.), *Clinical Manual of Emergency Pediatrics.* Norwalk, Conn.: Appleton-Century-Crofts, 1986, p. 1.
3. Kettrick, R.G., & Ludwig, S. Resuscitation: Pediatric basic and advanced life support. In G. Fleisher, & S. Ludwig (Eds.), *Textbook of Pediatric Emergency Medicine.* Baltimore: Williams & Wilkins, 1983, p. 5.
4. Coffey, Cardiopulmonary resuscitation, p. 1.
5. Ibid., p. 5.
6. American Heart Association, Standards, p. 2955.
7. Kettrick, & Ludwig, Resuscitation, p. 12.
8. American Heart Association, Standards, p. 2956.
9. Kettrick, & Ludwig, Resuscitation, p. 14.
10. American Heart Association, Standards, p. 2958.
11. Ibid.
12. Kettrick, & Ludwig, Resuscitation, p. 7.
13. American Heart Association, Standards, p. 2963.
14. Kettrick, & Ludwig, Resuscitation, pp. 10–11.
15. American Heart Association, Standards, p. 2964.
16. Kettrick, & Ludwig, Resuscitation, pp. 12–13.
17. American Heart Association, Standards, p. 2964.
18. Turbel, H. Intraosseus infusion. *American Journal of Diseases in Children* 137, no. 7(1983):706.
19. American Heart Association, Standards, p. 2964.
20. Ibid., p. 2965.
21. Kettrick, & Ludwig, Resuscitation, p. 24.
22. Ibid., p. 23.
23. American Heart Association, Standards, p. 2967.
24. Kettrick, & Ludwig, Resuscitation, p. 25.
25. Ibid., p. 23.
26. American Heart Association, Standards, p. 2967.
27. Kettrick, & Ludwig, Resuscitation, p. 23.
28. American Heart Association, Standards, p. 2967.

29. Ibid.
30. Ibid.
31. American Heart Association, Standards, p. 2967.
32. Kettrick, & Ludwig, Resuscitation, p. 26.
33. Ibid.
34. Hazinski, M.F. New guidelines for pediatric and neonatal cardiopulmonary resuscitation and advanced life support. *Pediatric Nursing* 12, no. 6(1986):448.

BIBLIOGRAPHY

Agostino, S.D. Set Your Mind at Ease on O$_2$ Toxicity. *Nursing 83* 12(1983):54–56.

American Heart Association. Standards and guidelines for cardiopulmonary resuscitation and emergency cardiac care. *Journal of the American Medical Association* 225(1986):2841–3044.

Cantwell, R., Hallis, R., & Rogers, M. Think fast—what do you know about cardiac drugs for a code. *Nursing 82* 12(1982):34–42.

Coffey, R.J. Cardiopulmonary resuscitation in infants and children. In Crain, E.F., & Gershel, J.C. (Eds.), *A Clinical Manual of Emergency Pediatrics*. Norwalk, Conn.: Appleton-Century-Crofts, 1986, pp. 1–15.

Crowley, C.P., & Marrow, A.L. A comprehensive approach to the child in respiratory failure. *Critical Care Quarterly* June 1980, pp. 27–43.

Greenberg, M., Baskin, S., & Roberts, J. Endotracheal administration of epinephrine during cardiopulmonary resuscitation. *American Journal of Diseases of Children* 136(1982):753–754.

Haller, J.A. Pediatric Trauma: The number one killer of children. *Journal of the American Medical Association* 249(1983):47.

Halpern, J.S. Pediatric resuscitation: Making the task easier. *Journal of Emergency Nursing* 10(1984):47–49.

Hazinski, M.F. Sudden cardiac death in children. *Critical Care Quarterly* September 1984, pp. 59–69.

Hazinski, M.F. New guidelines for pediatric and neonatal cardiopulmonary resuscitation and advanced life support. *Pediatric Nursing* 12, no. 6(1986):445–448.

Kettrick, R., & Ludwig, S. Resuscitation: Pediatric basic and advanced life support. In Fleisher, G., & Ludwig, S. (Eds.), *Textbook of Pediatric Emergency Medicine*. Baltimore: Williams and Wilkins, 1983.

McIntyre, K., & Lewis, A. (Eds.). *Textbook of Advanced Cardiac Life Support*. Dallas: American Heart Association, 1981.

Mendelson, J. Pediatric respiratory emergencies. *Topics in Emergency Medicine* April 1981, pp. 53–66.

Orlowski, J.P. Cardiopulmonary resuscitation of children. *Pediatric Clinics of North America* 27, no. 3(August 1980):495–512.

Orthersen, R.B., Jr. Intubation injuries of the trachea in children, management and prevention. *Annals of Surgery* 89(1979):601.

Pfister, S. Respiratory arrest—are you prepared? *Nursing 82* 12(1982):34–41.

Tomita, T., & McLone, D.G. Acute respiratory arrest. *American Journal of Diseases of Children* 137(1983):142–144.

Turbel, H. Intraosseous infusion. *American Journal of Diseases of Children* 137(July 1983):706.

Whaley, L.F., & Wong, D.L. Respiratory failure. In *Nursing Care of Infants and Children*. St. Louis: Mosby, 1983, pp. 1173–1179.

Whaley, L.F., & Wong, D.L. Physical assessment of the child: The chest and lungs. In *Nursing Care of Infants and Children*. St. Louis: Mosby, 1983, pp. 204–215.

EMERGENCY DEPARTMENT CARE GUIDE FOR THE CHILD IN CARDIOPULMONARY ARREST

Nursing Diagnosis	Interventions	Evaluation
Ineffective airway clearance related to obstruction by tongue and secretions	Perform chin-lift maneuver to deliver tongue anteriorly	Child's airway remains patent

(Continued)

Nursing Diagnosis	Interventions	Evaluation
	Maintain head in a neutral position Insert oropharyngeal airway Suction oral and nasal passages as needed to remove mucus and blood	
Ineffective breathing patterns related to respiratory arrest	Determine whether the child is breathing; look, listen, and feel for exhaled air flow Provide artificial ventilations with mouth-to-mouth breathing or use of bag-valve-mask device Assist or perform endotracheal intubation Administer 100 percent humidifed oxygen	Spontaneous respirations resume Balanced chest excursion is at normal rate for age
Impaired gas exchange related to cardio-pulmonary arrest	Provide artificial ventilations by mouth-to-mouth resuscitation and then bag-valve-mask device. Administer 100 percent oxygen Perform cardiopulmonary resuscitation Assist or perform endotracheal intubation Administer sodium bicarbonate as needed	Arterial blood gases are within normal limits
Ineffective cardiac output related to cardio-pulmonary arrest	Palpate the carotid, brachial, and femoral arteries Place child in supine position on a bedboard If pulselessness is established, perform chest compressions Obtain continuous electro-cardiogram Coordinate cardiac compressions with artificial respirations Administer drugs used to increase cardiac output and blood pressure Administer drugs used to control heart rate and rhythm Continually monitor blood pressure	Carotid, brachial, or femoral pulse is palpable Spontaneous heart beats resume Cardiac rate and rhythm are normal

Nursing Diagnosis	Interventions	Evaluation
Fluid volume deficit related to bleeding	Administer intravenous solution such as Ringer's lactate or dextrose 5 percent normal saline according to prescribed rate Administer blood products as needed Utilize pediatric chamber and microdrip for intravenous fluid administration Carefully measure fluid intake and output Continually monitor vital signs	Expansion of circulating blood volume is achieved Child is normotensive Tissue perfusion is adequate
Alteration in cardiopulmonary tissue perfusion related to cardiopulmonary arrest	Administer basic life support Administer advanced cardiac life support Carefully monitor arterial blood gases Continually assess pulses for strength Continually assess skin color and temperature	Spontaneous normal cardiac rhythm resumes Spontaneous respirations and heart beats resume Cardiac output improves, as evidenced by systolic blood pressure within normal limits for age
Alteration in cerebral tissue perfusion related to decreased cerebral blood flow	Continually assess pupil size and reactivity Continually assess child's neurologic status and level of responsiveness Hyperventilate patient if there is evidence of cerebral edema	Child's pupils are reactive and of normal diameter Child responds to verbal and tactile stimuli
Hypothermia related to decreased tissue perfusion	Continually monitor child's rectal temperature Warm intravenous fluids and blood products prior to administration Utilize overhead radiant heat lamps Utilize warming blanket	Child's body temperature returns to normal and stabilizes Decrease in peripheral cyanosis and mottling is observed
Anticipatory grieving related to child's cardiopulmonary arrest and possibility of death	Parents need continual reassurance that everything possible is being done to resuscitate their child Parents should be brought to a private area where they can express their fears and concerns Provide emotional support utilizing crisis intervention skills	Parents are able to comprehend the seriousness of their child's condition Parents feel supported and comforted by emergency department staff Parents actively begin grief work Parents can establish short-term goals

(Continued)

Nursing Diagnosis	Interventions	Evaluation
	Assign one member of emergency department staff to remain with parents	
Knowledge deficit related to child's condition and resuscitation procedures	Continually inform parents of child's progress and resuscitation procedures	Parents demonstrate comprehension of child's condition and treatments performed

7 | Multiple Trauma

Susan J. Kelley

Accidental injuries have replaced communicable diseases as the leading cause of childhood morbidity and disability in the United States. Pediatric trauma is responsible for 25,000 deaths in the United States each year. Half of these deaths are due to motor vehicle accidents, while drownings, burns, and accidents in the home are responsible for the remaining fatalities.[1] Almost one half of all deaths in children aged 1 to 14 years are the result of major trauma, as compared to one death in ten in the general population. Pediatric trauma claims almost five times as many lives as cancer, the second leading cause of death in children. Pediatric trauma also claims more lives than the next nine leading causes of death combined.

More than 100,000 children are seriously disabled in the United States each year, and another 2 million are incapacitated for 2 or more weeks by their injuries. Because injuries from accidents occur primarily to young people, they result in the loss of more productive years of life before the age of 65 than heart disease, cancer, or stroke.[2]

The peak accidental age range is between 4 and 12 years, with the highest frequency at age 8. Boys are involved in accidents more often than girls. There are patterns in the types of accidents according to age groups. Trauma to child passengers in motor vehicles is the leading cause of death in children after the first few months of life.[3] In the age group of 0 to 5 years, fall-related injuries occur at a rate 1½ to 2 times greater than with older children. One of every 12 children under 6 years require hospital treatment for a fall, with falls occurring most frequently in the home and usually being associated with furniture and stairs. Outside the home most falls are associated with playground equipment or strollers.[4] The risk in elementary school-aged children (6 to 12 years) of a pedestrian injury is twice that of younger children. More than one out of every 80 elementary school-aged children require hospital treatment for a non-motor vehicle-involved accident. This injury rate is twice the rate for teenagers and is 4 times that of preschoolers.[5]

In the adolescent age group (13 to 19 years), one out of every 14 adolescents requires hospitalization for a sports-related injury. The largest proportion of sports injuries are from football, basketball, roller skating, and baseball. Adolescents have a motor vehicle accident injury rate 6 times the rate of younger children; one of every 50 teenagers is injured as a motor vehicle occupant each year. Adolescents are also twice as likely as school-aged children to collide with a motor vehicle while riding a bicycle.[6]

TYPES OF INJURIES

The most common childhood injuries involve children as passengers in motor vehicles; children struck by cars while walking, playing, or riding bicycles; and children who fall from considerable heights.

Motor Vehicle Accidents

Most trauma in motor vehicle accidents is associated with the movement of occupants against interior surfaces within the vehicle or injuries from ejection. Collisions among occupants also contribute to injury, particularly in younger children. In a moving vehicle that is stopped by a sudden impact, an unrestrained child will continue to move at the original speed until impact with the interior of the vehicle.[7] Forty-one states have instituted mandatory car safety-restraint devices for young children. As a result of mandatory use of child-restraint devices, serious injuries and fatalities in the 0- to 4-year-old population have decreased significantly in states that require use of such devices.

The nature and extent of injury in a motor vehicle accident is a function of the mass of the occupant, the speed of travel, the tolerance of the impacted tissues to mechanical energy, and the degree of energy absorbed by the impacting surfaces, their configuration, and the area and length of contact.[8]

Falls

Falls are the second leading cause of death from trauma (excluding drownings and burns) in children in the United States. Falls are the most frequent cause of injury that bring children to the emergency department. The highest incidence of falls occurs among young children and the elderly. Falls have been found to be more frequent among boys, and the injury ratio of boys to girls living in urban areas increases with age. Falls in the home for children under 1 year are found more frequently in lower socioeconomic populations. Deficiencies in the environment,

such as deteriorating housing, windows that do not close or lock, and windows without secure screens, greatly contribute to the higher rates in low income groups. Falls occur half as often in suburban and rural areas in contrast to urban areas in all age groups.[9]

Falls do not occur uniformly throughout the day. The peak rate appears to be between noon and early evening. The objects or areas from which children fall vary. Injuries from stairs and steps predominate, while beds, tables, and chairs are also common injury sites. Regarding falls from considerable heights, windows are the predominant cause. Older children and adolescents tend to fall more often from trees, roofs, and ladders.[10]

The surface upon which children land contributes to their prognosis. Concrete and asphalt are associated with more severe injuries than other surfaces. Children who land on hard ground or concrete sustain greater injury than those who hit grass, even when the heights of the falls are similar.

Head trauma is responsible for the majority of deaths resulting from falls. Multiple trauma is also associated with death from falls.[11]

Pedestrian Injuries

Each year in the United States 2000 children are fatally injured when as pedestrians they are struck by motor vehicles. Another 110,000 children are injured as pedestrians.[12] Most fatal and nonfatal pedestrian injuries to children occur between the ages of 4 and 9 years. For fatal injuries a second peak occurs at 18 to 19 years. Twenty-four percent of injured child pedestrians suffer intracranial injury, while 13 percent sustain other fractures.[13]

Eighty percent of pedestrian injuries to children occur during daylight hours, with most between noon and 6 PM. The majority of pedestrian injuries occur on local through streets in urban areas. The mortality rate of pedestrian injuries increases proportionately as the speed limit at the site of injury increases. Injuries at intersections account for less than 15 percent of fatal and less than 30 percent of nonfatal injuries in children under 15 years. Children are more likely to be injured while darting or running into the street.[14]

Bicycle Injuries

Over 600 children and adolescents are killed annually in the United States while riding bicycles. There are also an estimated 554,000 injuries related to bicycle accidents each year that are serious enough to warrant treatment in the emergency department.[15]

Boys are at higher risk than girls for bicycle injuries and are 3.6 times more likely to die from a bicycle injury than females. Boys aged 10 to 14 years have the highest risk of death. Motor vehicles are involved in 95 percent of deaths among children injured on their bicycles. Most of these fatal injuries involve the central nervous system, head, and face.[16] Since most of these fatal injuries involve the head, the use of helmets should be encouraged.

MULTIPLE TRAUMA

Multiple trauma involves injury to more than one body system. Any child who presents with traumatic injury to one or more body systems, however, should be treated as a multiple trauma victim until proven otherwise. The first 20 minutes of management are crucial in determining the outcome for the multiple-injured child. The prompt assessment and treatment of the multiple-injured child requires a systematic, coordinated approach. Failure to rapidly assess and treat life-threatening injuries may preclude the child's survival. Initial resuscitation must begin the mo-

ment the child arrives in the emergency department, if it has not already been initiated in the prehospital setting.

The most common traumatic injuries seen in children are blunt, as opposed to penetrating, and often result in multiple organ injuries.[17] Pediatric trauma is therefore a special challenge to emergency personnel, since blunt trauma usually leaves minimal external evidence as to the location or severity of potentially life-threatening injuries.

History. While the trauma team is assessing and treating the injuries of the pediatric trauma patient, a nurse or physician should obtain a history from the parent or witness to the accident. The prehospital personnel who brought the child to the emergency department may provide some basic information related to the accident. If the parents have not already been notified, they should be called immediately. Information obtained from parents should include any past medical history, details of immunizations, medication allergies, and any medication the child is currently taking.

If witnesses to the accident are available, the information obtained should include time and type of accident. If the child was an occupant in a motor vehicle, the interviewer should ask how fast the motor vehicle was traveling at the time of impact, where the child was seated, if the child was wearing a safety restraint, and what the child struck. If the child was struck by a motor vehicle, the interviewer should determine how far the child was thrown, what type of surface the child landed on, where the child was struck (e.g., right side), and how fast the motor vehicle was travelling. If the child fell, the height of the fall and surface landed on should be determined.

Assessment: Primary Survey. Figure 7–1 provides an outline for the assessment and

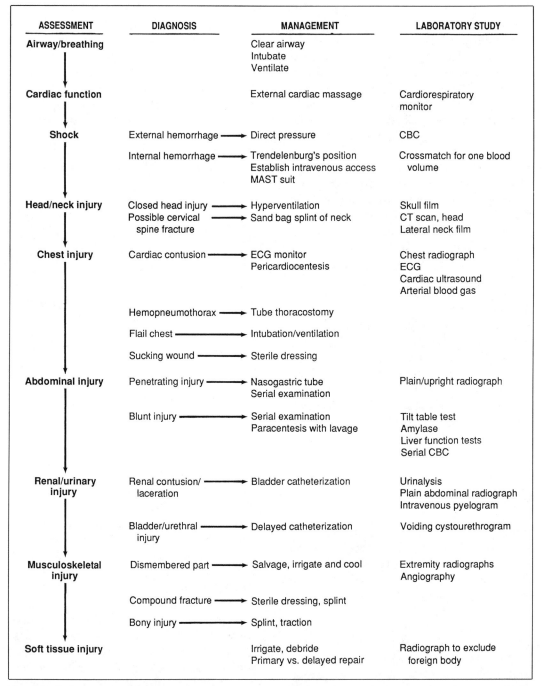

ASSESSMENT	DIAGNOSIS	MANAGEMENT	LABORATORY STUDY
Airway/breathing		Clear airway Intubate Ventilate	
Cardiac function		External cardiac massage	Cardiorespiratory monitor
Shock	External hemorrhage →	Direct pressure	CBC
	Internal hemorrhage →	Trendelenburg's position Establish intravenous access MAST suit	Crossmatch for one blood volume
Head/neck injury	Closed head injury → Possible cervical spine fracture →	Hyperventilation Sand bag splint of neck	Skull film CT scan, head Lateral neck film
Chest injury	Cardiac contusion →	ECG monitor Pericardiocentesis	Chest radiograph ECG Cardiac ultrasound Arterial blood gas
	Hemopneumothorax →	Tube thoracostomy	
	Flail chest →	Intubation/ventilation	
	Sucking wound →	Sterile dressing	
Abdominal injury	Penetrating injury →	Nasogastric tube Serial examination	Plain/upright radiograph
	Blunt injury →	Serial examination Paracentesis with lavage	Tilt table test Amylase Liver function tests Serial CBC
Renal/urinary injury	Renal contusion/ laceration →	Bladder catheterization	Urinalysis Plain abdominal radiograph Intravenous pyelogram
	Bladder/urethral injury →	Delayed catheterization	Voiding cystourethrogram
Musculoskeletal injury	Dismembered part →	Salvage, irrigate and cool	Extremity radiographs Angiography
	Compound fracture →	Sterile dressing, splint	
	Bony injury →	Splint, traction	
Soft tissue injury		Irrigate, debride Primary vs. delayed repair	Radiograph to exclude foreign body

Figure 7–1. Emergency department assessment and management plan for the injured child. *Reproduced with permission from G.R. Fleisher, & S. Ludwig (Eds.). Textbook of Pediatric Emergency Medicine. Baltimore: Williams & Wilkins, 1983, p. 782.*

management of the multiple-injured pediatric patient in the emergency department.

Airway. The airway should be carefully assessed for patency. Any foreign objects, vomitus, or blood should be carefully cleared from the airway. The use of oropharyngeal suctioning should be used sparingly, however, particularly in the patient with an intact gag reflex, since this may precipitate gagging, vomiting, and aspiration.

Airway obstruction is the most frequent source of ventilatory insufficiency in the pediatric trauma patient. Airway obstruction is commonly observed in unconscious children following severe head trauma. Most cases of pediatric airway obstruction result from obstruction of the oropharynx. The oral cavity in children is relatively small, and the upper airway is easily compromised by the lax oropharyngeal musculature in an obtunded supine patient. Upper airway obstruction is promptly relieved by manual positioning with the chin lift (jaw lift), a maneuver that delivers the mandible-tongue unit anteriorly.[18] The chin lift should be conducted with careful attention to avoiding hyperextension of the cervical spine, and therefore should not be performed on a child with obvious facial fractures or suspected cervical injury. If this does not improve the airway, the obstruction is likely to be in the lower airway, beyond the larynx.

Lower airway obstruction is often treated with percutaneous cricothyroidotomy using a 14-gauge Angiocath inserted by the physician through the cricothyroid membrane into the lumen of the trachea.

Breathing. Ventilation is determined by assessing the presence, rate, and depth of breathing. If the child is apneic or respirations are slow or shallow, artificial ventilation should be initiated with a bag-valve-mask and supplemental oxygen until an artificial airway can be inserted. If the patient is breathing spontaneously, supplemental oxygen should be administered. The lungs should be auscultated for bilateral diminished breath sounds, wheezing, stridor, rales, or rhonchi.

Clinical conditions that are most likely to produce life-threatening ventilatory insufficiency, in addition to airway obstruction, are open pneumothorax, tension pneumothorax, massive hemothorax, flail chest, and cardiac tamponade. Unequal bilateral breath sounds indicate a pneumothorax on the diminished or nonmoving side. This may necessitate rapid insertion of a needle and syringe by a physician to relieve the pneumothorax.

Circulation. Circulation should be assessed by auscultating heart sounds and palpating carotid and femoral pulses. If pulses are absent, chest compressions should immediately be instituted. The adequacy of circulation is judged by strength of peripheral pulses, skin color, and the time required for capillary refill of the nailbeds. Capillary filling times longer than two seconds are considered abnormal.[19] Any major external hemorrhage should be controlled by application of direct pressure.

The child should be rapidly assessed for signs of hypovolemic shock. The blood pressure and pulse should be continually monitored. Early indicators of hypovolemic shock include apprehension, pallor, irritability, slight tachycardia, slight decrease in blood pressure, and decreased urinary output. Indicators of advanced hypovolemic shock include decreased level of consciousness; dusky skin color; cool, clammy extremities; weak, thready pulses; poor capillary filling; tachycardia; tachypnea; and hypotension.

Consciousness. The child's level of consciousness should be rapidly assessed during the primary survey. This brief neuro-logic examination includes the child's level of activity; orientation to person, place, and time; pupillary responses and extraocular movements; sensation to extremities; and ability to follow simple commands.

Assessment: Secondary Survey. Next the pediatric trauma patient should be rapidly but thoroughly assessed in a head-to-toe order.

Head. The head should be examined for hematomas, depressions, and scalp lacerations. The anterior and posterior fontanels in infants should be palpated to detect fullness or bulging.

Face. The face should be examined for lacerations, foreign bodies, asymmetry, and obvious fractures.

Eyes. The eyes should be assessed for pupil responsiveness and symmetry, extraocular movements, hemorrhage, and foreign bodies. Periorbital bruising or racoon's sign is an indicator of basilar skull fracture.

Ears. The ears should be examined for presence of cerebrospinal fluid or bloody drainage. Ecchymosis over the mastoid process, or Battle's sign, is a late indicator of a basilar skull fracture. The presence of Battle's sign while in the emergency department indicates a head injury that is more than 12 hours old.

Nose. The nose should be examined for presence of cerebrospinal fluid or bloody drainage, nasal flaring, or obvious deformity. Because infants are obligate nose breathers, the nasal passages of infants should be kept as clear as possible.

Mouth. Circumoral cyanosis should be observed. The tongue, mucous membranes,

and teeth should be examined for injury. Loosened teeth can be aspirated, especially during insertion of airways.

Throat. The airway should be continually assessed. The larynx should be palpated for possible fracture. A fractured larynx is easier to palpate than to visualize.

Neck. The neck should be examined for pain, tenderness, lacerations, swelling, deformities, vein distention, and possible fracture of the larynx. The location of the trachea with respect to the midline should be noted. A cervical collar should be in place and should be removed only after cervical radiographs have ruled out any cervical fracture.

Chest. The heart sounds should be clear and distinct. The chest should be observed for symmetry of movements, wounds, fractures, flail chest, tension pneumothorax, or hemothorax. The anterior and posterior chest should be examined for contusions and abrasions that may indicate underlying pulmonary or cardiac contusions.

Abdomen. Observe for pain, rigidity, tenderness, distention, bruising, and penetrating wounds. Bowel sounds should be auscultated. The abdominal girth should be measured as a baseline and then remeasured every 5 to 10 minutes to note any increase in abdominal distention. A nasogastric tube should be inserted to prevent the child from swallowing air, which can lead to gastric distention, vomiting, and aspiration.

Pelvis and Hips. Assess femoral pulses while observing for femoral swelling or hematomas. Palpate the pelvic girdle for tenderness or deformities. The bladder should be palpated for distention. Inspect the genitalia and perineum for signs of trauma, and inspect the urinary meatus for bleeding. The rectum should be examined for bleeding. A flaccid rectal sphincter indicates spinal cord injury.

Extremities. Inspect the extremities for any deformities, lacerations, swelling, or open fractures. Assess presence and quality of pulses, especially those distal to an injury; capillary filling; sensation; skin color; and temperature. All suspected fractures should be immobilized.

Back. Carefully logroll the patient to observe for any deformities, lacerations, hematomas, or abrasions on the back and spine.

Injury Severity Scale. After the primary and secondary assessments are completed, an injury severity score should be assigned to the patient. Refer to Table 7–1.

Management

ABCs. As indicated earlier, the patient's airway, breathing, and circulation (ABCs) should be continually assessed and supported. Supplemental oxygen should be administered through nasal prongs, as children tolerate this better than a facial mask. A cardiac monitor should be placed on the child immediately. A standard 12-lead cardiogram should also be obtained. A catheter with the largest diameter possible should be inserted in the peripheral vein of an uninjured extremity. If unsuccessful, a peripheral venous cutdown should be performed by a physician. Lactated Ringer's with dextrose is administered at two-thirds maintenance rate unless the child appears hypovolemic. Overhydration should be avoided until the likelihood of a significant head injury with accompanying cerebral edema has been eliminated. Table 7–2 summarizes the nursing management priorities in the care of the critically injured child.

Hypovolemic Shock Resuscitation. All trauma patients need initial and continual assessment for hypovolemic shock. Shock following trauma is most often secondary to blood loss. Head trauma alone does not cause shock. If shock is thought to be present in a child with known head trauma, additional injuries such as abdominal hemorrhage are invariably present.

Shock, or circulatory failure, is characterized by decreased tissue perfusion that is inadequate to meet the metabolic demands of the body. The physiologic consequences of shock include hypotension, hypoxia, and metabolic acidosis. Hypovolemic shock is the most common type of shock seen in the pediatric trauma patient. The blood pressure in the pediatric trauma patient in impending or actual hypovolemic shock often remains stable until the shock state is advanced. The probability of survival after shock is directly related to its duration and therefore must be treated promptly.

Pediatric patients have an estimated blood volume of 80 ml/kg of ideal body weight. The pediatric patient in hypovolemic shock has lost between 25 and 50 percent of total blood volume. A fluid bolus of 20 ml/kg should therefore be infused. Resuscitation is initiated with D5 Ringer's lactate. The first bolus (20 ml/kg) is administered rapidly over 5 to 10 minutes. The patient's pulse rate, blood pressure, pulse pressure, and peripheral perfusion are reassessed. If hypotension persists, a second bolus of D5 Ringer's lactate at 20 ml/kg should be given. If the patient does not respond to this second bolus, a blood transfusion will be required, as any further dilution of the patient's remaining blood will reduce its oxygen-

TABLE 7-1. MODIFIED INJURY SEVERITY SCALE

	Minor—1	Moderate—2	Severe, Not Life-threatening—3	Severe, Life-threatening—4	Critical, Survival Uncertain—5
Neurologic	GCS[a] 15	GCS 13–14	GCS 9–12	GCS 5–8	GCS 4
Face and neck	Abrasion/contusion ocular apparatus; vitreous, conjunctival hemorrhage; fractured teeth	Undisplaced facial bone fracture; laceration of eye, disfiguring laceration; retinal detachment	Loss of eye, avulsion optic nerve, displaced facial fractures, "blowout" fractures of orbit	Bony or soft tissue injury with minor destruction	Injuries with major airway obstruction
Chest	Muscle ache or chest wall stiffness	Simple rib or sternal fracture	Multiple rib fractures; hemothorax or pneumothorax; diaphragmatic rupture; pulmonary contusion	Open chest wounds; pneumomediastinum, myocardial contusion	Laceration of trachea; hemomediastinum; aortic laceration or rupture
Abdomen	Muscle ache, seat belt abrasion	Major abdominal wall contusion	Contusion of abdominal organ; retroperitoneal hematoma; extraperitoneal bladder rupture; thoracic/lumbar spine fractures	Minor laceration of abdominal organs; intraperitoneal bladder rupture; spine fractures with paraplegia	Rupture or laceration of abdominal vessels or organs
Extremities	Minor sprains; simple fractures/dislocations	Compound fracture of digits, displaced long bone or pelvic fracture	Displaced long bone or multiple hand/foot fractures; single, open, long-bone fractures; pelvic fracture with displacement; laceration of major nerves/vessels	Multiple, closed, long-bone fractures; amputation of limbs	Multiple, open, long-bone fractures

[a]GCS = Glascow Coma Scale.
Reproduced with permission from G. Fleisher, & S. Ludwig (Eds.). Textbook of Pediatric Emergency Medicine. Baltimore: Williams & Wilkins, 1983, p. 780.

TABLE 7-2. PRIORITIES IN THE NURSING MANAGEMENT OF PEDIATRIC TRAUMA PATIENTS

Primary assessment: assessment and support of airway, breathing, and circulation (ABCs)

Assessment and treatment of hypovolemic shock

Cerebral resuscitation

Secondary assessment: head-to-toe assessment with stabilization of injuries

Application of cervical collar

Insertion of nasogastric tube, intravenous catheter, urinary catheter

Careful monitoring of vital signs

Psychosocial support of child and family

---

carrying capacity. If crossmatched-and-typed blood is not available immediately, 20 ml/kg of uncross-matched O-negative blood should be administered.

MAST Suit. The application of a pediatric pneumatic antishock garment, often referred to as military antishock trousers (MAST) may be indicated if hypotension persists. The MAST suit consists of a three-chambered trouser made of heavy-duty nylon or polyvinyl fabric capable of being inflated to an external pressure of approximately 105 mm Hg.[20] The chambers are inflated by a foot pump, resulting in circumferential pressure to the underlying body areas from the ankles to just below the diaphragm. The MAST suit increases systemic vascular resistance peripherally and translocates venous blood from the extremities into the central circulation. Application of the abdominal portion of the garment may be particularly helpful in tamponading retroperitoneal bleeding in patients with pelvic fractures.[21]

Pediatric MAST devices are generally designed for children 6 to 12 years of age, or 18 to 45 kg body weight. Adult MAST suits are used for children 13 years and older.[22] If the MAST suit is used for a very small child or infant and the abdominal chamber extends up over the rib cage, indicating that the suit is too large, the child

may be placed in one leg of the suit.[23] The application of the trousers may cause vomiting, urination, or defecation because of the increased pressure on the diaphragm and the abdominal organs.[24] Pedal pulses and vital signs should be continually monitored during use of the MAST suit. The MAST suit may be slowly deflated after the patient has been stabilized.

Vital Signs. The normal parameters for vital signs in the pediatric patient can vary appreciably (Table 7-3). It is important to be knowledgeable of the normal parameters of vital signs for the different age groups.

Heart rates should always be obtained apically in children and for 1 full minute to detect any irregular beats. Tachycardia may be found in conditions of fever, shock, and as an initial response to stress. The heart rate in a crying child can increase by as much as 40 to 80 beats per minute. The heart rate should be obtained again as soon as the child becomes quiet. Bradycardia in children can result from hypoxia, hypoglycemia, increased intracranial pressure, or hypothermia.

Children's respirations are often irregular, especially in a frightened or crying child, and therefore the respiratory rate should be obtained for 1 full minute. Tachypnea is a normal response to stress. The respiratory rate should be reassessed once the child has regained composure. When a stressed child has a slow respiratory rate, injury to the brain, spinal cord, phrenic nerves, and diaphragm should be considered.

Obtaining accurate blood pressure readings is critical in monitoring the pediatric trauma patient. It is extremely important to use the appropriately sized blood pressure cuff. If a cuff that is too large is used, the reading obtained will be inaccurately low. Likewise, if a cuff that is too small is used, the reading obtained will be

TABLE 7-3. NORMAL PEDIATRIC VITAL SIGNS

	Pulse	Respiratory Rate	Blood Pressure
Newborn–6 wk	100–170	30–50	70/40
6 wk–6 mo	100–150	28–40	74/44
6 mo–1 yr	90–140	24–32	80/50
1 yr–3 yr	80–130	24–32	90/60
4 yr–7 yr	80–120	22–28	100/60
8 yr–12 yr	80–110	20–24	110/60
13 yr–16 yr	70–100	16–22	120/70

inaccurately high. The cuff should cover two thirds of the upper arm. It is often difficult or impossible to auscultate both the systolic and diastolic blood pressures in infants and toddlers. In these cases it may be possible to obtain only the systolic pressure using a Doppler machine or palpation. The normal diastolic pressure is roughly two thirds the normal systolic pressure.

Thermoregulation. Temperature regulation in children, especially infants and toddlers, is more labile than in adults. Children are particularly susceptible to heat loss because of their large body surface area relative to their size. Major heat loss in an unclothed child in an emergency department during resuscitation may interfere with already compromised metabolic processes. A child left exposed in a cold room can quickly become hypothermic, which may lead to bradycardia, and possibly cardiac arrest. It is advisable to increase the room temperature or use overhead radiant heaters. Only expose the portion of the child that is necessary after the initial assessment. Rapid infusions of cold blood can also produce hypothermia. Measures should be taken to warm refrigerated blood and intravenous fluids before infusion is begun.

Standard Procedures for the Pediatric Trauma Patient. A hard cervical collar such as the Philadelphia collar should be used to immobilize the neck until radiographs have ruled out the presence of a cervical vertebral fracture. If a hard collar is not available, a soft neck collar may be used. Sandbags may also be placed on either side of the child's head to further decrease mobility.

A nasogastric tube should be inserted to decrease the likelihood of vomiting and aspiration. The alert, uncooperative, or combative child who attempts to resist the insertion of the nasogastric tube may thrash about and jerk the neck, however. In such cases it may be necessary to consider waiting for cervical spine radiograph results prior to insertion of the nasogastric tube.

A urinary catheter should be inserted after injury to the urethra has been ruled out. Blood at the meatus or hematuria contraindicate catheterization until further tests are conducted.

If there are any open fractures, lacerations, or wounds, the child may require tetanus prophylaxis. A careful history of the child's immunization record will indicate if there is a need for tetanus prophylaxis. The proper schedule for childhood immunizations is described in Appendix D.

Laboratory Data

Venipuncture. A complete blood count (CBC) with differential, coagulation profiles, crossmatch and type, and serum electrolytes, including glucose and amylase levels, should be obtained. Particularly young children easily become hypoglycemic under conditions of stress. An elevation in serum amylase may indicate a pancreatic injury. An arterial blood gas should be obtained if there is indication of hypovolemic shock or respiratory compromise.

Urinalysis. A urinalysis should be obtained prior to catheterization to rule out hematuria or injury to the urinary tract or renal system.

Radiographs. Cervical spine and chest films are obtained routinely on multiple trauma patients. Other films are obtained as indicated by history or physical findings. Computed tomography (CT) should be considered if significant head trauma is suspected.

Peritoneal Lavage. Peritoneal lavage is a relatively safe procedure for evaluation of abdominal hemorrhage and perforation of the intestine. Abdominal x-rays should be obtained prior to the procedure due to the possibility of air entering the abdomen during the procedure and interfering with the interpretation of later films. The bladder is emptied with a Foley catheter so that a distended bladder is not perforated.

A small incision is made midline between the umbilicus and pubis. A pediatric peritoneal lavage catheter is then inserted into the peritoneal cavity. Next a syringe is attached, and any fluid present is aspirated. If gross nonclotted blood is returned, the procedure is considered positive, indicating an intra-abdominal bleed, and the procedure is terminated. If there is no evidence of blood, however, an intravenous solution of normal saline is infused by gravity at a rate of 15 cc/kg. The fluid is then allowed to pool in the abdominal cavity. It may be necessary to roll the pa-

tient from side to side to facilitate mixing of the solution with peritoneal fluids. Next the fluid is drained from the abdominal cavity, the catheter removed, and the incision site sutured. If the fluid obtained is clear, the tap is considered negative; however, if the red blood cell count exceeds 100,000 rbc/mm^3, the white blood cell count exceeds 500 wbc/ml, newspaper print cannot be read through it, or stool is present, the procedure is considered to be positive. Lavage fluid should be sent to the laboratory for analysis of complete blood count, hematocrit, amylase, bile, gram stain, and culture.

SPECIFIC INJURIES IN PEDIATRIC TRAUMA

Central Nervous System Trauma

Head Trauma. Head injuries are particularly difficult to evaluate in the multiple-injured child, who may be anxious, afraid, or combative. Brain injuries are classified as either primary or secondary. Primary injuries to central nervous system (CNS) tissue occur at the time of initial trauma. This includes cerebral contusions, lacerations, and skull fractures that result from blunt impact, deceleration, and shearing forces. Secondary CNS damage occurs as a result of hypoxia, hypotension, or hypercarbia. Protection from this source of CNS disability is the responsibility of the emergency department trauma resuscitation team.[25]

Control of intracerebral pressure, maintenance of adequate CNS profusion, and prevention of hypoxia are the goals of cerebral resuscitation. Prevention of cerebral edema is achieved by hyperventilation. Destructive increases of intracerebral pressure occur with hypercarbia, and hypoventilation must be corrected. Control of seizures is important because convulsive activity frequently raises carbon dioxide production and impairs respiratory gas exchange.[26]

The head of the bed should be elevated to decrease venous pressure, and intravenous fluids should be restricted to two thirds of maintenance levels. Steroids may be administered to patients with significant head injury in the emergency department.

Continued neurologic assessment using the Glasgow Coma Scale is critical. (Refer to the chapter on head trauma for detailed information on the assessment and treatment of head trauma in children.)

Spinal Cord Injuries. Spinal cord injuries are less common in children than in adults because children's spines are more mobile. The vertebral columns of children are capable of considerable elongation. The cords themselves, however, are unable to withstand the same degree of trauma. Fracture dislocation is the most frequent cause of spinal cord injury. The lower cervical spine is at particular risk of injury because of the marked mobility of the neck. Common sites of spinal cord injuries in children are levels C-1, C-2, C-5, C-6, T-12, and L-1.

Most spinal cord injuries that children sustain in motor vehicle accidents are the result of indirect trauma. These injuries are caused by sudden hyperflexion or hyperextension of the neck, often combined with a rotational force. When proper seat restraints are not used, there will often be trauma to the spinal cord without evidence of vertebral fracture or dislocation. An unrestrained child becomes a projectile during sudden deceleration. The child is also subject to injury from objects inside and outside the car. Vertebral compression of the spine may also occur in falls.

The patient with possible spinal cord injury should be protected from further injury by stabilizing the spine. Special interventions include airway management, immobilization, and gentle traction, if indicated. The patient's neurologic status should be continually assessed. (Refer to the chapter on head trauma and spinal cord injuries for detailed information on assessment and management of spinal cord injuries.)

Chest Trauma

Most chest trauma in children is blunt, as opposed to penetrating. The significance of thoracic trauma is directly related to its impact upon the underlying cardiopulmonary structures. Chest wall mobility is increased in children, making them less susceptible to rib and sternal fractures. Fractured ribs occur following crushing and direct blow injuries. Pulmonary and cardiac lacerations and contusions, pneumothorax, hemothorax, and flail chest are severe sequelae that can complicate fractured ribs by causing additional distress to the cardiovascular and respiratory systems. Smaller lung volumes and narrower respiratory passages make children less tolerant than adults of any interference in gas exchange.

Open Pneumothorax. Since penetrating injuries are unusual in the pediatric population, open pneumothorax is relatively rare. An open pneumothorax is characterized by a "sucking" chest wound during inspiration and a "frothing or bubbling" wound with expiration.

An airtight dressing made with a petroleum gauze is placed on the chest wound. This should produce immediate improvement in the efficiency of the respiratory gas exchange. A chest tube should be inserted by the physician at the fifth intercostal space in the midaxillary line as soon as possible and should be attached to an underwater seal drainage (Fig. 7–2). A functioning chest tube should fluctuate with respiration.

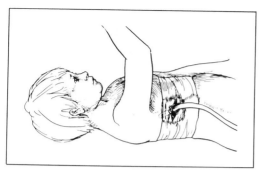

Figure 7–2. Open pneumothorax treated with insertion of intercostal tube through chest wound followed by occlusive dressing. *(Reprinted with permission from J.E. Pierog, & L.J. Pierog (Eds.). Pediatric Critical Illness and Injury: Assessment and Care. Rockville, Md.: Aspen, 1984, p. 189.)*

Tension Pneumothorax. A tension pneumothorax is produced when there is progressive accumulation of air in the pleural space with a shift of mediastinal structures to the opposite hemothorax and compression of the mediastinum and contralateral lung. Tension pneumothorax can progressively decrease cardiac output. Massive shunting of blood occurs from perfused but nonventilated areas, resulting from lung compression, atelectasis, and collapse.[27]

Physical findings typically observed include cyanosis, distended neck veins, decreased breath sounds, displacement of the trachea toward the contralateral lung, and a shift in cardiac sounds toward the contralateral side.[28]

Management includes needle aspiration in the second intercostal space at the midclavicular line to relieve the positive intrathoracic pressure. Next a tube thoracostomy should be performed to provide drainage of the pleural space.[29]

Hemothorax. A hemothorax occurs when, as a result of blunt or penetrating trauma, large amounts of blood accumulate in the pleural space, with secondary injury to intercostal and internal mammary arteries,

the heart, the great vessels, or the hilar vessels.[30] Massive hemothorax produces both circulatory collapse and respiratory failure from compression of the lung.

Indicators of hemothorax include tachycardia, pallor, restlessness, hypotension, decreased breath sounds, tracheal deviation, and a shift of heart sounds.

Management includes treatment of hypotension with fluid resuscitation and tube thoracostomy. The chest tubes are placed in the fourth or fifth intercostal space in midaxillary line. The chest tube should be connected to underwater seal drainage and 15- to 25-cm water suction. An emergency thoracotomy is performed in some rare cases.

Flail Chest. Flail chest occurs from blunt trauma in which multiple ribs are fractured, resulting in a movable chest-wall segment. Once a flail chest develops, there is a compromise in respiratory gas exchange. There is a paradoxic movement on respiration, which may compress lung tissue, decrease ventilation, and cause mediastinal shift to the opposite side.

Clinical indicators include tenderness over the ribs with crepitus and ecchymosis, tachycardia, tachypnea, hypotension, and paradoxic chest movements. The possibility of associated pulmonary and myocardial contusions should be considered.

Management includes stabilization of the flail chest with sandbags and pressure over the unstable segment of the chest. Intubation and mechanical ventilation are usually required to achieve sufficient respiratory gas exchange.

Cardiac Tamponade. Cardiac tamponade is usually the result of a penetrating thoracic injury (Fig. 7–3). The patient typically presents with Beck's triad, which includes an elevation of venous pressure, a decrease in arterial pressure, and muffled or

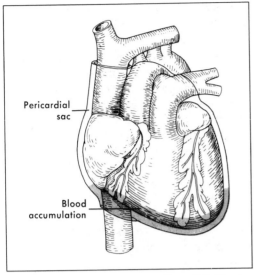

Figure 7–3. Cardiac tamponade. *(From S.B. Sheehy, & J. Barber (Eds.). Emergency Nursing: Principles and Practice (2nd ed.). St. Louis: Mosby, 1985, p. 317.)*

distant heart sounds. External jugular venous distention is prominent. The patient is often agitated, hypoxic, and has poor peripheral circulation. Pulsus paradoxis, or a 10- to 15-mm Hg decrease in systolic blood pressure with inspiration may be observed if the patient is not already in circulatory collapse.

Cardiac tamponade must be relieved immediately with pericardiocentesis, which involves a needle aspiration of the pericardial sac (Fig. 7–4). During this procedure continuous cardiac monitoring and vital sign monitoring are essential. An initial bolus of intravenous fluids with 0.9 normal saline, 10 to 20 ml/kg over 20 minutes, may be given prior to pericardiocentesis to provide support of blood pressure. A thoracotomy may be performed on the pulseless patient.

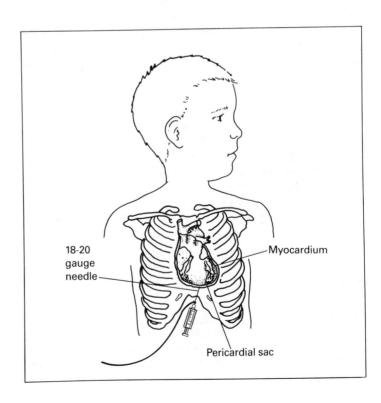

Figure 7–4. Pericardiocentesis.

Myocardial Contusion. Myocardial contusion results from blunt trauma to the anterior midchest from motor vehicle accidents, falls, or other blunt trauma. The injury causes a cardiac concussion with sudden disruption of cardiac activity, ventricular fibrillation, or arrhythmia from edema. The diagnosis is often difficult because of the presence of other conditions such as hypovolemic shock and pneumothorax.

Clinical indicators of myocardial contusion include tachycardia, dysrhythmias, chest pain, murmur, rales, hypotension, and contusion or tenderness over the anterior chest wall.

Treatment includes administration of oxygen, intravenous fluids, cardiac monitoring, and treatment of arrhythmias.

Abdominal Trauma

A significant number of pediatric deaths are the result of blunt abdominal trauma. Blunt abdominal trauma often leaves little external evidence of the location or severity of the trauma. Abdominal trauma is the leading cause of major blood loss in pediatric multiple trauma victims (Fig. 7–5).

Gastric and intestinal dilatation are common in children. Children who are crying swallow large amounts of air. Excessive gastric dilatation and abdominal distention can elevate the diaphragm and interfere with pulmonary functioning. A

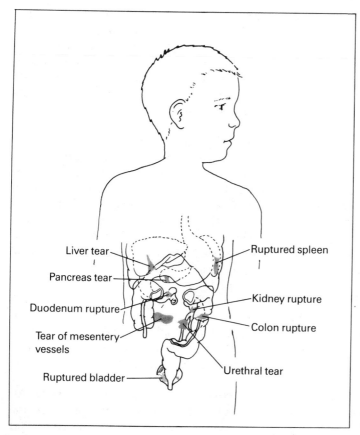

Liver tear
Pancreas tear
Duodenum rupture
Tear of mesentery vessels
Ruptured bladder
Ruptured spleen
Kidney rupture
Colon rupture
Urethral tear

Figure 7–5. Some possible consequences of blunt abdominal trauma.

nasogastric tube should therefore be inserted in all multiple trauma patients, unless contraindicated by facial, head, or spinal trauma.

Traumatic Diaphragmatic Hernia. Blunt trauma to the upper abdomen or lower chest can cause a tear in the diaphragm, resulting in the herniation of intra-abdominal contents into the chest cavity and severe respiratory distress. The patient may complain of abdominal and chest pain, nausea, and vomiting. Tachycardia, hypotension, abdominal distension, or tachypnea may be present. Diaphragmatic hernia on x-ray can be mistaken for hemothorax, pneumothorax, or pneumomediastinum.

Morbidity and mortality are usually related to an associated injury, such as head trauma, pulmonary contusion, or intra-abdominal organ injury, rather than the diaphragmatic lesion itself.

Management includes airway support and treatment of hypotension, respiratory distress, decompression of the stomach with a nasogastric tube, and surgery.

Liver. Trauma to the liver is a leading cause of morbidity and mortality in pediatric trauma. Although partially protected by the rib cage, the liver remains vulnerable to injury due to its large size and fragility. The thoracic cage in children is not a rigid structure and the liver remains vulnerable to crush or compression injury. A firm blow to the right upper quadrant can result in injury to the liver. The absence of bruises or abrasions in that area does not rule out the possibility of serious laceration or rupture. Even such seemingly minor trauma as falling against a rigid object or falling from low heights and landing on the right side can cause major hepatic injury and blood loss.

Children with trauma to the liver often complain of right upper quadrant pain or diffuse abdominal pain. Peritoneal lavage is useful in diagnosing intraperitoneal bleeding but is not specific for liver trauma and therefore necessitates either a laparotomy or radiologic study such as the liver scan. The liver scan can demonstrate laceration, rupture, or intrahepatic hematoma (Fig. 7–6).

Management is aimed at prevention or treatment of hypovolemic shock. Vital signs should be carefully monitored. Children with known or suspected liver trauma should be rapidly resuscitated and transferred to a medical facility equipped to perform major hepatic surgical procedures as well as provide pediatric intensive care.

Spleen. The spleen is the intra-abdominal organ most commonly injured following blunt abdominal trauma (Fig. 7–7). An injured spleen usually results in intraperitoneal hemorrhage, which produces pain and nausea. The most common physical finding in splenic injury is left upper quadrant tenderness with occasional referred pain to the shoulder, known as Kehr's sign. Peritoneal lavage, liver-spleen scans, and CT are excellent diagnostic tests for detecting splenic trauma.

Splenic rupture may be treated surgically or supportively. The unstable child or the child with suspected, serious, associated abdominal injuries will need to undergo immediate laparotomy. Children who appear quite stable can be safely observed with frequent monitoring of vital signs and hemoglobin and hematocrit values.

If surgery is necessary, it is directed toward preservation of the spleen. Nonsurgical and splenic salvage procedures have replaced splenectomy as the treatment of choice in traumatic splenic injuries.

Pancreatic and Duodenal Trauma. Although pancreatic and duodenal trauma are relatively rare in children, as compared

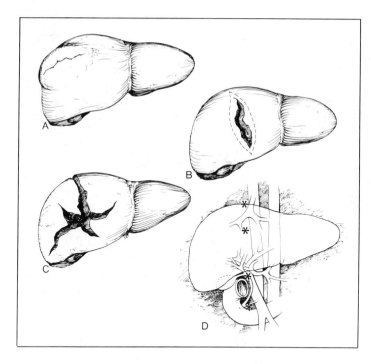

Figure 7-6. Pathophysiology of blunt injury to the liver. **(A)** Subcapsular liver hematoma. **(B)** Laceration of liver lobe with adjacent devitalized tissue. **(C)** Stellate burst laceration of liver lobe. **(D)** Liver injury may include suprahepatic vena cava, retrohepatic vena cava, and portal venous injury (*) and also extrahepatic biliary tree injury (*). *(From G.R. Fleisher, & S. Ludwig (Eds.). Textbook of Pediatric Emergency Medicine. Baltimore: Williams & Wilkins, 1983, p. 788.)*

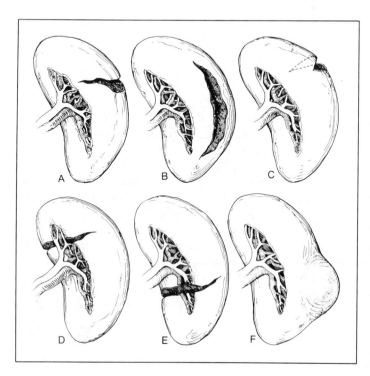

Figure 7-7. Pathophysiology of blunt injury to the spleen. **(A)** Single transverse laceration of free margin. **(B)** Vertical laceration of free margin. **(C)** Posterior laceration on diaphragmatic splenic surface. **(D)** Laceration of splenic hilar surface. **(E)** Hilar laceration involving major vascular branches. **(F)** Subcapsular splenic hematoma. *(From G.R. Fleisher, & S. Ludwig (Eds.). Textbook of Pediatric Emergency Medicine. Baltimore: Williams & Wilkins, 1983, p. 786.)*

to liver and splenic injuries, they remain a cause of morbidity and mortality in children. The pancreas and duodenum, lying in a retroperitoneal location, are relatively protected from abdominal trauma. They are susceptible, however, to anterior blows to the abdomen, which compress these structures against the rigid vertebrae behind them.

Injury to the pancreas and duodenum are difficult to diagnose due to lack of specific signs and symptoms and because frequently there is no blood loss, which would be detected by peritoneal lavage or a falling hematocrit.

Contusion is the most frequent pancreatic injury. Clinical presentation may include midepigastric pain, diffuse abdominal pain, nausea, vomiting, and back pain. Pancreatic laceration produces a much more serious injury, with leakage of pancreatic juice into the retroperitoneum. Unrecognized pancreatic injuries can progress to pancreatic pseudocyst formation. Trauma is the leading cause of pancreatic pseudocysts in children and may occur days or even months after trauma.[31]

Pancreatic injury is often associated with injury of the spleen, liver, and duodenum. The most reliable test for pancreatic injury is an elevated serum amylase level. Serial amylase determinations, obtained every 24 hours, are especially useful. Also urinary amylase levels are of value in diagnosing pancreatic trauma and may be elevated even with normal serum values. Other injuries that can result in elevated serum or urinary amylase levels are head and neck trauma with injury to the salivary glands and small bowel perforation. The radiologic evaluation of the child with suspected pancreatic or duodenal trauma should include flat and upright abdominal films and CT.

Vascular Injury. The most common intraabdominal great-vessel injury in children is to the hepatic veins and is associated with severe liver laceration. Injury to retroperitoneal vessels, particularly rupture of the pelvic vein, associated with a pelvic fracture can cause major blood loss. Due to the closed space involved, the bleeding will usually stop spontaneously by tamponade.

Renal System Trauma

Renal Trauma. Children are more susceptible to renal injuries than adults because their kidneys are more mobile and not as well protected by the large quantity of perinephritic fat found in adults. Ectopic kidneys, the result of congenital anomaly, are predisposed to traumatic injury because of their relatively superficial position. The kidney is injured more frequently than any other abdominal organ. Most renal injuries are caused by blunt trauma, such as an external blow to the abdomen or flank. Penetrating trauma to the kidneys, such as gunshot or stab wounds, occurs much less frequently in children than in adults.

The volume per minute of blood flow to the kidney is greater than to any other abdominal organ. The blood flow to the kidney is 25 percent of the cardiac output. Consequently injury to a kidney may result in rapid blood loss. Signs of hypovolemic shock should therefore be carefully monitored.

Children with renal trauma may present with abrasions, ecchymosis, or pain or tenderness over the lower back or abdomen. Associated injuries, especially to the abdomen, are often present.

Eighty percent of renal injuries are relatively mild (type I) and involve injury to the parenchyma of the kidney without damage to a major renal vessel or collecting system of the kidney. These contusions may present with hematuria or flank pain. Type I injuries are usually detected with an intravenous ureogram. The condition is usually self-limited, without specific treatment.

Type II injuries include laceration of the kidney, injury to a major renal vessel, or injury to the collecting system. Type III injuries include multiple renal lacerations or injury to the main renal artery. Patients with type II and type III injuries may present with flank tenderness, hematuria, nausea, or abdominal pain. There may also be a palpable abdominal or flank mass due to blood or urine loss into the retroperitoneum. Patients with type II injuries are often admitted to the hospital for bedrest. Type III injuries require immediate surgical repair[32] (Fig. 7–8).

Ureter, Bladder, and Urethral Trauma.
There are few acute manifestations of ureteral, bladder, or urethral injuries. When trauma does occur to these structures, it is rarely life threatening and is therefore of

secondary concern in management of the multiple-injured child with life-threatening injuries.[33]

Ureteral injuries are usually caused by penetrating trauma. In pediatric patients, however, because of the increased mobility of the renal unit, a forceful blow to the abdomen or flank can result in separation of the ureter at the juncture with the renal pelvis. Symptoms of ureteral injuries may not be manifest for several days. Ureteral injuries are often associated with a fracture of a vertebral transverse process.[34]

The bladder in the pediatric patient is less vulnerable to injury than in the adult patient because of its higher position. Significant blood loss may result from trauma to the bladder. Blood may accumulate in the bony pelvis and lead to hypotension. Hematuria is not always present with a ruptured bladder. Diagnosis is based on the result of a cystogram.[35]

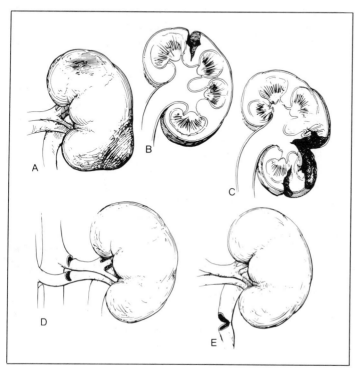

Figure 7–8. Pathophysiology of renal trauma. **(A)** Renal contusion with or without parenchymal hemorrhage. **(B)** Parenchymal laceration not involving the collecting system. **(C)** Parenchymal laceration extending into the collecting system. **(D)** Renal pedicle injury involving the renal artery and vein. **(E)** Ureteric disruption. *(From G.R. Fleisher, & S. Ludwig (Eds.). Textbook of Pediatric Emergency Medicine. Baltimore: Williams & Wilkins, 1983, p. 795.)*

Trauma to the urethra can be a serious problem. Complete or partial transection of the urethra can result from direct trauma to the perineum or secondary to a crush injury of the pelvis. Urethral injuries are more common in males. When urethral injuries occur in females, it is usually the result of penetrating trauma.

Blood may or may not be evident at the urethral meatus. Other indicators of urethral trauma include bladder distention, inability to void, irregularity of the pubis due to fracture, ecchymosis over the perineum and buttocks, and pelvic fracture. If any of these indicators are present, a urethral catheter should not be inserted until a retrograde urethrogram can be performed. Catheterization of a traumatized urethra may convert a lesser injury into a complete disruption.[36]

Musculoskeletal Trauma

The musculosketetal system is most frequently involved in multisystem pediatric trauma. Certain orthopaedic injuries in the pediatric trauma patient warrant close monitoring and immediate intervention.

Orthopaedic injuries in children can result in significant blood loss. For instance, a closed fracture of the femur can be responsible for 300 to 400 cc of lost blood. This may be 15 to 25 percent of the total circulating blood volume in a child and may contribute to hypovolemic shock. A fractured pelvis can cause significant blood loss in children. It is important to keep in mind that abdominal injury often accompanies a fractured pelvis. A considerable amount of blood can also be lost from open or compound fractures. It is therefore important to stablize any open fractures. Fractured extremities will need to be repaired within 6 hours. (Refer to Chapter 21 for further information on the management of specific orthopaedic injuries.)

PSYCHOSOCIAL SUPPORT AND PARENT EDUCATION

The pediatric trauma patient is usually experiencing fear, apprehension, and a great deal of pain. The pediatric patient in a trauma room is also subjected to sensory overload due to staff conversing loudly and moving about hurriedly, invasive and painful procedures, and unfamiliar surroundings. Consequently the pediatric trauma patient requires the emotional support of a calm, reassuring emergency nurse. Children are generally more cooperative when spoken to softly, in simple terms they can easily comprehend.

When appropriate, children need reassurance that they will survive their injuries. Many children, especially when brought to the hospital by ambulance, fear that they are going to die. During the initial phases of trauma resuscitation, emergency department staff often overlook the child's emotional needs. Explanations of procedures are often inadequate in the immediate lifesaving phases of resuscitation. Nurses must make every effort to provide the child with as many explanations as possible in clear, simple terms.

Because parents are not permitted in the trauma room until a seriously injured child has been stabilized, the child needs reassurance that his or her parents are nearby in the emergency department or in route to the hospital.

Since childhood accidents are unexpected, parents do not have time to prepare or adjust to their child's serious condition. Parents often experience feelings of shock, denial, disbelief, and guilt. They often fear that their child will die or be permanently disabled. Parents need reassurance that everything possible is being done for their child. They should be kept continually informed of the child's condition and of all procedures and treatments. Ideally a member of the resuscitation team is assigned as the liaison to the parents, providing them with as much information as possible. Once the child has been stabilized, parents should be allowed in the trauma room as soon as possible to visit their child. This visit is reassuring to both the child and parents. When possible parents should be allowed to accompany their child during transportation to such places as radiology or the operating room.

Most childhood accidents are preventable. The emergency department nurse therefore has an ongoing responsibility to teach accident prevention to parents at every possible and appropriate opportunity. It would be inappropriate to teach accident prevention while a child is being treated for a serious injury. Not only are parents incapable of absorbing information during this time of crisis, but such advice would increase their existing feelings of guilt and responsibility for the accident. Accident prevention teaching is most appropriate when children are treated in the emergency department for minor injuries.

NOTES

1. F.C. Ryckman, & J. Noseworthy. Multisystem trauma. *Surgical Clinics of North America* 65(1985):1287.
2. U.S. Department of Health and Human Services, Division of Maternal and Child Health. *Developing Childhood Injury Prevention Programs*, 1983.
3. L.S. Robertson. Motor Vehicles. *Pediatric Clinics of North America* 32(1985):87.
4. B. Guyer, & S.S. Gallagher. An approach to the epidemiology of childhood injuries. *Pediatric Clinics of North America* 32(1985):11.
5. Ibid., p. 12.
6. Ibid., pp. 12–13.
7. Robertson, Motor vehicles, p. 88.
8. Ibid.
9. L.K. Garrettson, & S.S. Gallagher. Falls in children and youth. *Pediatric Clinics of North America* 32(1985):154.
10. Ibid., p. 155.
11. Ibid, p 157.
12. National Safety Council. *Accident Facts.* Chicago: National Safety Council, 1983.
13. B. Guyer, A.M. Talbot, & I.B. Pless. Pedestrian injuries to children and youth. *Pediatric Clinics of North America* 32(1985):165.
14. Ibid., p. 166.
15. A.M. Fried, C.V. Azzara, S.S. Gallagher, & B. Guyer. The epidemiology of injuries to bicycle riders. *Pediatric Clinics of North America* 32(1985):141.
16. Ibid., p. 145.
17. D.D. King. Trauma in infancy and childhood: Initial evaluation and management. *Pediatric Clinics of North America* 32 (1985):1299.
18. B.H. Harris. Management of multiple trauma. *Pediatric Clinics of North America* 32 (1985):176.
19. King, Trauma in infancy and childhood, p. 1306.
20. V.D. Cardona. *Trauma Reference Manual.* Bowie, Md: Brady, 1985, p. 150.
21. King, Trauma in infancy and childhood, p. 1307.
22. J.E. Concannon, W.M. Matre, & A.D. Verhagen. Antishock trousers in pediatrics: A case management report. *Clinical Pediatrics* 32(1984):78–80.
23. N. Beckwith, & S.R. Carriere. Fluid resuscitation in trauma: An update. *Journal of Emergency Nursing* 11(1985):298.
24. S.B. Sheehy, & J. Barber. *Emergency Nursing: Principles and Practice* (2nd ed.). St. Louis: Mosby, 1985, p. 246.
25. King, Trauma in infancy and childhood, p. 1308.
26. Ibid.
27. R.M. Barkin, & P. Rosen. *Emergency Pediatrics.* St. Louis: Mosby, 1984, p. 365.
28. King, Trauma in infancy and childhood, p. 1303.
29. Ibid.
30. Barkin, & Rosen, *Emergency Pediatrics,* p. 369.
31. Ibid., p. 386.

32. D.L. Hoover. Genitourinary trauma. *Topics in Emergency Medicine* 4(1982):55–56.
33. Ibid., p. 58.
34. Ibid.
35. Ibid.
36. Ibid., p. 59.

BIBLIOGRAPHY

Barkin, R.M., & Rosen, P., eds. *Emergency Pediatrics*. St. Louis: Mosby, 1984.

Bass, J.L., Gallagher, S.S., & Mehta, K.A. Injuries to adolescents and young adults. *Pediatric Clinics of North America* 32(1985):31–39.

Beckwith, N., & Carriere, S.R. Fluid resuscitation in trauma: An update. *Journal of Emergency Nursing* 11(1985):293–299.

Cardona, V.D. *Trauma Reference Manual.* Bowie, Md.: Brady, 1985.

Concannon, J.E., Matre, W.M., & Verhagen, A.D. Antishock trousers in pediatrics: A case management report. *Clinical Pediatrics* 32(1984):78–80.

Dean, D.F. The child with possible spinal cord injury. *Emergency Medicine* 5(1982):123–151.

Feins, N.R. Multiple trauma. In Reece, R.M. (Ed.), *Manual of Emergency Pediatrics* (3rd ed.). Philadelphia: W.B. Saunders, 1984, pp. 198–200.

Fried, A.M., Azzara, C.V., Gallagher, S.S., & Guyer, B. The epidemiology of injuries to bicycle riders. *Pediatric Clinics of North America* 32(1985):141–151.

Garrettson, L.K., & Gallagher, S.S. Falls in children and youth. *Pediatric Clinics of North America* 32(1985):153–162.

Greensher, J., & Mofenson, H.C. Injuries at play. *Pediatric Clinics of North America* 32(1985):127–139.

Guyer, B., & Gallagher, S.S. An approach to the epidemiology of childhood injuries. *Pediatric Clinics of North America* 32(1985):3–15.

Guyer, B., Talbot, A.M., & Pless, I.B. Pedestrian injuries to children and youth. *Pediatric Clinics of North America* 32(1985):163–174.

Harris, B.H. Management of multiple trauma. *Pediatric Clinics of North America* 32(1985):175–181.

Hausman, K.A. Critical care of the child with increased intracranial pressure. *Nursing Clinics of North America* 16(1981):647–656.

Hoover, D.L. Genitourinary trauma. *Topics in Emergency Medicine* 4(1982):55–60.

King, D.R. Trauma in infancy and childhood: Initial evaluation and management. *Pediatric Clinics of North America* 32(1985):1299–1309.

Lyon, S.H. Critical care of the child with multitrauma. *Nursing Clinics of North America* 4(1981):657–670.

Manley, L.K. Pediatric trauma: Initial assessment and management. *Journal of Emergency Nursing* 13(1987):77–87.

Meier, E. Evaluating head trauma in infants and children. *Maternal Child Nursing* 8(1983):54–57.

National Safety Council. *Accident Facts.* Chicago: National Safety Council, 1983.

Pashley, J., & Wahlstrom, M.L. Polytrauma: The patient, the family, the nurse, and the health team. *Nursing Clinics of North America* 16(1981):721–728.

Robertson, L.S. Motor vehicles. *Pediatric Clinics of North America* 32(1985):87–94.

Ryckman, F.C. & Noseworthy, J. Multisystem trauma. *Surgical Clinics of North America* 65(1985):1287–1302.

Salzberg, A., & Brooks, J. Thoracic trauma. *Topics in Emergency Medicine* 4(1982):1–7.

Sheehy, S.B. Trauma patient guidelines. *Journal of Emergency Nursing* 11(1985):209–210.

Sheehy, S.B., & Barber, J. *Emergency Nursing: Principles and Practice* (2nd ed.). St. Louis: Mosby, 1985.

U.S. Department of Health and Human Services, Division of Maternal and Child Health. *Developing Childhood Injury Prevention Programs.* Washington, D.C.: U.S. Department of Health and Human Services, 1983.

Weber, R., & Grosfeld, J.L. Abdominal injuries in children. *Topics in Emergency Medicine* 4(1982):41–53.

Wong, D.L. Childhood trauma: Its developmental aspects and nursing interventions. *Critical Care Quarterly* 5(1982): 47–59.

Zeidelman, C. Increased Intracranial pressure in the pediatric patient: Nursing assessment and intervention. *Journal of Neurosurgical Nursing* 3(1980): 7–10.

EMERGENCY DEPARTMENT CARE GUIDE FOR THE MULTIPLE-INJURED CHILD

Nursing Diagnosis	Interventions	Evaluation
Ineffective airway clearance related to mucus and blood in the respiratory tract	Continually assess and support airway Clear airway with sterile suctioning Perform jaw-thrust maneuver to prevent tongue from obstructing airway Immobilize cervical vertebrae with neck collar until injury is ruled out Insert oropharyngeal airway Prepare equipment for intubation and tracheostomy	Child's airway is patent Child's neck remains immobile
Ineffective breathing pattern related to thoracic trauma	Continually assess and support breathing Observe chest for retractions and symmetry of movement Assess bilateral breath sounds Administer humidified oxygen Provide artificial ventilation if necessary Prepare and monitor chest tubes Monitor arterial blood gas values	Child's respirations are of adequate rate and quality Breath sounds are equal bilaterally Blood gas values are normal Skin color and temperature are normal
Decreased cardiac output related to hypovolemia	Continually assess and support circulation Continually monitor vital signs Assess femoral and carotid pulses Initiate cardiac monitoring Administer intravenous fluids or blood products Monitor urinary output carefully Administer symphathomimetic drugs as ordered	Child is normotensive Peripheral circulation is adequate Skin is warm and pink Urinary output is sufficient (>1 ml/kg/hr)
Fluid volume deficit related to hypovolemia	Continually monitor vital signs Administer intravenous fluids or blood products	Child's vital signs are stable Child tolerates fluid administration and blood products

(Continued)

Nursing Diagnosis	Interventions	Evaluation
	Carefully monitor intake and output	
	Monitor electrolyte balance	
	Assess skin for temperature and color	
Alteration in cerebral tissue perfusion related to head injury	Continually assess child's neurologic status	Child's level of consciousness is unaltered, and child is alert, cooperative
	Elevate head of bed 30 degrees	Child is normotensive
	Restrict fluid intake	Child does not have any seizure activity
	Carefully record output	Serum electrolytes remain balanced
	Monitor for increased intracranial pressure	
	Institute seizure precautions	
	Monitor serum electrolytes	
Alteration in cardiopulmonary perfusion related to hypovolemia	Continually assess patient for hypovolemic shock	Child is normotensive
	Administer intravenous fluids or blood products	Peripheral circulation is normal
	Inflate MAST suit as indicated	Skin temperature is warm
	Control any external bleeding with application of pressure	
Hypothermia related to resuscitation procedures	Continually monitor child's rectal temperature	Child's temperature returns to normal and stabilizes
	Utilize overhead radiant warmers	
	Warm intravenous fluids, blood products, and peritoneal lavage solutions prior to infusion	
	Cover child with warm blankets where possible	
Potential for infection related to multiple injuries	Administer tetanus prophylaxis as needed by immunization status	Child remains free of infection
	Administer antibiotics as ordered	
Fear related to injuries and emergency department procedures	Use developmental approach to explain all procedures and treatments to child	Child is able to understand procedures
	Reassure child that parents are nearby	Child is reassured by presence of parents
	Allow parents into the trauma room as soon as child is stabilized	

Nursing Diagnosis	**Interventions**	**Evaluation**
Alteration in comfort: pain related to injuries	Position child to make child as comfortable as possible Administer analgesics only in absence of head trauma	Child experiences an increase in comfort

8 | Burns

Catherine Kneut

According to the National Safety Council, burn injuries are the third leading cause of accidental death in childhood. Fires and burns are the leading cause of death for children between the ages of 0 to 5 years. Children constitute one third of the more than 8000 people who die each year from burn injuries.

More than 80 percent of the burn injuries in children occur in the home. A brief lapse in adult supervision is frequently cited as the cause of burn injury in young children. Accidental burns in children are related to age and developmental stage. Scald burns and electrical burns are generally more common in infants and toddlers, while flame injuries more frequently occur in older children and adolescents.

Many children with thermal injuries can be effectively treated in community hospitals either as inpatients or outpatients. The more severely burned child requires more intensive care, which can be found in a burn center. It is imperative, however, that nurses working in emergency departments in both community and urban centers be knowledgeable about the emergency care of children with thermal injuries to intervene effectively during the initial assessment and treatment phase.

THERMAL INJURIES

Physiologic Aspects. To fully comprehend the systemic effects thermal injuries can produce, it is necessary for the nurse to understand the structure and function of the integumentary system. The skin is the largest organ of the human body. It functions to protect against bacterial invasion, mechanical injury, and the loss of body fluids.

The skin is composed of two layers: the epidermis and the dermis. The epidermis, the outer layer of skin, consists of four layers: the stratum corneum, stratum granulosum, stratum spinosum, and stratum germinativum. The stratum corneum contains fibers and cells responsible for creating a vapor barrier. The stratum germinativum produces epidermal cells that are responsible for skin regeneration. The stratum granulosum provides a transition into the stratum germinativum and is active in keratinization. The stratum spinosum consists of several rows of prickly cells.

The dermis contains hair follicles and sebaceous and sweat glands. Epithelial cells are also found within the dermis. Peripheral nerve fibers lie deeper in the dermis and are responsible for relaying information to the central nervous system about the external environment. Subcutaneous tissue lies below the dermis and consists of areolar and adipose tissue. This layer contains vascular networks, lymphatics, and nerves and acts as a heat insulator.

Burn injuries disrupt skin integrity and therefore impede its functions. Physiologically the thermal injury results in cellular damage to the skin and the tissues and structures below it. The capillaries dilate, and permeability increases, allowing fluids, electrolytes, and plasma proteins to readily infiltrate the interstitial tissue. This causes edema at the injured site. The heat from the burn frequently causes blood vessel thromboses, thereby impeding circulation to the burn site.

Systemic reactions to thermal injuries are largely dependent on the extent of the burn. Destruction of the skin results in increased insensible water loss as the body's protective barrier is injured. Insensible water losses are higher in children. Fluid shifts from the intravascular space to the interstitial space, producing hypovolemia and hypoperfusion of major internal organs. To further compound the problem, fluid from undamaged tissue is pulled into the circulation as a compensatory mechanism. In major burns, however, this compensatory system is not totally effective. Peak fluid losses in burn edema occur within the first 6 to 8 hours.

Electrolyte imbalances also occur in thermal injuries. Hyponatremia is the result of sodium loss into the edema fluid. Hyperkalemia is the result of cellular destruction, which allows the intracellular cation to enter the vascular space.

Acid-base imbalance occurs in severe thermal injuries. The hypovolemia, vessel thromboses, and poor microcirculation lead to decreased tissue perfusion. The cells become hypoxic and revert to anaerobic metabolism. Anaerobic metabolism leads to an increase in lactic acid, which in turn causes metabolic acidosis. Respiratory alkalosis may also occur in thermal injuries. The pain and anxiety experienced by the pediatric patient frequently causes him or her to hyperventilate, thereby blowing off excess carbon dioxide. This results in respiratory alkalosis. (Respiratory problems associated with smoke inhalation are discussed in Chapter 17.)

The renal system attempts to compensate for the hypovolemia and electrolyte imbalances. Antidiuretic hormone and aldosterone, secreted in response to these alterations, cause the kidneys to conserve sodium and water. The hemolysis of red blood cells and muscle tissue leads to the release of free hemoglobin and myoglobin. These hemochromogens are filtered by the renal system and turn the urine deep red or brown (hemoglobinuria). These substances are found in the presence of deep tissue damage, electrical burns, and extensive red blood cell destruction. It should be noted, however, that the extent of red blood cell destruction is masked initially by the hemoconcentration due to hypovolemia.

A hypermetabolic state occurs as a result of thermal injury. Evaporative water losses are high, causing a commensurate loss of body heat. The glucose and fat stores are mobilized to meet energy needs. These stores are rapidly depleted, necessitating protein catabolism. Negative nitrogen balance soon develops not only as a result of protein catabolism but also through direct thermal destruction of protein and its loss through the burn exudate.

All of these systemic reactions are determined by the severity of the burn wound. Minor burns result in only small local reactions, without overwhelming systemic reactions. (The categorization of thermal injuries as to their severity is found later in this chapter.)

Classification of Burn Depth and Extent. It is imperative that all health care personnel involved with the treatment of burned children be aware of the terminology used to assess and determine the severity of the injury. A common framework helps to determine the most appropriate treatment modality and the most appropriate treatment site (community hospital or burn center).

Thermal injuries are typically described according to the depth of injury to the epidermis and dermis. Burns may be classified as first-, second-, and third-degree burns or as partial- and full-thickness burns (Fig. 8–1). A first-degree burn is a partial-thickness burn characterized by erythema with little or no edema. Blisters are not present, and the area is painful. A sunburn is a typical example of a first-degree burn.

A second-degree burn is also a partial-thickness injury. The burn involves the epidermis and extends into the dermis. It is mottled pink to red in color, and vesicles are apparent. Edema formation is mild to moderate, and the area is very painful.

A third-degree, or full-thickness, burn, involves destruction of the epidermis and dermis. The full-thickness injury is avascular and therefore is pale white to black in appearance. Nerve endings are destroyed; therefore little or no pain is experienced. A fourth-degree burn extends down to underlying structures such as muscle and bone. It has the same characteristics as third-degree injuries.

Extent of the burn refers to the per-

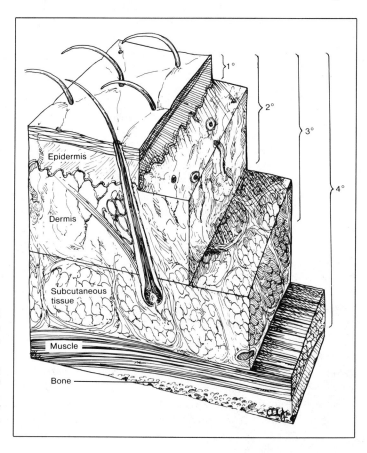

Figure 8–1. Degree of burn wound depth. First degree involves only epidermis; second degree extends into the dermis; third degree into subcutaneous tissue; and fourth degree to muscle, tendons, or bone. *(From G.R. Fleisher, & S. Ludwig (Eds.). Textbook of Pediatric Emergency Medicine. Baltimore: Williams & Wilkins, 1983, p. 945.)*

centage of the total body surface area (BSA) involved. The most accurate means of determining this for burned children is the Lund-Browder chart (Table 8-1, Fig. 8-2). The "rule of nines" with modifications for children can also be used but is not as accurate. The depth and extent of the burn as well as the child's age, burn site, past medical history, and presence of other concurrent injuries are used to determine the severity of the burn injury.

Categories of Severity of Burn Injury. The American Burn Association (ABA) divides burns into three categories, taking into account all the factors mentioned previously. These categories are as follows (includes adults and children):

1. Major Burn Injury: Second degree burns greater than 25 percent BSA (greater than 20 percent in children); all third degree burns 10 percent or greater BSA; all burns involving the hands, face, eyes, ears, feet, or genitalia; all inhalation injury, electrical burns, and burn injuries complicated by fractures or other major trauma; all poor risk patients.

2. Moderate, uncomplicated burn injury: Second degree burns of 15 to 25 percent BSA (10 to 20 percent in children); third degree burns less than 10 percent BSA that do not involve the hands, face, eyes, ears, feet, or genitalia.

3. Minor burn injury: Second degree burns less than 15 percent BSA (less than 10 percent in children); third degree burns less than 2 percent not involving the hands, face, eyes, ears, feet, or genitalia.[1]

These categories are used to initially triage patients to the most appropriate health care facility. It is preferable that children with greater than 15 percent partial-

TABLE 8-1. LUND-BROWDER CHART FOR ESTIMATING PERCENTAGE OF BURNS ACCORDING TO BODY AREA

Area	Birth–1 yr	1–4 yr	5–9 yr	10–14 yr	15 yr	Adult	Partial Thick- ness 2°	Full Thick- ness 3°	Total
Head	19	17	13	11	9	7	_____	_____	_____
Neck	2	2	2	2	2	2	_____	_____	_____
Anterior trunk	13	13	13	13	13	13	_____	_____	_____
Posterior trunk	13	13	13	13	13	13	_____	_____	_____
Right buttock	2½	2½	2½	2½	2½	2½	_____	_____	_____
Left buttock	2½	2½	2½	2½	2½	2½	_____	_____	_____
Genitalia	1	1	1	1	1	1	_____	_____	_____
Right upper arm	4	4	4	4	4	4	_____	_____	_____
Left upper arm	4	4	4	4	4	4	_____	_____	_____
Right lower arm	3	3	3	3	3	3	_____	_____	_____
Left lower arm	3	3	3	3	3	3	_____	_____	_____
Right hand	2½	2½	2½	2½	2½	2½	_____	_____	_____
Left hand	2½	2½	2½	2½	2½	2½	_____	_____	_____
Right thigh	5½	6½	8	8½	9	9½	_____	_____	_____
Left thigh	5½	6½	8	8½	9	9½	_____	_____	_____
Right leg	5	5	5½	6	6½	7	_____	_____	_____
Left leg	5	5	5½	6	6½	8	_____	_____	_____
Right foot	3½	3½	3½	3½	3½	3½	_____	_____	_____
Left foot	3½	3½	3½	3½	3½	3½	_____	_____	_____
						Total	_____	_____	_____

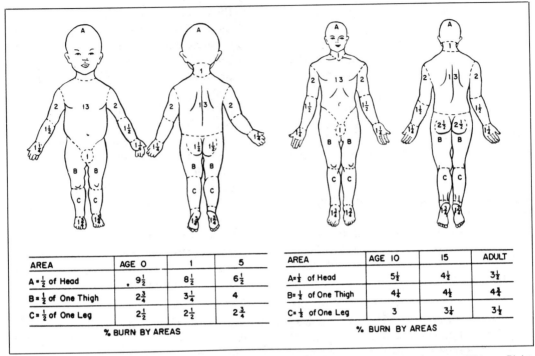

AREA	AGE 0	1	5
A = ½ of Head	9½	8½	6½
B = ½ of One Thigh	2¾	3¼	4
C = ½ of One Leg	2½	2½	2¾
% BURN BY AREAS			

AREA	AGE 10	15	ADULT
A = ½ of Head	5½	4½	3½
B = ½ of One Thigh	4¼	4½	4¾
C = ½ of One Leg	3	3¼	3½
% BURN BY AREAS			

Figure 8–2. Burn assessment chart as modified by Lund and Browder. *Left:* Infants and young children. *Right:* Older children and young adults. *(From A.M. Rudolph (Ed.). Pediatrics (18th ed.). Norwalk, Conn.: Appleton & Lange, 1987, p. 707.)*

thickness burns or greater than 10 percent full-thickness burns be admitted to a burn center. Less serious burns can be managed in a burn unit of a general hospital or on an outpatient basis if the injury is truly minor.

History. An accurate and thorough history is necessary to alert health care personnel to potential problems. It is important to ascertain the mechanism of thermal injury, including a description of the burn source (wet or dry heat). One should also note exposure time to the heat and its approximate temperature. A description of the events leading up to the injury or associated with it are important to include in the history. If the thermal injury is due to flame, ascertain if the fire occurred in a closed space, as smoke inhalation injury could be a potential problem. Determine if the child was exposed to any noxious

gases and the amount of exposure to them.

In addition to a history of the thermal injury, other factors need to be ascertained. The child's general health status, past medical history, and any allergies must be documented. The child's age is important in determining the extent of the burn. Any medications the child currently uses or has used in the recent past should be noted in the history. The child's immunization status, particularly in regard to tetanus, is also necessary.

Thermal injuries in the pediatric population are, tragically, often due to abuse. If the history of the thermal injury does not correlate with the burn wound, then further inquiry must be made about the exact circumstances of the injury. The types of burns that should arouse suspicion of emergency department staff members are circumferential burns of the feet, circumferential burns of the buttocks, cigarette burns, extensive scalding injuries, and areas of scarring that may be the result of previous intentionally inflicted burns.[2]

Assessment. Assessment of the thermally injured pediatric patient does not begin with the burn wound itself. The first priority is maintaining a patent airway and observing for any signs of obstruction. The child's respiratory effort and the adequacy of his or her ventilations must be assessed. Lung sounds are evaluated for the presence of rales, rhonchi, wheezing, and stridor. The chest is observed for symmetry of movement and the use of accessory muscles. Airway obstruction can occur if there are burns of the nose, mouth, face, or neck. Smoke or noxious gas inhalation injuries can also produce respiratory distress. A more detailed assessment for smoke inhalation injuries is provided further in this chapter.

The child's circulatory status is assessed by measuring the apical pulse and blood pressure. Peripheral circulation is assessed by checking the color, pulses, capillary filling, sensation, and movement of the extremities and burned areas.

The head and neck region is examined for areas of tenderness and pain. The head should also be examined for burns. In an emergency situation burns of the scalp may be missed if a thorough examination is not performed. In addition, if the child has sustained his thermal injury due to a car accident, a closed-head injury may exist. The child's neurologic status is determined by pupillary reaction to light, level of consciousness, reflexes, and motor strength. The eyes are also examined for conjunctivitis, and the cornea is examined for thermal injury.

The abdomen is examined for distention, rigidity, areas of tenderness, and the presence or absence of bowel sounds. Any

nausea or vomiting is also noted. The liver and spleen are palpated to check for enlargement.

The extremities are examined for any fractures. Edema of the extremities is also noted. As cited previously, a neurovascular assessment is performed. It may be necessary to use an ultrasonic flowmeter to assess peripheral pulses, particularly if the burn is circumferential.

When all of the preceding assessments have been made and any complicating factors (fractures, internal injuries, head injuries) have been evaluated, the thermal injury is examined. The depth of the burn is determined as best as possible and is recorded. A completely accurate burn depth determination is not possible in all situations. The extent of the burn is determined by using the Lund-Browder chart. Information about the depth and size of the thermal injury can be recorded directly on this chart. The body sites affected by the burn are also noted on the Lund-Browder chart. When the burn has been evaluated and any other associated injuries have been considered, the physician is the health care provider who determines whether the injury is minor, moderate, or major, according to established guidelines. It is also his or her responsibility to triage the child to the most appropriate health care facility according to the resources available.

Management

Airway, Breathing, and Circulation Support. Nursing interventions in the emergency department are based on an accurate and comprehensive assessment. Interventions should be performed in a systematic manner. The ABC approach (airway, breathing, and circulation) is the best one to use. Ascertain if the child has a patent airway and can maintain effective respirations. It may be necessary to provide oxygen. Endotracheal intubation and ventilator support may be required for children with smoke inhalation, head and neck burns, major thermal injuries, or circumferential burns of the thorax.

Vital signs are obtained immediately upon admission to establish baseline data. The child's temperature, apical pulse, blood pressure, and respirations are monitored and recorded frequently. Cardiac monitoring is necessary for children with major burns or electrical injury. Laboratory tests obtained on admission include a complete blood count, hematocrit, hemoglobin, blood chemistries (BUN, creatinine, serum electrolyte levels, blood sugar, albumin and globulin levels, osmolality), and coagulation studies. An arterial blood gas may also be drawn to ascertain acid-base balance. The child is weighed to provide a basis for fluid resuscitation. An indwelling urinary catheter is inserted to measure hourly urine outputs.

Fluid Resuscitation. Several fluid resuscitation formulas are used for pediatric clients. The differences in the resuscitation formulas are in the use of colloids (e.g., albumin, blood products) and the amount of crystalloid (e.g., saline, lactated Ringer's, dextrose) used. The present trend is to use formulas that do not use colloids in the first 24 hours. Not all authorities, however, agree with the postponement of colloid use; thus nurses in an emergency department must be familiar with the major resuscitation formulas (Table 8–2).

The goal of fluid resuscitation, regardless of the formula used, is to maintain perfusion until the capillary permeability resolves and plasma volumes are restored to normal or near normal. Modifications in fluid replacement are made according to the individual child's response. The hourly urine output is one important measure for judging the adequacy of fluid resuscitation. The urine output desired is 1

ml/kg/hr for children weighing less than 30 kg. Children larger than 30 kg should have an hourly urine output of 30 to 50 ml. If the urine output is below or above these parameters, adjustments are made accordingly.

Fluids are administered through a large intravenous catheter inserted either percutaneously or by cutdown. The intravenous site should be in an unburned area if possible. A central venous catheter may also be inserted to measure the adequacy of fluid replacement.

Pain Management. Pain in the thermally injured pediatric patient ranges from mild to severe, depending on the nature of the burn. Anxiety and fear can also contribute to the child's expressions of pain. The usual agents employed in pain management are Demerol and morphine sulfate. They are administered in small increments intravenously as needed to control pain. The use of small frequent doses rather than a large bolus of narcotics seems to avoid many of the side effects associated with narcotic analgesics.[3] Narcotics should not be administered intramuscularly due to their incomplete and unpredictable absorption in children with moderate and major burns. Narcotic analgesics are used in the emergency department treatment of thermal injuries. They are not used for the entire duration of hospitalization. Other less potent analgesics are employed for long-term pain management in burned children.

Wound Treatment. After the ABCs of treatment have been instituted, attention is focused on the burn injury. Burned or smoldering clothing should have been removed at the accident site. Remaining clothing should be removed on admission to the emergency department. All dirt and debris is removed from burned areas by washing with a providone-iodine solution.

TABLE 8–2. FLUID RESUSCITATION FORMULAS

	Evans	Brooke	Parkland	Modified Brooke
Day 1				
Colloid	1 ml/kg/% burn	0.5 ml/kg/% burn	None	None
Crystalloid	Lactated Ringer's solution: 1 ml/kg/% burn	Lactated Ringer's solution: 1.5 ml/kg/% burn	Lactated Ringer's solution: 4 ml/kg/% burn	Lactated Ringer's solution: 2 ml/kg/% burn (adult) 3 ml/kg/% burn (child)
5% D/W	2000 ml/meter²	2000 ml/meter²	None	None
Rate	½ total in first 8 hr ¼ total in next 8 hr ¼ total in next 8 hr	½ total in first 8 hr ¼ total in next 8 hr ¼ total in next 8 hr	½ total in first 8 hr ¼ total in next 8 hr ¼ total in next 8 hr	Same as Brooke
Volume calculation	Use burn area up to a total of 50% TBSA; if greater than 50%, calculate as a 50% burn	Same as Evans	Use total burn area regardless of size	Same as Parkland
Day 2				
Colloid	0.5 ml/kg/% burn	0.25 ml/kg/% burn	Only if needed to maintain plasma volume	0.3–0.5 ml/kg/% burn
Crystalloid	Lactated Ringer's 0.5 ml/kg/% burn	Lactated Ringer's 0.75 ml/kg/% burn	None	None
5% D/W	1500–2000 ml	1500–2000 ml	Sufficient to maintain urine output	Sufficient to maintain urine output

Loose tissue is removed, and blisters are excised. If scalp burns are present, the hair is shaved around the burn area. The true extent of the burn can be more accurately determined once the wound has been cleaned. The depth of the burn is not always easy to determine. Superficial partial-thickness burns or deep, charred, full-thickness burns are readily identified. The problem in determining burn depth arises with whether the wound is a deep partial-thickness burn or a mixed partial-/full-thickness burn.[4] With burns of questionable depth, the area is observed initially and is examined carefully for the next 72 hours, as these wounds frequently demonstrate increasing depth.[5]

Several topical agents can be used for burn wound treatment. Silver sulfadiazine is a bacteriocidal agent available as a white cream. It does not burn or cause pain when applied. It can be applied directly to the burn wound or to a fine-mesh gauze dressing that is then placed on the wound.

Mafenide acetate (Sulfamylon) is also a bacteriocidal agent available as a white cream. It is applied in the same fashion as silver sulfadiazine. The disadvantages of this agent are that it causes pain when applied and it is a carbonic-anhydrase inhibitor that can lead to metabolic acidosis as the kidney's ability to secrete hydrogen ions is interfered with. Both silver sulfadiazine and Sulfamylon can be used in either the open (no dressing) or closed (dressing) method of treatment.

Silver nitrate is used in a hypotonic solution (0.5 percent) that is applied to the burn wound by means of thick layers of gauze that have been saturated with the solution. Since silver nitrate is hypotonic, it leeches sodium, chloride, and potassium from the body, necessitating electrolyte replacement. The solution also discolors anything it comes in contact with, turning it black.

Other agents employed include providone-iodine cream and gentamicin. Their use at present, however, is limited. Most emergency treatment modalities use the three agents discussed above. All burn wound care is carried out using aseptic technique. In all situations sterile gloves are worn to clean the wound and to apply a topical agent. Sterile gowns, masks, and head caps are indicated for moderate and major burns. Sterile sheets are used to cover the pediatric client. It is imperative that these precautions be observed to protect the child from subsequent infection.

Tetanus Prophylaxis. In addition to the interventions already discussed, there are other measures to be undertaken. Tetanus toxoid is given if the child has not received a tetanus immunization within the past year, as burns are considered ''dirty'' wounds. If the child has never been immunized, then tetanus immune globulin is given.

Gastric Decompression. A paralytic ileus frequently develops in children with major burns. A nasogastric tube is frequently inserted in the emergency department when this entity is present. Gastric decompression may also be necessary to prevent vomiting and aspiration. Hemorrhagic gastritis is due to bleeding from congested gastric mucosal capillaries. It is often present in the first 24 hours following thermal injury. A nasogastric tube may be necessary if hemorrhagic gastritis occurs.

Minor Thermal Injuries. Most of the nursing interventions discussed have focused on the pediatric client with a moderate or major thermal injury. The differences in treatment of minor burns are few. Children with burns of less than 10 percent total body surface area (TBSA) partial-thickness burn (excluding hands, feet, face, perineum, and other major illness or trauma) do not require fluid resuscitation. These burns are considered minor and can be treated on an outpatient basis. Children with less than a 2 percent full-thickness burn (with the same exclusions previously cited) can also be treated on an outpatient basis. Infants are considered poor risk patients and should, in most situations, be hospitalized for burn treatment.

The topical agents used for burn care on an outpatient basis are silver sulfadiazine, mafenide acetate, Xeroform or Adaptic gauze. The latter two are generally used for burns covering less than 2 percent of TBSA, while the former two are employed for larger burns. All are used with closed, dry dressings. Parents can be instructed in dressing changes and in the signs and symptoms of infection. Parents are also told when to return to clinic for follow-up care and evaluation of their child's burn.

Psychosocial Support and Parent Education. Children who sustain burns, whether mild, moderate, or major, experience anxiety and fear in addition to their burn injuries. Nursing interventions should also focus on alleviating these anxieties. Emergency department nurses should take into account the child's developmental stage when providing nursing care. Explanations of the care provided should be geared to the child's level of understanding. Parents can also benefit from an explanation of the treatment methods.

They also need reassurance and support in such a crisis situation. Nurses practicing in emergency departments must be as cognizant of these psychosocial needs as of the physical ones.

ELECTRICAL BURNS

Physiologic Aspects. Flow of electrical current generates heat as it encounters resistance. In the human body this resistance to flow varies in different tissues. Bones and fat are the most resistant, while nerves and blood vessels are the least resistant. Bone therefore has the potential for the highest heat generation. Tissue surrounding the bone may be more severely damaged than the skin surface.

Alternating current is more dangerous than direct current, as it tends to cause ventricular fibrillation. Alternating current in the range between 40 and 200 cycles per second is the most likely to cause myocardial fibrillation and is therefore the most dangerous.[6] Ordinary house current is 60 cycles per second.

The electrical current pathways through the body cannot be exactly determined because of the varying resistance offered by different structures. Entrance and exit sites may be present, however, which may aid in identifying an approximate current pathway. Currents that course through vital organs cause more damage. The longer the duration of contact with the electrical current the greater the injury sustained. The duration of contact may be prolonged by tetanic contractions of the flexor muscles in the forearms.

History. The information to collect on admission to the emergency department has previously been discussed. Specific data, however, are relevant to the electrical injury. It is necessary to know the duration of contact with the electrical current, the voltage amount, and the type of electrical force (alternating or direct current). These factors, as well as tissue resistance and surface area of contact, have an impact on the severity of the injury.

It is also important to obtain a history of the events surrounding the injury. Associated injuries (e.g., fractures, head trauma) may be present if the child's electrical burn is due to contact with elevated high-voltage wires. A history of unconsciousness at the accident site, and the duration of unconsciousness, should also be noted.

Assessment. The assessment is performed in the same manner as previously described. The ABC approach is again used. The visible damage from electrical burns may be small, while the internal damage may be quite significant. It is therefore imperative that the assessment be comprehensive. Major assessment factors to be considered are discussed here with the understanding that factors discussed previously are to be included in actual clinical practice.

A thorough neurologic assessment is conducted. Electrical injuries can cause seizures, disorientation, psychotic behavior, paralysis, and a host of other neurologic problems. Skull fractures or other head injuries may also be present if the electrical injury was accompanied by a fall.

A complete neurovascular assessment is performed on all extremities. Extensive subfascial edema can cause vascular compromise. The presence or absence of pulses should be determined on admission. The extremities are examined for any fractures. These can result either from a fall or from severe tetanic contractions.

Internal injuries are frequently associated with electrical burns. The abdomen is examined for any signs of distention or rigidity. The child is also observed for any signs of internal hemorrhage. Nausea, vomiting, and paralytic ileus are other potential problems.

Cardiac or respiratory arrest are always a potential danger. Vital signs are continually assessed and evaluated. Respiratory arrest can occur due to either direct brain-stem damage or asphyxiation due to tetanic contractions of respiratory muscles.

The color of the urine is examined. A dark red color indicates extensive muscle injury and the presence of myoglobin in the systemic circulation. Myoglobinuria can potentially result in acute renal failure.

The surface burns caused by the electrical contact are evaluated using the Lund-Browder chart. It must be kept in mind, however, that the surface wounds do not correlate with the internal damage. Progressive thrombosis occurs, and it may be several days before the true extent of tissue damage is revealed. An entry and exit site of the electrical current may be identifiable in some (but not all) children.

The diagnostic tests used for evaluation in electrical burns include an electrocardiogram; x-rays of long bones, cervical and spinal regions; urine for hemochromogen quantitation; and all the hematologic tests previously cited. Additional diagnostic tests may be indicated if the child has sustained other injuries along with the electrical burn.

Management. Nursing priorities are airway, breathing, and circulation. High-voltage injuries frequently result in cardiopulmonary arrest, thereby necessitating resuscitation. An airway is established by intubation (if necessary), and oxygen or ventilator support is provided as needed. Since electrical burns cause ventricular fibrillation and other cardiac arrhythmias, cardiac monitoring is initiated in the emergency department. A nasogastric tube is inserted to observe for any bleeding and for decompression.

There is no specific fluid resuscitation formula for use in electrical injuries. The extent of the tissue injured cannot be accurately ascertained from the surface wounds. Close attention must therefore be paid to the parameters that indicate adequate hydration (urine output, serum and urine sodium and osmolality, and blood volume). Intravenous fluid, usually Ringer's lactate, is infused to maintain a urine output of 1.5 to 2.0 ml/kg/hr. If myoglobinuria is present, an osmotic diuretic (e.g., mannitol) may be used in addition to the intravenous fluids to promote diuresis of myoglobin and to prevent acute tubular necrosis.[7] The administration of intravenous fluids is titrated according to the individual child's response and hourly urine output.

Neurovascular monitoring is an ongoing intervention. Fluid resuscitation may promote the collection of edema fluid under the fascia and subsequently cause neurovascular compromise. If neurovascular compromise is suspected, an escharotomy and fasciotomy of the affected extremity are performed immediately.

Care of the surface burns is the same as for thermal injuries. The wounds are cleaned and dressed with an appropriate agent. A tetanus immunization is also administered as necessary. Systemic antibiotics are also initiated in the emergency department.

These interventions are directed toward the care of a child who has sustained a high-voltage injury. Preadolescent and adolescent boys are the most likely to receive these injuries from climbing around high-tension wires. Children between the ages of 6 months and 2 years sustain the majority of low-voltage burns from chewing or sucking on electrical cords. Burns of the mouth and oral cavity can result in serious bleeding within 3 weeks of the injury. Burns of the mouth are assessed according to the same protocol as for severe electrical injury. Interventions are modified to the child's needs.

Electrical burns are *never* considered

minor. All children should be hospitalized for observation and treatment. Internal damage may not be readily apparent for several days. Progressive thrombosis of tissue occurs over several days; therefore the true extent of damage is not evident in the emergency department. Complications and later sequelae of electrical burns mandate hospitalization rather than outpatient care.

INHALATION INJURIES

Physiologic Aspects. The three major respiratory problems in the early postburn period are smoke inhalation, carbon monoxide poisoning, and upper airway burns. Children who sustain their thermal injuries in smoke-filled, enclosed areas are susceptible to smoke inhalation. The smoke causes a chemical injury to the lungs. There is an immediate loss of bronchial epithelial cilia and decreased alveolar surfactant. Atelectasis results and is compounded by mucosal edema in small airways. In a few hours a hemorrhagic tracheobronchitis develops.[8] The chemical mechanisms of injury may differ with the various toxic products produced by the fire; however, the resultant injury to the respiratory tract is the same.

Carbon monoxide is a colorless, odorless gas that is a component of the gaseous part of smoke and is a byproduct of combustion. Carbon monoxide poisoning is another problem experienced by children who have suffered burns in an enclosed space. Carbon monoxide displaces oxygen on the hemoglobin molecule, thereby producing hypoxia and tissue ischemia. Cerebral hypoxia can lead to stupor, coma, and brain death. The levels of carboxyhemoglobin in the blood measure the degree of carbon monoxide poisoning. Normal levels of carboxyhemoglobin are 0 to 10 percent. Levels greater than 15 percent are indicative of carbon monoxide poisoning.

Levels greater than 50 percent are usually fatal.

Upper airway burns are usually associated with facial burns. The inhalation of super-heated air produces thermal injury to the mouth, nasopharynx, pharynx, and larynx. Edema formation produces rapid narrowing and obstruction of the airway. Children, with their smaller airways, are very vulnerable to rapid airway occlusion.

History. The history should include an accurate description of the thermal injury. How and where the burn occurred should be documented as well as any exposure to smoke, fumes from chemicals, or steam. It must be kept in mind that furniture, carpets, housing materials, and other household items contain synthetic agents that can produce noxious gases.

It must be determined whether the child was trapped in an enclosed space. A confined space can increase the concentration of toxic fumes in a short span of time. The length of time the child was exposed to the smoke, carbon monoxide, or noxious fumes should be determined. Any history of previous respiratory problems experienced by the child should also be documented. All other factors cited in the section on obtaining a history for thermal burns should also be included.

Assessment. An early and comprehensive assessment of the child's respiratory status is mandatory. Hypoxia or carbon monoxide poisoning may exist but may go undetected unless a careful assessment is performed. Some of the clinical features associated with inhalation injuries are facial burns, singed nasal hair, perioral edema, pharyngeal edema, hoarseness, wheezing, and carbonaceous sputum.

The child's oral cavity and pharynx are examined for erythema and blistering, which can indicate potential upper airway obstruction. The child's respiratory rate is determined as well as the respiratory pattern. Auscultation will reveal the presence of rales, rhonchi, wheezing, or stridor. The chest is percussed for any areas of dullness.

Signs of respiratory distress include hoarseness, labored respirations, nasal flaring, retractions, and abdominal respirations. Children with smoke inhalation injuries frequently have carbonaceous sputum. Signs of hypoxia in children include confusion, restlessness, agitation, and combativeness.

Laboratory data gathered to assist in the diagnosis and treatment of inhalation injuries are arterial blood gases, carboxyhemoglobin levels, and a chext x-ray. A bronchoscopy may be performed to determine if smoke inhalation has occurred or the extent of tissue damage. This procedure can ascertain inhalation injury even in the absence of clinical signs and symptoms.

Management. On admission to the emergency department a set of baseline vital signs are obtained (temperature, pulse, respirations, and blood pressure) and are monitored every 15 to 30 minutes. The respiratory status is thoroughly assessed and interventions executed to maintain adequate oxygenation.

Carbon monoxide poisoning is treated by the administration of 100 percent oxygen until the level of carboxyhemoglobin is decreased to an acceptable point. Oxygen can be administered through mask or endotracheal tube. It is also necessary to determine if oxygen was administered at the injury site to ascertain the approximate level of carbon monoxide poisoning.

If a facial burn is present, upper airway obstruction is a potential problem. Significant pharyngeal burns necessitate early endotracheal intubation before progressive edema occludes the airway. A humidified oxygen source is also employed to provide mist and oxygen as needed.

The child should be prepared for intubation if he or she is old enough and is reasonably alert to what is happening. Parents are also prepared and are given an explanation of events.

Smoke inhalation injuries in children require intubation with either complete or assisted ventilator support. High humidification is needed to prevent drying of the secretions and mucosa. Suctioning is performed using sterile technique. Frequent suctioning may be necessary initially due to copious secretions.

For all children with inhalation injuries, arterial blood gases are drawn to determine their acid-base balance and oxygenation status. Intravenous fluids are administered according to the extent of the child's surface burn injury. Children who have inhalation injuries may require additional fluids. Caution must be used to avoid fluid volume overload and the development of pulmonary edema, which can exacerbate pulmonary injuries.

Children with hypoxia demonstrate a neurologic response that is vastly different from that of adults. After the hypoxic period a rapid onset of cerebral edema or vascular congestion occurs, causing a sudden significant increase in intracranial pressure. These children may demonstrate agitation, high-pitched screams, and seizures. Respiratory arrest can occur suddenly. All children with smoke inhalation injuries should therefore be observed carefully for changes in neurologic status. Narcotics are avoided until hypoxia has been corrected so as not to obscure neurologic changes.

Respiratory tract injuries are a major cause of mortality, morbidity, and extended hospitalization. In many instances the inhalation injury causes greater damage than the surface injury itself. Any child who has sustained a thermal injury should also be observed carefully for any signs of respiratory distress.

NOTES

1. R.T. Fitzgerald. Prehospital care of burned patients. *Critical Care Quarterly.* 1(1978):16.
2. American College of Emergency Physicians. *Minor Burns: Evaluation and Treatment.* Kansas City, Mo.: Marion Laboratories, 1979, p. 26.
3. J. Marvin. Acute care of the burned patient. *Critical Care Quarterly.* 1(1978):32.
4. Ibid., p. 33
5. Ibid.
6. R.E. Salisbury, and G.P. Dingeldein. Specific burn injuries. In R.E. Salisbury, N.M. Newman, & G.P. Dingeldein (Eds.), *Manual of Burn Therapeutics.* Boston: Little, Brown, 1983, p. 82.
7. Ibid., p. 85.
8. D.M. Heimbach. Smoke inhalation: Current concepts. In T.L. Wachtel, V. Kahn, & H.A. Frank (Eds.). *Current Topics in Burn Care.* Rockville, Md.: Aspen Systems, 1983, p. 34.

BIBLIOGRAPHY

American College of Emergency Physicians. *Minor Burns: Evaluation and Treatment,* Kansas City, Mo.: Marion Laboratories, 1979, p. 26.

Bayley, E.W., & Martin, M.T. (Eds.). *A Curriculum for Basic Burn Nursing Practice* (4th ed.). Galveston, Tex.: American Burn Association/ Shriners Burn Institute, 1985.

Deitch, E.A., & Statts, M. Child abuse through burning. *Journal of Burn Care and Rehabilitation* March-April 1982, pp. 89–94.

Fitzgerald, R.T. Prehospital care of burned patients. *Critical Care Quarterly* 1(1978):13–24.

Heimbach, D.M. Smoke inhalation: Current concepts. In Wachtel, T.L., Kahn, V., & Franks, H.A. (Eds.), *Current Topics in Burn Care.* Rockville, Md. Aspen Systems, 1983.

Hummel, R.P. *Clinical Burn Therapy.* Boston: John Wright, PSG, 1982.

Lushbaugh, M. Critical care of the child with burns. Symposium on Pediatric Critical Care. *Nursing Clinics of North America* 16(1981):635–646.

Marvin, J. Acute care of the burned patient. *Critical Care Quarterly* 1(1978):24–35.

Philbin, P., et al. Management of the pediatric patient with a major burn. *Journal of Burn Care and Rehabilitation* 3(1982):118–121, 123–125.

Salisbury, R.E., & Dingeldein, G.P. Specific burn injuries. In Salisbury, R.E., Newman, N.M., & Dingeldein, G.P. (Eds.), *Manual of Burn Therapeutics.* Boston: Little, Brown, 1983.

Shires, T.J., & Black, E.A. (Eds.). Proceedings from the Second Conference on Supportive Therapy in Burn Care. *The Journal of Trauma* (Special Supplement) August 1981, pp. 686–724.

EMERGENCY DEPARTMENT CARE GUIDE FOR THE CHILD WITH BURNS

Nursing Diagnosis	Interventions	Evaluation
Ineffective airway clearance related to edema from burns of face and neck	Assess and support airway, breathing, and circulation Clear airway of mucus or blood with suctioning Insert oropharyngeal airway Administer 100 percent humidified oxygen	Airway remains patent

(Continued)

Nursing Diagnosis	Interventions	Evaluation
Ineffective breathing patterns related to circumferential burns to chest	Continually assess child's respiratory status Continually assess arterial blood gas values Assist with escharotomy as needed Prepare for endotracheal intubation and artificial ventilation	Breath sounds are normal Arterial blood gas values are adequate
Fluid volume deficit related to shift of fluid from vascular to interstitial spaces during first 6 to 12 hours	Administer intravenous fluids as calculated based on size of burn through large bore intravenous line Continually assess vital signs with special attention to signs of hypovolemic shock Insert indwelling urinary catheter Carefully measure and record fluid intake and urinary output Continually monitor serum electrolytes	Vital signs remain stable Urinary output is sufficient (>1 ml/kg/hr) Serum electrolytes remain within normal limits
Impairment of skin integrity related to loss of protective layer secondary to thermal injury	Estimate and record the size and depth of burns Cleanse the wounds with surgical soap solution Assist in debridement of dead skin from broken blisters Apply topical antimicrobial agent Dress burn wounds loosely so as not to impede circulation Check sensation and circulation below areas of burns on extremities	Depth and extent of burns are recorded Wounds are cleansed and dressed Circulation remains adequate distal to areas of extremity burns
Potential for infection related to loss of protective layer of skin, secondary to thermal injury	Wear sterile gowns, mask, caps, and gloves when providing care to prevent contamination of wounds Obtain wound culture Cleanse wounds with antiseptic agent Apply topical agents and sterile dressing	Wounds are cleansed and dressed Sterile environment is maintained

Nursing Diagnosis	Interventions	Evaluation
	Administer tetanus prophylaxis as indicated by immunization status Administer systemic antibiotics as ordered	
Hypothermia related to impairment in skin integrity	Continually monitor temperature Use overhead radiant warmers during resuscitation Elevate room temperature and humidity Warm intravenous fluids prior to infusion	Child maintains normal body temperature
Fear related to burn accident and painful hospital procedures	Explain all procedures to child Reassure child in a calm, supportive manner Allow parents to be with child as soon as child is stabilized and wounds are dressed Prepare child for hospital admission or transfer to burn treatment center	Child remains calm
Pain related to burns and painful treatment procedures	Observe child for verbal and nonverbal signs of pain Administer pain medication as ordered Position child to make him or her as comfortable as possible	Child is able to tolerate treatments in emergency department
Alteration in family processes related to hospitalization of child	Assess for possibility of child abuse Continually inform parents of child's condition and treatments Prepare parents for child's admission to hospital or transfer to burn center	Parents demonstrate appropriate concern

9 | Poisonings and Ingestions

Elena Hopkins-Lotz

In this age of pharmaceutical and chemical sophistication, every home has a multitude of lethal preparations available for various purposes. Ingestion of these toxic and even nontoxic materials is a common occurrence. It is estimated that annually about 6,000,000 children ingest toxic products,[1] making poisoning one of the most common medical emergencies among children and adolescents. While less than 1 percent of these visits are life threatening,[2] they are emergencies from the perspective of the child and his or her parents.

Upon entering the fast-paced emergency department, the child and parents often turn to the nurse for information, support, and guidance. A biological/psychologic/social approach is invaluable as the child and parents deal with fear and anxiety as well as the postingestion sequelae. The parents may experience a sense of guilt, which may decrease their coping skills. As a result the parents must also be treated as patients.

Poisoning is a significant cause of morbidity and mortality in the United States; it is the fourth leading cause of death in children.[3] Approximately 80 percent of accidental ingestions occur in children under 5 years of age, with the peak incidence being between 1½ and 3 years.[4-6]

Ingestions may be either accidental or intentional. Accidental poisonings make up some 80 to 85 percent or more of all poisoning exposures, while intentional poisoning comprises the other 10 to 15 per-

cent.[7] Among children aged 5 and under essentially all poisonings are accidents related to exploratory behavior stemming from their newly discovered mobility and curiosity. Accidental poisoning should be suspected as a suicide gesture in children who are over 5 years of age and of normal intelligence and therefore warrants a psychologic evaluation. The incidence of ingestions drops significantly after 5 years until ages 15 to 24, when it again rises.[8] This may represent a reflection of the adolescent's depression or fascination with experimentation. Manipulative behavior and suicide again become important motivators to be examined in such cases. (Refer to Chapter 4 for further discussion on suicidal behavior.)

Poisonings apparently occur with greater frequency whenever there is a disturbance in the household or a deviation from the ordinary routine, such as during any period of stress or tension.[9] In most cases the child is in his or her own home at the time of ingestion, with the most common areas involved being the kitchen and bedroom.

Poisoning has been defined as exposure to an amount of substance likely to produce untoward effects in a substantial fraction of exposed subjects. In children it is usually the result of the interaction of a susceptible host, an available poison, and a temporarily unstable environment. The nurse's first contact with the results of such an interaction may be when a panic-stricken mother arrives in the emergency department with her infant or young child, who has ingested a toxic (or nontoxic) substance. At other times the nurse is forced to deal with evidence that is merely suggestive of an ingestion.

An accidential poisoning can be suspected if the child has been involved in previous episodes, since some children repeat this behavior. Suspicion is also warranted if there has been a sudden change in behavior in a previously well child who is under 5 years old.[10] Another important consideration in dealing with poisonings in the infant age group is the possibility of child abuse. This should be suspected if the history is sketchy or does not correlate with the physical presentation.

Regardless of the overt presentation, the major thrust of nursing intervention is to deal appropriately with life-threatening problems, to terminate the exposure of the patient to the poison, and to provide psychosocial support to the child and parents. Figure 9–1 summarizes the initial management of the child who has ingested a poison.

ASSESSMENT

The child who has ingested or is suspected of ingesting any potentially toxic substance should *never* be relegated to the waiting room of the emergency department. In addition to any abrupt change in behavior or personality, the triage nurse should also be alerted to the possibility of a poisoning by a change in the child's state of consciousness or by lethargy, stupor, or coma. Other clinical manifestations that may indicate overdose include unexplained cyanosis, seizures, and vascular collapse.

As in all critically ill patients, the initial assessment and management should include establishment of an airway, artifi-

cial ventilation, and appropriate measures to restore circulation. These basic steps must not be underplayed by the intense concern with learning the specific treatment for the poison. Acute attention should be paid to the heart rate, blood pressure, central nervous system function (reflexes, response to verbal and painful stimuli, pupil size, and response to light), and hydration. Most patients in a toxic condition also have the potential for seizures and therefore must be observed for seizure activity.

Observation and documentation of the child's behavior upon arrival in the emergency department is vital before triage is completed. The poisoned patient may appear lethargic, controlled, withdrawn, agitated, or combative. The patient out of control must be placed in an appropriate area where safety is provided for himself or herself as well as for the care providers. During the triage assessment the nurse also needs to assess the need for physical restraint or observation for the intentionally overdosed or suicidal patient.

At this unstable, preliminary stage it may be necessary for the triage nurse to ask the parents or guardians of the child to wait in another area. Overwhelmed by the experience itself, they will need support and guidance while thinking over the series of events that will help to clarify the poisoning episode.

HISTORY

The nurse should be prepared to ask three simple questions that will aid greatly in diagnosis and subsequent management: What was ingested? When was it ingested? How much was ingested? It is wise to limit questions to the available facts.

Since estimating amounts is difficult, it may be more effective to ask: How much

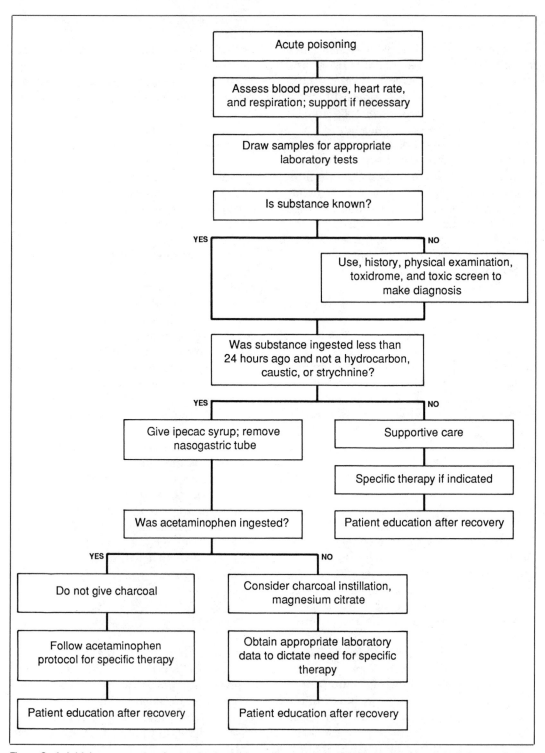

Figure 9-1. Initial management of poisoning in children. *(Reproduced with permission from D.X. Driggers. Pediatric poisoning—The first 30 minutes. Postgraduate Medicine 72, no. 2(1982):55.)*

was in the bottle originally? How much remains? What symptoms did the patient show? How long ago did the ingestion take place? Was any treatment performed at home? It is also always important to ask if the patient has any chronic or current illnesses and if he or she is taking any medications.

MANAGEMENT

Once the patient has been stabilized and vital functions are intact, five basic principles must be followed: (1) identify the poison; (2) stop absorption; (3) hasten elimination; (4) give symptomatic care; and (5) give appropriate antidote.[11]

Identify the Poison

In addition to identifying the toxic agent, the health care team also needs to determine the time and rate of exposure and to estimate the amount ingested. The accuracy of the clinical history is often difficult to ascertain following an acute poisoning, especially when the episode is the result of a suicide gesture or street drug abuse. When dealing with young children, there is often greater difficulty in identifying the offending agent because of the lack of a witness to the episode, lack of circumstantial evidence, and the inability of the child to express the vital details.

Determining the exact name of the ingested product is essential because products with similar names often contain different chemical constituents. For example, Anacin contains aspirin and caffeine, whereas Anacin 3 contains acetaminophen and caffeine.[12]

An inventory of toxins and chemicals in the home may provide a clue. Have the patient or a family member recall all possible products in the home. If the product found with the child has not been brought to the emergency department, the nurse could suggest that someone retrieve the remainder (or even the empty bottle or container). While helping to maximize the quality of intervention their child receives, parents then also feel productive and helpful in an otherwise frustrating situation.

In cases in which the poisoning agent is unknown, the health care team must rely on the characteristic signs and symptoms of specific types of poisoning, or toxidromes (Table 9–1) and on laboratory tests to aid in the diagnosis and planning of care.

Laboratory Data. When qualitative and quantitative tests are used in conjunction with clinical assessment and pharmacologic data on the ingested substance, a logical approach to management is possible. Laboratory analysis should be performed to confirm the substance ingested and to evaluate the biochemical status of the patient. Several techniques such as rapid screening tests and the toxic screen may be used to identify the toxic agents. Qualitative tests performed on blood, urine, or gastric contents can help to identify the specific toxin, and a quantitative measurement using blood can then help in assessing the severity of the intoxication. The care of the poisoned patient, however, should be based on clinical status and not on drug levels.

In addition to the general toxicology screen, baseline blood samples for glucose, complete blood count, BUN, and electrolyte values should be obtained to monitor potential acidosis where applicable.

Stopping Absorption

Specific care should be directed initially at minimizing the duration of exposure and at reducing the opportunity for continued absorption of the toxin. The next goal is elimination of the toxin that has already been absorbed. The method used to minimize this exposure depends on the type of exposure. More than 80 percent of poison-

TABLE 9-1. TOXIDROMES: CLINICAL MANIFESTATIONS BY SYSTEM WITH
ASSOCIATED TOXIC SUBSTANCES

Manifestations	Substances
Central Nervous System	
Depression and coma	Sedatives-hypnotics, narcotics, anticonvulsants, tranquilizers, tricyclic antidepressants, phenothiazines, antimuscarinic agents, hypoglycemic agents, alcohols, aromatic hydrocarbons, carbon monoxide, lead, mercury, lithium, cyanide, gases, solvents
Stimulation and/or seizures	Amphetamines, xanthines, sympathomimetic agents, psychotropic drugs (phencyclidine, lysergic acid diethylamine, mescaline), cocaine, nicotine, salicylates, ergot, camphor, lead, strychnine, organophosphates, carbonates, chlorinated insecticides
Hallucinations	Psychotropic drugs, amphetamines, alcohol withdrawal, antihistamines, antimuscarinic agents, cocaine, camphor, tricyclic antidepressants
Hyperpyrexia	Salicylates, atropine
Ocular System	
Mydriasis	Antimuscarinic agents, sympathomimetic agents, psychotropic drugs, cocaine, amphetamines
Miosis	Narcotics, organophosphate insecticides, parasympathomimetic drugs
Blurred vision	Antimuscarinic agents, alcohols
Colored vision	Digitalis, quinine
Scotomas	Quinine, salicylates
Red eye	Marijuana
Nystagmus	Dilantin, phencyclidine
Auditory System	
Tinnitus	Salicylates, streptomycin, ergot, quinine
Cardiovascular System	
Arrhythmias	Digitalis, quinidine, tricyclic antidepressants, phenothiazines
Tachycardia	Amphetamines, sympathomimetic agents, xanthines, cocaine, tricyclic antidepressants
Cardiovascular System	
Bradycardia	Beta blockers, cardiac glycosides, quinine
Hypotension	Narcotics, phenothiazines, antihypertensive agents, tricyclic antidepressants
Hypertension	Cocaine, amphetamines
Respiratory System	
Hypoventilation	Central nervous system depressants
Hyperventilation	Salicylates, cocaine, nicotine, carbon dioxide
Abnormal odor on breath of:	
Alcohol	Alcohols, phenols, chloral hydrate
Acetone	Alcohol, acetone, lacquer
Wintergreen	Methyl salicylate
Garlic	Phosphorous, arsenic
Bitter almonds	Cyanide
Pears	Chloral hydrate, turpentine, camphor
Gastrointestinal System	
Nausea, vomiting and diarrhea	Almost any toxic substance can produce these signs or symptoms
Increased salivation	Organophosphate insecticides, mushrooms
Decreased salivation	Antimuscarinic agents, antihistamines
Genitourinary System	
Urine retention	Tricyclic antidepressants, anticholinergic agents
Dark green urine	Phenol, resorcinol

TABLE 9-1. *(Continued)*

Manifestations	Substances
Skin and Teguments	
Cyanosis	Nitrites, nitrobenzene, aniline dyes
Jaundice	Carbon tetrachloride, benzene, aniline dyes, chromates, phenothiazines,
Staining	quinacrine
Black	Bismuth
Flushed face	Atropine
Discoloration of gums	Lead, bismuth, arsenic
Hematologic System	
Pink blood	Carbon monoxide or cyanide
Brown blood	Methemoglobinemia

Reproduced with permission from P. Gaudreault, & F.H. Lovejoy. Acute poisoning. In J.D. Dickerman, & J.S. Lucey (Eds.), The Critically Ill Child: Diagnosis and Medical Management. Philadelphia: W.B. Saunders, 1985.

ings in children 5 years old or younger involve ingestion, with ocular and topical exposures being the next most common route.[13]

In the case of topical, ocular, or inhalation exposures, the child should be removed from the toxic environment immediately. The eyes should be irrigated with copious amounts of normal saline for a steady 15 to 20 minutes. Skin exposed to insecticides or acid or alkali agents should be flooded with tepid water and washed well with soap and a soft wash cloth or sponge.

Oral Ingestion. In the case of acute oral intoxication, the time of ingestion is of special importance. Most patients will develop symptoms within 2 to 4 hours of ingestion. The majority of patients who do not show signs or symptoms within 6 to 8 hours of ingestion will remain asymptomatic. Some toxins, however, such as acetaminophen, diphenoxylate hydrochloride, and paraquat, produce symptoms that may be delayed from 12 hours to a few days.

Another important factor is the amount ingested. Although an accurate estimate is difficult to obtain following a suicidal gesture, the amount accidentally ingested by young children can often be determined with the assistance of the parent. In the child, one swallow is equivalent to 10 to 15 ml.[14] When determining therapy it is important to use the largest estimated amount and to always relate the amount taken to the patient's weight.

The next step is to determine whether the ingested substance is a hydrocarbon, a caustic, or a strychnine. If it is any of these the general rule of thumb is to initiate supportive therapy.[15]

Because of their potential for causing esophagitis, caustics, hydrocarbons, and strychnine should not be treated by emesis. Any acid or alkali ingestion should be diluted with milk or water. In addition to receiving supportive care, the patient should be observed for development of pulmonary complications secondary to esophageal mucosal injury. Other situations in which emesis should not be induced include (1) the comatose patient or the patient who has taken medication that will probably cause drowsiness within half an hour, (2) the convulsing patient, and (3) the patient who has been given activated charcoal.

Hasten Elimination

Ipecac Syrup. The speed, effectiveness, and safety of ipecac syrup make it the method of choice for removing toxic material from the stomach of the awake, alert, pediatric patient. The dose of ipecac syrup for children is as follows:

9 to 12 months	10 cc
12 months to 12 years	15 to 30 cc
Over 12 years	30 cc

This dose is followed by 150 to 250 cc of clear fluids. Milk or heavily sugared drinks should not be used, since they delay the time to onset of emesis.

If vomiting does not occur within 20 minutes, the same dose may be repeated once. Emesis should be induced up to 6 hours after ingestion. Once the syrup of ipecac is administered, the child should be carefully observed and should never be left alone. After vomiting starts the patient should be supported in a sitting position to prevent aspiration. Three to four episodes of vomiting occur over 30 to 60 minutes following the administration of ipecac syrup. It effectively induces emesis of all ingested toxins, including antiemetic drugs such as the phenothiazines.

Gastric Lavage. If emesis does not occur within 20 minutes of the administration of the second dose, removal of the ingested product by gastric lavage may be indicated. Gastric lavage is less effective than ipecac-induced emesis, especially for the removal of whole or partially dissolved tablets or capsules. This procedure should therefore be reserved for the obtunded or comatose patient only. This must be done very carefully, with a cuffed endotracheal tube in place because of the increased risk of lung aspiration in the unconscious patient due to a depressed gag reflex. Using the largest nasogastric tube possible and

with the patient in the head-down position, lavage should be performed with one-half normal or normal saline (volume determined by child's weight) and should be continued until the return is clear.

Activated Charcoal. Once the stomach has been emptied, activated charcoal may minimize further absorption of toxins in the gastrointestinal tract. It is indicated in almost all serious oral overdoses except those of cyanides, alcohols, caustic substances, heavy metals, and hydrocarbons. Although it should be given as soon as possible after ingestion, the emergency nurse should wait 60 minutes following ipecac-induced emesis, since ipecac is inactivated by the charcoal.

Activated charcoal (15 to 30 g) is mixed with water (50 ml for a 1-year-old to 300 ml for an adolescent) or with an ionic cathartic such as magnesium citrate to form a liquid of milkshake-like consistency that may be administered orally or through a nasogastric tube after gastric lavage. Activated charcoal should *not* be mixed with jam, milk, or ice cream. The mixture can be made a bit more tolerable by covering the cup with paper and inserting a straw through the middle.

Even if the charcoal does not absorb the ingested substance, its black color will serve to identify complete evacuation of the gastrointestinal tract. Charcoal is ineffective with inorganic compounds such as acids, bases, cyanide, or iron salts.

Give Appropriate Antidote

Unfortunately, no effective antidote specific to each poisoning exists.* In the management of acetaminophen ingestion,

---

*Emergency department staff should always contact the Poison Control Center in their area (refer to Table 9-2) for information on the appropriate management, including possible antidote for the specific substance ingested.

N-acetylcysteine (Mucomyst) has emerged as the treatment of choice.

Acetaminophen has become increasingly popular as an analgesic and antipyretic drug in the home. It is therefore becoming a more common cause of poisoning as well. Although therapeutic doses of the drug are relatively safe, accidental or suicidal dose ingestions are life threatening. Early symptoms may not appear for 4 to 6 hours after ingestion, and symptoms of the risk of developing hepatotoxicity may not be visible until 48 hours or more after ingestion.

Once it has been decided that acetaminophen was taken, therapy is based mainly on acetaminophen serum concentration at different times after ingestion. Activated charcoal should not be instilled, and a specific protocol for Tylenol or acetaminophen poisoning should be followed, which includes determination of serum levels, use of a nomogram to determine possible toxicity, and N-acetylcysteine (Mucomyst), 140 mg/kg therapy. If given early enough, either orally (mixed with juice or soft drink) or through a nasogastric tube, Mucomyst will detoxify acetaminophen metabolites, preventing eventual liver damage.[16]

DISCHARGE PLANNING

The decision to admit or discharge a poisoned pediatric patient from the emergency department is based on the patient's clinical condition, predicted severity of the poisoning, and the parents' ability to cope effectively and appropriately at the given time. Several different types of ingestion require reevaluation hours after ingestion (e.g., tricyclic antidepressants) and thus warrant the child's admission. Other types of poisons most likely to require hospitalization are (1) salicylates, (2) acetaminophen, (3) iron, (4) petroleum distillates,

(5) sedative-hypnotic and antidepressant drugs, and (6) corrosive acids and alkalies.[17]

Psychiatric evaluation is another important consideration in dealing with overdose patients, as suicide attempts involving drugs and other toxic substances are on the increase among adolescents and school-aged children.

If the poisoning is accidental, the nurse and other members of the interdisciplinary team need to assess the parents' ability to maintain the child if discharged and to prevent such accidents from happening in the future. Often the involvement of a social worker at the initial entry stage into the emergency department can be quite helpful in making this assessment or in making appropriate referrals. A referral to a public health nurse who will conduct a home visit to assess the home situation and provide teaching is often indicated.

PSYCHOSOCIAL SUPPORT AND PARENT EDUCATION

In any poisoning episode involving a young child, parents are invariably overwhelmed by their sense of guilt and are often paralyzed by their fear of the potential outcome for their child. Once the patient is stabilized and out of danger, the nurse should attempt to sit with the parents in a quiet, nonthreatening area to discuss these issues. If the child is to be discharged, appropriate family teaching regarding safety in the home and poison prevention should be initiated. Because of the crisis orientation of the situation, this teaching needs to be basic. In addition to any discussion, the parents should receive written information about poison prevention and written care instructions for their child. Poison control center information and phone numbers are also pertinent at this time. Refer to Table 9–2 for a listing of

TABLE 9-2. POISON CONTROL CENTERS

Alabama	Alabama Poison Center, (800) 462-0800 (statewide)	Louisiana	Louisiana Regional Poison Control Center, (800) 535-0525
Alaska	Anchorage Poison Center, (907) 563-3393	Maine	Maine Poison Control Center, (800) 442-6305
Arizona	Arizona Regional Poison Control System, (800) 362-0101	Maryland	Maryland Poison Center, (800) 492-2414
Arkansas	Statewide Poison Control Drug Information Center, (800) 428-8948 (statewide)	Massachusetts	Massachusetts Poison Control System, (800) 682-9211
California	Los Angeles County Medical Association, Regional Poison Information Center, (213) 484-5151	Michigan	Poison Control Center, (800) 572-1655, 462-6642
	San Diego Regional Poison Center, (619) 294-6000		Blodgett Regional Poison Center, (800) 632-2727
	San Francisco Bay Area Regional Poison Center, (415) 666-2845	Minnesota	Hennepin Poison Center, (612) 347-3141
			Minnesota Poison Control System, (800) 222-1222
Colorado	Rocky Mountain Poison Center, (800) 332-3073	Mississippi	Regional Poison Control Center, (601) 354-7660
Connecticut	Connecticut Poison Control Center, (203) 674-3456, 674-3457	Missouri	Cardinal Glennon Children's Hospital Regional Poison Center, (800) 392-9111
Delaware	Poison Information Center, (302) 655-3389		Mid-Plains Poison Control Center, (800) 228-9515
District of Columbia	National Capital Poison Center, (202) 625-3333	Montana	Rocky Mountain Poison Center, (800) 525-5042
Florida	Tampa Bay Regional Poison Control Center, (800) 282-3171	Nebraska	Mid-Plains Poison Control Center, (800) 642-9999 (outside Omaha); (800) 228-9515 (Idaho, Iowa, Kansas, Missouri, South Dakota)
Georgia	Georgia Poison Control Center, (800) 282-5846	Nevada	Southern Nevada Memorial Hospital, (702) 385-1277
Hawaii	Hawaii Poison Center, (800) 362-3585	New Hampshire	New Hampshire Poison Center, (800) 562-8236
Idaho	Mid-Plains Poison Control Center, (800) 228-9515	New Jersey	New Jersey Poison Information and Education System, (800) 962-1253
Illinois	Chicago Area Poison Resource Center, (800) 942-5969	New Mexico	New Mexico Poison and Drug Information Center, (800) 432-6866
	Central & Southern Illinois Regional Poison Resource Center, (800) 252-2022	New York	Binghamton: Southern Tier Poison Center, (607) 723-8929
Indiana	Poison Center, (800) 382-9087		Buffalo: Western New York Poison Center, (716) 878-7654, 878-7655
Iowa	Mid-Plains Poison Control Center, (800) 228-9515		East Meadow: Long Island Regional Poison Control Center, (516) 542-2324, 542-2325, 542-2323
	University of Iowa Hospital and Clinics, Poison Control Center, (800) 272-6477		New York: New York City Poison Center, (212) 340-4494, 764-7667
Kansas	Mid-American Poison Center, (800) 332-6633	North Carolina	Duke Poison Control Center, (800) 672-1697
	Mid-Plains Poison Control Center, (800) 228-9515	North Dakota	North Dakota Poison Information Center, (800) 732-2200
Kentucky	Louisville: Kentucky Regional Poison Center of Kosair-Children's Hospital, (800) 722-5725		

TABLE 9-2. *(Continued)*

Ohio	Central Ohio Poison Control Center, (800) 682-7625	Texas	Texas State Poison Center, (800) 392-8548
Oklahoma	Oklahoma Poison Control Center, (800) 522-4611	Utah	Intermountain Regional Poison Control Center, (800) 662-0062
Oregon	Oregon Poison Center and Drug Information Center, (800) 452-7165	Vermont	Vermont Poison Center, (802) 658-3456
Pennsylvania	Allentown: Lehigh Valley Poison Center, (215) 433-2311 Hershey: Capital Area Poison Center, (717) 534-6111 Philadelphia: Philadelphia Poison Information, (215) 922-5523, 922-5524 Pittsburgh: Pittsburgh Poison Center, (412) 681-6669 (emergency); 647-5600 (Administration/Consultation)	Virginia	Charlottesville: Blue Ridge Poison Center, (800) 552-3723 (Virginia only); (800) 446-9876 (out of state) Norfolk: Tidewater Poison Center, (804) 489-5288 Richmond: Central Virginia Poison Center, (804) 786-4780
		Washington	Seattle Poison Center, (800) 732-6985 (statewide)
		West Virginia	West Virginia Poison System, (800) 642-3625
Puerto Rico	Poison Control Center, (809) 754-8535	Wisconsin	Green Bay Poison Control Center, (414) 433-8100 Milwaukee Poison Center, (414) 931-4114
Rhode Island	Rhode Island Poison Control Center, (401) 277-5906		
South Carolina	Palmetto Poison Center, (800) 922-1117	Wyoming	Wyoming Poison Center, (307) 777-7955
South Dakota	Mid-Plains Poison Control Center, (800) 228-9515		
Tennessee	Memphis: Southern Poison Center, (901) 528-6048 Nashville: Vanderbilt University Hospital, (615) 322-6435		

many of the poison conrol centers in the United States.

Once social service is involved, a decision often needs to be made regarding the parents' ability to maintain a safe environment for the child. Multiple ingestions should alert the health care team that neglect or other forms of child abuse should be investigated.

The ultimate goal of the emergency nurse caring for a pediatric patient who has ingested a toxic or nontoxic substance is to care for the patient, not the poison. The nurse's efforts may take the form of early crisis management, maintenance of family systems, or long-term patient/family teaching.

Although there has been a recent decline in mortality from pediatric poisoning secondary to increased consumer education, legislation and broad scale investigations, children are still exposed annually to an overwhelming number of noxious agents. The ultimate solution to the problem of childhood poisoning lies in prevention. Poison prevention education by health care providers and through programs sponsored by poison control centers has had a tremendous impact on the public's knowledge.

NOTES

1. P. Gaudreault, & F.H. Lovejoy. Acute poisoning. In J.D. Dickerman, & J.S. Lucey (Eds.) *The Critically Ill Child: Diagnosis and*

Medical Management. Philadelphia: W.B. Saunders, 1985, pp. 78–111.

2. S. Fought, & A. Throne. The pediatric patient. In *Psychosocial Nursing Care of the Emergency Patient.* New York: Wiley, 1984, pp. 51–63.

3. R.M. Barkin, K.W. Kulig, & B.H. Rumock. Poisoning and overdose. In R. Barkin, & D. Rosen (Eds.), *Emergency Pediatrics.* St. Louis: Mosby, 1984, pp. 266–298.

4. T.M. Deeths, & J.T. Breeden. Poisoning in children—A statistical study of 1,057 cases. *Journal of Pediatrics* 78, no. 2(1971):299–305.

5. H. Jacobziner. Accidental poisoning in children. *Medical Times* 94, no. 2(1966):221–241.

6. R.C. Nelson, M.I. Faw, D.J. Brancato, B.I. Cohen, & G.D. Armstrong. Poisoning among young children. *Journal of the American Medical Association* 251, no. 3(1981):1660–1664.

7. F.M. Henretig, G.C. Cupit, & A.R. Temper. Toxicologic emergencies. In G. Fleisher, & S. Ludwig, (Eds.), *Textbook of Pediatric Emergency Medicine.* Baltimore: Williams & Wilkins, 1984, pp. 489–531.

8. M. Ochs. Poisons. In C.G. Warner (Ed.), *Emergency Care.* St. Louis: Mosby, 1983, pp. 397–412.

9. D.J. Turbeville, & R.G. Fearnow. Is it possible to identify the child who is a high risk candidate for the accidental ingestion of a poison? *Clinical Pediatrics* 15, no. 10(1976): 918–920.

10. F. Simon. Poisoning in children. *American Family Physician* 25, no. 2(1982):206–211.

11. Ochs, Poisons, pp. 397–412.

12. Gaudreault, & Lovejoy, Acute poisoning, pp. 78–111.

13. Simon, Poisoning in children, pp. 206–211.

14. R.H. Jackson. Poisoning in childhood. *The Practitioner* 227(1983):1451–1457.

15. D.X. Driggers. Pediatric poisoning—The first 30 minutes. *Postgraduate Medicine* 72, no. 2(1982):53–60.

16. L. Goldfrank, R. Kirstein, & R.S. Weisman. Acute acetaminophen overdose. *Hospital Physician* 11(1980):52–60.

17. C. Cahn. Care of the poisoned child. *Critical Care Quarterly* 3, no. 1(1980):55–61.

BIBLIOGRAPHY

Barkin, R.M., Kulig, K.W., & Rumock, B.H. Poisoning and overdose. In Barkin, R., & Rosen, D. (Eds.), *Emergency Pediatrics.* St. Louis: Mosby, 1984, pp. 266–298.

Cahn, C. Care of the poisoned child. *Critical Care Quarterly* 3, no. 1(1980):55–61.

Deeths, T.M., & Breeden, J.T. Poisoning in children—A statistical study of 1,057 cases. *Journal of Pediatrics* 78, no. 2(1971):299–305.

Driggers, D.X. Pediatric poisoning—The first 30 minutes. *Postgraduate Medicine* 72, no. 2(1982):53–60.

Fought, S., & Throne, A. The pediatric patient. In *Psychosocial Nursing Care of the Emergency Patient.* New York: Wiley, 1984, pp. 51–63.

Gaudreault, P., & Lovejoy, F.H. Acute poisoning. In Dickerman, J.D., & Lucey, J.S. (Eds.), *The Critically Ill Child: Diagnosis and Medical Management.* Philadelphia: W.B. Saunders, 1985, pp. 78–111.

Goldfrank, L., Kirstein, R., & Weisman, R.S. Acute acetaminophen overdose. *Hospital Physician* 11(1980):52–60.

Henretig, F.M., Cupit, G.C., & Temper, A.R. Toxicologic emergencies. In Fleisher, G., & Ludwig, S. (Eds.), *Textbook of Pediatric Emergency Medicine.* Baltimore: Williams & Wilkins, 1984 pp. 489–531.

Jackson, R.H. Poisoning in childhood. *The Practitioner* 227(1983):1451–1457.

Jacobziner, H. Accidental poisoning in children. *Medical Times* 94, no. 2(1966):221–241.

Nelson, R.C., Faw, M.I., Brancato, D.J., Cohen, B.I., & Armstrong, G.D. Poisoning among young children. *Journal of the American Medical Association* 251, no. 3(1981):1660–1664.

Ochs, M. Poisons. In Warner, C.G. (Ed.), *Emergency Care.* St. Louis: Mosby, 1983, pp. 397–412.

Simon, F. Poisoning in children. *American Family Physician* 25, no. 2(1982):206–211.

Turbeville, D.J., & Fearnow, R.G. Is it possible to identify the child who is a high risk candidate for the accidental ingestion of a poison? *Clinical Pediatrics* 15, no. 10(1976):918–920.

EMERGENCY DEPARTMENT CARE GUIDE FOR THE CHILD WHO HAS INGESTED A POISON OR TOXIC SUBSTANCE

Nursing Diagnosis	Interventions	Evaluation
Ineffective airway clearance	Continually assess and support airway Insert oropharyngeal airway in unconscious patient Perform oropharyngeal suctioning as necessary Assist in endotracheal intubation if indicated	Airway remains patent
Ineffective breathing patterns related to depressed central nervous system	Continually assess and support breathing Artificially ventilate patient as needed Monitor arterial blood gas values	Respirations are adequate to provide oxygenation Blood gas values are normal
Potential for injury related to ingestion of toxic substance	Continually assess vital signs Identify the substance ingested through history or laboratory tests Interrupt absorption of toxic substance through gastric lavage and administration of cathartic and activated charcoal Contact poison control center Administer appropriate antidote	Vital signs are stable Ingested substance is identified Poison is removed and absorption is slowed Poison control center provides consultation on patient management
Alteration in comfort related to emergency procedures	Carefully explain all procedures to child Allow parents to remain with child as much as possible	Child remains calm and cooperative Parents provide reassurance to child
Anxiety (parental) related to uncertainty of child's condition and feelings of guilt	Inform parents of all treatment procedures Continually update parents on child's condition Reassure parents that all that is possible is being done for their child Maintain a nonjudgmental approach toward parents Alleviate parent's feelings of guilt	Parents are informed of all treatment procedures Parents understand child's condition Parents do not feel criticized by emergency department staff

(Continued)

Nursing Diagnosis	Interventions	Evaluation
Knowledge deficit related to poison prevention	Teach parents ways to provide a safe environment for their child in the future Encourage practices that decrease chances of accidental poisoning Instruct parents to notify their poison control center when ingestions occur Instruct parents to keep ipecac syrup in home but use only when instructed	Parents provide a safe environment for their child The child does not have exposure to poisonous substances in future Parents keep phone number of poison control center in ready access Parents follow directions of poison control center

10 | Head Trauma and Spinal Cord Injuries

Nancy Sullivan Flint

Approximately 5 million children and infants are evaluated for head trauma each year.[1] There are 200,000 hospital admissions annually, of which 4000 children die.[2,3] Many children die within hours after the injury has occurred.[4] Of the children admitted, it is estimated that nearly 15,000 children require prolonged hospitalization.[5]

The leading causes of head trauma are falls, followed by motor vehicle accidents.[6] Head injuries can be caused by gunshot wounds, stabbings, diving accidents, or blows to the head. Frequently children fall while standing, running, skating, or bicycling. Children may also fall from fences, trees, furniture, or swings. Head injuries may be sustained from falling out of a parent's arms, out of windows, or down a flight of stairs. Child battering or even vigorous shaking of the infant can potentially cause central nervous system damage.[7] The infant or younger child is particularly vulnerable to child abuse. Head injuries that are seen most commonly among adolescents are caused by athletic injuries, penetrating wounds, and motorcycle and automobile accidents.[8]

The head and neck may sustain a significant injury due to head trauma. Before discussing the different types of head injuries, a brief review of the anatomy and physiology of the head and spinal cord will be presented. Figures 10–1, 10–2, and 10–3 depict diagrams of the head, brain, and surrounding structures, which the reader may refer to when reviewing the anatomy of the head and spinal cord with a discussion on the brain and cranial nerve function.

REVIEW OF ANATOMY AND PHYSIOLOGY

The scalp is composed of three layers: the dermal layer, which is well supplied with blood containing connective tissue; the sebaceous glands, and hair follicles; the vascular, fatty, subcutaneous layer; and the galea.

The skull is composed of the cranial vault, commonly referred to as the bony framework of the head. The skull is made up of the eight bones of the cranium. The skeleton of the face is composed of 14 bones. The cranium lodges and provides a protective vault for the brain. In an infant the bones of the skull are separated by sutures, which are membranous tissue spaces. The points of junction where the major sutures intersect in both the anterior and posterior portions of the skull are referred to as fontanelles. There are two major fontanelles, the anterior and the posterior. The anterior is the largest and

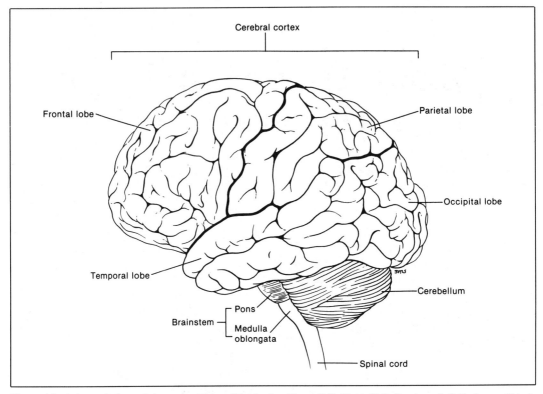

Figure 10-1. Lateral view of the major areas of the brain. *(From S.R. Mott, N.R. Fazekas, & S.R. James (Eds.). Nursing Care of Children and Families. Menlo Park, Calif.: Addison-Wesley, 1985, p. 1518.)*

measures 4 to 6 cm in diameter at birth. The anterior fontanelle normally closes between 4 and 26 months of age (90 percent close between 7 and 19 months of age).[9] The posterior fontanelle is triangular in form and measures 1 to 2 cm at birth. The posterior fontanelle is obliterated within a month or two after birth.[10]

The meninges are membranes that specifically cover the brain and spinal cord to protect it. There are three membranes: the dura mater, the arachnoid mater, and the pia mater. The dura mater is a tough, fibrous membrane forming the outer envelope of the brain. The dura mater adheres to the inside of the skull bones. There are two layers of the dura mater that separate in places to provide space for the venous sinuses. They are called the outer endos-

teal dura and the inner meningeal duras. The space between the bone of the skull and the endosteal dura is called the epidural or extradural space. The middle membrane is termed the arachnoid mater. The arachnoid mater is an avascular, more delicate, fibrous membrane. It is separated from the dura mater by a potential space called the subdural space. The pia mater is the innermost membrane. It is so thin that it is almost transparent. The pia mater is a vascular layer through which blood vessels nourish the cerebrum and spinal cord. The pia mater hugs the brain and spinal tissue and follows every contour of their structure. The space between the arachnoid and the pia mater is called the subarachnoid space. It is a common site for hemorrhage because it contains cerebral

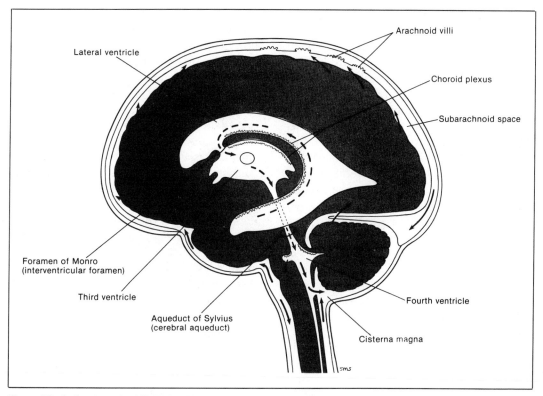

Figure 10-2. Cerebrospinal fluid circulation. *(From S.R. Mott, N.R. Fazekas, & S.R. James (Eds.). Nursing Care of Children and Families. Menlo Park, Calif.: Addison-Wesley, 1985, p. 1521.)*

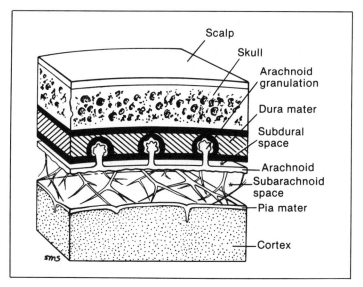

Figure 10-3. Meningeal layers covering the brain surface. *(From S.R. Mott, N.R. Fazekas, & S.R. James (Eds.). Nursing Care of Children and Families. Menlo Park, Calif.: Addison-Wesley, 1985, p. 1517.)*

arteries, veins, arachnoid trabeculae, and cerebrospinal fluid (CSF).

The brain has four ventricles, which are cavities that lie primarily within the cerebrum. There is one lateral ventricle in each cerebral hemisphere, the third ventricle is in the diencephalon, and the fourth ventricle is in the pons of the medulla. The ventricles, the subarachnoid space of the brain, and the spinal cord are filled with CSF. CSF is produced in the ventricles by a specialized secretory structure known as the choroid plexus. The choroid plexus secretes the clear, colorless, and odorless CSF, which serves as a protective shock absorber for the brain and spinal cord.

The cerebrum is the most prominent part of the brain. It is divided by the longitudinal fissure into the left and right hemispheres. The two hemispheres are then further divided into the following lobes: frontal, parietal, temporal, and occipital. The frontal lobe is the largest, occupying part of the lateral, medial, and inferior surfaces. This lobe is responsible for personality and complex intellectual function, and it controls voluntary movement. The parietal lobe occupies part of the lateral and medial surfaces of the hemisphere. It contains a sensory area that receives messages, such as pain, pressure, heat, and cold, as well as position of body parts. The temporal lobe is separated from the frontal lobe by the lateral sulcus. This lobe is responsible for receiving impulses related to hearing, taste, and smell. Wernicke's area, which is the major speech and language center, is contained in the temporal lobe. The occipital lobe is the portion of the brain responsible for interpretation of vision.

The cerebellum lies above the pons and medulla and beneath the posterior portion of the cerebrum. The tentorium separates the cerebellum from the posterior part of the cerebrum. The cerebellum consists of two lateral hemispheres united by a narrow middle portion called the vermis. The main function of the cerebellum is that of a reflex center. The cerebellum maintains coordination in movement, posture, and equilibrium.

The brain stem is the part of the brain that connects the cerebrum and the cerebellum to the spinal cord. The brain stem is a vital relay and reflex center of the central nervous system and contains insertion sites for the cranial nerves. The brain stem consists of the medulla oblongata, the pons, and the midbrain. The medulla oblongata's dorsal surface fits into the fossa between the hemispheres of the cerebellum. It is the center for respiratory, cardiac, vasoconstrictor, sneezing, coughing, swallowing, salivation, and vomiting reflexes. It is therefore considered a vital organ in itself. The medulla contains the point of origin for four cranial nerves: the glossopharyngeal (ninth), vagus (tenth), spinal accessory (eleventh), and hypoglossal (twelfth). The pons is located between the midbrain and the medulla. The lower portion of the pons contains a vital center for respiratory functioning. The nuclei of the trigeminal (fifth), abducens (sixth), facial (seventh), and auditory (eighth) cranial nerves are located in the pons. The midbrain is the short portion of the brain stem and is situated above the pons. The midbrain is involved in visual reflexes and the coordination of visual tracking movements and is the implantation site for the oculomotor (third) and trochlear (fourth) cranial nerves.

The spinal column, also referred to as the vertebral column, is a formation of a series of 33 bones called vertebrae (Fig. 10–4). The vertebrae are classified according to the regions they occupy. There are five regions comprised of 7 cervical vertebrae, 12 thoracic vertebrae, 5 lumbar vertebrae, 5 sacral vertebrae, and 4 coccygeal vertebrae.

The spinal cord is located within the vertebral column in the vertebral canal. It

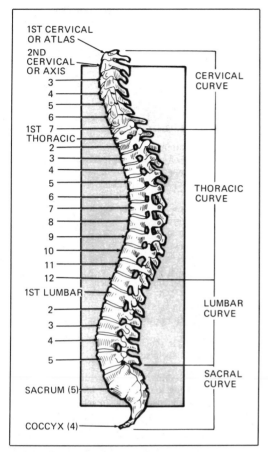

1ST CERVICAL
OR ATLAS
2ND
CERVICAL
OR AXIS
3
4
5
6
1ST 7
THORACIC
2
3
4
5
6
7
8
9
10
11
12
1ST LUMBAR
2
3
4
5
SACRUM (5)
COCCYX (4)

CERVICAL
CURVE

THORACIC
CURVE

LUMBAR
CURVE

SACRAL
CURVE

Figure 10–4. Lateral view of the vertebral column. *(From E.B. Rudy, & V.R. Gray. Handbook of Health Assessment (2nd ed.). Norwalk, Conn.: Appleton-Century-Crofts, 1986, p. 142.)*

extends from the medulla oblongata down through the vertebral canal to the level of the second lumbar vertebra in adults and to the sacral region in infants. There are 31 nerves of the spinal cord, which are divided into five segments: 8 cervical, 12 thoracic, 5 lumbar, 5 sacral, and 1 coccygeal. These 31 nerves of the spinal cord do not match anatomically by number the 33 associated vertebrae, since the vertebral column grows faster and becomes longer than the spinal cord. The 31 spinal nerves exit from successive levels from the spinal column at the numerically corresponding vertebrae.

The spinal cord is submerged in CSF and is protected by the three layers of membrane called meninges: dura mater, arachnoid, and pia mater. The spinal cord is composed of white matter and gray matter. The white matter, or myelinated nerve fibers, is the outside layer of the spinal cord. Its purpose is to serve as a conducting pathway for impulses connecting the spinal cord and the brain. The gray matter, or unmyelinated neuronal tissue, contains the cell bodies for spinal nerves. It can be found in the internal core of the spinal cord and is considered the integrative area for the cord reflexes.

The 31 spinal nerves contain two roots, a posterior and an anterior root. The posterior root is also known as the sensory root because the fibers of the spinal nerve root transmit impulses to the cord. Conversely, the anterior root is called the motor root because the fibers of the spinal nerve root dispatch impulses from the spinal cord to muscles and various structures.

TYPES OF HEAD INJURIES

Types of Skull Fractures

Fractures are categorized into two broad classifications: open or closed. In an open (or compound) fracture there is communication between the inside of the skull and the outside. Either blunt or penetrating trauma can be a cause of an open skull fracture. In a closed (or simple) fracture there is no communication between the external environment and the cranial cavity.

The six types of skull fractures that may result from head trauma during childhood are linear, depressed, compound, basal, diastatic, and "growing." Skull fractures are commonly caused by a significant force delivered to the head. This siz-

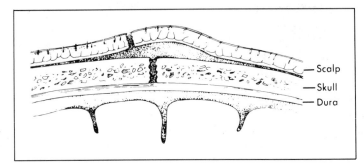

Figure 10-5. Simple skull fracture. *(From J. Barber, L. Stokes, & D. Billings. Adult and Child Care (2nd ed.). St. Louis, Mosby, 1977.)*

able force may cause both the fracture and injury to the brain.

Linear Skull Fracture. Approximately 75 percent of all skull fractures seen in pediatric patients are linear skull fractures.[11] This type of skull fracture often is identified as a lucent line on the skull x-ray. It resembles a single crack in the skull and is frequently called a simple fracture (Fig. 10-5).

Linear fractures heal in 3 to 4 months and require no special treatment. Management of a linear skull fracture is directed toward that of the underlying brain injury. The location of the linear skull fracture provides invaluable clues as to the possibility of any complications. Fractures that cross the vascular arterial grooves (undersurface of the skull) may tear an artery and can potentially lead to a severe hemorrhage.

Depressed Skull Fracture. A depressed skull fracture (Fig. 10-6) occurs when there is a disruption of the integrity of the bone, which is usually broken into many fragments. A depressed skull fracture may be associated with bone fragments penetrating into the substance of the brain, thus causing pressure on the brain.

In young infants or newborns the skull bones are immature and somewhat flexible. If there is a sufficient amount of force, of if delivery is difficult, the malleable bone may become indented, or a "ping pong ball" depression without a laceration may be seen. A depressed skull fracture is usually palpable and may be diagnosed with x-rays. The brain tissue underneath the fracture can sustain a contusion or laceration. Elevation of the skull fracture is indicated if the depression exceeds 5 mm in depth or if fragments are below the in-

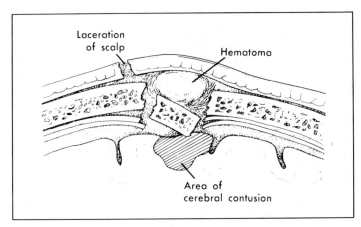

Figure 10-6. Depressed skull fracture. *(From J. Barber, L. Stokes, & D. Billings. Adult and Child Care (2nd ed.). St. Louis: Mosby, 1977.)*

ner table of the skull. Surgical intervention may be essential within 24 hours after the injury. Management is directed toward exploring and removing the debris.

Compound Skull Fracture. Compound or open skull fractures have a direct communication between the scalp laceration and the cerebral substance. The integrity of the skin is broken down to the site of the fracture. It indicates that a scalp laceration and a depressed skull fracture exist. This type of fracture requires early operative intervention with surgical debridement and elevation of the depressed bone. Antibiotic and tetanus prophylaxis are indicated with a compound skull fracture.

Diastatic Skull Fracture. A traumatic separation of the cranial bones at one or more sites caused by blunt trauma with sizable force may result in a diastatic skull fracture. This type of skull fracture generally affects the lambdoid suture. It is usually seen in children under the age of 4. A diastatic skull fracture is relatively uncommon and requires no specific therapy. Close observation for the development of arterial or venous epidural hemorrhage is recommended.

Growing Skull Fracture. "Growing" skull fractures are generally seen in children under the age of 3. A "growing" fracture occurs when a cyst develops at the site of a linear or diastatic skull fracture, thus preventing fusion of the cranial bones. The cyst usually develops within 6 months after the head injury occurred and quite often affects the parietal bone. Treatment of the "growing" skull fracture includes surgically removing the cyst and repairing the underlying dural tear. A cranioplasty must also be performed.

Basal Skull Fracture. A basal skull fracture is not often visualized on skull x-rays be-

cause the fracture involves the base of the skull, particularly the anterior and middle fossae. Basal skull fractures may involve a crack or fracture in the basal portions of frontal, ethmoid, sphenoid, temporal, or occipital bones. The diagnosis of a basal skull fracture is based upon the characteristics of the physical findings. These coexisting signs may include drainage of CSF and blood from both the nose (rhinorrhea) and ear (otorrhea). This is an extremely serious problem because it creates a potential avenue for a meningeal infection to occur. Meningitis can possibly result from pathogens such as *Staphylococcus pneumoniae* and *Hemophilus influenzae*, type B, which may gain access through the dural tear by entering through the nose or ear.[12]

It may be difficult to detect CSF when it is mixed with blood. When blood is encircled by a yellowish stain, it is called the halo sign. This should be compared to a drop of blood. The yellowish, or halo, sign should resemble blood components in the center, and one or more clear rings of clear fluid will develop around the center. If this occurs it is highly indicative of blood encircled by CSF.

Another common physical finding suggesting a basal skull fracture is hemorrhage into the nose, nasopharynx, or middle ear. Ecchymosis, or bruising, in the mastoid region (Battle's sign) also indicates the presence of a basal skull fracture. Other signs are bleeding behind the tympanic membrane (hemotympanum) and periorbital hematomas, known as "racoon eyes." Other characteristics indicating a basal skull fracture include injuries to various cranial nerves. Some of the signs and symptoms of cranial nerve damage that may be found during the initial assessment or that can develop later include:

- A loss of vision (blurry vision or blindness)—cranial nerve II
- A loss of hearing and difficulty with bal-

ance (auditory nerve damage)—cranial nerve VIII

- A loss of eye movements, a squint, or fixed dilated pupil (oculomotor nerve damage)—cranial nerve III
- A loss of sense of smell (olfactory nerve damage)—cranial nerve I
- A partial facial paresis or paralysis (facial nerve damage)—cranial nerve VII

The clinical indicators of a basal skull fracture are summarized in Table 10–1.

Treatment of a patient with a basal skull fracture includes strict bed rest (with the bed flat), which is done to decrease intracranial pressure and the amount of CSF draining from the dural tear. It is possible for the dural tear to close spontaneously while the child is on strict bedrest. The patient should be frequently observed, and neurologic signs should be carefully assessed. If a CSF leak is suspected, then the patient should be placed on a course of prophylactic antibiotics to prevent infection. If the CSF continues to leak, then a craniotomy must be performed to repair the dural tear.

A basal skull fracture is a serious head injury because of the close proximity of the fracture line to the structures surrounding the brain stem. The patient must be carefully watched and consistently evaluated for signs of increased intracranial pressure, which can possibly lead to respiratory and cardiac arrest.

TABLE 10–1. CLINICAL INDICATORS OF A BASAL SKULL FRACTURE

Leakage of CSF
Hemorrhage into the nose, nasopharynx, or middle ear
Battle's sign
Hemotympanum
Periorbital hematomas
Cranial nerve palsies

Cerebral Contusion and Laceration

A cerebral contusion is a bruising of part of the brain associated with damage to the brain substance itself. In addition to a portion of the brain being bruised, there can be multiple areas of petechial and punctate hemorrhages present. A cerebral laceration occurs when there is a tearing of the cortical surface of the brain tissue.

A cerebral contusion and laceration generally result from severe blunt trauma to the head. A sizable blow to the head causes massive movement of the intracranial contents, which may produce a cerebral contusion or cerebral laceration. A coup injury or bruising will occur directly beneath the site of impact.[13] In contrast, contrecoup injuries occur in the regions of the brain opposite the site of impact.[14] Contrecoup injuries are the direct result of the massive movement of the brain contents at the time of the initial injury. A cerebral laceration is caused by a penetrating wound (such as a gunshot) resulting from depressed skull fragments or debris. On the initial evaluation a contusion is frequently clinically indistinguishable from a cerebral laceration. A cerebral contusion or a laceration, however, is identifiable and can be seen on a computed tomographic (CT) scan.

During the initial evaluation in the emergency department, only alert patients may be diagnosed as having a cerebral contusion. The diagnosis of cerebral contusion or cerebral laceration cannot be made in a semicomatose or comatose patient because the results of the neurologic examination will not be accurate. The child must be able to cooperate with the examiner for proper testing of cerebral function.[15]

The result of a patient receiving a cerebral contusion is lack of nerve function to the part of the brain that is bruised. A patient with a cerebral contusion or cerebral laceration with hematoma formation and possible punctate hemorrhage may possess a variety of neurologic signs and symptoms.

An alert patient with a frontal or temporal lobe contusion may be aphasic (loss of the faculty of transmission of ideas) or confused, agitated, and uncooperative. A patient who displays a slight paralysis affecting one side only may be showing the effects of a frontal contusion. This may vary from slight hemiparesis to a history of unconsciousness and paralysis. Other neurologic signs and symptoms include disturbances in strength, sensation, visual awareness, or even focal seizures.

The areas of brain that are the major sites for a cerebral contusion or laceration to occur are the occipital, frontal, and temporal lobes; the orbital surfaces of the frontal lobes; the anterior temporal lobes; and the frontal temporal junctions. The anterior and middle fossae at the base of the skull possess irregular surfaces. When the brain is forcefully impacted upon these surfaces, it is capable of sustaining bruises or lacerations.

The initial medical management is directed toward obtaining an accurate diagnosis. Frequent assessment of the neurologic status is essential for successful management of a patient suspected of having a cerebral contusion or laceration. Depending upon the severity of the injury, steroids may be used to decrease brain swelling. If a cerebral laceration is present, surgical intervention, including exploration, debridement, and closure of the dura, may be necessary to prevent herniation of the edematous brain and leakage of CSF.

Concussion

A cerebral concussion is the most common type of head injury. A concussion is caused by a violent shaking or jarring of the brain resulting from a blow to the head. A cerebral concussion implies no significant or structural damage to the brain. It typically occurs most frequently with blunt, nonpenetrating, minor trauma to the head.

The pathogenesis of the symptoms of concussion are still unclear. It may, however, be the result of acceleration-deceleration force on the brain and the shearing forces causing stretching, compression, and tearing of nerve fibers. The shearing stress occurs on the reticular formation, which is the area responsible for consciousness.[16,17]

A cerebral concussion is characterized by a transient period of unconsciousness, including a temporary loss of awareness and responsiveness. This period of unconsciousness can persist for a relatively short period, lasting less than 5 minutes to hours. After the transient loss of consciousness, the patient may be confused or may lose memory. This type of amnesia can include loss of memory from the moment the injury was sustained and for a variable period before the injury. The two components of posttraumatic amnesia are retrograde amnesia and anterograde amnesia. Retrograde amnesia occurs when there is loss of memory of events that happened several years prior to the head injury. This type of anmesia will lessen with time, possibly within a few hours after the head injury was sustained, and eventually will disappear. Anterograde amnesia is the period of memory loss after the head injury. The patient will be unable to acquire or retain information anywhere from minutes to hours after the occurrence of the head injury. The patient with anterograde amnesia will typically resolve spontaneously within 24 hours.[18,19]

Other clinical manifestations may include a depression or suppression of reflexes, a temporary cessation of respirations (lasting a few seconds), a brief period of bradycardia, and hypotension. After the instantaneous loss of awareness, the patient will open his or her eyes but will not be oriented. The patient's reflexes will return as the patient becomes oriented, and he or she will follow simple commands. The clinical manifestations accompanying a patient who has temporary neurogenic dysfunction may persist, in some instances, for minutes to hours. A majority of the symptoms will disappear spontaneously within a few hours. Depending upon the severity of the head injury, consciousness may be regained slowly through the successive stages.[20]

The pediatric patient with a documented loss of consciousness should be admitted to the hospital for 24 hours of observation. The length of amnesia must also be evaluated. The child may continue to have persistent vomiting, or seizures may occur.

Cephalhematoma

A cephalhematoma occurs when blood vessels rupture and produce bleeding into the area between the surface of a cranial bone and the periosteum membrane. Cephalhematomas occur frequently in vertex deliveries.[21] During the labor and delivery process the pressure of the fetal head against the bony prominences of the pelvis causes the blood vessels to rupture, resulting in a cephalhematoma. Upon palpation the boundaries of the cephalhematoma are well defined, do not extend beyond the bone, and do not cross over suture lines. The edematous scalp may become apparent at birth or may develop in the next 2 days. The swelling may be minimal at birth, since the subperiosteal bleeding is a slow process. The cephalhematoma may occur in the parietal region; however, the occipital and frontal bones are seldomly affected.

Most cephalhematomas are absorbed and disappear within 2 weeks to 3 months without special treatment. The nursing care is directed toward observing the infant and explaining to the parents the etiology and treatment of a cephalhematoma.

Caput Succedaneum

Caput succedaneum is a diffuse swelling of the soft tissue of the scalp. This edematous area of the scalp is evident at birth. It involves the portion of the scalp that presented during delivery and that was encircled by the cervix. Caput succedaneum is usually the result of a long and hard labor. The portion of the scalp encircled by the cervix results in compression of local vessels, and therefore venous return is slowed, causing an increase in fluids and a swelling of the scalp. The fluid is accumulated above the bone, and it is not sharply demarcated. The swelling may be palpated in a small area, or it may extend beyond the bone margins. Pressure on the affected area will cause pitting of the edema. Caput succedaneum may contain a general or localized ecchymotic discoloration as well as petechiae.[22]

Swelling generally subsides within a few days after the birth and requires no special treatment. The nurse should discuss the etiology of caput succedaneum with the parents, however, and offer some reassurance.

Scalp Injuries and Lacerations

Trauma to the head should not be treated lightly, for even an insignificant blow to the head may result in severe cerebral damage. When a child sustains a scalp injury, the velocity of the force and the characteristics of the impact are important factors in determining the severity of the injury. The impact to the head may or may not result in compression, tension, and tearing of the scalp.

A scalp injury may occur when there is any damage to the surface of the scalp such as a contusion, abrasion, or puncture wound. A scalp laceration may result from a traumatic loss of continuity of the dermis (a tearing of the scalp).

The mechanism of injury as well as length of time since the injury occurred must be identified. Lacerations more than 12 hours old are often not sutured because of the high incidence of infection. The nurse should assess the scalp wound, determining the location, size and depth, degree of contamination, other structures involved, signs of skull fracture, and the amount of tissue loss. The wound should also be inspected for any CSF leaks.[23]

The wound should be irrigated with copious amounts of saline. Scalp wounds should be explored, specifically assessing for a fracture or foreign body. The presence of bone chips indicates the need for the wound to be explored or surgically repaired. Bone chips should never be removed in the emergency department. Any debris, including hair, must be removed. All hair around the laceration should be shaved to decrease the risk of infection. Scalp lacerations should then be sutured using sterile technique.

Abrasions are associated with the loss of epidermis and frequently a partial loss of dermis. The wound should be irrigated with copious amounts of saline. It should be cleansed thoroughly and any foreign material removed with forceps.

A contusion is caused by blunt trauma to the skin without penetrating the tissues. The area should be cleansed and an ice pack applied to reduce the pain and swelling.

A puncture wound results from a penetrating object. The area should be debrided, carefully cleansed, and irrigated with copious amounts of saline. A fracture or foreign body should be ruled out.

The nurse should apply sterile dressing over the wound to prevent infection and to promote optimal healing. When the patient has sustained a laceration, abrasion, or puncture wound, tetanus prophylaxis is recommended. The nurse should instruct the patient and family on wound healing, tissue swelling, dressing changes, suture removal, medications (if applicable), signs and symptoms of infection, and expected reaction to tetanus toxoid.[24]

Acute Epidural Hematoma

An epidural hematoma, also known as an extradural hematoma, refers to bleeding that occurs between the skull and the dura mater. Epidural bleeding is commonly caused by a lacerating or rupturing of the middle meningeal artery.[25] It can also be caused by a tear in the dural veins or the dural sinuses, resulting in a hemorrhage. An acute epidural hematoma most frequently occurs in the parietotemporal region from a laceration of the artery caused by a skull fracture in the squamous portion of the temporal bone.[26]

Approximately 25 percent of all epidural hematomas seen in the pediatric population have no associated skull fractures.[27] Acute epidural hematomas are seen more frequently in the pediatric age group than in adults because the dura is not firmly attached to the bone table. Acute epidural hematomas occur in 1 to 2 percent of all head trauma patients.[28]

The hemorrhage is often associated with an arterial bleed; therefore the signs and symptoms of an epidural hematoma are acute. The classical description of a patient who has sustained an acute epidural hematoma begins with a period of momentary unconsciousness immediately following the head injury. The patient then awakens and is in a phase in which he or she is lucid before lapsing into a coma. This intervening lucid interval can last for a few hours to 1 to 2 days. If venous bleeding occurs, this phase can last for 2 days to a week. In the pediatric population the dominant signs and symptoms of an acute epidural hematoma are similar to the characteristics of increased intracranial pressure. The various signs and symptoms indicating an acute epidural hematoma may include vomiting; lethargy; separation of the cranial sutures; fullness of the anterior fontanelle; headache; papilledema; paresis of the third and sixth cranial nerves; slow, labored, shallow and irregular respirations; and increased systolic blood pressure with a decrease in patient's bounding pulse.[29]

Focal signs will frequently appear first, consisting of a dilated pupil and a ptosis of the eyelid on the same side caused by a compression of the oculomotor nerve (third cranial nerve). Contralateral hemiparesis, brisk or hyperactive reflexes, and a positive Babinski's sign may be present, resulting from cerebral peduncle compression on the herniation side. As the hematoma increases in size, the brain is forced toward the opposite side, thus causing severe increased intracranial pressure. These late signs include decerebrate rigidity and severe changes in the vital signs. Decerebrate posture consists of clenched jaws and extended neck and adducted arms extended at the elbows, with the forearms pronated and wrists and fingers flexed.[30] A complication that can potentially develop is temporal lobe herniation with paralysis of the oculomotor cranial nerve, hemiparesis, and hemianopsis. The patient may continue to rapidly deteriorate, and seizures may occur.

The diagnosis of an acute epidural hematoma is made by a careful history, clinical signs and symptoms, skull x-ray, CT scan, and arteriograms, which will localize the lesion. Treatment is directed to surgical intervention by emergency burr holes or twist drills into the skull to evacuate the hematoma and to ligate the bleeding vessel. Surgical intervention must be prompt to prevent serious compression of the brain tissue. In addition, osmotic diuretics may be given to lower the intra-cranial pressure. If the diagnosis and treatment are delayed, secondary brain injury will occur rapidly, and death may result.

Subdural Hematoma

An epidural hematoma is generally caused by an arterial bleed. Conversely, a subdural hematoma is more frequently caused by a rupture of the veins in the subdural space. The hemorrhage is therefore much slower in comparison to an epidural hematoma. A subdural hematoma consists of a collection of blood possibly mixed with blood pigments and protein between the dura mater (outer meninges) and the arachnoid layer of the meninges in the subdural space (Fig. 10–7). The subdural bleed may be caused by a rupture of laceration of the small vessels of the bridging veins or branches of the cerebral arteries. The subdural hematoma may also be the result of bleeding from a cerebral contusion or may be caused by a tear in the brain. Head trauma related to the birth process, resulting in a subdural hematoma, is a fairly common occurrence in newborns.[31]

Subdural hematomas are divided into three categories distinguished by the time interval between the head injury and the onset of signs and symptoms of the lesion. The classifications of subdural hematomas are: (1) acute, (2) subacute, and (3) chronic.

The approximate time frame in which the onset of symptoms commences is: (1) acute: within 24 hours of injury; (2) subacute: from 2 days to 2 weeks; and (3) chronic: greater than 2 weeks to months.

Acute Subdural Hematoma. Acute subdural hematomas are generally found in children less than 2 years of age, with a peak frequency at approximately 6 months of age.[32] It is common in about 75 percent of pediatric cases to find bilateral acute subdural hematomas.[33] Acute epidural

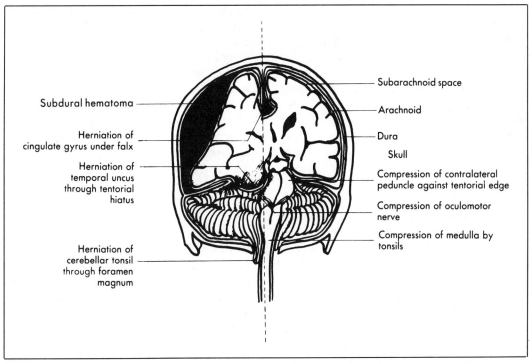

Figure 10-7. Mechanism of injury in subdural hematoma. *(From S.A. Budassi. Journal of Emergency Nursing, May, 1979, p. 45.)*

hematomas are usually unilateral.[34] Seizures may occur in 75 percent of the pediatric age group with an acute subdural hematoma.[35]

An acute subdural hematoma is often attributed to a severe head injury and is generally associated with a cerebral contusion and lacerations. The clinical manifestations seen in children with a subdural hematoma vary greatly depending upon the amount of damage sustained and the age of the child.

Significant neurologic signs and symptoms will occur within the first 24 to 48 hours postinjury. Acute subdural hematomas are caused by bleeding from a lacerated brain consistent with a tear in the arachnoid, thus allowing both blood and CSF to collect in the subdural space.

The onset of signs and symptoms of an acute subdural hematoma are slower due to the fact that subdural hematomas are commonly caused by venous rather than arterial bleeds. The characteristics of an acute subdural hematoma are considerably the same as those evident with an acute epidural hematoma. The symptoms of increasing intracranial pressure may occur. The most frequent signs are complaints of a headache, bulging fontanelles (in infants), retinal hemorrhage, confusion, drowsiness, slow cerebration, and, commonly, agitation, vomiting, seizures, and fever. If the bleeding is extensive it can possibly lower the hematocrit of an infant. All of the symptoms previously mentioned gradually worsen, and focal signs commence.[36]

The ipsilateral pupil becomes fixed and dilated. The patient should be closely monitored for subtle and progressive changes in the signs and symptoms. The child's level of consciousness, hemiparesis, pupillary dilatation, and extraocular eye movements (EOMs) should be carefully monitored and documented for any gradual changes. The child's death is inevitable following the progression of hemorrhage, compression, edema, and herniation if emergency surgical intervention is not performed to evacuate the hematoma.

Subacute Subdural Hematoma. A subacute subdural hematoma often develops after a patient has been discharged from the hospital. The patient generally becomes symptomatic within 2 to 10 days after the head injury has occurred. A significant neurologic deficit is detected during this time. The classic history obtained from a patient with a subacute subdural hematoma begins with a gradual improvement after the initial head injury. The patient then begins to develop a decreasing level of consciousness and finally becomes difficult to arouse. The patient will not respond to verbal or painful stimuli at this time. The patient with a subacute subdural hematoma may be found to be drowsy and inattentive and to demonstrate personality changes. The increase in intracranial pressure and the shift of intracranial contents related to the accumulation of blood will eventually lead to herniation of the uncus. In turn, focal or lateralizing signs will appear, such as hemiparesis and pupillary signs.[37]

Chronic Subdural Hematoma. A chronic subdural hematoma may develop from minor head trauma. A patient who has sustained a chronic subdural hematoma may be unaware of or may have even forgotten the incident. A chronic subdural hematoma may occur weeks, months, and possibly years after the head injury.

Slow bleeding occurs into the sub-dural space from trauma resulting in a rupture of one of the veins. The blood becomes organized as a clot and is then surrounded by a fibrous membrane easily separated from the arachnoid and dura mater. The hematoma slowly increases in size due to repeated small hemorrhages. The hematoma finally becomes so enlarged that compression of the brain tissue results.[38]

The most common signs and symptoms manifested from a chronic subdural hematoma are a headache (which increases in severity), disturbances in consciousness, slow cerebration, drowsiness, confusion, personality changes, possibly seizures, and hemiparesis. The ipsilateral pupil will be dilated and sluggish to light. Papilledema may also be the symptom of a chronic subdural hematoma. The child with a chronic subdural hematoma may develop a variety of symptoms that fluctuate daily. This can be related to gradual spatial compensation and decompensation of neural and vascular structures surrounding the tentorial notch.[39]

Diagnosis and treatment of subdural hematomas are similar to that of epidural hematomas. A diagnosis can be made by obtaining a careful history along with a CT scan, carotid arteriogram, and echoencephalogram. The purpose of an echoencephalogram is to indicate a shift of midline structure. It does not, however, discriminate the type of lesion responsible.

It is vitally important to mention that bilateral subdural hematomas are frequently present. Diagnostic measures therefore should be used to detect and rule out this possibility.

Surgical evacuation and prompt removal of the hematoma is the treatment of choice. Without evacuation of the clot, death will result secondary to increased intracranial pressure and tentorial herniation. A craniotomy may be indicated for treatment of subacute and all chronic subdural hematomas because of the inaccessible gelatinous hematoma through a burr hole.

Subarachnoid Hemorrhage

Severe head trauma may result in a subarachnoid hemorrhage or hematoma. A head injury may cause damage to the vasculature of the brain, resulting in bleeding into the epidural space, subdural space, subarachnoid space, or beneath the pia mater into the brain itself. A rupture of the cerebral artery supplying the base of the brain causes bleeding between the pia mater and arachnoid membrane (subarachnoid space), resulting in a subarachnoid hemorrhage.

Severe head trauma, ruptured aneurysm of the cerebral artery, hemorrhage into brain tumors, and bleeding from arteriovenous malformations are the causes of a subarachnoid hemorrhage. The most common type of intracranial hemorrhage following severe head trauma is a subarachnoid bleed. The most frequent cause in fatal cases is a massive subarachnoid hemorrhage.[40]

The signs and symptoms of a subarachnoid hemorrhage may vary depending upon the significance of the head trauma, size and extent of the bleeding, areas involved in the bleeding, and the presence and degree of vasospasm. Nuchal rigidity, headache, deteriorating level of consciousness, mental dysfunction, such as restlessness or irritability, nausea and vomiting, hemiparesis and focal neurologic signs are most commonly found with a subarachnoid hemorrhage. The focal neurologic signs include sensory disturbances, diplopia, ipsilateral dilated pupil, and seizures. This type of hemorrhage may result in meningeal irritation from blood in the spinal fluid.[41]

The immediate treatment of a subarachnoid hemorrhage depends upon the cause. The fear of brain stem herniation from increased intracranial pressure contraindicates a lumbar puncture. Surgical intervention may be used in an emergency situation.

Increased Intracranial Pressure

Another complication of head trauma is an increase in intracranial pressure (ICP). The major causes of increased ICP in head trauma are cerebral edema and expanding lesions such as hematomas. Increased ICP is attributed to the swelling or pressure exerted by the constituents of the brain. The contents of the brain include the brain tissue, CSF, and intravascular blood. These constituents are contained within the rigid skull, which cannot expand. To understand the pathophysiology related to increased intracranial pressure, one should be familiar with the Monro-Kellie hypothesis. This hypothesis, simply stated, contends that the skull is a rigid compartment filled to capacity with brain matter, intravascular blood, and CSF. The contents of the skull are basically noncompressible, and the volume remains nearly constant. If there is an alteration in any one of the three intracranial components, the change in the cranial volume will lead to pressure changes. If one of the constituents increases in volume, another component must decrease, or the result will be a rise in the intracranial pressure. This hypothesis does not apply to an infant, however, because an infant's skull is not rigid.[42]

ICP ranges between 40 to 200 mm H_2O or 4 to 15 mm Hg. Pressures elevated above 200 mg H_2O or 20 mm Hg are considered abnormal and frequently signify increasing ICP. To ensure adequate blood supply to the brain if increased ICP exists, compensatory mechanisms are triggered by the body. Cushing's reflex (increased blood pressure, decreased pulse, and respiratory changes) is involved when there is increased intracranial pressure. This reflex helps to decrease the amount of blood in the cranial vault without decreasing adequate perfusion of the brain tissue.[43,44]

A continuous intracranial monitoring device is the most suitable instrument for obtaining reliable data for evaluation on increased intracranial pressure. Continuous assessment of the patient's vital signs and neurologic signs, however, may reveal significant signs and symptoms of increased intracranial pressure. The "classical" signs and symptoms that may indicate increased intracranial pressure include (1) rising systolic blood pressure, (2) widening of the pulse pressure, and (3) bradycardia.

Other signs and symptoms are headache, vomiting, deterioration in the level of consciousness, papilledema, dilated or constricted pupils, sluggish to nonreactive response to light in one or both pupils, alteration in the characteristics of the respiratory pattern, change in motor function progressing from hemiparesis to hemiplegia, blurred vision, and less responsiveness to light and deep touch, pain, temperature, and proprioception. In addition to altered vital signs, children and infants may demonstrate palsies of cranial nerves VI and VIII and an altered mental status. Other signs and symptoms found in infants are a full fontanelle or separated sutures.[45,46] Table 10-2 summarizes the clinical indicators of increased ICP.

TABLE 10-2. CLINICAL INDICATORS OF INCREASED INTRACRANIAL PRESSURE

Increased blood pressure
Widening pulse pressure
Bradycardia
Headache
Vomiting
Decreasing level of consciousness
Papilledema
Pupillary changes
Changing respiratory pattern
Loss of motor and sensory functions
Cranial nerve palsies

The signs and symptoms discussed above are not entirely reliable indications of increased ICP. These signs and symptoms do occur when there is cerebral edema or an expanding lesion relating to brain stem dysfunction.

The treatment of increased intracranial pressure will be discussed in the section on emergency management of head trauma and spinal cord injuries.

SPINAL CORD INJURY

Spinal cord injuries (SCI) do not occur as frequently in children as in adults. The highest incidence of spinal cord injuries is in young adults, with the most vulnerable age group being between 12 and 15 years.[47,48] Leading rehabilitation centers have reported two to four new cases per year of spinal cord injuries in children.[49]

Cervical injuries in children tend to occur high in the cervical spine between C-3 through C-5, whereas, over 80 percent of the cervical injuries in adults occur below C-5. This difference can be related to the fact that a child's head size is disproportionately large for his or her body size. The child's center of gravity is therefore closer to the brain.[50]

In children and young adults spinal cord injuries occur most commonly as a result of automobile accidents. In infants congenital defects (e.g., a myelomeningocele) are the most common causes of spinal cord damage. Spinal cord injuries may also occur during sporting events such as diving or skiing or even with accidental falls. In addition spinal cord damage may be the sequela of traumatic injuries resulting from child abuse or gunshot or stab wounds.[51]

The mechanisms of spinal cord injuries include flexion, extension, and rotation (individually or in combination). Subluxation or dislocation, compression fractures or other simple fractures without displacement, fracture dislocations, and compound fractures may affect only the vertebral column.

The most common mechanism of spinal cord injury in children involved in car accidents is a sudden hyperflexion or hyperextension of the neck that may be combined with rotation. The head is bent forward in a hyperflexion injury. The spinal cord is angulated acutely in a hyperextension injury when the head is bent backward suddenly. Direct trauma to the forehead or a whiplash injury also causes an unexpected hyperflexion of the neck. When a hypoflexion-hyperextension injury is sustained, it is often combined with a rotational force, causing a rotation of the neck and thus producing a more complex injury. There may be a compression of one side of the body more than the other if rotation accompanies flexion. Vertebral compression of the spine may be the result of blows to the occiput or buttocks, which occur in athletic activities such as diving or skiing.[52]

Compression of the spinal cord and its roots may produce edema. The treatment of spinal cord injuries will also be discussed in the section on emergency management of head trauma and spinal cord injuries.

Spinal Shock

Spinal shock syndrome is caused by the immediate loss of autonomic and reflex activity in addition to loss of voluntary activity and sensation below the level of the cord lesion. This may be the result of either an acute physiologic or anatomic transection of the spinal cord. Spinal shock is consistent with sympathetic collapse, paralysis, anesthesia, areflexia, and the loss of sphincter function below the level of the damage.[53]

Most children who have sustained a spinal cord injury will experience spinal shock. The signs and symptoms of spinal shock vary depending upon the severity and the location of the injury. One of the results of spinal shock is vasodilation, which produces immediate and severe hypotension. The child will not be able to conserve heat through vasoconstriction; therefore high (hyperthermia) or low (hypothermia) body temperatures may develop. Other signs and symptoms suggestive of spinal shock include absence of reflexes at or below the level of the cord lesion, loss of bladder and bowel control, and loss of sensory and motor function in the body parts innervated by the affected spinal nerves below the injury.

The period of spinal shock may last for many months. This period varies and depends upon the individual. Relatively soon after the spinal cord injury was sustained the symptoms will appear and may last from 1 to 6 weeks. The neurologic deficits one may see following compression may resolve slowly or can possibly be permanent. If there is a sufficient amount of force available to compress the cord, then the result is total disruption of the cord. All functions below the segment of the compressed spinal cord are destroyed.[54]

A concussion of the spinal cord and its roots may result in transient neurologic symptoms. These neurologic symptoms usually resolve within hours. A contusion or bruising of the spinal cord may result in changes within the tissues, producing a surface hemorrhage, vascular damage, and edema.

Occasionally the spinal cord itself may become either partially or completely transected. If a partial or incomplete transection occurs, loss of sensory and motor function will be present below the level of the spinal cord lesion at varying degrees. When the spinal cord is completely severed, it results in loss of all voluntary movements and sensation below the level of the lesion. A complete transection of the spinal cord produces immediate deficits that are permanent and irreversible.[55]

Patients who have sustained severe multiple trauma or head trauma must be thoroughly assessed for the presence of a spinal cord injury or spinal fracture. Assessment for spinal damage includes a careful neurologic examination. If a spinal fracture exists, the patient may complain of local pain that radiates into the arm, thorax, abdomen, or legs. If these symptoms are present, the patient should not be moved until a complete medical examination is performed and the appropriate x-rays are completed. The anatomic and reflex activity may then return in approximately 3 weeks. The reappearance of any reflex activity that was previously lost due to the cord lesion is indicative of a sign of recovery. Relatedly, if the period of spinal shock is short, then additional voluntary activity and sensation may be expected.[56]

MANAGEMENT

Initial treatment given to a child with a severe head injury or suspected spinal cord injury in the emergency department should be rendered in an organized and systematic manner. The initial management during the first stage consists of supportive efforts directed toward (1) preventing further neurologic damage, (2) monitoring vital signs, and (3) preventing any complications. The priorities in the nursing management of children with head trauma or spinal cord injuries are summarized in Table 10-3.

History. It is imperative that either the emergency nurse or physician obtain an accurate history of events. The information should be elicited from the child, if possible, and then from observers, such as friends, parents, or emergency medical technicians (EMTs). The EMTs should in-

TABLE 10-3. PRIORITIES IN THE NURSING MANAGEMENT OF PEDIATRIC HEAD TRAUMA AND SPINAL CORD INJURIES

Airway, breathing, and circulation—ABCs
Immobilization of the head, neck, and spinal column
Monitoring of vital signs every 5 to 15 minutes
Initiation of intravenous therapy at one-half to two-thirds normal maintenance; necessary blood samples obtained
Nasogastric tube placement (if indicated)
Insertion of Foley catheter (if indicated)
Ongoing neurologic assessment

quire about and document on the patient's prehospital record specific observations of the patient's condition immediately after the accident. The EMTs or observers should provide hospital personnel with details of the incident, particularly noting the child's level of consciousness; orientation to person, place, and time; any visual disturbances; vomiting; headache; and memory loss. The EMTs or other observers should also note any changes in vital signs. It is crucial to have accurate data available regarding the incident. The importance of the initial assessment and examination lies in the continual reassessment of the child, which will enable the health care providers to detect and evaluate any subtle changes.

Whenever possible the parents or guardians should provide the nurse or physician with a detailed history, including the past medical history as well as the present. The history should include information regarding drug allergy, significant medical problems such as diabetes mellitus, seizure disorder, and a history of any medications the child is taking.[57]

Assessment

Airway. The first priority in the treatment of head trauma or spinal cord injury is to establish that the airway is patent and that the child's ventilations are adequate (airway, breathing, and circulation: ABCs).

All pediatric patients with a head injury must be simultaneously evaluated for the presence of a spinal cord injury. Until proven otherwise it is assumed that *all* pediatric head trauma patients may have an associated cervical spine injury. Hyperextension of the head therefore must *not* be performed to open the airway. The chin-lift or jaw-thrust method should be used. The head and neck should be gently placed in the "sniffing" position. If the airway remains blocked, the nurse may displace the mandible forward by gripping the angles of the jaw. If the patient is unable to maintain a patent airway, nasotracheal intubation or cricothyroidotomy may be performed. If the cervical spine radiographs are negative, orotracheal intubation may be performed.

Vomiting is a common occurrence following a head injury. In a semiconscious or unconscious patient it is essential to insert a nasogastric tube to empty the stomach contents to prevent possible aspiration. Nasogastric tube insertion should be performed after the patient is intubated, as passage of a nasogastric tube (NG-tube) may induce vomiting. The nasogastic tube should not be inserted until the presence of a cervical spine injury has been ruled out. Also if a frontal basal skull fracture is suspected, oral insertion of the nasogastric tube may be preferred, since there could be a danger of inadvertent intracranial intubation with nasal insertion.

Careful attention to the child's neck immobilization is mandatory. The child should be immobilized so proper alignment will be maintained during any transportation of the patient. This includes transporting the patient from the scene of the accident to the hospital in addition to any transportation that may be required in the hospital facility (i.e., to radiology or CT scan). The child should be placed on either a short or long backboard, depending on the size of the child. A cervical collar or sandbags may be applied to hold the head in alignment if a cervical spine injury is suspected. The cervical collar must fit correctly or the result can be hyperextension of the neck with a compromise of the airway. A strap or a piece of tape can be applied to the child's forehead (with sandbags placed on both sides of the head and neck). This will help to properly immobilize the head and neck while maintaining body alignment. If indicated, other extremity fractures should be splinted.

Breathing. Head injuries typically produce abnormal respiratory patterns. Cheyne-Stokes respirations may suggest central nervous system difficulties. Initially a slowing of the respiratory rate may indicate an acute rise in intracranial pressure. As the ICP increases, the respiratory rate becomes more rapid. The patient may have had cervical spine trauma, which may produce respiratory embarrassment or total arrest.

The respiratory rates of infants or children are more responsive to illness, exercise, and emotion than are adult respiratory rates. The respiratory rates in infants and children also have a greater range than adult rates. In an infant or child the nurse should observe the abdominal excursions when ascertaining the respiratory rate because diaphragmatic breathing is predominant. In older children the thoracic movement should be observed to calculate the respiratory rate.[58]

The nurse should observe the rate, rhythm, and effort of breathing. The shape of the chest should be noted, paying attention to any deformities of the thorax. Any abnormal retraction of the interspaces or abnormal bulging of the interspaces should be noted. The nurse should palpate the chest to identify areas of tenderness, to assess observed abnormalities, to assess respiratory excursion, and to elicit vocal or tactile fremitus. The nurse may also percuss the chest to determine if the underlying tissues are air filled, fluid filled, or solid. The chest should then be auscultated to note breath sounds or any abnormal sounds such as crackles, wheezes, or rales.

Circulation. The patient's blood pressure should be checked frequently. A rise in ICP may be reflected in an elevated blood pressure. There may be a rise in systolic blood pressure with a widening of the pulse pressure. Preexisting hypertension as well as pain or anxiety must also be evaluated. Variations in a child's blood pressure may be caused by exercise, crying, or an emotional upset. Severe hypotension may occur as a result of spinal shock.

Throughout infancy and childhood the systolic blood pressure gradually increases. At approximately 1 year of age the diastolic pressure reaches 60 mm Hg and gradually increases to approximately 75 mm Hg. Normal systolic pressures are approximately 50 mm Hg at birth, 60 mm Hg at 1 month, 70 mm Hg at 6 months, 95 mm Hg at 1 year, 100 mm Hg at 6 years, 110 mm Hg at 10 years, and 120 mm Hg at 16 years.[59]

With severe head trauma the pulse will initially slow down and may become irregular. An increase in ICP may produce bradycardia. If bradycardia follows a period of tachycardia, it indicates an increase in the ICP. If these signs coexist with a rising systolic blood pressure and a widening pulse pressure, this also reflects a rise in ICP. The child should be placed on a cardiac monitor for at least the first 24 hours after admission to detect any irregularities.

Similar to the blood pressure and respiratory rate in infants and children, the heart rate is also more sensitive to illness, exercise, and emotion than in adults. The heart rate should be obtained by directly auscultating the heart in infants. The

nurse may palpate the radial artery in older children. The nurse should identify the heart rate, rhythm, amplitude, and contour. Any abnormalities should be noted.[60]

The child's vital signs should be monitored frequently (at least every 15 minutes). It is crucial to note and report any changes in the vital signs. These changes, if present, may provide valuable information to define the patient's systemic as well as neurologic status. Table 10–4 contains

TABLE 10–4. NORMAL PULSE, RESPIRATIONS AND BLOOD PRESSURE FOR INFANTS AND CHILDREN

Average Heart and Respiratory Rates of Infants and Children at Rest

Age	Average Heart Rate (beats/min)	Average Respiratory Rate (breaths/min)
Newborn	140	35
1–11 mo	120	30
1–2 yr	110	25
2–6 yr	103	23
6–10 yr	95	20
10–14 yr	85	19
14–16 yr	80	18
16–18 yr	75–80	16–18

Average Blood Pressure Readings in Infants and Children

Age	Average Normal Systolic Pressure (flush method*)
Birth	50 mm Hg
1 mo	60 mm Hg
6 mo	70 mm Hg
1 yr	95 mm Hg
6 yr	100 mm Hg
10 yr	110 mm Hg
16 yr	120 mm Hg

*Diastolic pressure reaches about 60 mm Hg at 1 year of age and increases throughout childhood to an average of 75 mm Hg.

Data from L.F. Whaley, & D.L. Wong. *Nursing Care of Infants and Children.* St. Louis: Mosby, 1983; and from B. Bates. *A Guide to Physical Examination* (3rd ed.). Philadelphia: Lippincott, 1983, pp. 457–458.

the normal vital signs for infants and children.

Temperature Regulation. The patient's body temperature frequently falls immediately after a head injury. Both hypothermia and hyperthermia can occur in the head trauma patient. These temperature changes may suggest injury to the central nervous system in the area of the hypothalamus. Hypothermia may develop from vasodilation; therefore, measures need to be instituted to conserve body heat. A temperature elevation may be seen when there is bleeding into the ventricles. Fever control measures would include tepid sponging, antipyretics, and a cooling blanket or mattress. The nurse must accurately monitor all vital signs and then document findings, noting any changes.

Neurologic Assessment. This next section will review the nursing assessment of a child in the emergency department with focus on the neurologic assessment. The initial nursing assessment of a child with a head injury or spinal cord injury consists of monitoring vital signs and assessing the child's level of consciousness and ocular function. A thorough neurologic assessment would include an assessment of the child's level of consciousness, orientation, memory functions, eye and pupillary examination, reflexes, and motor and sensory function.

After the airway has been determined to be patent and the child's ventilations and circulation are adequate, the child's level of consciousness should be assessed. The Glasgow Coma Scale (GCS) is one measurement tool that may accurately assess the child's level of consciousness. This information can be communicated to the nursing staff in the form of an easily produced scoring system.

The GCS is a widely used assessment tool that provides information to measure changes and to describe a patient's level of consciousness. It was developed in 1974 at the University of Glasgow. Purpose of the GCS is to standardize observations of neurologic status in patients who have sustained head trauma. A decreasing level of consciousness is vital to note because it is an early sign of increasing intracranial pressure.

The GCS includes three components: assessment of eye opening, verbal response, and best motor response (Table 10–5). The patient should be assessed hourly for any subtle changes. The information should be documented by charting the patient's responses, and the physician should be notified of any changes. The GCS will allow the nurse to note any signs of improvement or deterioration in the patient's level of consciousness.

The points assigned to each response should be added together. The total points are an objective indication of the patient's level of consciousness. The points can range from 14 to 3, with 14 being the score a normal individual would obtain. The lowest possible score is 3, which may be indicative of brain death. A total score of 7 or below is commonly referred to as the definition of coma.

The GCS can also be used to communicate at the change of shift and between various nursing units. Each staff member and nursing unit will have identical criteria to assess the level of consciousness in all patients who may be critically ill.

After the child's level of consciousness is determined, an eye examination should be performed to check eye and pupillary responses. The child's eye and pupillary responses should be incorporated into the cranial nerve assessment. Refer to Table 10–6 for an overview of the cranial nerves, functional classification (sensory or motor), and how to test for the function of each cranial nerve. The cranial nerve as-

TABLE 10-5. GLASGOW COMA SCALE

	Points	
I Eye Opening Response	4	The patient opens his or her eyes spontaneously (already open blinking)
	3	The patient opens his or her eyes to speech
	2	The patient only opens his or her eyes in response to a painful stimulus
	1	The patient does not open his or her eyes even with a painful stimulus. Note if the patient's eyes are swollen shut
II Verbal Response	5	The patient is oriented to person, place, and time
	4	The patient still answers questions but is confused and is not oriented to person, place, and time
	3	The patient uses inappropriate words that make little or no sense
	2	The patient responds with incomprehensible sounds
	1	The patient does not respond verbally. Note if the patient is intubated, which can prevent speech
III Motor Response	5	The patient obeys a command and pain is not required (i.e., patient moves a limb to command)
	4	The patient tries to change the location of the painful stimulus
	3	The patient flexes his or her arm or pulls away in response to a painful stimulus
	2	The patient's elbow extends and his or her wrist internally rotates in response to a painful stimulus. The response is not purposeful
	1	The patient has no motor response when a painful stimulus is applied in any limb
Total	____	

The total number of points is an objective indication of the patient's level of consciousness.
Adapted from C. Jones. Glascow coma scale. American Journal of Nursing, September 1979, p. 1552.

sessment can be performed quickly in a systematic and organized fashion.

Pupils should be checked frequently at regular intervals along with monitoring of vital signs and an assessment of the child's level of consciousness. The nurse should observe and record the size and equality of the pupils, the response to light, and the equality of the reaction to light. An inequality of the pupil size and reaction to light may suggest localization of the head injury on the side of the dilated fixed pupil.

The child's orientation and memory may be tested by asking the child his or her name, what day it is, where he or she

is being treated, and how the head injury occurred. The child may also be asked what events led to the incident. The child should be asked to repeat a digit span and to recall three items after 5 minutes. A child between 4 to 6 years of age can be expected to recall three digits, whereas a child 6 years or older should remember five digits. It is important to test a child in relation to his or her developmental stage.

The child's motor function, including muscle strength and tone, can be assessed as an adult's is assessed, with application of an in-depth knowledge of developmental milestones of the infant, toddler, and child. Depending upon the severity of the

TABLE 10-6. CRANIAL NERVE ASSESSMENT

	Cranial Nerve	Functional Class	Test
I	Olfactory	Sensory	Test the patient's sense of smell with eyes closed. Have patient identify a substance, one nostril at a time
II	Optic	Sensory	Test the patient's vision with Snellen chart. Check visual fields. An opthalmologic examination should be performed
III	Oculomotor	Motor	These cranial nerves are tested together. Check for pupillary con-
IV	Troclear	Motor	striction in reaction to light and accommodation. Also check
VI	Abducens	Motor	for convergence and extraocular movements (EOMs) in all directions, including downward-inward eye movement (tro-clear) and lateral eye movement (abducens)
V	Trigeminal	Motor	Muscles of mastication are tested (temporal and masseter mus-cles), also lateral movement of the jaw
		Sensory	Sensation of the head and face is tested by touching with a piece of cotton. Corneal reflex tested by a touching with wisp of cotton. Observe and note all three branches for sensation: ophthalmic, maxillary, and mandibular
VII	Facial	Sensory	Test taste on the anterior two thirds of the tongue
		Motor	Test muscles of facial expression (including wrinkling of fore-head, forceful closing of the eyes, puffing out of cheeks, and showing of teeth)
VIII	Acoustic	Sensory	Test hearing (air and bone conduction with a tuning fork) and equilibrium
IX	Glossopharyngeal	Sensory	Tested together. Taste on posterior one third of the tongue and
X	Vagus	and Motor	sensation in the pharynx. Check gag reflex movements of swallowing, palate on vocalization, and note position of uvula
XI	Spinal accessory	Motor	Test movements of head and shoulders (sternocleidomastoid and trapezius muscles) against resistance and shoulder shrugging
XII	Hypoglossal	Motor	Test the movement of the tongue. Note any deviations, atrophy, or fasciculations

Data from J. Ferholt, et al. *Clinical Assessment of Children: A Comprehensive Approach to Primary Pediatric Care.* Philadelphia: Lippincott, 1981, p. 60; and from B. Bates. *A Guide to Physical Examination* (3rd ed.). Philadelphia: Lippincott, 1983, p. 378.

head or neck injury, the child should be evaluated for voluntary movements of the extremities, muscular development, strength, resistance to passive movement, atrophy, fasciculations, and tremors. The child's posture, gait, and symmetry of muscle strength should be observed for any abnormalities. Hand grasps are checked for strength and equality. Decorti-cate, decerebrate, or any other abnormal position should be carefully noted in a co-matose patient.

Each major muscle group can be tested through range of motion, noting whether muscle tone, spasticity, or flaccid-ity are present. If additional data are nec-essary, an age-appropriate Denver Devel-opmental screening test may be used for specific gross and fine motor coordination testing.

To test a child's sensory function, the examiner should recall that a child's thresholds of touch, pain, and temper-ature are higher in older children. In an in-fant the examiner should gently touch the baby's arms and legs with a pin and ob-serve for movement or change in the facial expression. The child may be tested for sensory function by noting sensation to pinprick, light touch, temperature, and vibration in all four extremities and in trunk and face; for position sense in toes and fingers; for tactile localization; for two-point discrimination; and for stereognosis (ability to identify objects by touch).

In addition, deep tendon reflexes should be tested and compared on both sides. The examiner should note the following reflexes: clonus, plantar (Babinski's), abdominal and cremasteric, grasp, suck, Moro's, tonic neck, blinking, and an anal sphincter reflex to touch. The nurse should note any abnormal localized findings, failure to elicit appropriate responses, any asymmetry of normal responses, late persistence of normal responses, and any developmental delays.

Incorporated into the neurologic assessment is the assessment of the total body for any abnormalities that may have been sustained from the incident, such as bumps, bruises, abrasions, lacerations, and contusions. In particular the nurse should note any ecchymosis on the mastoid area (Battle's sign), periorbital ecchymosis (raccoon eyes), or conjunctival hemorrhages. These signs may indicate a basal skull fracture. All the assessment findings should be properly documented in the nurses' notes so that an accurate data base may be obtained. The data base should be used to help in the development of a comprehensive and sensitive nursing care plan that meets the individual needs of the child and family.

Fluid Management. An intravenous line must be rapidly started either at the scene of the accident by paramedics or immediately upon arrival at the emergency department. Blood samples should be drawn at the time the intravenous line is started. Samples should be sent to the laboratory and should include a complete blood count, measurement of electrolytes, blood for type and crossmatching, and, if appropriate, toxicology and drug screening and arterial blood gases.

Continuous intravenous infusion should be closely monitored and maintained to establish adequate circulation. Depending upon the specific injury, isotonic fluids, blood, and blood products may be used to maintain adequate perfusion pressure to the brain. The next useful isotonic solution would be to administer 5 percent dextrose in 0.2 percent saline at one half to two thirds the normal maintenance rate. Overhydration should be avoided if the child is not in shock. Fluid overload may aggravate nervous system injuries. Fluids should be calculated according to the age of the child to keep the blood pressure within normal limits.[61]

A Foley catheter should be inserted to check for hematuria, to ascertain the adequacy of renal perfusion, and to closely monitor urine output in case osmotic agents need to be administered. Hourly measurement of urine output is recommended to check the adequacy of the circulatory system. Fluid intake and output must be strictly monitored.

A complication of severe head trauma is the syndrome of inappropriate secretion of antidiuretic hormone (SIADH). This is a metabolic imbalance characterized by low serum sodium, high urinary sodium output, high urinary specific gravity, and low urine volume.[62] As the treatment of SIADH is fluid restriction, it is essential that accurate intake and output and electrolyte monitoring be continued in all patients with a severe head injury.

Medications and Treatments. Medication administration plays a vital role in the treatment and management of a child with a head or spinal cord injury. Tables 10–7 and 10–8 contain a synopsis of the medica-

TABLE 10–7. MEDICATIONS AND TREATMENTS FOR PEDIATRIC HEAD TRAUMA AND SPINAL CORD INJURIES

Medication	Dosage	Administration or Route	Peak Level	Actions and Indications
Acetaminophen (Tylenol)	1 g/yr of age or 10 mg/kg/dose	Give per rectum initially (repeat every 4 to 6 hr)	30–60 min	Analgesic, useful in fever control and in reducing pain
Ampicillin	300 mg/kg/day	Give intravenously every 4 hr for 4 days	At the end of infusion	Useful in prophylaxis treatment for basilar skull fractures, open fractures, or penetrating injuries
Antacid	Variable (depending on neutralizing capacity of the product)	Give orally by nasogastric tube every 2 hr	Prompt	Antacid, useful in preventing gastric irritation
Dexamethasone (Decadron)	0.2 mg/kg (loading dose: 1.5 mg/kg)	Give intravenously every 6 hr	12–24 hr	Reduces cord inflammation, cerebral edema
Diazepam (Valium)	0.2–0.5 mg/kg (total dosage for infants is 2–4 mg); (total dosage for older child is 5–10 mg)	Give intravenously. To be infused no faster than 1 mg/min (may be repeated every 15 to 30 min, to a total of 3 doses if necessary)	15 min	Useful in the treatment of post-traumatic convulsions. It is a rapid acting anticonvulsant. Side effects may include hypotension and respiratory depression
Mannitol	0.25 g–1.0 g/kg	Give intravenously every 4 to 8 hr	15–90 min	Produces a shift in water; therefore decreases brain volume and ICP. Side effects may include dehydration, renal failure, and intracranial bleeding. Mannitol is used to "buy time". Reduces ICP and decreases edema
Methylprednisolone (Medrol)	0.5 for ages less than 5 yr, 1 g for ages 5–15 yr	Give intravenously (repeat dose in 6 hr if no improvement is evident)	6 hr	
Phenytoin (Dilantin)	15–18 mg/kg	Give intravenously at a rate of 25 to 50 mg per min	Therapeutic blood level is reached almost immediately	Used in treatment of post-traumatic convulsions. Side effects may include occasional hypotension or supraventricular arrhythmias. Does not significantly depress consciousness
Tetanus (prophylaxis)	If not up to date less than 6 yr of age, 0.5 cc DPT; greater than 6 yr of age 0.5 cc Td; 14–16 yr of age, 0.5 cc Td	Give intramuscularly		For active immunization and prevention of tetany. Side effects may include fever within 24 to 48 hr, soreness, and swelling at the site of injection

TABLE 10—8. OTHER TREATMENTS

Treatment	Goal	Actions and Interventions
Passive hyperventilation	Reduce $PaCO_2$ from 40 to 20–25 torr	Decreases intracranial pressure by reducing cerebral blood flow and thus cerebral blood volume
Hypothermia	Reduce core body temperature	Decreases cerebral metabolism and blood flow; used in treating elevated intracranial pressure

tions and treatments used in the emergency management of head or spinal cord injuries in children.

Laboratory Data. Extensive laboratory studies must be completed. A complete blood count, electrolytes, BUN, glucose, type and crossmatch, toxicology, drug screening, and blood gases may be drawn. A complete x-ray series of the skull and spine are mandatory. A chest x-ray may be performed to rule out any suspected injuries to thoracic structures. Due to danger of brain stem herniation, a spinal tap is contraindicated in a child with head trauma. Additional diagnostic procedures may include a CT scan, radionucleotide scan, echogram, arteriography, and an electroencephalogram.

PSYCHOSOCIAL SUPPORT AND PARENT EDUCATION

Parents and family members are often left alone while the child is being evaluated. They frequently relive the events that led up to the accident. During this time the parents and family members feel guilty and blame themselves for the accident.

The emergency department nurse should consistently provide them with as much information as possible regarding the child's condition. The nurse should allow the parents to visit the child as soon as the child is stable. Before this occurs the nurse should explain any type of equipment or procedures to help allay any fear or anxiety.

To be completely effective the nurse should focus the reporting of the child's condition to the entire family unit. This will aid the family's ability to understand and accept the difficult situation. The emergency nurse can have an integral role in helping the family cope with the realities of individual situations and in assisting in the development of plans for the immediate future.

Appendix A contains discharge instructions for the home management of children following evaluation for head trauma.

NOTES

1. R.C. Raphaely, D.B. Swedlow, J.J. Downes, & D.A. Bruce. Management of severe pediatric head trauma. *Pediatric Clinics of North America* 27, no. 3(August 1980):715.
2. Ibid.
3. L.F. Whaley, & D.L. Wong. *Nursing Care of Infants and Children.* St. Louis: Mosby, 1983, p. 1395.
4. Raphaely, Swedlow, Downes, & Bruce, Management of severe pediatric head trauma, p. 715.
5. Ibid.
6. Whaley, & Wong, *Nursing Care of Infants and Children,* p. 1395.
7. Ibid.
8. D.F. Dean. The child with possible spinal cord injury. *Emergency Medicine* May 15, 1982, p. 124.

9. B. Bates. *A Guide to Physical Examination* (3rd ed.). Philadelphia: Lippincott, 1983, p. 465.
10. Ibid.
11. N.P. Rosman, J. Herskowitz, A.P. Carter, & J.F. O'Conner. Acute head trauma in infancy and childhood. *Pediatric Clinics of North America* 26(1979):717.
12. Ibid., p. 721.
13. Whaley, & Wong, *Nursing Care of Infants and Children*, p. 1396.
14. Ibid.
15. C. Warner. *Emergency Care: Assessment & Intervention*. St. Louis: Mosby, 1983, p. 285.
16. Ibid., p. 279.
17. Whaley, & Wong, *Nursing Care of Infants and Children*, p. 1397.
18. Ibid., p. 1396.
19. Rosman, Herskowitz, Carter, & O'Connor, Acute head trauma in infancy and childhood, p. 723.
20. Ibid.
21. S.B. Olds, M.L. London, P.A. Ladewig, & S.V. Davidson. *Obstetric Nursing*. Reading, Mass.: Addison-Wesley, 1980, p. 669.
22. Ibid.
23. J. Luckmann, & K. Sorensen. *Medical-Surgical Nursing* (2nd ed.). Philadelphia: W.B. Saunders, 1980, p. 2187.
24. Ibid., p. 2185.
25. R.M. Reece (Ed.). *Manual of Emergency Pediatrics* (2nd ed.). Philadelphia: W.B. Saunders, 1978, p. 153.
26. Rosman, Herskowitz, Carter, & O'Connor. Acute head trauma in infancy and childhood, p. 728.
27. Reece, *Manual of Emergency Pediatrics*, p. 153.
28. Luckmann, & Sorensen, *Medical-Sugical Nursing*, p. 662.
29. Whaley, & Wong, *Nursing Care of Infants and Children*, p. 1398.
30. Bates, *A Guide to Physical Examination*, p. 427.
31. J.V. Hickey. *The Clinical Practice of Neurological and Neurosurgical Nursing*. Philadelphia: Lippincott, 1981, p. 236.
32. Reece (Ed.), *Manual of Emergency Pediatrics*, p. 153.
33. Ibid., p. 154.

34. Rosman, Herskowitz, Carter, & O'Connor, Acute head trauma in infancy and childhood, p. 728.
35. Ibid.
36. Whaley, & Wong, *Nursing Care of Infants and Children*, p. 1398.
37. S. Price, & L. McCarty Wilson. *Pathophysiology: Clinical Concepts of Disease Processes* (2nd ed.). New York: McGraw-Hill, 1982, p. 674.
38. Ibid.
39. Ibid.
40. B.C. Johanson, C.U. Dungca, D. Hoffmeister, & J.J. Wells. *Standards for Critical Care*. St. Louis: Mosby, 1981, p. 215.
41. Ibid.
42. Raphaely, Swedlow, Downes, & Bruce, Management of severe pediatric head trauma, p. 716.
43. Johanson, Dungca, Hoffmeister, & Wells, *Standards for Critical Care* (St. Louis: The C.V. Mosby Company, 1981), p. 193.
44. C. Zeidelman. Increased intracranial pressure in the pediatric patient: Nursing assessment and intervention. *Journal of Neurosurgical Nursing* March, 1980, p. 7.
45. Johanson, Dungca, Hoffmeister, & Wells, *Standards for Critical Care*, p. 193.
46. Whaley, & Wong, *Nursing Care of Infants and Children*, p. 1380.
47. Ibid., p. 1562.
48. Dean, The child with possible spinal cord injury, p. 124.
49. Whaley, & Wong, *Nursing Care of Infants and Children*, p. 1562.
50. Dean. The child with possible spinal cord injury, p. 137.
51. Ibid., p. 124.
52. Whaley, & Wong, *Nursing Care of Infants and Children*, p. 1565.
53. Ibid., p. 1566.
54. Price, & Wilson, *Pathophysiology: Clinical Concepts of Disease Process*, p. 675.
55. Ibid., p. 675.
56. Whaley, & Wong, *Nursing Care of Infants and Children*, p. 1566.
57. Ibid., p. 1399.
58. Bates, *A Guide to Physical Examination*, p. 458.
59. Ibid.

60. Ibid., p. 457.
61. Raphaely, Swedlow, Downes, & Bruce, Management of severe pediatric head trauma, p. 716.
62. W.B. Schwartz, W. Bennett, S. Curelop, & F.C. Bartter. A syndrome of renal sodium loss and hyponatremia probably resulting from inappropriate secretion of antidiuretic hormone. *American Journal of Medicine* 23 (1957):529.

BIBLIOGRAPHY

Agee, B.L., & Herman, C. Cervical logrolling on a standard hospital bed. *American Journal of Nursing* March, 1984, pp. 314–318.

Alexander, M.M., & Brown, M.S. *Pediatric History Taking and Physical Diagnosis for Nurses.* New York: McGraw-Hill, 1979.

Allmond, B.J. Management of cervical and thoracic spine/cord injured patients. *Journal of Neurosurgical Nursing* April 1981, pp. 97–101.

Bates, B. *A Guide to Physical Examination* (3rd ed.). Philadelphia: Lippincott, 1983.

Berk, J., & Sampliner, J. *Handbook of Critical Care.* Boston: Little, Brown, 1982.

Brigman, C., Dickey, C., & Zegeer, L.J. The agitated-aggressive patient. *American Journal of Nursing* October 1983, pp. 1409–1412.

Brunner, L.S., & Suddarth, D.S. *Textbook of Medical-Surgical Nursing* (4th ed.). Philadelphia: Lippincott, 1980.

Burrell, L., & Burrell, Z. *Critical Care* (4th ed.). St. Louis: Mosby, 1982.

Cobb, B., & Williams, D. Test your neurologic nursing skills. *Nursing 80* January 1980, pp. 40–43.

Coffey, R.J. Pediatric neurological emergencies. *Topics in Emergency Medicine* July 1982, pp. 67–80.

Dean, D.F. The child with possible spinal cord injury. *Emergency Medicine* May 15, 1982, pp. 123–151.

DeYoung, S. *The Neurologic Patient: A Nursing Perspective.* Englewood Cliffs, N.J.: Prentice Hall, 1983.

Farrell, J. *Illustrated Guide to Orthopedic Nursing* (2nd ed.). Philadelphia: Lippincott, 1982.

Ferholt, J.D.L. *Clinical Assessment of Children: A Comprehensive Approach to Primary Pediatric Care.* Philadelphia: Lippincott, 1980.

Gray, H. *Anatomy of the Human Body* (36th ed.). Philadelphia: Lea & Febiger, 1980.

Hahn, A.B., Barkin, R., & Oestreich, S.J.K. *Pharmacology in Nursing* (15th ed.). St. Louis: Mosby, 1982.

Hausman, K.A. Critical care of the child with increased intracranial pressure. *Nursing Clinics of North America* 16(December 1981):647–656.

Hickey, J.V. *The Clinical Practice of Neurological & Neurosurgical Nursing.* Philadelphia: Lippincott, 1981.

Howry, L., Bindler, R., & Tso, Y. *Pediatric Medications.* Philadelphia: Lippincott, 1981.

Johanson, B.C., Dungca, C.U., Hoffmeister, D., & Wells, S.J. *Standards for Critical Care.* St. Louis: Mosby, 1981.

Jones, C. Glasgow coma scale. *American Journal of Nursing* September 1979, pp. 1551–1553.

Kaktis, J.V. An introduction to monitoring intracranial pressure in critically ill children. *Critical Care Quarterly* June 1980, pp. 1–8.

Kenner, C.V., Guzzetta, C.E., & Dossey, B.M. *Critical Care Nursing.* Boston: Little, Brown, 1981.

Kunkel, J. Nursing management of the head injured patient. *Critical Care Update* 8, no. 3(1981):22–23.

Kunkel, J., & Wiley, J. Acute head injury: What to do when . . . and why. *Nursing 79* March 1979, pp. 22–23.

Luckman, J., & Sorensen, K. *Medical-Surgical Nursing* (2nd ed.). Philadelphia: W.B. Saunders, 1980.

Malasanos, L., Barkauskas, V., Moss, M., & Stoltenberg-Allen, K. *Health Assessment* (2nd ed.). St. Louis: Mosby, 1981.

Meir, E. Evaluating head trauma in infants and children. *Maternal Child Nursing* 8(January/February 1983):54–57.

Miller, L. Neurological assessment: A practical approach for the critical care nurse. *Journal of Neurosurgical Nursing* March 1979, pp. 2–5.

Nelson, W.E. *Textbook of Pediatrics* (12th ed.). Philadelphia: W.B. Saunders, 1983.

Nezamis, F. The child with a head injury. *Issues in Comprehensive Pediatric Nursing* July/August 1977, pp. 30–37.

Olds, S.B., London, M.L., Ladewig, P.A., &

Davidson, S.V. *Obstetric Nursing.* Reading, Mass.: Addison-Wesley, 1980.

Pantell, R., *Taking Care of Your Child: A Parent's Guide to Medical Care.* Reading, Mass.: Addison-Wesley, 1977.

Perloff, J.K. *Physical Examination of the Heart and Circulation.* Philadelphia: W.B. Saunders, 1982.

Price, S., & Wilson, L.M. *Pathophysiology: Clinical Concepts of Disease Processes* (2nd ed.). New York: McGraw-Hill, 1982.

Raphaely, R.C., Swedlow, D.B., Downes, J.J., & Bruce, D.A. Management of severe pediatric head trauma. *Pediatric Clinics of North America* August 1980, pp. 715–727.

Reece, R.M. (Ed.), *Manual of Emergency Pediatrics* (3rd ed.). Philadelphia: W.B. Saunders, 1984.

Rosman, N.P., Herskowitz, J., Carter, A.P., & O'Connor, J.F. Acute head trauma in infancy and childhood. *Pediatric Clinics of North America* 26(1979):707–736.

Rosman, N.P., Oppenheimer, E.Y., and O'Connor, J.F. Emergency management of pediatric head injuries. *Emergency Medicine Clinics of North America* April 1983, pp. 141–174.

Schwartz, W.B., Bennett, W., Curelop, S., & Bartter, F.C. A syndrome of renal sodium loss and hyponatremia probably resulting from inappropriate secretion of antidiuretic hormone. *American Journal of Medicine* 23(1957):529.

Scipien, G.M., Barnard, M.U., Chard, M.A., et al. *Comprehensive Pediatric Nursing* (2nd ed.). New York: McGraw-Hill, 1979.

Tackett, J.J.M., & Hunsberger, M. *Family-Centered Care of Children and Adolescents: Nursing Concepts in Child Health.* Philadelphia: W.B. Saunders, 1981.

Thompson, J., & Bowers, A.C. *Clinical Manual of Health Assessment.* St. Louis: Mosby, 1980.

Tyson, G.W., Remel, R.W., Winn, H.R., et al. Acute care of the spinal cord injured patient. *Critical Care Quarterly* June 1979, pp. 45–60.

Tyson, G.W., Remel, R.W., Winn, H.R., et al. Acute care of the head injured patient. *Critical Care Quarterly* June 1979, pp. 23–44.

Vestal, K.W. *Pediatric Critical Care Nursing.* New York: J. Wiley, 1981.

Ward, J. Central nervous system trauma. *Trauma* October 1981, pp. 11–18.

Warner, C. *Emergency Care: Assessment & Intervention.* St. Louis: Mosby, 1983.

Whaley, L.F., & Wong, D.L. *Nursing Care of Infants and Children* (2nd ed.). St. Louis: Mosby, 1983.

Wieczorek, R.R., & Natapoff, J.N. *A Conceptual Approach to the Nursing of Children: Health Care from Birth Through Adolescence.* Philadelphia: Lippincott, 1981.

Zeidelman, C. Increased intracranial pressure in the pediatric patient: Nursing assessment and intervention. *Journal of Neurosurgical Nursing* March 1980, pp. 7–10.

EMERGENCY DEPARTMENT CARE GUIDE FOR THE HEAD-INJURED CHILD

Nursing Diagnosis	Interventions	Evaluation
Ineffective airway clearance related to decreased level of consciousness	Continually assess and support airway Insert oropharyngeal airway in unconscious child Suction oropharyngeal airway as needed Immobilize neck with cervical collar until injury to cervical vertebrae has been ruled out	Airway remains patent Cervical spine radiographs are negative
Ineffective breathing pattern related to decreased level	Continually assess and support child's breathing	Child's respiratory rate is adequate

(Continued)

Nursing Diagnosis	Interventions	Evaluation
of consciouness and insult to respiratory center of brain	Artificially ventilate child as needed Monitor arterial blood gases Monitor breath sounds, chest symmetry, and rate Continually assess vital signs	Arterial blood gases are normal Skin temperature is warm and color is good Breath sounds are clear Vital signs remain stable
Potential alteration in body temperature related to fluid volume deficit	Decrease body temperature in patients with increased ICP to decrease tissue oxygen requirements, and decrease cerebral blood flow through administration of antipyretics and use of cooling mattress Continually monitor rectal temperature	Hypothermia is achieved, body rectal temperature is gradually reduced to 33C
Fear related to emergency procedures	Carefully explain all procedures to child who is alert Allow parent to remain with child once child has been stabilized Prepare child and parents for admission to hospital	Child remains calm and cooperative
Alteration in cerebral tissue perfusion related to increased ICP	Continually assess neurologic status Restrict fluid intake to two-thirds maintenance Elevate head of bed to 30° to increase cerebral venous drainage Maintain head in neutral position Assist in endotracheal intubation Hyperventilate patient to decrease cerebral carbon dioxide content Administer corticosteroids as ordered Administer osmotic diuretics as ordered Insert Foley catheter and measure urinary output Assess patient for presence of Cushing's triad (slowed pulse, altered respiratory rate, and elevated blood pressure)	Child remains alert and oriented Fluid intake is restricted Venous drainage increases Child's respiratory rate is maintained at a higher than normal rate Osmotic diuretics result in increased urinary output Vital signs remain stable Child tolerates insertion of ICP monitoring device

Nursing Diagnosis	Interventions	Evaluation
	Assist in insertion of intracranial monitoring device	
Anxiety (parental) related to child's serious condition	Explain all procedures to parents	Parents are kept informed of child's condition
	Continually report child's condition to parents	Parents are allowed to remain with child
	Allow parents to remain with child once child has been stabilized	Parents feel supported by emergency department staff
	Use nonjudgmental approach and provide emotional support to decrease feelings of parental guilt	
Knowledge deficit related to child safety and accident prevention	Assess parental knowledge of accident prevention	Parents express knowledge of accident prevention and child safety
	Provide anticipatory guidance related to injury prevention according to child's developmental stage	

11 | Seizure Disorders

Susan J. Kelley

Seizure disorders are among the most frequently encountered neurologic emergencies in childhood. A number of studies indicate that 4 to 6 percent of children will have at least one seizure in the first 16 years of life. Seizures can occur in a wide variety of conditions involving the central nervous system. Seizures occur in children of all ages, from newborns to adolescents. Most seizure disorders do not persist into adulthood. In adults the frequency of seizure disorders becomes approximately 1 in 200 or one fifteenth that found in children. The disappearance of seizures in many children as they grow older can in part be explained by the increasing functional maturity of the brain.[1]

Etiology. Seizure disorders have numerous and varied causes. Seizure disorders are diagnosed as idiopathic if the cause is unknown and as organic or symptomatic if the cause was acquired and therefore identifiable. Idiopathic epilepsy is usually familial, with possible genetic factors that lower the seizure threshold. A seizure disorder may also be acquired as the result of perinatal injuries, birth trauma, head trauma, hypoxia, central nervous system infections, acute cerebral edema, occupying lesions in the brain, metabolic disorders, endogenous or exogenous toxins, and a variety of other causes. Table 11–1 summarizes the etiologic classification of seizure disorders.

Pathophysiology. Seizures result from abnormal electrical discharges initiated by a group of hyperexcitable cells that may arise from central areas in the brain that affect consciousness immediately; may be restricted to one area of the cerebral cortex, producing manifestations characteristic of the particular anatomic focus; or may begin in a localized area of the cortex and spread to other positions of the brain, which may produce generalized neurologic manifestations.[2] During a seizure there is an increase of oxygen and glucose consumption, cerebral blood flow, carbon dioxide, lactic acid, and pyruvate production.

TYPES OF SEIZURES

Children are brought to the emergency department with many types of seizures. Seizures are classified according to seizure type. Generalized seizures include grand mal, petit mal, atonic, and myoclonic seizures.

Partial or focal seizures include motor, sensory, and psychomotor seizures (partial complex, temporal lobe). Partial seizures can evolve into generalized seizures, especially in patients not taking anticonvulsant medications.[3]

Other types of seizures seen in the emergency department include neonatal seizures and febrile seizures.

TABLE 11-1. ETIOLOGIC CLASSIFICATION OF CONVULSIVE DISORDERS

I. *Acute*	C. Intracranial hemorrhage
A. Infections	D. Anoxia
1. Simple febrile seizures	E. Hypertension
2. Intracranial infections (meningitis, encephalitis,	F. Trauma
cerebral abscess, sinus thrombophlebitis)	G. Brain tumors
3. Shigellosis	H. Miscellaneous
B. Toxic/metabolic disturbances	II. *Chronic*
1. Hypernatremia	A. Idiopathic
2. Hyponatremia	B. Postanoxic injury
3. Hypocalcemia	C. Postinfectious injury
4. Hypomagnesemia	D. Posttraumatic injury
5. Hypoglycemia	E. Posthemorrhagic injury
6. Pyridoxine deficiency	F. Posttoxic injury
7. Renal diseases	G. Degenerative diseases
8. Liver diseases	H. Congenital disorders
9. Exogenous toxins	
10. Inherited metabolic disorders	

Reproduced with permission from R.J. Packer, & P.H. Berman. Neurologic emergencies. In G. Fleisher, & S. Ludwig (Eds.), Textbook of Pediatric Emergency Medicine. Baltimore: Williams & Wilkins, 1983, p. 334.

Rapid identification of the cause and type of seizure activity is critical for immediate and appropriate intervention. Brief seizures rarely produce lasting neurologic damage. Prolonged and serial seizures, however, especially status epilepticus, may be associated with permanent neurologic damage.

Grand Mal Seizures

Grand mal, or major motor seizures, can occur at any age and may be focal or generalized. The patient with focal seizures is usually conscious, whereas the patient with generalized seizures is unconscious. These are the most common and most dramatic of all seizure manifestations in children. Grand mal seizures often occur without warning; however, 20 to 30 percent of children may experience a sensory or motor aura. This type of seizure may involve an immediate loss of consciousness, falling to the ground, dilated pupils, eye deviation upward or outward, and a tonic phase lasting 10 to 30 seconds. The tonic rigidity is then followed by a clonic phase with violent jerking movements of the extremities.[4] It is often associated with incontinence of urine or stool. This phase may last anywhere from 30 seconds to 30 minutes, followed by a postictal state in which the child may remain semiconscious or unconscious for anywhere from a few minutes to several hours. Upon awakening from the postictal state the child may be disoriented, with ataxia and impaired speech. The child will usually have no recollection of the seizure.

Petite Mal Seizures

Petite mal seizures (absences) are associated with very brief losses of consciousness, with minimal or no alteration in muscle tone, and often go unrecognized. The onset of petit mal seizures is abrupt, usually starting between 5 and 9 years of age. There may be associated automatisms, such as lip smacking, twitching of the face and blinking of eyelids, or slight hand movements. Petit mal seizures are often mistaken for inattentiveness or daydreaming and may result in behavioral or learning difficulties.

Atonic Seizures

Atonic, or akinetic, seizures are manifested as a sudden momentary loss of muscle tone and posture control. In children who are sitting, the seizure is manifested by a sudden dropping forward of the head. In children who are standing, the seizure is manifested by a very sudden loss of muscle tone and posture control, resulting in a fall to the ground. These may occur at any age but are unusual before 18 months of age.

Myoclonic Seizures (Infantile Spasms)

Myoclonic seizures, or infantile spasms, occur most commonly between 3 and 12 months of age. In one third of these cases no cause can be identified. In the other two thirds the seizures are the result of a definable brain disease. Perinatal causes are most common. Infantile spasms usually consist of a series of sudden, brief, symmetric contractions during which the head is flexed, the arms and legs are extended, and the hips are flexed. The eyes may roll upward or inward. The seizure is often preceded by a cry. There may or may not be loss of consciousness and change in color. These seizures tend to occur in a series and as often as several hundred times a day.

Infants who present to the emergency department with a history consistent with infantile spasms but who have been previously undiagnosed are usually admitted for a complete neurologic evaluation. Treatment for infantile spasms includes intramuscular adrenocorticotropic hormone (ACTH) or oral corticosteroids, valproic acid, clonazepam, and dietary measures such as the ketogenic or medium chain triglyceride diets.

The prognosis for normal intellectual development is poor. Between 55 and 98 percent of the patients with infantile spasms will ultimately be mentally deficient. About 50 percent of children with infantile spasms develop another form of seizure, most frequently grand mal seizures.[5]

Complex Partial (Psychomotor) Seizures

Psychomotor seizures usually manifest as purposeful but inappropriate repetitive movements. Psychomotor seizures are associated with an altered state of consciousness and automatisms. The automatisms may include lip smacking, eye blinking, and purposeless hand or body movements. Psychomotor seizures are often preceded by an aura that is sensory (i.e., visual, auditory, or olfactory). Although the child does not lose consciousness during the seizure, he or she does not remember the seizure. Postictal confusion or sleep may follow the seizure. Psychomotor seizures are associated with focal lesions of the temporal lobe and are therefore often referred to as temporal lobe seizures.

Neonatal Seizures

Neonatal seizures occur during the first month of life, with the majority occurring in the first 2 days. Neonatal seizures may be caused by perinatal anoxia or trauma, metabolic disorders, acute infectious processes, or drug withdrawal. Clinical presentations may include altered respiratory rate, eye deviations or blinking, and brief jerking movements of the extremities.

Febrile Seizures

Febrile seizures are divided into two categories: simple and complex. Simple febrile seizures are brief, lasting from 10 to 15 minutes, and are generalized. Complex febrile seizures are prolonged and may have focal features.[6]

Simple febrile seizures usually occur

between the ages of 6 months and 5 years in previously well children and within the first 24 hours of a febrile illness. There is often a positive family history for febrile seizures and a negative family history for other types of seizure disorders. Approximately 5 percent of all children experience a febrile seizure by age 5.[7] In the majority of cases the seizure activity occurred at home and has ceased upon arrival in the emergency department. The child will usually present in a postictal state that will lighten during the stay in the emergency department.

Febrile seizures are associated with an acute, benign febrile illness. Children with one simple febrile seizure have a 30 percent chance of having a second febrile seizure.[8] The rate of recurrence appears to be dependent on the age at the time of the first febrile seizure. The younger the patient at the time of the first febrile seizure the greater the chance for recurrence. Fifty percent of recurrences take place within the first year. Normally children have a convulsive threshold that is high enough to suppress excessive neuronal discharges. Febrile seizures occur when a febrile illness lowers the convulsive threshold temporarily.

STATUS EPILEPTICUS

In most cases involving a brief, self-limiting seizure, the seizure activity will have ceased prior to arrival in the emergency department, since by definition these seizures last less than 15 mintues. The actively seizing child seen in the emergency department is already in a state of prolonged or serial seizure activity.[9]

Status epilepticus is a state of continual seizure acitvity lasting more than 30 minutes or a series of shorter seizures occurring repetitively, so that recovery between seizures is incomplete. It is esti-mated that 3 to 10 percent of children with seizure disorders will experience at least one episode of status epilepticus.[10]

Status epilepticus may be caused by inadequate anticonvulsant therapy that occurs with a rapid or sudden withdrawal of anticonvulsants, central nervous system infections, head trauma, metabolic disturbances, or ingestion of a toxic substance. The precipitant must be identified early in the course of treatment. A careful history and evaluation are critical.

The patient in status epilepticus will present with continual seizure activity that is usually generalized and bilaterally symmetrical or, occasionally, unilateral. The patient is generally unresponsive, with increased secretions and depressed respirations. Status epilepticus is followed by a postictal state of relative mental and motor impairment.

History. A rapid but thorough history should be obtained from the parents or caretaker. A history of known seizure disorder, febrile illness, ingestion of a toxic substance, lead poisoning, or recent head trauma should be sought. If a past history of seizure disorder exists, a careful medication history should be obtained. Many parents are reluctant to admit that they discontinued anticonvulsant therapy against their physician's orders, missed doses, or ran out of medication. This information should be carefully elicited. Parents should be asked to describe the child's activity prior to the onset of the seizure. A careful description of the onset, type, and duration of seizure activity should be obtained. Other important information to be obtained includes any problems in the prenatal or perinatal period and any history of developmental delay. A family history of seizure disorders should also be ascertained.

If the seizure activity has stopped prior to arrival in the emergency department, elicit the following information from the parents: child's activity prior to the onset of the seizure, child's color, eye movements, description of movements of the extremities, history of incontinence, length and pattern of seizure activity, and child's level of responsiveness during and immediately after the seizure. When obtaining the history from the parents, keep in mind how frightening it may have been for them to witness this seizure. Parents will often overestimate the duration of the seizure due to their fear and anxiety at the time of occurrence. A careful history and assessment will help to differentiate between a simple febrile seizure, generalized seizure with increased temperature due to an increased muscle activity, meningitis, or encephalitis. Identification of infants with meningitis or encephalitis can be most difficult. The infant with meningitis or encephalitis may have a recent history of irritability, a high-pitched cry, poor feeding, fever, and vomiting. In children 1 to 5 years old with meningitis or encephalitis, there may be a preceding history of headache, nuchal rigidity, and vomiting. Lethargy observed in the emergency department can be the result of a postictal state or the presence of meningitis or enchephalitis.

Assessment. The patient's airway, breathing, and circulation (ABCs) should be rapidly and continually assessed. The respirations of the patient who is actively seizing are irregular, and their rate is lower than normal. Respirations in the postictal patient are often shallow.

Vital signs should be carefully monitored. Blood pressure and heart rate may increase during seizure activity. Anticonvulsant therapy can cause hypotension, cardiac arrhythmias, and apnea. A cardiac monitor should be placed on all patients in status epilepticus. Carefully monitor the patient's temperature throughout the sei-

zure. Increased muscle activity during a prolonged seizure may cause an increase in body temperature.

Carefully observe and record all seizure characteristics. Describe movements of the extremities, trunk, head, face, and eyes. Carefully time the length of all seizure activity. Continually assess the patient's level of consciousness, pupillary response and purposeful movements, and monitor for signs of increased intracranial pressure (ICP).

Level of consciousness and purposeful movements of the extremities should be observed. Pupil size and reaction to light should be noted. The child should be carefully examined for evidence of head trauma, even in the absence of a history of trauma. The skin should be examined for petechiae or purpura, which is often seen in meningitis or septicemia, and for the hypopigmented macules seen in tuberous sclerosis. Anterior and posterior fontanelles in infants should be evaluated for fullness or bulging. Describe and record the termination of the seizure along with the postictal level of consciousness and any purposeful movements. Record the length and depth of postictal sleep.

Laboratory Data. Some or all of these tests may be indicated based on history, previously diagnosed seizure disorder, and physical findings.

LUMBAR PUNCTURE. A lumbar puncture should be performed as soon as possible on all infants and children who present with a first-time history of seizure activity to rule out the presence of meningitis or encephalitis, increased ICP, or intracranial bleeding.

COMPLETE BLOOD COUNT. A complete blood count (CBC) should be obtained to rule out an acute bacterial infection, or sepsis. An increase in leukocytes (over 10,000) may be found, as in response to the stress of the seizure, and does not necessarily imply the presence of an infection. Anemia may be seen with lead poisoning, sickle cell anemia, and leukemia, each of which may be associated with seizures.

BLOOD CULTURE. A blood culture should be obtained to rule out sepsis or bacteremia.

URINE CULTURE AND URINALYSIS. Urinary tract infections are a common cause of hyperthermia in children. A suprapubic bladder tap may be performed to obtain a sterile urine culture in infants.

TOXIC SCREEN. Toxic screens (serum, gastric contents, and urine) should be obtained to rule out the possibility of an ingestion or lead poisoning.

ANTICONVULSANT LEVELS. If the child has a known seizure disorder and is on medication, anticonvulsant levels should be obtained.

SERUM ELECTROLYTES. Serum glucose, sodium, potassium, calcium, phosphorus, magnesium, and BUN levels should be obtained. A dextrostick will provide a rapid glucose value.

SKULL X-RAYS. X-rays of the skull may be indicated if a history of trauma is suspected. Evidence of chronically raised ICP may be seen.

Management

ABCs. The airway, breathing, and circulation should be assessed rapidly and supported. Establish and maintain a patent airway and adequate ventilation. An oropharyngeal airway should be inserted. Secretions should be suctioned judiciously. Clothing around the neck should be loosened. Oxygen should be administered

to prevent hypoxic damage to the central nervous system. Apnea or depressed respirations may occur. Assisted ventilation by face mask or endotracheal intubation may be necessary.

The child should be placed in a semi-prone position and a nasogastric tube inserted to decompress the stomach and minimize the danger of aspiration.

Protect the Patient. Carefully protect all body parts, particularly the head, while the patient seizes. Never restrain or hold extremities, as a fracture could result. Pad all side rails.

Thermoregulation. Carefully monitor the patient's temperature every 15 minutes. Administer acetaminophen or aspirin orally only if the patient is totally alert, rectally if the patient is seizing or is postictal. All clothing should be removed immediately to allow release of body heat through the skin. A tepid sponge bath should be given if the patient is stable. Alcohol should never be used in sponge baths because it is rapidly absorbed through the skin and can be toxic and even cause death.

Intravenous Therapy. An intravenous line should be inserted as soon as possible to establish a route for anticonvulsant therapy and intravenous fluid administration. Fluid intake and output should be recorded. Fluid intake should be restricted until cerebral edema has been ruled out.

Anticonvulsant Therapy. The goal of anticonvulsant therapy in status epilepticus and other forms of seizure activity is the prompt cessation of seizure activity without significant respiratory or cardiovascular depression. A number of anticonvulsant drugs are currently used for status epilepticus, each with its own advantage and disadvantage. These drugs and their

TABLE 11-2. ANTICONVULSANTS USED TO TREAT STATUS EPILEPTICUS

Drug	Dosage	Administration	Special Nursing Concerns	Advantages	Disadvantages
Phenobarbital (Luminal)	8–15 mg/kg Maximum: 300 mg One half the initial dose may be repeated 1 hr later if seizure continues	30–50 mg/min intravenously or intramuscularly	May produce sedation, respiratory, and cardiovascular depression. Vital signs must be closely monitored	Produces prolonged anticonvulsant effect due to long half-life (40 to 80 hr)	Effective brain concentrations are achieved slowly (20 to 60 min)
Diazepam (Valium)	0.2–0.5 mg/kg Maximum: 2 to 4 mg in infants; 5 to 10 mg in older children May be repeated every 15 to 30 min. Do not dilute in intravenous solution	Intravenously at a rate of 1 mg/min	May cause respiratory depression or arrest. Ambu bag and facial mask should be readily available	Very effective in status epilepticus. Can stop seizure activity in seconds	Anticonvulsant effect is poorly sustained due to short half-life (30 to 60 min). A second longer-acting anticonvulsant is usually required
Phenytoin (Dilantin)	15–18 mg/kg Maximum: 1 g Begin maintenance in 12 hr	25–50 mg per min intravenously; line must be flushed with normal saline before and after injection, or precipitation of drug will occur	May cause cardiac arrythmias. Cardiac monitor must be used. Observe for allergic reactions.	Effective in about 80 percent of patients with status epilepticus; penetrates the brain rapidly and stops the seizures in 5 to 30 min	Can precipitate cardiac arrythmias
Paraldehyde	0.1–0.25 ml/kg Maximum: 7 ml May be repeated in 1 hr and then every 2 to 4 hr	Usually given per rectum through rectal tube. May be given through nasogastric tube, intramuscularly or intravenously	Must be mixed with equal amounts of mineral oil when given rectally. Rectal tube should be clamped and buttocks held together past administration so patient can retain medication	Generally safe	Slow onset of action

proper dosages, routes, advantages, disadvantages, and special nursing concerns are listed in Table 11–2. Anticonvulsant therapies for other types of seizure disorders are listed in Table 11–3.

Whether the patient is admitted to the hospital or is discharged home depends on the patient's history, laboratory findings, and physical findings. Children with first-time febrile seizures are often admitted to the hospital for further observation and diagnostic testing. Children with previously undiagnosed afebrile generalized seizures are often admitted for further evaluation and anticonvulsant therapy. Children with previously diagnosed seizure disorders

who are stabilized are often discharged home.

PSYCHOSOCIAL SUPPORT AND PARENT EDUCATION

Parents are often extremely distressed by the occurrence of a seizure in their child, especially if it is the first seizure. They often fear their child is dying and feel helpless. Parents need a tremendous amount of support and teaching. Teaching should include medication administration and signs of drug reactions or toxicity. Protecting the child, especially his or her head,

TABLE 11–3. ANTICONVULSANT THERAPY FOR VARIOUS TYPES OF SEIZURES

Type of Seizure	Drug	Initial Dosage	Administration	Special Nursing Concerns
Neonatal Seizures				
Metabolic cause	Glucose 25%	2–4 mg/kg	IV push	Measure blood glucose level with dextrostick before and after administration
	Magnesium sulfate 50%	0.2 ml/kg	IM	
Varied cause	Phenobarbital	2–8 mg/kg daily	IV or IM	May produce respiratory and cardiovascular depression
	Dilantin	5–15 mg/kg	IV slow push	May cause cardiac arrhythmias Cardiac monitor necessary
	Valium	0.2–0.5 mg/kg	IV slow push	May cause respiratory depression or arrest
Petit mal seizures	Valium	0.15–0.3 mg/kg	IV slow push	May cause respiratory depression or arrest
Psychomotor seizures (temporal lobe)	Phenobarbital	2–8 mg/kg	IV slow push or IM	May produce cardiovascular or respiratory depression
Minor motor seizures (atonic and myoclonic)	Valium	0.15–0.3 mg/kg	IV slow push	May cause respiratory depression or arrest
Major motor seizures	Phenobarbital or	2–8 mg/kg	IV slow push or IM	May produce cardiovascular or respiratory depression
	Valium	0.15–0.3 mg/kg	IV slow push	Never give valium and phenobarbital together

Abbreviations: IV = intravenous; IM = intramuscularly.

during subsequent seizures should be stressed. Parents should be instructed never to place an object or fingers into a seizing child's mouth. Instead they should be instructed to turn the child's head to the side to prevent aspiration. If a fever is associated with the seizure, fever control should be taught.

NOTES

1. E.Y. Oppenheimer, & N.P. Rosman. Seizures in childhood, an approach to emergency management. *Pediatric Clinics of North America* 26(November 1979):837.
2. L.F. Whaley, & D.L. Wong. *Nursing Care of Infants and Children* (2nd ed.). St. Louis: Mosby, 1983, p. 1404.
3. R.J. Packer, & P.H. Berman. Seizures. In G. Fleisher, & S. Ludwig (Eds.), *Textbook of Pediatric Emergency Medicine.* Baltimore: Williams & Wilkins, 1983, p. 335.
4. Ibid.
5. Oppenheimer, & Rosman, Seizures in childhood, p. 846.
6. Packer, & Berman, Seizures, p. 334.
7. E.M. Ouellette. Seizures. In R.M. Reece (Ed.), *Manual of Emergency Pediatrics* (2nd ed.). Philadelphia: W.B. Saunders, 1979, p. 259.
8. Packer, & Berman, Seizures, p. 334.
9. Ibid., p. 336.
10. E.Y. Oppenheimer, & N.P. Rosman. Seizures. In R.M. Reece (Ed.), *Manual of Emergency Pediatrics* (3rd. ed.). Philadelphia: W.B. Saunders, 1984, p. 278.

BIBLIOGRAPHY

Barkin, R.N., & Rosen, P., Eds. Seizures. In *Emergency Pediatrics.* St. Louis: Mosby, 1984, pp. 600–610.

Bindler, R.N., & Howrez, L.B. Nursing care of children with febrile seizures. *American Journal of Maternal Child Nursing* 3(1978):270–273.

Coughlin, M.K. Teaching children about their seizures and medications. *American Journal of Nursing* 4:(1979):161–162.

Holmes, G.L. Anticonvulsants in management of seizure disorders of childhood. *Urban Health* (1982):39–44.

Johnson, M.V., & Freeman, J.M. Pharmacological advances in seizure control. *Pediatric Clinics of North America* 28(1981):179–191.

Meuhl, J.N. Seizure disorders in children: Prevention and care. *American Journal of Maternal Child Nursing* 4(1979):154–160.

Nelson, K.B. & Ellenberg, J.H. Prognosis in children with afebrile seizures. *Pediatrics* 61(1978):720–727.

Norman, S.E., & Browne, T.R. Seizure disorders. *American Journal of Nursing* 81(1981): 985–994.

Oppenheimer, E.Y., & Rosman, N.P. Seizures in childhood, an approach to emergency management. *Pediatric Clinics of North America* 26(1979):837–856.

Oppenheimer, E.Y., & Rosman, N.P. Seizures. In Reece, R.M. (Ed.), *Manual of Emergency Pediatrics* (3rd ed.). Philadelphia: W.B. Saunders, 1984, pp. 277–288.

Packer, R.J., & Berman, P. Seizures. In Fleisher, G., & Ludwig, S. (Eds.), *Textbook of Pediatric Emergency Medicine.* Baltimore: Williams & Wilkins, 1984, pp. 333–338.

Rothner, A.D., & Erenberg, G. Status epilepticus. *Pediatric Clinics of North America* 27(1980):593–602.

Santilli, N., & Tonelson, S. Screening for seizures. *Pediatric Nursing* 7(1981):11–15.

Taylor, J.W., & Ballinger, S. *Neurological Dysfunction and Nursing Intervention.* New York: McGraw-Hill, 1980.

Tucker, C.A. Complex partial seizures. *American Journal of Nursing* 81(1981):996–1000.

Willis, J.K., & Oppenheimer, E.Y. Children's seizures and their management. *Issues in Comprehensive Pediatric Nursing* 2(1977):56–57.

**EMERGENCY DEPARTMENT CARE GUIDE FOR THE CHILD
WHO IS ACTIVELY SEIZING**

Nursing Diagnosis	Interventions	Evaluation
Ineffective airway clearance related to increased respiratory secretions	Continually assess and support child's airway Insert oropharyngeal airway in unconscious child Suction oropharyngeal cavity to clear secretions Remove or loosen any clothing around child's neck	Airway remains patent
Ineffective breathing pattern related to prolonged seizure activity	Continually assess and support child's breathing Administer humidified oxygen during prolonged seizure Provide artificial ventilations if respiratory rate is inadequate or respiratory arrest occurs	Respirations remain adequate to oxygenate body tissue Breath sounds are clear
Impaired gas exchange related to altered respiratory status and prolonged seizure activity	Obtain arterial blood gases Assess child's color and capillary refill Administer humidified oxygen through face mask Assist in endotracheal intubation if necessary Provide artificial ventilations if necessary Continually assess vital signs	Arterial blood gases remain within normal range Child's color remains normal Capillary refill is normal Vital signs remain stable
Alteration in cerebral tissue perfusion related to prolonged seizure activity	Continually assess child's neurologic status Administer humidified oxygen Hyperventilate patient if there is evidence of increased ICP Insert intravenous line Administer anticonvulsant as ordered Restrict intravenous fluid volume to prevent increased ICP	Child's pupils remain reactive and are of a normal size Child regains consciousness following seizure and postictal period Seizure activity ceases Fluid intake and output are carefully measured and recorded
Potential for injury related to uncontrolled body movements during seizure activity	Prevent child from striking head or extremities during seizure activity by placing padding around side rails	Child remains free from injury during seizure

(Continued)

Nursing Diagnosis	Interventions	Evaluation
Hyperthermia related to increased muscle activity or infection	Continually assess child's rectal temperature Remove heavy clothing to allow body temperature to escape Administer antipyretic Assess child for any infections that may have precipitated febrile episode Collect necessary laboratory specimens and cultures	Childs body temperature returns to normal Source of fever is identified
Alteration in patterns of urinary elimination: incontinence	Assess child for urinary incontinence during seizure activity Provide proper cleansing to perineum after seizure ends	Child is clean, dry, and comfortable following incontinence episode
Altered growth and development related to seizure disorder	Obtain child's developmental history from parents Assess child's ability to comprehend verbal explanations for emergency department procedures	Child comprehends explanations at an appropriate level
Fear related to emergency department and procedures	Upon child's awakening from postictal state, carefully explain what has happened and all procedures to follow Allow parents to remain with child once child's condition has stabilized	Child remains calm and cooperative
Knowledge deficit (parental) related to child's seizure disorder	Continually inform parents of child's condition and all procedures Instruct parents on how to care for their child during a seizure Instruct parents on proper medication administration Teach parents methods for fever control Stress to parents the importance of regular visits to the child's primary care provider or neurologist for ongoing management of seizure disorder	Parents demonstrate understanding of child's condition and all procedures Parents demonstrate an understanding of safety precautions to be taken during a seizure Parents administer medications properly Parents demonstrate awareness of fever control Parents attend regular visits to primary care provider

Disorders of the Ear, Nose, and Throat

Wendy J. Liston

DISORDERS OF THE EAR

Acute Otitis Media

Acute otitis media (AOM) is an inflammation of the middle ear that is characterized by effusion. It is the most common ear problem in infants and children. In most cases otitis media can be successfully treated. If otitis media is not treated promptly and effectively, however, possible complications that can arise include chronic serous otitis media, hearing loss, mastoiditis, meningitis, and cholesteatoma.

Etiology. Bacterial sources account for close to 70 percent of diagnosed AOM. Causative agents seem to vary with the age of the child[1] (Table 12–1).

Viral organisms such as parainfluenza, respiratory syncytial virus, adenovirus, enterovirus, and coxsackievirus are sometimes mentioned in conjunction with AOM but have rarely been isolated from the middle ear.[2,3]

Pathophysiology. The middle ear is connected to the nasopharynx by the eustachian tube. The eustachian tube has three basic functions. It protects the middle ear from secretions originating in the nasopharynx, drains secretions from the middle ear into the nasopharynx, and ventilates the middle ear to equalize middle ear pressure and atmospheric pressure.

Adult eustachian tubes are long and flat, but children have eustachian tubes that are short, wide, and lie horizontally (Fig. 12–1). As a result of this anatomic difference, children are much more likely to develop eustachian tube dysfunction. Such dysfunction causes inadequate ventilation, producing negative pressure in the middle ear. Eventually this negative pressure produces sterile transudate within the middle ear and pulls organisms from the nasopharaynx into the middle ear, which becomes contaminated. Once in the middle ear these organisms proliferate rapidly and invade the mucosa.

Additional factors that can contribute to eustachian tube dysfunction include upper respiratory infection, allergies, and cleft palate.

History. Fluid accumulation in the middle ear causes a build-up of pressure on the tympanic membrane (TM) and surrounding structures, causing the pain that is classically associated with AOM.

Infants are irritable, pull at the affected ear, and rub their heads from side to side in the crib. Anorexia, high fever (up to 40C), diarrhea, rhinitis, and cough may be found.

Older children will complain of in-

TABLE 12-1. ACUTE OTITIS MEDIA: COMMON PATHOGENS AND TREATMENT

Age Group/Condition	Common Pathogens	Antibiotics[a]	Dosage (mg/kg/24 hr)	Frequency Route	Duration	Comments
<2 mo	S. pneumoniae, H. influenzae, group A streptococci, S. aureus, gram-neg enteric	Ampicillin and gentamicin	100–200 5.0–7.5	q 4 hr IV q 8 hr IV	3–7 days, then appropriate PO	Appropriate if signs of systemic illness; tympanocentesis indicated; hospitalize; if no signs or symptoms, use 2 mo–8 yr regimen
2 mo–8 yr	S. pneumoniae, H. influenzae, group A streptococci	Amoxicillin; or erythromycin and sulfisoxazole[b], or erythromycin and trimethoprim-sulfamethoxazole	30–50 30–50 100–150 30–50 8.0/40	q 8 hr PO q 6 hr PO q 6 hr PO q 6 hr PO q 12 hr PO	10 days 10 days 10 days 10 days 10 days	
9 yr and older	S. pneumoniae, group A streptococci	Penicillin V or erythromycin	25,000–50,000 U/kg/24 hr 35–50	q 6 hr PO q 6 hr PO	10 days 10 days	
Persistent		Sulfisoxazole or trimethoprim-sulfamethoxazole	100–150 8.0/40	q 6 hr PO q 12 hr PO	14 days 14 days	Use after initial course of amoxicillin; if no resolution consider tympanocentesis
Recurrent		Sulfisoxazole or trimethoprim-sulfamethoxazole	50–75 8.0–40	q 12 hr PO q 12 hr PO	2 mo 2.4 mo	Should be done in conjunction with otolaryngologist

Abbreviations: q = every; IV = intravenous; PO = orally.

[a] Additional acceptable antibiotics are available but are either broader in spectrum or more costly.

[b] Available as a single combination (Pedizole).

Reproduced with permission from Ear, nose, and throat disorders. In R.M. Barkin, & P. Rosen, Emergency Pediatrics. St. Louis, Mosby, 1984.

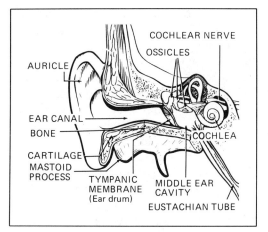

COCHLEAR NERVE
OSSICLES
AURICLE
EAR CANAL
BONE
COCHLEA
CARTILAGE
MASTOID
PROCESS
TYMPANIC
MEMBRANE
(Ear drum)
MIDDLE EAR
CAVITY
EUSTACHIAN TUBE

Figure 12-1. Ear canal, middle ear, and inner ear. *(From E.B. Rudy, & V.R. Gray. Handbook of Health Assessment (2nd ed.). Norwalk, Conn.: Appleton-Century-Crofts, 1986, p. 79.)*

tense pain in the ear. They may have a history of fever, vomiting, diarrhea, hearing loss, anorexia, cough, nasal congestion, and irritability.

Also significant is a history of severe pain followed by relief. Drainage is found on the pillow. This usually indicates perforation of the ear drum.

Assessment. Full visualization of the ear canal with an otoscope is required. Removal of cerumen or debris may be necessary, either with a curette or through irrigation (if it is certain that perforation is not present). Examination reveals a red bulging tympanic membrane with absence of the light reflex. Landmarks are partially or completely obstructed. Mobility of the tympanic membrane is impaired. Purulent discharge may be found in the ear canal.

Inflammation of the tympanic membrane alone is not considered to be diagnostic because crying can produce an inflamed tympanic membrane. Whenever purulent discharge is present it should be cultured to identify the causative organism. If discharge is not present but it is

essential to identify the causative organism, tympanocentesis (aspiration of middle ear fluid) may be performed. Indications for tympanocentesis include children who are seriously ill, who do not respond to antibiotic treatment, who develop a complication of AOM, or who are newborn.[4]

Tympanometry tests the compliance of the tympanic membrane to measure middle ear pressure. Normally the TM moves easily when either positive or negative pressure is applied. If tympanometry indicates abnormal compliance of the TM, middle ear effusion is usually present. An irregular tympanometry alone does not indicate the diagnosis of AOM.

On complete physical examination enlargement of cervical and postauricular lymph glands may be found.

Management. Treatment of AOM begins immediately upon diagnosis.

Antibiotics are prescribed for all symptomatic children and include axmoxicillin, ampicillin, erythromycin, gentamicin, penicillin V, sulfisoxazole, and trimethoprim-sulfamethoxazole. The drug of choice depends upon the most likely causative agent (Table 12-1).

Antihistamines and decongestants have been prescribed in the past, but there is little data to support their effectiveness. It would not be wrong to prescribe them, however, when the history indicates a child who has obtained relief from them in the past.

Analgesics may be used to promote comfort. Acetaminophen is usually sufficient. In extreme cases codeine may be indicated.

Ear drops should not be used, even though they may promote comfort, because they distort visualization of the tympanic membrane.

A hot water bottle or heating pad wrapped in a towel may reduce pain. The child should lie on the affected side. Ice packs placed on the affected ear will reduce swelling and pressure, thereby relieving pain. Each method should be tried and the most effective one continued.

Fever control is achieved with acetaminophen. Persistently high fevers may require sponging the child.

Myringotomy (incision of the TM) is indicated in the child who does not respond to antibiotic therapy after 48 to 72 hours. It may also be appropriate in the seriously ill child, the child with a severe earache who needs immediate relief, and the child with decreased defenses.[5]

Follow-up care is essential to determine if therapy has been effective. The child should be checked in 2 weeks for persistence of effusion, hearing loss, and complications.

Recurrent episodes of AOM are managed by prophylactic antibiotics for several months to 1 year.[6] These children are given either trimethoprim-sulfamethoxazole or sulfisoxazole.[7]

Psychosocial Support and Parent Education. During otoscopic examination of the ears, proper restraint is essential. It is quite helpful to enlist the aid of the parent. A very young child may be most comfortable lying across the parent's lap. An uncooperative older child can be placed on the examination table wrapped mummy style in a sheet. Remember to rest the examination instruments against the child's head so that the instruments will move with the child.

In addition to emotional support, the nurse provides teaching in several areas. Initially the main concern of parent and child will be relief of pain. Once pain is alleviated the tendency to forget to administer antibiotics will be great. Parents must be reminded of the importance of finishing the full antibiotic regimen. They should be told to return with the child for a follow-up appointment in 2 to 3 weeks but to call

sooner if the child's condition does not improve within 36 to 48 hours of treatment.

Parents should also be assessed for the need for education related to fever control, safety when using either heat or cold therapy, and antibiotic side effects.

Draining ears should be kept dry when the child is being bathed or is having his or her hair shampooed.

Teach parents of infants that placing their child in the supine position during and after feedings causes formula to pool in the nasopharynx and to move into the middle ear with swallowing. This position should therefore be avoided.

Bullous Myringitis

Bullous myringitis is vesicular inflammation of the TM and adjacent wall. The vesicles may be serous or hemorrhagic. This condition is often associated with upper respiratory infection.

Etiology. Usually the causative agent is *Mycoplasma pneumoniae.* Influenza viruses are also suspected.[8] Bullous myringitis may also be found in conjunction with acute bacterial otitis media.[9]

Assessment. This condition presents itself in the same way as acute otitis media. Acute pain is the most frequently identified complaint.

Otoscopy reveals blister(s) on the TM. The remainder of the TM is usually normal. Effusion may or may not be present in the middle ear. Thorough otoscopic examination is necessary because initial inspection may reveal a bulging TM, which is actually a cluster of blisters.

Culture of a draining bulla is always carried out. When exact identification of the causative organism is needed, an intact bulla may be incised and cultured.

Management. In general treatment is the same as that for acute otitis media. The drug of choice for antibiotic therapy is usually erythromycin 30 to 50 mg/kg/day in four equal doses. A heating pad and analgesics may be recommended for relief of pain. Following otoscopic diagnosis Auralgan ear drops may be used.[10] When pain is particularly intense, the blister may be incised to relieve discomfort.[11]

Psychosocial Support and Parent Education. Emotional support and teaching is the same as for acute otitis media. In addition, it is important for nurses to prepare the parents and child for the possibility of serous or sanguinous drainage from the ear canal following rupture of the bullae. Appearance of unexpected bloody drainage from the ear is quite frightening.

Otitis Externa

Otitis externa, also known as "swimmer's ear," is painful inflammation of the external auditory canal. This condition is usually found in children over the age of 5.[12] Pain due to otitis externa should be differentiated from pain caused by acute otitis media, dental infections, mastoiditis, and posterior auricular lymphadenopathy. Complications of otitis externa are rare,[13] but invasive otitis externa can cause cranial nerve palsies, osteomyelitis of the skull, and death.

Etiology. In the condition known as swimmer's ear, *Pseudomonas aeruginosa* is the organism most frequently cultured, but the infectious process is usually of mixed origin.[14]

It is possible for otitis externa to occur secondary to a foreign body in the ear canal or as a result of drainage of pus from a perforated tympanic membrane. Impetigo, herpes simplex, and *Staphylococcus aureus* furunculosis are all infectious organisms that have also been found to cause otitis externa.[15]

Pathophysiology. In the case of swimmer's ear, a diffuse dermatitis, it is thought that chlorine found in swimming pool water kills normal bacterial flora in the ear canal, allowing other bacteria and fungi to flourish. Inadequate drying of the ear canal after swimming may also contribute to the problem.[16]

Assessment. The child complains of severe pain, especially when the tragus is manipulated. Drainage is usually present in conjunction with erythema and edema of the external ear canal.

Otoscopy of the external canal and TM is necessary. Removal of cerumen and exudate is done to fully visualize the involved structure. Irrigation with warm saline or Burrow's solution is helpful (in the absence of perforation).

A diagnosis of otitis externa is made when the external canal is swollen, inflamed, and is draining exudate. If otitis externa is not secondary to a perforation, the TM will be intact, mobile, and pearly grey.

Management. Foreign bodies are removed. Eardrops containing cortisone and antibiotics effective against *Pseudomonas* and *Staphylococcus* (Cortisporin) are used for 1 to 2 weeks. If the ear canal is occluded by edema, a wick is inserted into the canal as far as possible and is saturated with the otic solution as prescribed. Irrigation with saline to cleanse the canal may be done 1 to 2 times per week as needed, and swimming is contraindicated. Cotton is placed in draining ears to prevent damage to the pinna. Analgesics such as acetaminophen or codeine are given for comfort. Systemic antibiotics are prescribed when an underlying condition has caused otitis externa.

The child should be treated at home but should be reevaluated if resolution is not seen in 4 to 5 days.[17]

Psychosocial Support and Parent Education. Parents should be taught the correct procedure for instilling ear drops.

The need to refrain from swimming is reinforced. Upon resolution of otitis externa ear plugs are recommended for swimming, and the need for thorough drying of the ears is emphasized. Instillation of 2 to 3 drops of white vinegar (5 percent acetic acid) has been recommended as a prophylactic before and after swimming.

The child should return for a follow-up appointment in 2 to 3 weeks to check for complete resolution.

Foreign Bodies in the Ear

The old adage that nothing smaller than the elbow should be placed in the ear is correct. Anything found in the ear other than cerumen is considered to be a foreign body. Complications of foreign bodies in the ear include perforation of the ear drum and infection.

Etiology. Young children have been known to place a variety of foreign objects into their ears, including beads, peas, corn, paper clips, small toys, and pebbles. The child may have placed the object into his own ear or a friend may have "helped" him out. Insects have been found to have flown or crawled into the ear canal. The child may be brought for treatment after a family member has seen the child place the object in his ear.

Assessment. An insect in the ear canal will be quite bothersome as it moves and buzzes, so the child will probably complain immediately after the occurrence. But in many cases the foreign body may not be found for quite some time until pain, discharge, and signs of inflammation are present. Sometimes the only complaint is that of hearing loss.

Otoscopic visualization of the ear canal is essential (refer to acute otitis media for a description of immobilization of the child). Examination seeks to identify the nature of the material and to determine whether or not the TM has been perforated. Management depends upon both findings.

Management. Removal of the object should only be done if it is clearly visible and if the child can be properly restrained. The majority of foreign objects can be removed by irrigation. The stream of water is directed beyond the object to flush it out. A water pik or syringe may be used. A 10-cc syringe with scalp-vein needle tubing cut 1 to 1½ inches from the hub is recommended.[19] Insects should be killed prior to irrigation by instillation of either alcohol or mineral oil.

The ear canal should *not* be irrigated when the foreign body is vegetable matter because the vegetation will absorb the water and swell even further. Vegetable matter should be removed with a curette or alligator forceps. Never irrigate an ear canal when the TM has been perforated. Again, remove the object with curette or alligator forceps, and treat the child for ear drum perforation. When the object cannot be easily removed or when the child cannot cooperate, a referral should be made to an otolaryngologist. General anesthesia may be necessary to remove the object without causing further damage to the canal wall.

Superficial trauma to the external canal should be treated in the same manner as otitis externa.

Psychosocial Support and Parent Education. The nurse comforts and restrains the child during the removal process. An older child should be taught the importance of keeping objects out of body orifices. It should be emphasized to the child that the removal process was not performed as punishment.

Support for the family includes helping parents deal with guilt feelings associated with the incident. Parents may also need to be taught not to put objects such as cotton swabs into the ear for cleaning.

Ear Drum Perforation

Ear drum perforation is rupture of the TM. With proper treatment perforations heal rapidly, but it is possible for scarring and adhesions to occur, causing permanent hearing loss. Perforations that do not heal leave the middle ear open to bacteria and potential mastoiditis, meningitis, labyrinthitis, and cholesteatoma.

Etiology. Ear drums can be ruptured by (1) purulent infections caused by acute otitis media (25 percent of AOM results in perforation),[20] (2) direct trauma caused by foreign body insertion, (3) a sharp blow to the ear, (4) skull fracture, or (5) barotrauma.

Pathophysiology. In otitis media, as both purulent exudate and pressure increase the tympanic membrane ruptures, allowing the exudate to drain.

Direct blows to the head compress the column of air in the ear canal, causing a sudden change of the ear pressure-regulating mechanism. Barotrauma caused by airplane ascents and descents and diving into water affect the same regulating mechanisms. Children with large adenoids or compromised eustachian tubes are at a greater risk to be affected by pressure changes.

Assessment. At the time of perforation pain is severe. Other symptoms include nausea, vomiting, vertigo, tinnitus, and hearing loss. Clinical signs may include the presence of purulent drainage, blood, or cerebrospinal fluid.

Pneumatic otoscopy reveals perforation, drainage, and an immobile TM. Drainage should be identified and cultured. A dipstix is used to test clear drainage for the presence of glucose, which would identify it as cerebrospinal fluid.

Consultation with an otolaryngologist or neurosurgeon may be indicated because of potential complications associated with ear drum perforation.

Management. Both medical and nursing management depend upon the cause of perforation:

1. Acute otitis media is treated with antibiotic therapy.
2. Foreign bodies are removed and treatment instituted as required.
3. Traumatic perforations generally require no treatment because they will heal on their own. Traumatic diving injuries are treated with antibiotics because water may bring organisms into the middle ear.
4. Skull fractures are referred to a neurosurgeon after sterile cotton has been inserted into the external meatus.

Never irrigate the ear canal or instill ear drops into a perforated ear. All draining ears should be cleansed with sterile cotton or pledgets soaked in hydrogen peroxide. When drainage is profuse, the auricle and skin surrounding the ear are protected from breakdown by frequent cleansing and application of petroleum or zinc oxide.

Hospitalization of the child is necessary when the injury has been severe enough to cause damage to inner ear structures (oval window, round window, and cochlea).

Psychosocial Support and Parent Education. The child and family are likely to be frightened by the appearance of drainage, especially if it is bloody. Explanations should be calm, direct, and specific. If the injury is a result of a blow to the ear, counseling about effective discipline techniques is in order. Remember that parents will probably be dealing with feelings of guilt.

Other teaching should include information about:

1. Positioning the child on the affected side to promote drainage
2. Complying with antibiotic regimen
3. Preventing skin breakdown
4. Preventing nose blowing
5. Keeping water out of the ear until healing has occurred
6. Keeping all objects out of the ear
7. The need for a follow-up appointment in 2 to 3 weeks to assess healing and to check for hearing loss

DISORDERS OF THE NOSE

Foreign Body in the Nose

Etiology and Pathophysiology. As young children explore their bodies, they discover that it is easy to place small objects into the nostrils, such as peanuts, popcorn, peas, beads, erasers, and pebbles. The child usually does not push the object very far into the nose, but an unskilled person can push it in deeper in an attempt to remove it.

Objects may also be found in the nasal cavity following an episode of vomiting. The presence of a foreign body irritates the nasal mucosa, causing inflammation, obstruction, and potential infection.

Assessment. Vegetable matter will increase in size rapidly as it absorbs moisture, causing the child to complain of discomfort. Other foreign bodies may not cause symptoms for several weeks or months. A foreign body should be suspected in children who present with unilateral obstruction of the nare in conjunction with foul smelling, purulent discharge that is unresponsive to antimicrobial therapy.

The child complains of tenderness when the nose is touched. A history might reveal frequent sneezing.

Examine the child with a nasal speculum or nasoscope to confirm the presence of the object. X-rays may be needed if the object has been pushed in posteriorly.

Management. Cooperation of the child is essential to prevent further damage to the nasal mucosa or aspiration of the object. The child is assessed and either immobilized, sedated, or anesthetized.

The following steps are then carried out:

1. The nose is anesthetized with 4 percent lidocaine drops.
2. Mucosa vessels are constricted with phenylephrine drops or spray, which requires 5 minutes to take effect.[21]
3. The object is removed using nasal suction, alligator forceps, or a blunt darning hook that is passed behind the object and then pulled forward. Be sure to check for the presence of more than one object.

Less frequently used maneuvers for removal of an object include:

1. Obstructing the unaffected nare with the finger and blowing into the mouth, as in mouth-to-mouth resuscitation. This moves the object into the anterior nasal chamber.[22]
2. Passing a lubricated No. 8 Foley catheter beyond the object and inflating it with 2 to 3 ml of water. The Foley is then withdrawn. The child should be in reverse Trendelenburg's position as this is done.[23]

If bleeding becomes a problem or if the foreign body is very difficult to remove, the child should be referred to an otolaryngologist.

Psychosocial Support and Parent Education. The nurse offers comfort while helping to immobilize the child. She emphasizes that restraint is not being used as punishment. Child and family are taught the importance of keeping foreign objects out of body orifices.

Acute Sinusitis

Acute sinusitis is an inflammatory reaction within the sinuses. Maxillary, ethmoid, sphenoid, or frontal sinuses may be involved (Fig. 12–2).

Potential complications include periorbital infections; blindness; osteomyelitis of the wall of the sinus; abscess of the brain, subdura, or epidura; facial cellulitis; oral-antral fistula; cavernous sinus thrombosis; otitis media; and meningitis.

Etiology. Acute sinusitis is usually seen as a complication of viral nasopharyngitis. Sinuses become occluded by swollen nasal mucosa, and bacteria proliferate. Offending organisms include *Hemophilus influenzae* (32 percent), *S. pneumoniae* (9 to 18 per-

cent), Group A streptococci (17 to 27 percent), and *S. aureus* (6 to 21 percent). Fungal infections have been identified in diabetics and in immunocompromised patients.[24]

Children who have hypertrophied adenoids, nasal polyps, cleft palate, or allergies are at higher risk for developing acute sinusitis. Trauma and dental infections can also produce sinusitis.

Assessment. Generally the child has purulent nasal discharge with congestion, mouth breathing, headache, fever, malodorous breath, and postnasal drip that produces a chronic cough.

Some children complain of pain and swelling over the involved sinus. Pain in the upper cheeks and teeth is associated with maxillary sinusitis. Frontal sinusitis often causes pain when bending the head forward. More than one sinus may be involved.

Physical examination reveals red

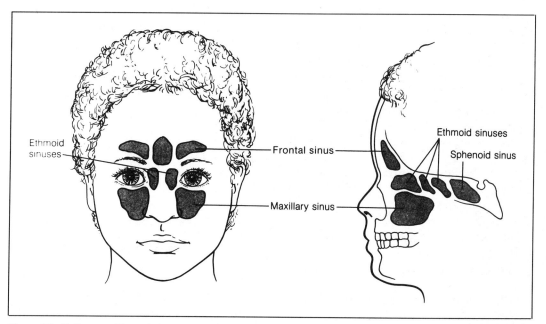

Figure 12–2. Front and lateral views of the facial sinuses. *(From S.R. Mott, N.R. Fazekas, & S.R. James (Eds.). Nursing Care of Children and Families. Menlo Park, Calif.: Addison-Wesley, 1985, p. 398.)*

swollen turbinates and purulent nasal discharge. Postnasal drip can be seen in the pharynx.

Cultures and smears of the nasal discharge are obtained but do not always correlate with the offending organism.

X-rays may help to identify the area and extent of infections but are difficult to interpret in a child under the age of 5. Sinusitis appears as thickening mucosa, clouding, or air-fluid levels within the sinuses.

Transillumination is accomplished by placing a light into the child's mouth in a dark room. Paranasal sinuses should light up equally, and both pupils should appear red. Unequal or poor transillumination is found in 76 percent of sinusitis.[25]

Management. Antibiotics are given for at least 10 days. The child is started on ampicillin 100 mg/kg/day in four equal doses until culture results are available. If *S. aureus* is suspected dicloxacillin 50 mg/kg/day is added.[26]

Nasal decongestion is achieved with phenylephrine drops or spray or 0.05 percent Afrin spray every 8 hours.[27] Systemic decongestants and antihistamines are of questionable value because their drying effects can impede drainage.

Comfort is attempted through an analgesic such as acetaminophen and warm compresses. Acetaminophen and cool sponges are used for fever control. Secretions are liquified with cool mist and increased fluids.

If any of the complications of sinusitis listed above are present, the child will require hospitalization for intravenous antibiotic therapy. Drainage and irrigation of the affected cavity may become necessary.

Psychosocial Support and Patient Education. Compliance with antibiotic regimen is emphasized. Correct application of nose drops is demonstrated. The child's head is kept low and turned to one side.

Signs and symptoms of possible complications are listed. Parents are told to return if symptoms worsen, have not significantly improved within a week, or are still present in 2 to 3 weeks.

Epistaxis

Epistaxis, commonly called a nosebleed, is a hemorrhage from the nose. Ninety percent of epistaxis originates in the anterior portion of the nasal septum, called Kiesselbach's plexus.[28] It is usually a self-limiting condition but can cause anemia or shock if extensive.

Less frequently nasal bleeding can arise from a portion of the posterior septum. This condition requires hospitalization because it may be fatal if improperly treated.

Etiology. Epistaxis is most common in childhood and occurs more frequently in winter months.

Possible causes include:

- Nose picking
- Consistent exposure to dry air
- Foreign bodies
- Forceful nose blowing during an upper respiratory infection or allergies
- Direct trauma to the nose
- Polyps/neoplasms
- Bleeding dyscrasias (idiopathic thrombocytopenic purpura, von Willebrand's disease, hemophilia)
- Aspirin ingestion
- Anticoagulants
- Telangiectasis
- Leukemia
- Hemangioma
- Severe hypertension
- Renal failure

Assessment. Active bleeding from one or both nostrils is seen. Bleeding from both nostrils is more indicative of posterior involvement.

The child who has had a nosebleed

during the night may vomit coffee-ground-like matter or have tarry stools.

In a posterior nosebleed the only sign may be frequent swallowing and the presence of blood in the pharynx. Persistent bleeding will lead to signs of shock (pallor, restlessness, increased pulse and respirations, and decreased blood pressure).

Diagnostic Evaluation. Vital signs are taken. A review of systems is done to determine etiology of the epistaxis. The nose is examined to identify the bleeding site. First the child is asked to gently blow his nose to dislodge any clots, or the nose is suctioned if the child is unable to cooperate.

In the case of prolonged bleeding a hematocrit is ordered and the child is evaluated for signs of hypovolemic shock. When systemic disease is suspected as the cause of epistaxis, a bleeding screen is done and the child is referred for a differential diagnosis.

Management. Management of epistaxis involves the following principles:

1. Have the child sit quietly with his head tilted forward. Pinch the nose by applying firm pressure to the cheek bones on either side of the nose with thumb and forefinger for at least 10 minutes. Ice may also be applied to the nose, lips, and back of the neck. Pressure should not be applied to a fractured nose. If bleeding does not stop, continue with steps 2 through 6.
2. Constrict the vessels of the nose and apply topical anesthesia with (1) 4 percent cocaine (not to exceed 2.5 mg/kg/hr) and (2) 4 percent lidocaine and 0.50 percent phenylephrine (drops or spray).[29]
3. Suction blood and wait 5 minutes.
4. Hold a silver nitrate stick to the bleeding vessel for 15 minutes. Be careful that the silver nitrate only comes in con-

tact with the bleeding site. Do not use this step in children with bleeding problems.
5. If bleeding is still not controlled, packing is placed inside the nose against the vessel. Cotton or one-quarter–inch packing gauze covered with bacitracin or neomycin ointment is used. Both ends of the packing are placed anteriorly to prevent aspiration. Both nares should be solidly packed so that pressure is applied equally throughout. Packing is left in place for 3 to 7 days.
6. Vital signs are monitored throughout the process.

Posterior bleeding and bleeding due to underlying systemic disease should be referred to an otolaryngologist or other appropriate specialist.

Psychosocial Support and Parent Education. A nosebleed is a frightening experience for a child. Calm, simple explanations are needed to allay some of the child's fear.

Parent-child teaching should include information related to:

1. Proper nose blowing
2. Preventing objects from being placed in the nose, including fingers
3. Increasing humidity in the home
4. Applying vaseline to the nares for 4 to 5 days
5. The need to sneeze through the mouth
6. Proper method of applying pressure to the nose to stop recurrent bleeding
7. Expecting the possibility of coffee ground-like vomitus or tarry stools if a large amount of blood was swallowed
8. Calling if bleeding cannot be controlled, if large amounts of blood are lost, or if unexplained bruises appear.[30]

If packing is left in place, a follow-up appointment should be scheduled.

Nasal Fracture

A fracture occurs when resistance to a stress being exerted gives way to the force of the stress. Fractures are most common in children and in the elderly.[31]

A nasal fracture usually can easily be treated. Possible complications include hemorrhage, airway occlusion, and associated trauma to the head and spinal column. Long-range complications include scarring and angulation deformities.

Etiology. Accidents are the leading cause of death in children. There are many factors that predispose the child to traumatic injuries. Injury to the nose is no exception.

Children are very active but lack gross motor coordination. They participate in contact sports, especially during school-age years. Falling, colliding with another child, motor vehicle accidents, being hit by a baseball, and child abuse are just a few examples of how a nose chould be fractured.

In addition, the bony structures of the nose and midface are smaller in children, placing them at higher risk for cartilaginous injury and fractures.

Assessment. Following a traumatic incident, pain, bruising and swelling are found over the nose and can extend to the areas under the eyes.

Epistaxis frequently occurs. If the fracture is not treated, one side of the nares may be occluded, causing breathing difficulties, rhinitis, and chronic sinusitis.

An intranasal examination is carried out to look for hematomas and intranasal lacerations. The nose is palpated to identify irregularities. Diagnosis is often confirmed by x-ray.

Additional injury to facial bones, skull, and spinal column should be ruled out. Drainage from the nose is tested for the presence of glucose, which would indicate cerebrospinal fluid leakage.

The oropharynx is examined, and blood clots or foreign bodies that could occlude the airway are removed.

Management. Once airway maintenance is assured and more serious injuries are managed, treatment is begun:

1. If bleeding is present it is treated first (refer to the section on epistaxis).
2. Ice is applied to the nose to reduce swelling.
3. The fracture is reduced, stabilized, and immobilized as soon as possible.
   a. Malaligned bones are reduced to their proper position using a surgical knife handle, nasal elevator, or Walsham forceps.[32]
   b. Significant deformity requires closed or open reduction under general anesthesia. This procedure is often delayed for 3 to 7 days while swelling decreases.
4. Following reduction the nose is immobilized by nasal packing and an external splint. The nasal packing also prevents reaccumulation of blood. It is left in place for 3 to 4 days. External splints are made of plaster, dental compound, or preformed metal. A splint is kept in place for 7 to 10 days.
5. Ice is also used following reduction to decrease swelling and pain.

Psychosocial Support and Parent Education. Families will be concerned about possible permanent effects on the physical appearance of the child. It is helpful to provide information regarding successful repair of nasal fractures.

Teaching should focus on:

1. Proper application of ice
2. Use of acetaminophen for discomfort rather than aspirin to prevent bleeding problems
3. Identification of signs of infection such

as an increased temperature or purulent discharge

4. The need to refrain from sneezing or blowing the nose. Sneezing is done with the mouth open, and the nose is wiped rather than blown. This is necessary to prevent nasal flora from being forced through lacerations into facial and orbital tissue[33]

5. Discouraging the use of decongestant sprays, which decrease the blood supply needed for healing

A follow-up appointment is made to remove the splint and to check the healing process.

DISORDERS OF THE THROAT

Pharyngitis

An infectious condition in which the throat is the principle site of involvement is called acute pharyngitis. Pharyngitis includes the conditions of tonsillitis and pharyngotonsillitis. It may be of either bacterial or viral origin, and its peak incidence is between the ages of 4 and 7.

Complications of viral pharyngitis are rare, but bacterial pharyngitis may lead to acute rheumatic fever, acute glomerulonephritis, otitis media, cervical adenitis, peritonsillar abscess, sinusitis, and meningitis.

Etiology and Pathophysiology. The late preschool and early school years are the logical time for the incidence of pharyngitis to peak. The child is exposed to more organisms outside the home while at the same time hypertrophy of the lymphoid tissue is naturally occurring, causing enlarged tonsils and adenoids.

Approximately 80 to 90 percent of pharyngitis is of viral origin (adenovirus, enterovirus, influenza, parainfluenza, Epstein-Barr virus, and herpes simplex).[34]

Group A beta-hemolytic streptococci (strep throat) account for the majority of other cases. Before the age of 3, however, strep throat is quite rare. It is the bacterium *H. influenzae* that is more commonly found in the child under 3.[35]

Bacterial and viral pharyngitis develop similarly, but some identifying factors can help in their differentiation (Table 12–2).

Assessment. Physical examination focuses on identifying the differentiating signs and symptoms found in Table 12–2.

Laboratory data include the following:

1. Throat cultures obtained on every child with a sore throat, with or without fe-

TABLE 12–2. CLINICAL PRESENTATIONS OF VIRAL AND STREPTOCOCCAL PHARYNGITIS

	Viral Pharyngitis	Streptococcal Pharyngitis
Age	Any age	Over age 2–3 years
Onset	Gradual	Sudden
Fever	Slight to moderate	Moderate to high
Symptoms	Sore throat, rhinitis, conjunctivitis, cough, hoarseness, headache, general malaise	*Severe* sore throat, headache, abdominal pain, vomiting, dysphagia
Clinical signs	Slight to moderate: erythema of pharynx, enlargement of tonsils, and tenderness and enlargement of cervical nodes; normal to slightly elevated WBC	Moderate to severe: erythema of pharynx, tenderness and enlargement of cervical nodes, enlargement of tonsils, petechiae on soft palate, and white exudate on tonsils and pharynx; scarletiniform rash; elevated WBC

ver, and evaluated for Group A streptococci (culture infants through the nose rather than the throat)
2. White blood cell (WBC) count
3. Monospot, if necessary
4. Culture for *Corynebacterium diptheriae*, if indicated

Additional data may include:

1. Examination of the abdomen for signs of organomegaly, which could be related to infectious mononucleosis
2. Careful auscultation of the heart to rule out the possibility of rheumatic complications

Management. Treatment for viral pharyngitis is symptomatic and consists of:

1. Warm saline gargles as often as every 2 hours (1 tsp. salt in 8 oz. water)
2. Sucking hard candy
3. Acetaminophen (10 to 15 mg/kg/dose orally every 6 hours as needed)
4. Increased rest and mild, cool fluids
5. Cool mist humidity in the child's room
6. Hot or cold compresses to tender cervical nodes

If culture results are positive for streptococcus, the child begins antibiotic therapy. Antibiotics are not begun until culture results return because a 48-hour delay in treatment has not been found to increase the incidence of rheumatic fever or glomerulonephritis. The delay also enables the child to develop an antibody response.[36]

Antibiotics must be taken for a 10-day period:

1. Penicillin: 40,000 to 80,000 units/kg/24 hours every 6 hours orally
2. Erythromycin: 30 to 50 mg/kg/24 hours every 8 hours orally for the child who is allergic to pencillin
3. Benzathine penicillin G: As a one-time dose intramuscularly if noncompliance

is suspected.[37] This is extremely painful; the child will require immobilization and emotional support.

Symptomatic treatment used for viral pharyngitis is also recommended for strep pharyngitis.

Psychosocial Support and Parent Education. Following a diagnosis of strep throat, symptomatic family members should also be cultured.

Teaching focuses on:

1. Medication compliance
2. Directions for symptomatic treatment
3. Sending the child back to school 24 hours after treatment is instituted if he or she feels well enough
4. Providing warm baths or moist heat to the injection site if benzathine penicillin G has been used
5. Follow-up care. The child should return in 2 to 3 weeks for a follow-up visit. Parents should call if the fever lasts over 48 hours; the child develops severe pain, dysphagia, or large lymph glands; or the infection develops elsewhere.

Peritonsillar Abscess

Peritonsillar abscess is an infection of the tonsils that has suppurated beyond the tonsillar capsule into the surrounding tissue. It is a medical emergency requiring prompt diagnosis and treatment to prevent the serious complications of sepsis, extension of the abscess, thrombophlebitis, and spontaneous rupture leading to aspiration pneumonia and death.

Etiology. Peritonsillar abscesses are caused by beta-hemolytic streptococci in about 50 percent of cases.[38] *S. aureus, H. influenzae, S. pneumoniae,* and normal mouth flora have also been implicated.[39] Peritonsillar abscesses occur most frequently in adolescents and young adults and are uncommon in toddlers.[40]

Assessment. The child complains of severe pain on the involved side and of dysphagia. Drooling of saliva, trismus, alterations in speech ("hot potato voice"), and high fever are present.

The pharynx is inflamed anterior and superior to the tonsil. A bulge is seen on the soft palate that may be yellow in color and fluctuant. The uvula is deviated to the opposite side. Cervical lymphadenitis is present as well as an elevated WBC.

Culture and gram stain may be required for diagnosis. Aspiration of the abscess to obtain culture and gram stain is done by an otolaryngologist.

Management. Airway maintenance is the first priority. The child is hospitalized for intravenous antibiotic therapy of:

1. Ampicillin: 100 to 200 mg/kg/day every 4 hours intravenously,[41] or
2. Oxacillin: 100 to 200 mg/kg/day every 6 hours intravenously,[42] or
3. Other antibiotic selected on the basis of culture and sensitivity results.

Initially the child is restricted from oral ingestion and receives intravenous fluid hydration. The head of the bed is elevated 30 degrees, and cool mist is provided by mask or tent.

Meperidine 1 to 2 mg/kg/dose is given every 4 to 6 hours intramuscularly for relief of severe pain.

If resolution does not occur within 48 hours, incision and drainage (I & D) will be necessary. Large bore needle aspiration can be both therapeutic and diagnostic. Full scale I & D is carried out in the operating room.

A tonsillectomy may be performed if the condition continues to resist resolution.

Psychosocial Support and Parent Education. Hospitalization comes as a surprise to the family. They will need time to adjust to such a rapid admission.

This is an extremely painful condition. The child should be medicated appropriately. Parents may not realize the extent of the discomfort experienced by the child and may question the use of meperidine.

A referral is made to an otolaryngologist upon discharge, at which time an elective tonsillectomy may be discussed.

Cervical Adenitis

Cervical adenitis is a localized infection of the cervical lymph node(s). It can be present as a result of both infectious and noninfectious conditions. Possible complications occur as a result of spontaneous drainage and include:

1. Cosmetic problems due to exterior drainage
2. Nodes that drain chronically (especially those caused by chronic mycobacteria)
3. Interior drainage with subsequent involvement of multiple neck structures

Pathophysiology. Cervical lymph glands are found along the carotid sheath and drain the head and neck. Afferents are present from the nose, tonsils, tongue, teeth, and back of the head and neck. Nodes can become inflamed with suppuration if infection is present in any of these areas.

Etiology. The most frequent causes of cervical adenitis are *S. aureus* and group A beta-hemolytic streptococci. Cervical adenitis can develop, however, in association with a large number of additional conditions. Some of the more common ones include atypical mycobacteria, infectious mononucleosis, enterovirus, rubella, cat scratch fever, toxoplasmosis, and Kawasaki disease.

Assessment. If adenitis is due to staphylococcus or streptococcus, the child has tender, firm, discrete swelling along one side of the sternocleidomastoid muscle in the neck. Tenderness and swelling may be present over a wider area if inflammation extends outside of the node into soft tissue. Erythema is also present. Fever is usually found but is rarely higher than 101F (38.5C).

Lesions containing pus eventually become fluctuant, and the child becomes increasingly toxic. Nonpyogenic lesions have a more insidious course.

Additional symptomatology depends upon the underlying disease process.

A detailed history focuses on progression of symptoms, recent travel, exposure to cats or tuberculosis, and concurrent signs and symptoms. A complete physical examination is performed to identify the underlying disease process.

Laboratory data that might help to identify the causative agent include:

1. CBC with differential
2. Throat culture for group A streptococci
3. Heterophil and Monospot tests
4. Antistreptolysin titer
5. Intermediate strength purified protein derivative (tuberculin)
6. Aspiration, culture, and gram stain of a fluctuant node
7. Culture of any other lesions or infectious processes found in the body
8. Other diagnostic tests indicated by history and epidemiology

Management. Treatment of cervical adenitis depends upon underlying pathology. For adenitis associated with local reactions to what seems to be either staphylococcus or streptococcus, cultures are obtained and antibiotics prescribed for 10 days. Antibiotic choices are:

1. Penicillin G: 50,000 units/kg/day in four doses; or penicillin V: 50 mg/kg/day in four doses

2. Erythromycin: 50 mg/kg/day in four doses; or clindamycin: 10 to 20 mg/kg/day in 3 doses; or cephalexin: 50 to 100 mg/kg/day in four doses if the child has a penicillin allergy
3. Oxacillin, nafcillin, or cloxacillin: 50 to 100 mg/kg/day in four doses; or dicloxacillin: 25 to 50 mg/kg/day in four doses if the organism is penicillinase producing.[43]

Other antibiotics may be used depending upon culture and sensitivity results.

Warm, moist soaks are applied continuously to the affected node to promote localization of suppuration. When the node is fluctuant, I & D is performed. This is a painful process requiring both physical and emotional support.

With significant toxicity the child is hospitalized for I & D. The node is then irrigated and packed daily with iodophorm gauze while healing progresses. Parenteral antibiotic therapy is used.

Acetaminophen, codeine, and warm packs are used for comfort. Additional treatment depends upon the disease process.

Psychosocial Support and Parent Education. Children treated at home require close follow-up. Parents should understand that complete resolution may require several months.

Teaching includes:

1. Antibiotic compliance
2. Correct use of analgesics
3. Need for increased rest
4. Application of sterile gauze soaked in warm saline to provide comfort and to promote healing.

Foreign Body in the Throat

Aspiration of foreign bodies is a leading cause of death by accident in infants and toddlers. Complications of a swallowed foreign body depend upon its location. The object can cause airway obstruction if it lodges in the larynx. This leads to death when complete obstruction is present. Secondary infection is seen when foreign bodies lodge in pharyngeal tissue.

Etiology. Young children are quite likely to place foreign objects in the mouth. The child from 1 to 3 years is most likely to put nonfood substances in the mouth, such as coins, safety pins, nails, balloons, and small toys. Another source of difficulty for this age group is age-inappropriate foods, such as peanuts, popcorn, hard candy, and tough meats. The ability to thoroughly chew foods is not completely mastered until the preschool years.

History. Signs and symptoms depend upon whether or not obstruction is present. When the object is lodged in pharyngeal tissue, the child will be irritable or will complain of pain and a feeling of fullness upon swallowing. In many cases pain is present even after the object has been swallowed because tissue has been scratched.

If the foreign body is lodged in the larynx, the child usually presents with choking, gagging, high-pitched wheezing, dysphonia, or aphonia.

Parents may or may not have seen the child ingest the object.

Assessment. The diagnostic evaluation of a foreign body aspiration involves the following principles:

1. Adequacy of the airway should be established.
2. Physical examination and history should focus on differentiating a foreign body aspiration from an infectious process, such as croup.

3. X-rays (anteroposterior and lateral neck and chest) may reveal the presence of a radiopaque object.
4. Indirect laryngoscopy with adequate illumination may reveal the location of the object.
5. Arterial blood gases should be measured if the child is experiencing respiratory distress.

Management. If the child is stable and is in no acute respiratory distress, a laryngeal foreign body is removed by direct laryngoscopy in the operating room. Foreign bodies lodged in pharyngeal or tonsillar tissue are removed by indirect laryngoscopy using large, curved forceps.

Acute respiratory distress requires immediate attention. For infants under 1 year old, deliver four back blows between the scapulae with the infant lying down across the rescuer's thighs. Next, use four chest thrusts (identical to those used in standard cardiopulmonary resuscitation [CPR]) if back blows are unsuccessful. If the child is over 1 year old, the Heimlich maneuver should be utilized by a series of subdiaphragmatic abdominal thrusts. If the above manuevers are unsuccessful, lift the jaw and open the mouth to remove any object that can be visualized. A blind finger sweep should never be used because the object may be pushed further into the airway.

An unconscious child will usually require emergency cricothyrotomy and tracheostomy. Oxygen is provided by face mask.

Following traumatic removal of a foreign body the child is usually hospitalized and placed in a mist tent. Clear fluids will be offered cautiously at first, followed by encouragement of large amounts of fluids to decrease pain. The child is closely observed for the presence of laryngeal edema, which could compromise the airway.

Psychosocial Support and Parent Education. A tremendous amount of support will be needed for the entire family if the child's life is in danger. Parental guilt will usually be acute.

Once the child is stable, teaching should focus on

1. Keeping floors clear of all small objects
2. Inspecting toys for small removable parts
3. Not placing dangerous small items into waste baskets to which the child has access
4. Refraining from feeding the child "fun foods," such as popcorn, peanuts, and whole hot dogs, until developmentally ready.

Thrush

Thrush is a fungal infection of the mouth or throat found most frequently in young children. It is also called candidiasis or moniliasis. Thrush is found in 5 percent of neonates.[44] It is self-limiting but if untreated can result in lesions of the face, respiratory tract, gastrointestinal tract, and perineum. High-risk neonates have developed cases of renal candidiasis, which lead to death.[45]

Etiology. Thrush is caused by the yeast *Candida albicans.* When this monilial infection is present in a mother's vagina, her infant contracts the disease during descent through the birth canal. *C. albicans* can also be transmitted via contaminated breasts, hands, bottles, nipples, and pacifiers.

At-risk children include those with facial anomalies and children who have had their natural oral flora suppressed by antibiotics or immunologic deficiencies. Diabetic mothers are more likely to be carriers of *Candida* because the high glucose content of their urine provides a favorable environment for yeast growth.

Assessment. The child has white to white-grey patches on the oral mucosa that resemble milk or cheese curds. If these patches are scraped, the underlying mucosa is raw and may bleed.

Thrush is sometimes painful. Pain is manifested by decreased sucking.

The above findings on physical examination are diagnostic for *C. albicans.* Culture or microscopic examination of the scraped lesions reveal the *Candida* organism.

At-risk infants (premature neonates who have been treated for sepsis) should have a urine culture for yeasts.[46]

Management. Antifugal agents are prescribed. Nystatin (Mycostatin) mouthwash 100,000 units/ml is given until 3 to 4 days after resolution of lesions; 1 to 5 ml is placed in both cheeks four times a day (after feedings) and is then swallowed. Another successful method is to allow an older child to suck on a nystatin tablet or suppository. A suppository can also be placed in an infant's pacifier that has been split.

Mouth rinses are recommended every 2 hours. Normal saline, half-strength vinegar, or half-strength hydrogen peroxide are appropriate agents.

Psychosocial Support and Parent Education. Remind parents to use frequent, thorough handwashing and to boil nipples for 20 minutes after they have been washed because spores are resistant to heat. Rinsing the infant's mouth with clear water after feedings helps prevent recurrence.

Sources of infection must be identified. If it is the mother, she is treated. Contaminated objects are discarded. Correct administration of nystatin is taught and compliance encouraged.

Gingivostomatitis

Inflammation of the mouth and gums can be caused by a variety of organisms. Most cases of gingivostomatitis are self-limiting and cause few complications. Severe cases can lead to decreased fluid consumption and dehydration.

Etiology. Herpes stomatitis is caused by the virus herpes simplex. Aphthous stomatitis (canker sores) has an unknown causative agent. Acute necrotizing gingivitis (trench mouth) is caused by spirochete *Borrelia vincentii.* This condition occurs infrequently but can lead to bone loss and loosened teeth.

Transmission of conditions with known causative agents is by direct contact with an affected individual. The organism enters through a break in the skin, so teething babies are particularly at risk.

Assessment. Herpes stomatitis has an abrupt onset. Fever, irritability, and anorexia may be present. Gums are swollen and often bleed. Painful vesicular lesions are found on mucous membranes. They are irregularly shaped yellow lesions with red rims that eventually rupture and ulcerate.

Aphthous stomatic lesions are light yellow, small, oval, and covered with fibrinous exudate. History reveals that they are painful and have recurred over a period of months, usually at a time of physical or emotional stress.

Acute necrotizing gingivitis is seen where there has been a history of recent physical or emotional stress. Intensely painful interdental ulcerations are seen, and the entire gingival mucosa is tender and fragile. A foul odor is present in the mouth. Severe cases can cause regional lymphadenopathy, malaise, and fever.

History and physical examination lead to diagnosis. Culture of the lesions attempts to confirm the diagnosis.

Management. Herpes and aphthous stomatitis are treated symptomatically, as they are self-limiting. Hydration status is closely monitored. Cool liquids are en-

couraged, but citrus juices are avoided. Analgesia is important to provide relief from pain and to improve hydration status. An oral analgesic such as acetaminophen may provide some relief but is not as effective as a topical solution.

Cepacol or 5 percent chloraseptic mouthwash is recommended every 2 hours.[47] Milder cases may be helped by rinses of normal saline or half-strength hydrogen peroxide. More severe cases are helped by viscous lidocaine, diclone, or a mixture of one-half benadryl and one-half kaopectate two to three times a day before meals.[48] Glycerine, Gly-oxide, or petroleum jelly is applied to the lips.

Acute necrotizing gingivitis requires antibiotic therapy. Penicillin V is given orally for 10 days. Follow-up by a dentist is required for tissue debridement and evaluation of dental status.

Psychosocial Support and Parent Education. Parents need reassurance that their child will improve. They should offer soft, bland foods but should not be upset if the child refuses to eat. Emphasize the importance of hydration status instead.

Proper oral hygiene is taught, and flossing is encouraged in the older child (following resolution of the problem).

Family members should wash hands thoroughly immediately after contact with the child's mouth.

A herpes virus may clear up but reappear during times of stress. Recurrences often appear at the vermillion border of the lips as "cold sores" and "fever blisters." Consistent adequate rest and nutrition are encouraged to diminish the chance of recurrence.

Traumatic Loss of Teeth

Tooth avulsion is the complete displacement of a tooth. Teeth lost as a result of trauma can cause occlusion problems and infection if treated improperly. Secondary teeth are traumatically lost during the childhood years for a variety of reasons, including falls, child abuse, sports injuries, fights, and bicycle and automobile accidents. Children with protruding teeth, craniofacial abnormalities, and muscular disorders are more prone to dental injuries.

Management. A displaced tooth should be replaced in the socket without waiting for dental consultation. Reimplanted teeth have been retained for periods ranging from 6 months to 12 years. Even those retained for a short period of time help to prevent malocclusion during the critical period of permanent tooth eruption. Prognosis is best when the tooth is replaced immediately.

The process for replacement is to:

1. Place the tooth in normal saline to cleanse it, being careful not to disturb periodontal fibers.
2. Gently remove blood clots and debris from the open socket.
3. Place the tooth back in the socket and gently press in place. The tooth is then immobilized in place for 3 weeks with a splint.

Following replacement of the tooth the child should be referred to a dentist for x-rays and follow-up.

Antibiotic therapy with penicillin V or erythromycin is usually given. If the tooth is contaminated, the child's immunization records should be checked. Tetanus toxoid is given if it has been more than 5 years since the last booster.

Psychosocial Support and Parent Education. Parents and older children will be very upset about the child's physical appearance. They need to be told that the tooth will eventually be replaced by a prosthetic device.

Remind children who play sports to protect their teeth with plastic mouth guards and emphasize the importance of follow-up dental care.

NOTES

1. R.M. Barkin, & P. Rosen. Ear, nose and throat disorders. In *Emergency Pediatrics.* St. Louis: Mosby, 1984, p. 568.
2. Ibid.
3. J. Graef, & T. Cone. *Manual of Pediatric Therapeutics* (2nd ed.). Boston: Little, Brown, 1980, p. 527.
4. G.M. Scipien, & M.A. Chard. The special senses. In G.M. Scipien, M.U. Barnard, M.A. Chard, et al. (Eds.), *Comprehensive Pediatric Nursing* (2nd ed.). New York: McGraw-Hill, 1979, p. 1013.
5. Ibid.
6. M.S. Brown, & M.A. Murphy. *Ambulatory Pediatrics for Nurses.* New York: McGraw-Hill, 1981, p. 371.
7. Graef, & Cone, *Manual of Pediatric Therapeutics*, p. 528.
8. Graef, & Cone, *Manual of Pediatric Therapeutics*, p. 527.
9. Brown, & Murphy, *Ambulatory Pediatrics for Nurses*, p. 370.
10. Graef, & Cone, *Manual of Pediatric Therapeutics*, p. 527.
11. R.R. Wieczorek, & J.N. Natapoff. *A Conceptual Approach to the Nursing of Children: Health Care From Birth Through Adolescence.* Philadelphia: Lippincott, 1981, p. 667.
12. Scipien, & Chard, The special senses, p. 1025.
13. Barkin, & Rosen, Ear, nose and throat disorders, p. 485.
14. G. Simpson. Otitis externa. In R.M. Reece (Ed.), *Manual of Emergency Pediatrics* (2nd ed.). Philadelphia: W.B. Saunders, 1984, p. 527.
15. Barkin, & Rosen, Ear, nose, and throat disorders, p. 484.
16. Simpson, Otitis externa, p. 527.
17. Barken, & Rosen, Ear, nose, and throat disorders, p. 485.
18. Scipien, & Chard, The special senses, p. 1025.
19. Graef, & Cone, *Manual of Pediatric Therapeutics*, p. 525.

20. Wieczorek, & Natapoff, *A. Conceptual Approach to the Nursing of Children*, p. 668.
21. Graef, & Cone, *Manual of Pediatric Therapeutics*, p. 530.
22. Scipien, & Chard, The special senses, p. 1019.
23. Barkin, & Rosen, Ear, nose and throat disorders, p. 477.
24. Barkin, & Rosen, Ear, nose and throat disorders, p. 494.
25. Ibid.
26. Graef, & Cone, *Manual of Pediatric Therapeutics*, p. 533.
27. Ibid.
28. Barkin, & Rosen, Ear, nose and throat disorders, p. 475.
29. Graef, & Cone, *Manual of Pediatric Therapeutics*, p. 531.
30. Barkin, & Rosen, Ear, nose and throat disorders, p. 476.
31. L.F. Whaley, & D.L. Wong. *Nursing Care of Infants and Children* (2nd ed.). St. Louis: Mosby, 1983, p. 1542.
32. J. Bertz. Maxilofacial injuries. *Clinical Symposia* no. 4(1981):26.
33. S.M. Black. Facial fractures. *American Journal of Nursing* 82(July 1982):1088.
34. Barkin, & Rosen, Ear, nose and throat disorders, pp. 488–489.
35. M. Hunsberger. Respiratory conditions and related problems. In J.J. Tackett, & M. Hunsberger (Eds.), *Family Centered Care of Children and Adolescents*. Philadelphia: W.B. Saunders, 1981, p. 940.
36. Ibid.
37. Barkin, & Rosen, Ear, nose and throat disorders, p. 490.
38. D. Teele. Peritonsillar abscess. In R.M. Reece (Ed.), *Manual of Emergency Pediatrics* (2nd ed.). Philadelphia: W.B. Saunders, 1984, p. 535.
39. Barkin, & Rosen, Ear, nose and throat disorders, p. 487.
40. Teele, Peritonsillar abscess, p. 534.
41. Barkin, & Rosen, Ear, nose and throat disorders, p. 488.
42. Graef, & Cone, *Manual of Pediatric Therapeutics*, p. 536.
43. J. Klein. Cervical adenitis. In R.M. Reece (Ed.), *Manual of Emergency Pediatrics* (2nd ed.). Philadelphia: W.B. Saunders, 1984, pp. 533–534.
44. J.J. Tackett. Potential stresses during infancy: Temporary alterations in health status. In J.J. Tackett, & M. Hunsberger (Eds.), *Family Centered Care of Children and Adolescents*. Philadelphia: W.B. Saunders, 1981, p. 508.
45. J.J. Tackett. More than a little thrush. *Emergency Medicine* 13(July 1981):59.
46. Ibid.
47. Graef, & Cone, *Manual of Pediatric Therapeutics*, p. 534.
48. Ibid.

BIBLIOGRAPHY

Barber, J., & Budassi, S. *Manual of Emergency Care*. St. Louis: Mosby, 1979.

Barkin, R.M., & Rosen, P. Ear, nose and throat disorders. In *Emergency Pediatrics*. St. Louis: Mosby, 1984, pp. 474–497.

Bertz, J.E. Maxilofacial injuries. *Clinical Symposia* 4(1981):2–32.

Black, S.M. Facial fractures. *American Journal of Nursing* 82(July 1982):1086–1088.

Blum, J. Dental emergencies. In Reece, R.M. (Ed.), *Manual of Emergency Pediatrics* (2nd ed.). Philadelphia: W.B. Saunders, 1984, pp. 94–100.

Brown, M.S., & Murphy, M.A. *Ambulatory Pediatrics for Nurses* (2nd ed.). New York: McGraw-Hill, 1981.

Bruch, W. Otitis media. *Pediatric Nursing* 5(January/February 1979):9–12.

Chow, M.P., Durand, B.A., Feldman, M.N., & Mills, M.A., eds. *Handbook of Pediatric Primary Care*. New York: Wiley, 1979.

Dupont, J. EENT emergencies. *Nursing 79* 9(November 1979):65–70.

Freeman, G. Ear, nose and throat emergencies. In Warner, C.G. (Ed.), *Emergency Care* (3rd ed.). St. Louis: Mosby, 1983, pp. 302–315.

Graef, J., & Cone, T. *Manual of Pediatric Therapeutics* (2nd ed.). Boston: Little, Brown, 1980.

Hunsberger, M. Respiratory conditions and related problems. In Tackett, J.J., & Hunsberger, M. (Eds.), *Family Centered Care of Children and Adolescents*. Philadelphia: W.B. Saunders, 1981, pp. 940–946.

Hunsberger, M. Infection in a youthful sinus. *Emergency Medicine* 13(July 15, 1981):83–84.

Ingram, N.M. Stanching nosebleeds: Your guide to all measures available. *RN* 45(September 1982):50–53.

Ingram, N.M. Trauma to ear, nose, face and neck. *Journal of Emergency Nursing* 6(July/August 1980):8–12.

Klein, J. Cervical adenitis. In Reece, R.M. (Ed.), *Manual of Emergency Pediatrics* (2nd ed.). Philadelphia: W.B. Saunders, 1984.

Malamed, S.F. Dental emergencies. In Warner, C.G. (Ed.), *Emergency Care* (3rd ed.). St. Louis: Mosby, 1983, pp. 324–347.

Manton, A. Epistaxis. *Journal of Emergency Nursing* 7(March/April 1981):66–67.

Moore, L.T. Emergency management of facial injuries. In Warner, C.G. (Ed.), *Emergency Care* (3rd ed.). St. Louis: Mosby, 1983, pp. 316–323.

More than a little thrush. *Emergency Medicine* 13(July 15, 1981):59.

Reiter, D. A primer of ENT emergencies. *Emergency Medicine* 15(January 1983):120–126.

Sataloff, R., & Colton, C. Otitis media: A common childhood infection. *American Journal of Nursing* 81(August 1981):1480–1483.

Scipien, G.M., & Chard, M. The special senses. In Scipien, G.M., Barnard, M.U., Chard, M.A., et al. (Eds.), *Comprehensive Pediatric Nursing* (2nd ed.). New York: McGraw-Hill, 1979, pp. 997–1030.

Simpson, G. Otitis externa. In Reece, R.M. (Ed.), *Manual of Emergency Pediatrics* (2nd ed.). Philadelphia: W.B. Saunders, 1984, pp. 423–425.

Sloane, P. Sore throats: They're common, but full of surprises. *Consultant* 22(May 1982): 110–127.

Tackett, J.J. Potential stresses during infancy: Temporary alterations in health status. In Tackett, J.J., & Hunsberger, M. (Eds.), *Family Centered Care of Children and Adolescents.* Philadelphia W.B. Saunders, 1981, pp. 493–521.

Teele, D. Peritonsillar abscess. In Reece, R.M. (Ed.), *Manual of Emergency Pediatrics* (2nd ed.). Philadelphia: W.B. Saunders, 1984, pp. 534–535.

Upchurch, D.T. Removing foreign bodies from ears, nose and throat. *Consultant* 22(March 1982):283–294.

Whaley, L.F., & Wong, D.L. *Nursing Care of Infants and Children* (2nd ed.). St. Louis: Mosby, 1983.

Wieczorek, R.R., & Natapoff, J.N. *A Conceptual Approach to the Nursing of Children: Health Care From Birth Through Adolescence.* Philadelphia: Lippincott, 1981.

Wolf, R. Pediatric epistaxis. *Nurse Practitioner* 10(November/December 1982):12–16.

EMERGENCY DEPARTMENT CARE GUIDE FOR THE CHILD WITH AN EAR, NOSE OR THROAT PROBLEM

Nursing Diagnosis	Interventions	Evaluation
Alteration in comfort: pain related to inflammation	Administer systemic or local analgesic as indicated Administer antibiotic as ordered to eliminate infection	Child's pain is alleviated Child's infection is treated effectively
Potential for fluid volume deficit related to child's discomfort and refusal to take adequate amounts of fluid	Assess child's hydration status Encourage child to take fluids by mouth Administer intravenous fluids if necessary Measure urinary output and obtain specific gravity Obtain serum electrolytes to	Child's hydration status is adequate Child demonstrates ability and willingness to consume adequate amounts of fluids by mouth Child's urinary output is adequate (>1ml/kg/hr)

Nursing Diagnosis	Interventions	Evaluation
	assess child's electrolyte balance	Child's specific gravity is within normal range
		Child's serum electrolytes are normal
Impaired swallowing related to pain	Encourage child to drink very cold, clear fluids	Child is able to drink clear fluids in adequate amounts to prevent dehydration
	Administer analgesics as indicated	
	Administer antibiotics as ordered	Analgesics provide relief from pain
Hyperthermia related to infection	Identify source of infection	Source of infection is identified and treated
	Administer antipyretics	
	Give tepid sponge bath to young child or infant	Fever returns to normal
Fear related to painful procedures and strange environment	Carefully explain all procedures to child at appropriate developmental level	Child remains calm and cooperative
	Allow parents to remain close to child during examinations and treatments	
Knowledge deficit (parental) related to child's illness/injury and treatments	Carefully explain all procedures and treatments to parents	Parents demonstrate comprehension of treatments and nature of child's illness or injury
	Teach parents regarding the cause of their child's illness or injury	Parents demonstrate an understanding of how to avoid similar accidents in the future
	Teach parents how to provide a safe environment for their child	
	Instruct parents on the administration of medications and treatments	Parents demonstrate an understanding of proper administration of prescribed medications
	Inform parents to contact their primary care provider or emergency department physician if child's condition worsens or if child is unable to retain medication	Parents understand the importance of contacting their physician if child's condition changes
	Instruct parents in techniques of fever control	Parents demonstrate an understanding of fever control

13 | Ophthalmic Emergencies

Linda S. Goodale

Ophthalmic problems in children are commonly seen in emergency departments. Generally they are evaluated and treated by nonophthalmologic personnel. Because of this fact it is important that providers are familiar with diagnosis and are comfortable with treating commonly seen pediatric ocular emergencies. Appropriate intervention by the initial caretakers can prevent unnecessary pain and worry and can save precious sight.

It is important to remember that the pediatric patient who arrives with an ocular emergency is usually accompanied by at least one adult. The nurse must therefore provide care and reassurance to both the child and accompanying adult(s). If time is taken initially to calm and reassure the child and parent, diagnosis and treatment will be much easier.

HISTORY

For any patient who arrives at the emergency department with an ocular injury, a very careful and thorough history of the event should be taken. This history should also include past and current treatment for any eye disorder, including amblyopia, any previous eye injuries, and whether or not the child wears corrective lenses. A complete medical history should also be obtained, taking care to inquire whether the child is currently taking medication for any reason.

ASSESSMENT

Prior to initiation of treatment a visual acuity is usually obtained of both eyes. The child should be wearing his or her glasses (if prescribed) for this procedure. This simple examination is frequently overlooked and can be critical to the ocular well-being of the patient.

Children younger than 3 years may be unable to participate in this examination using the traditional Snellen chart or "E" game but may respond to the use of Allen figures.

Each eye should be tested separately; usually the right eye is tested first. An ocular occluder should be used, taking care not to apply pressure to the eye while temporarily blocking the vision. Results should be recorded as follows: OD $^{20}/-$ OS $^{20}/-$. Or distances used during the examination can be recorded, such as OD $^{10}/- $ OS $^{10}-$.[1]

The accompanying adult can be a tremendous asset in examining children, specifically young, anxious children. The adult can frequently obtain the cooperation necessary to complete the examination.

The initial examination can be done without touching the patient. Simple inspection and observation can allow examination of lids, lashes, symmetry, conjunctiva, cornea, ocular motility, and pupillary responses (Fig. 13-1).[2]

Much of the examination may be car-

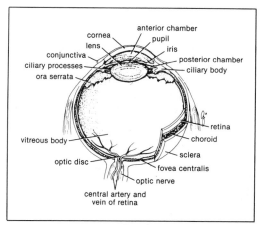

cornea — anterior chamber
lens — pupil
conjunctiva — iris
ciliary processes — posterior chamber
ora serrata — ciliary body
vitreous body — retina
— choroid
optic disc — sclera
— fovea centralis
optic nerve
central artery and
vein of retina

Figure 13–1. Anatomy of the eye. *(From R.S. Snell. Student's Aid to Gross Anatomy. Norwalk, Conn.: Appleton-Century-Crofts, 1986, p. 324.)*

ried out while the child is being held by a trusted adult, if necessary. A penlight, direct ophthalmoscope, and Wood's lamp are simple tools available in most emergency departments, and an adequate examination can be done using these tools. Ideally slit lamp microscopy is available for ocular emergencies and allows for a more complete examination.

Frequently health care providers, both nurses and physicians, are uncomfortable in caring for the patient with an ocular injury. This type of response should be recognized and evaluated so that optimal ex-

pertise and management can be provided to the patient and family. Any anxiety from the staff will be rapidly passed to the patient and may compound the existing problem. When staff remain calm and in control, the situation remains controlled.

Because the eye is such a delicate structure, a note of caution should be mentioned to limit the number of personnel examining an ocular injury. Any unnecessary repetition may cause the patient more anxiety and pain and with some injuries may cause further damage. All necessary equipment should be available so that a thorough examination can be done only as necessary. Table 13–1 sumarizes the equipment that should be available in the emergency department to treat pediatric ophthalmic emergencies. Table 13–2 contains ophthalmic medications that are frequently used in pediatric emergencies.

SPECIFIC OPHTHALMIC EMERGENCIES

Corneal Abrasions
Corneal abrasions are among the most common pediatric emergency eye problems. Causes frequently include fingernail scratches, foreign bodies, child abuse, and inappropriate use of contact lenses.

TABLE 13–1. OPHTHALMIC MEDICATIONS FOR PEDIATRIC EMERGENCIES

Topical anesthetic
  Proparacaine hydrochloride 0.5%
	Antibacterial ointment
	  Sodium sulfacetamide

Dilating drops
  Phenylephrine hydrochloride 2.5%, 10%
  Tropicamide 1% (Mydracil)
	Antibiotic drops
	  Gentamycin sulfate

Cycloplegic drops
  Cyclogel 1%
  Tropicamide 1%
  Atropine 0.5%, 1%
	Antibiotic ointment
	  Erythromycin
	  Gentamycin

Antibacterial drops
  Sodium sulfacetamide 10%
	Antihistamine—Decongestants
	  Naphazoline hydrochloride—Pheniramine maleate
	  Naphazoline hydrochloride—Antazoline phosphate

Adapted from G.R. Diamond, Ophthalmic emergencies. In G. Fleisher, & Ludwig (Eds.), Textbook of Pediatric Emergency Medicine. Baltimore: Williams & Wilkins, 1983, p. 879.

Adapted from G.R. Diamond. Ophthalmic emergencies. In G. Fleisher, & S. Ludwig (Eds.), Textbook of Pediatric Emergency Medicine. Baltimore: Williams & Wilkins, 1983, p. 879.

TABLE 13-2. OPHTHALMIC EQUIPMENT FOR PEDIATRIC EMERGENCIES

Visual acuity charts (Snellen chart, "E" game, Allen cards)
Lid speculum
Saline squeeze bottles for sterile irrigation
Fluorescein strips, sterile
Wood's lamp
Eye pads, sterile
Direct ophthalmoscope
Cotton swabs, sterile 6"
pH test strips
Paper tape
Silk tape

The abrasion occurs when the top layers of the cornea, only a six-cell–layer structure, are scratched or eroded. The abrasion can sometimes be seen with the unaided eye but is better visualized with fluorescein staining. Microscopic abrasions are frequently seen with poor fitting or over use of contact lenses.[3]

Assessment. Within a short time of injury, irritation and pain are usually present. The cornea is exquisitely sensitive to pain, and usually a child will complain readily.

Often, if the injury is not immediately recognized (which may happen with infants and very young children), the lid will swell, and the bulbar conjunctiva will appear reddened. The child may be photophobic, and the pupillary response may be sluggish in the affected eye. This may indicate the presence of ciliary spasm. When the eye is stained with fluorescein dye, the area of injury may become readily visible when examined with an ultraviolet (Wood's) lamp. This is because the subepithelial corneal cells pick up the bright green dye.

Management. When a corneal abrasion is suspected and corneal perforation has been ruled out, usually a topical anesthetic (proparacaine 0.5 percent) is instilled into the affected eye. The drop will burn on instillation, but an anesthetic effect is achieved immediately. Any pain and blepharospasm (uncontrollable lid spasm) will be eliminated for approximately 20 minutes. During this time the patient may be examined more thoroughly, and visual acuity may be obtained, if it was not possible to obtain earlier.

The patient should be instructed not to rub the eyes, as further damage may result.

Sometimes a topical anesthetic is not used in small children because of the greater danger of rubbing.

Treatment consists of a plan to allow the cornea to reepithelialize and to avoid infection. Since the constant opening and closing of the eyelids inhibits healing, the most commonly seen treatment plan includes the use of antibiotic ointment and application of a snug pressure patch.[4]

The use of ointment serves a dual purpose. It provides a protective emollient layer to the healing surface and provides antibiotic coverage to protect the cornea from infection. The application of ointment should be made to the lower conjunctival sac. It is easily instilled by gently pulling the lower lid down and squeezing a ribbon of ointment in along the palpebral conjunctival surface. The child will then blink it onto the corneal surface. Medication should never be instilled directly onto the corneal surface because of the possibility of trauma to cornea from contact with the ointment tube.

If the patient has ciliary spasm as well as abrasion, a cycloplegic agent may be instilled prior to instillation of ointment or application of a pressure patch. Ciliary spasm is seen when the patient is photophobic, the affected pupil reacts sluggishly, and the patient complains of pain even after the use of the topical anesthetic. For small children and infants, the installation of medication and application of a patch may require two people.[5]

The application of a pressure patch is most easily accomplished with the patient lying on his or her back. Usually two eye pads are used with paper or silk tape. The first pad should be placed against the lid and the second pad folded in thirds as a stint against the first patch. Tape is then applied from forehead to cheek. Each piece should be applied at the same angle. The ''X'' pattern should not be used in the application of a pressure patch.

Parent Education. Corneal abrasions generally heal rapidly without complications when properly treated. Usually a patch is necessary for only 24 hours. The patient should return to a health care provider for removal of the initial patch and should be reexamined every 24 hours until the abrasion is healed.

When treating infants and toddlers with corneal abrasions, frequently the patch is omitted. Most very small children will not tolerate the presence of a patch and are better managed by frequent instillation of antibiotic ointment.

Foreign Bodies in the Eye

Foreign bodies are also quite common in the pediatric age group. They may include small particles of metal, frequently iron, pencil graphite, or organic or vegetable matter, such as leaves, dirt, or wood. Foreign bodies may appear as superficial, imbedded, or intraocular.

Assessment. The presentation of a foreign body may be similar to that of a corneal abrasion, depending on the location of the foreign body.

A conjunctival foreign body may be easily visualized and may not cause any pain to the patient. A foreign body that is trapped under the upper or lower eyelid may be exquisitely painful as it is dragged across the cornea during blinking.

A corneal foreign body that is imbedded may cause minor irritation and may not bring a patient to the emergency department until a small ulcer is seen around the irritant. If a foreign body is metal, a rust ring may be observed 12 hours after it is embedded.

Management. Initial history of the incident will be helpful in identifying the nature of the foreign body. Knowing whether or not the object dropped into the eye (such as sand) or entered the eye with high velocity (such as metal) may be helpful to its removal.

Installation of proparacaine 0.5 percent will assist in examination and evaluation of the injury. Again, once blepharospasm has been alleviated, measuring visual acuity may be easier.

Superficial foreign bodies may be gently washed away with a stream of saline or may be removed by touching the foreign body with a moist, cotton-tipped applicator.

Imbedded foreign bodies (usually corneal) will not move with a saline irrigation and require removal with the tip of a 25-gauge needle or ophthalmologic spud. Topical anesthetic is used, and the procedure is painless. Such removal should be attempted only by a qualified practitioner.

Superficial and imbedded foreign bodies are treated as corneal abrasions after their removal.

These injuries are usually treated with a moderate acting cycloplegic agent prior to instillation of antibiotic ointment and patching. The injury should be evaluated 24 hours later to ensure that healing is taking place.

Occasionally patients will have all the signs and symptoms of foreign body or corneal abrasion and will give a history of a past event of corneal abrasion that was treated. Usually the injury was caused by a fingernail scratch or an organic foreign body. This may be recurrent erosion and should be referred to an ophthalmologist for follow-up. Treatment in the emergency department would be the same as for a corneal abrasion.

Intraocular foreign bodies may be caused by any material traveling at high velocity. Usually the offending agent is metal, and since metallic substances rust quickly in the eye, these foreign bodies are ophthalmologic emergencies. (For more details, see the section on penetrating trauma in this chapter.)

Parent Education. It is appropriate for nurses to determine the use of eye protection and to encourage its use as needed. Many ocular foreign bodies could be prevented if children used standard eye protection when indicated.

Encourage patients to return to their provider or ophthalmologist for follow-up even if the eye feels better when the patch is removed.

Blunt Trauma to the Eye

Blunt trauma is a frequent occurrence in the pediatric age group. It is most commonly seen with sports injuries involving small balls such as for tennis, racquet ball, field hockey, ice hockey, and street hockey. It is also seen as a result of inflicted injury from fists and may be seen with child abuse. In the school-aged child rubber bands may cause blunt trauma.

Assessment. A child who has experienced blunt trauma to the eye may have symptoms as mild as pain and redness or may develop decreased visual acuity or loss of vision in the affected eye along with systemic symptoms such as pain, headache, and vomiting. Systemic symptoms may indicate acute glaucoma.

Management. Children with blunt trauma to the eye may be classified as ocular emergencies. A thorough history and careful examination of visual acuity are critical in these patients. Intraocular bleeding or retinal hemorrhage may result in a lowered visual acuity and may be overlooked if not properly evaluated. These patients should be evaluated by direct ophthalmoscopy and should be hospitalized in the event of intraocular bleeding. They should be calmed and reassured while in the emergency department and encouraged not to cry. The bed or litter should be maintained at 30 degrees to avoid any increase in intraocular pressure, and a perforated metal or plastic eye shield should be put in place *without* an eye pad to prevent further damage to the eye.

Parent Education. If the patient is to be discharged, eye safety should be strongly reinforced. If the injury occurred at school, school authorities should be notified of the incident. Parents need to be included in any discharge teaching. Follow-up with an ophthalmologist should be planned.

Penetrating Trauma

Injuries that result in penetrating trauma are unfortunately seen too commonly in children. They may occur from knives, scissors, arrows, darts, sticks, and other sight-threatening objects. These injuries are frequently disabling and may result in significant or complete loss of sight if not managed expeditiously. Intraocular foreign bodies also fall into this category.

Assessment. Patients with a penetrating injury may appear with signs as minor as an abnormally shaped pupil or excessive fluid ''tearing'' from the eye. This fluid may be aqueous humor from the anterior chamber of the eye, indicating a penetrating injury. Patients may also present with pain, bleeding, and decreased visual acuity or visual loss.

Management. These patients and accompanying caretakers may need extensive reassurance. A visual acuity should be obtained. If severe injury is present, it will still be important to ascertain the perception of light or finger-counting capability.

Patients with any penetrating trauma should be maintained in a sitting position no lower than 30 degrees, and an eye shield should be placed over the affected eye without eye pad. They should be restricted from oral intake and it should be determined when they last ate or drank. An ophthalmologist should see the child as soon as possible, and at that point the injury should be surgically repaired. Ultimate restoration of sight may hinge upon initial treatment.

Penetrating foreign bodies should never be removed prior to evaluation by an ophthalmologist. Usually this removal, along with removal of intraocular foreign bodies, is performed under general anesthesia in a controlled environment. Pressure should never be applied to the eyeball if a penetrating injury has not been ruled out.

Parent Education. Penetrating trauma or foreign body injury usually results in admission to the hospital. Family members need to understand why the child is being admitted and why measures such as head elevation, eye shield, and sedation may be necessary. Family members or caretakers may feel tremendous guilt as a result of the accident and need support in regard to this issue.

Hyphema

A hyphema is obvious or microscopic bleeding into the anterior chambers of the eye almost always following direct trauma (Fig. 13–2). The bleeding frequently results from a torn iris root and may not have been present with initial injury. The patient will have a red and teary eye. Injuries that may result in hyphema include those

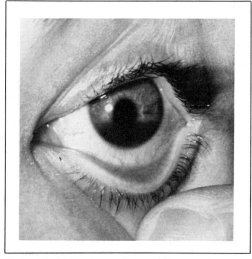

Figure 13–2. Hyphema. Note the presence of blood in the anterior chamber.

that are seen with blunt trauma as well as small missile injuries such as spit balls, elastic bands, and others. This injury differs from hemorrhage in the posterior chamber of the eye, but both injuries may be present.

Assessment. The patient presents with decreased visual acuity and a blood layer in the anterior chamber, which can best be seen in the upright position. There may be associated injuries to the iris, lens, retina, and filtration angle.

Management. Management and treatment of these children may differ depending on the severity of injury.

A microscopic hyphema seen in combination with a corneal abrasion may not be appreciated as such until subsequent evaluation 24 hours later by an ophthalmologist. In the emergency department if the patient complains of pain (over the brow) and decreased vision after topical anesthetic has been instilled, the child should be evaluated for traumatic iritis and microscopic hyphema. These patients are given a moderate- to long-acting cycloplegic agent. This is used to break the ciliary spasm and to rest the iris. Remember, visual acuity should not be tested after the instillation of cycloplegic or mydriatic agents. Visual acuity should be determined with initial examination. The microscopic hyphema may be managed as an outpatient.

A child with an obvious hyphema with bright bleeding into the anterior chambers of the eye will be admitted to the hospital for evaluation, rest, and possible sedation. In the emergency department the child should be maintained sitting or with the bed or litter at 30 degrees and an eye shield in place. The patient should be placed in a quiet room or area.

If the level of bleeding does not include the pupillary space, a visual acuity may be determined. Again, any perception of light or finger counting may eliminate the concern for possible bleeding in the posterior chamber. The posterior chamber cannot be easily evaluated if the anterior chamber is filled with blood.

Children are usually admitted because the incidence of rebleeding is quite common during the first few days after injury.[6] They are maintained on bedrest, and no reading is permitted. They may watch television with their eye shield in place at all times. It may be necessary to mildly sedate these children to maintain a quiet state. Parents and family need support and assistance in helping their child to rest during this critical period.

If a rebleed occurs, the presence of acute glaucoma should also be considered. This occurrence would limit a positive prognosis and resolution of the injury.

Parent Education. Teaching can be tailored to coincide with the injury but certainly will involve eye safety. Children who have eye shields in place need to understand why the shield is there and should be made aware of the risk of rein-

jury and rebleeding in the first few days after initial injury. Close follow-up by an ophthalmologist is important in promoting a resolution to this injury.

Rupture of the Eyeball
Rupture of the globe always occurs as the result of direct trauma such as a missile or a fall. Children with a global rupture are always treated as ophthalmic emergencies.

Assessment. The injured eye may appear as a red, bleeding pulp with corresponding history. The patient may be agitated, disoriented, and diaphoretic.

Management. These patients should be restricted from oral intake on arrival in the emergency facility and should be assessed for shock. An ophthalmologist should be called. These children should be prepared for the operating room.

Under anesthesia a detailed examination can be carried out and reconstructive procedures instituted. If the globe has been lost, muscles are sutured to the initial staged repair, and the orbit is prepared for prosthesis.

Fracture of the Orbital Walls
Orbital fractures are not uncommon and are seen most frequently in the adolescent age group. A fracture usually results from large-object impact such as a fist or brick.

Assessment. Lid swelling and bruising may be seen along with facial bruising and asymmetry. Diplopia may or may not be present. Proptosis may be present. History of the incident is useful in arriving at a diagnosis.

Management. These patients should be reassured and carefully examined to determine the location or locations of fractures.

The patient may be initially examined and scheduled for x-ray examination and computed tomography (CT).

Presence of subcutaneous emphysema may indicate fracture of the ethmoid air cell, while a cerebrospinal fluid (CSF) rhinorrhea may indicate fracture of the orbital roof. Lateral wall fractures may result in damage or transection of the optic nerve and visual loss.

The most common fractures are seen in the floor and lateral walls of the orbit. For floor fractures the orbital contents may be trapped in the cracks. Generally management is maintained on an outpatient basis for 10 days to 2 weeks to allow for resolution of edema. At that point, if indicated, surgery will be performed to correct asymmetry, entrapment, or defect.

Chemical Injuries to the Eye

Chemical burns, either acid or alkali, are among the most serious of ocular emergencies. Of the two types, alkali burns are far more disastrous to long-term prognosis. Cigarette burns should also be mentioned, as they are commonly seen in the infant and toddler age group. Usually these burns involve the cornea and may be accidental in nature.

Assessment. With any of the burns above the patient will have severe blepharospasm and pain. The child and caretakers may both be agitated and upset.

Management. The initial management step is *immediate* irrigation with whatever liquid is available. Use of a sink and tepid water from the tap is fine while saline irrigation is being set up. A saline irrigation with intravenous tubing allowing for at least 2 liters of fluid is ideal. Topical proparacaine 0.5 percent may be used to assist in reducing blepharospasm and to allow for a thorough irrigation of both conjunctival sacs. The pH should be measured and should be between 7 and 8 at the end of irrigation. Recheck pH in 10 minutes after lavage has stopped.

Alkali substances in the eye continue to destroy the ocular structures after the initial exposure. Rapid intervention can minimize the disastrous consequences of lye burns. Lye burns can damage internal ocular structures rapidly upon contact with the cornea. Acid burns are less common than lye and are usually related to chemistry class accidents or battery explosion. These injuries are severe but usually less so than lye burns. Cigarette burns are treated as corneal abrasions once the ash and debris has been flushed.

Careful attention should be paid to the history of the incident. This is very important when evaluating small children, as they may be at risk for further injury if they have access to lye- or acid-based household products or if they have been burned by cigarettes.

If a child is severely burned by heat or chemical and the cornea is badly damaged, the prognosis may be grim. Chemically damaged tissue does not lend itself well to repair, and the resulting eye may be both painful and blind.

The most important treatment is prompt and thorough lavage.

Parent Education. If injuries are minor and the patient is discharged, assist the family with follow-up plans. Parents or caretakers are likely to feel extreme guilt if they perceive themselves as negligent regarding this accident. They need the support and understanding of the health care team during this difficult time.

NOTES

1. L.D. Ervin-Nulvey, L.B. Nelson, & D. Freeley. Pediatric eye trauma. *Pediatric Clinics of North America* December 1983, p. 999.
2. Ibid., p. 1171.
3. Ibid., p. 1175.
4. Ibid., p. 1176.

5. Ibid., p. 1177.
6. J. Calhoun. Eye trauma. In R.M. Reece (Ed.), *Manual of Emergency Pediatrics* (3rd ed.). Philadelphia: W.B. Saunders, p. 545.

BIBLIOGRAPHY

Beauchamp, S. Causes of visual impairment in children. *Pediatric Annals* 9(1)(1980):16–22.

Boyd-Monk, H. (Ed.). Ophthalmic nursing. *Nursing Clinics of North America* September 1981, p. 381–485.

Calhoun, J. Eye disorders. In Reece, R.M. (Ed.), *Manual of Emergency Pediatrics*, 3rd ed. Philadelphia: W.B. Saunders, 1984, pp. 536–542.

Cardona, V.D. Ocular/orbital injuries. In *Trauma Reference Manual*. Bowie, Md.: Brady Co, 1985, pp. 101–108.

Cohen, S.A., & Walton, D. Eye trauma. In Cohen, S.A. (Ed.), *Pediatric Emergency Management*. Bowie, Md.: Brady Co, 1982, pp. 44–45.

Diamond, G.R. Ophthalmic emergencies. In Fleishner, G., & Ludwig S. (Eds.), *Textbook of Pediatric Emergency Medicine*. Baltimore: Williams & Wilkins, 1983.

Gigliotti, F., Williams, W.T., Hayden, F.G., &

Hendley, O. Etiology of acute conjunctivitis in children. *Journal of Pediatrics* 98(April 1981):531–536.

Harley, R.D. Ocular manifestations of child abuse. *Pediatric Ophthamology Strabismus* 17, no. 5(1980):5–13.

Helveston, E., & Ellis, F. *Pediatric Ophthamology Practice*. St. Louis: Mosby, 1980.

McNeer, K.W. Pediatric opthalmology. *Pediatric Nursing* 5, no. 6(1979):47–49.

Moore, R., & Schmitt, B. Conjunctivitis in children. *Clinical Pediatrics* 18, no. 1(1979):26–39.

Oglesby, R. Eye trauma in children. *Pediatric Annals* 6, no. 5(1977):5–22.

Pascoe, D.J., & Grossman, M. *Quick Reference to Pediatric Emergencies*. Philadelphia: Lippincott, 1978.

Sheehy, S.B. Eye emergencies. In Sheehy, S.B., & Barber, J. (Eds.), *Emergency Nursing: Principles and Techniques* (2nd ed.). St. Louis: Mosby, 1985, pp. 276–294.

Strafford, P.W., & Tepas, J.J. Triage and treatment of injuries of the eyes, ears, nose, and mouth in children. *Topics in Emergency Medicine* 4, no. 3(October 1982):19–27.

Wang, I.M. Ophthalmic emergencies. In Crain, E.F., & Gershel, J.C. (Eds.), *A Clinical Manual of Emergency Pediatrics*. Norwalk, Conn.: Appleton-Century-Crofts, 1986, pp. 405–414.

EMERGENCY DEPARTMENT CARE GUIDE FOR THE CHILD WITH AN OPHTHALMIC EMERGENCY

Nursing Diagnosis	Interventions	Evaluation
Sensory perceptual alterations: visual, related to eye injury	Assess eyes for signs of injury or orbital fractures Assess child's visual acuity Irrigate eyes with normal saline if there is a history of chemical injury Apply eye patch if indicated	Child's vision returns to normal Chemicals are removed from eyes Eye patch is applied and remains in place
Potential for infection related to eye injury	Instill ophthalmic antibiotic ointment or drops as ordered Instruct parents in proper method of instilling ophthalmic antibiotics Obtain history of child's immunization status	Child's eyes remain free from infection Child remains protected from tetanus

Nursing Diagnosis	Interventions	Evaluation
	Administer tetanus prophylaxis as indicated	
Alteration in comfort: pain related to eye injury	Administer topical ophthalmic anesthetic as ordered Administer systemic analgesic as ordered	Child describes a decrease in pain
Fear related to eye injury and treatment procedures	Carefully explain all procedures to child Reassure child that his or her vision should return to normal within a specified period of time Allow parents to remain with child throughout visit in emergency department Allow young children to sit on parent's lap during examination and treatment	Child demonstrates an understanding of procedure Child remains calm and cooperative
Knowledge deficit related to eye safety and discharge care	Instruct child and parents in eye safety precautions Instruct parents in administration of eye medications Instruct parents in changing eye pads Explain to parents the importance of follow-up appointment	Parents and child demonstrate knowledge of eye safety Parents demonstrate knowledge of administration of medications and use of eye pads Parents demonstrate an understanding of importance of keeping follow-up appointment

14 | Cardiac Dysrhythmias

Martha A.Q. Curley

Recently there has been increased recognition of cardiac dysrhythmias in the pediatric population. This phenomena can be attributed to several factors, such as widespread monitoring, improved assessment techniques, and increased survival of critically ill children. The emergency department nurse is responsible for identifying the pediatric patient at risk, correctly identifying the dysrhythmia in the pediatric population, assessing the hemodynamic effect of the dysrhythmia, assisting in the initiation and evaluation of treatment, and for child and family education.

Unlike the adult, the pediatric norms vary according to the patient's age. Abnormal rhythms among pediatric patients most frequently result from an abnormal quality, not quantity, of coronary artery blood flow (i.e., the pediatric patient usually has normal coronary arteries). This necessitates a change in the emergency department nurse's focus, as both of these factors—age and status of coronary arterial blood—must be considered whenever a pediatric rhythm strip is assessed for normalcy, cardiac dysrhythmias, electrolyte imbalance, and drug effects.

Improved diagnostic techniques have helped to define the pediatric norms. Southall, Johnson, et al.[1] and Southall, Richards, et al.[2] have identified transient significant sinus bradycardia, sinus arrest with junctional escape rhythms, first-degree heart block, second-degree–type 1 atrioventricular (AV) block, and premature atrial and ventricular contractions without hemodynamic compromise in healthy pediatric populations. Dysrhythmias occurring without hemodynamic compromise in those with morphological normal hearts are generally considered benign in pediatrics and do not require treatment.[3]

CLINICAL SIGNIFICANCE

Like the adult, the risks posed by cardiac dysrhythmias in the pediatric population include further deterioration in cardiac rhythm and decreased cardiac output. Note the rapid deterioration in cardiac rhythm that occurred in a 9-month-old (Fig. 14–1). This rhythm strip illustrates the equable potential for rapid electrical compromise in a pediatric patient.

The risk of dysrhythmia-related, decreased cardiac output is more significant in the pediatric population. Cardiac output is the product of stroke volume multiplied times the heart rate. Stroke volume is determined by three factors: preload, afterload, and contractility. Preload is determined by ventricular end-diastolic pressure or the quantity of blood in the ventricle just prior to systole. Frank Starling's law demonstrates the positive relationship between contraction force and end-diastolic pressure or volume. Afterload refers to the resistance or impedance faced by the ventricle during systole, while contractility is the speed and efficiency of

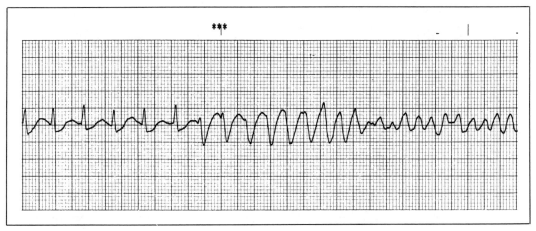

Figure 14–1. Rapid electrical compromise in a 9-month-old: supraventricular tachycardia to ventricular tachycardia to ventricular fibrillation.

myocardial shortening independent of preload and afterload.

Like adults, older children and adolescents are capable of increasing their stroke volumes to maintain cardiac output when their heart rate decreases, but infants and young children cannot. (Cardiac output is maintained by an increase in stroke volume, i.e., bradycardia increases diastolic filling time, thus increasing preload and the resultant contraction.) Infants have relatively "fixed" stroke volumes, so their cardiac outputs depend almost entirely upon their heart rate and rhythm. The limited capacity to increase stroke volume in this age group is due to their decreased ventricular compliance. This can be attributed to the greater proportion of noncontractile myocardial tissue to contractile myocardial mass.[4] This relationship is illustrated nicely in Figure 14–2. Note that point B, the normal infant and young

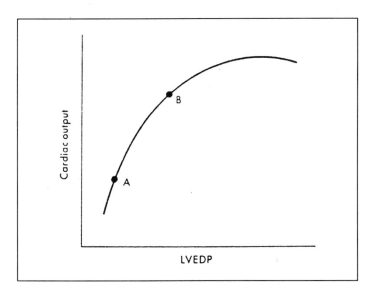

Figure 14–2. Frank Starling's ventricular function curve depicting the normal, resting adult state (point A). Infants and young children seem to have a resting point higher on the curve (point B) or perhaps have a slightly different curve altogether. The net difference represents decreased ventricular compliance in infants. *(Reproduced with permission from E.K. Daily, & J.S. Schroeder. Techniques in Bedside Hemodynamic Monitoring. St. Louis: Mosby, 1985, p. 167.)*

child's resting point, is higher on the volume pressure curve, illustrating their normal decreased ventricular compliance. Ventricular compliance and stroke volume will increase with growth and development, as illustrated in Figure 14–3, at which point the child is less dependent upon heart rate for cardiac output as illustrated in Figure 14–4.

While infants and young children are very much heart rate/rhythm dependent, ironically they are, at the same time, sympathetically immature. Infants have decreased sympathetic receptor density and responsiveness[5] and thus are more sensitive to parasympathetic or vagal stimulation. (Sympathetic stimulation provides a positive chronotropic, inotropic, and dromotropic [speed of impulse conduction] effect, while parasympathetic stimulation provides a negative chronotropic and dromotropic effect.) For this reason procedures that may induce vagal stimulation or valsalva induction should always be performed with care in the pediatric patient, i.e., suctioning, obtaining rectal temperatures, and invasive procedures. Maturation of sympathetic innervation occurs with time, as noted by an improved response to catecholamine administration.

ETIOLOGY

Immaturity of the conduction system and its autonomic innervation are contributing factors in the pathogenesis of cardiac dysrhythmias in the newborn and infant populations. It has been noted that cardiac dysrhythmias occur more frequently in the first week of life than in later infancy.[6] This can be attributed to the numerous metabolic and functional alterations taking place during the transition from intrauter-

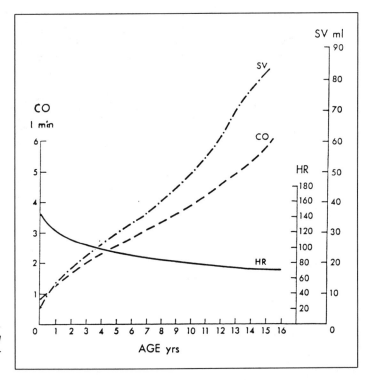

Figure 14–3. This shows diagrammatically the postnatal changes in cardiac output (CO), heart rate (HR), and stroke volume (SV) from birth to 16 years. *(Reproduced with permission from A.M. Rudolph. Congenital Diseases of the Heart. Chicago: Year Book, 1974, p. 27.)*

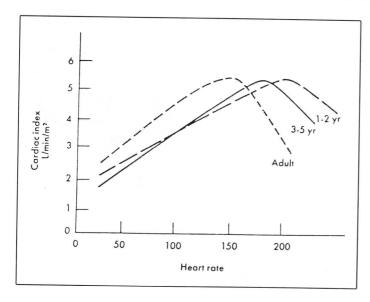

Figure 14-4. Heart rate versus cardiac index graph illustrating relative differences among age groups. Data for this figure are based on the 50th percentile norms for cardiac index and heart rate. *(Reproduced with permission from E.K. Daily, & J.S. Schroeder. Techniques in Bedside Hemodynamic Monitoring. St. Louis: Mosby, 1985, p. 142.)*

ine to extrauterine life. The parasympathetic dominance in this population also places newborns and infants at greater risk for vagal-induced dysrhythmias, e.g., significant sinus bradycardia, sinus arrest with junctional escape rhythms, first-degree heart block, second-degree–type 1 AV block.

Cardiac dysrhythmias occur more frequently in pediatric patients with structurally normal hearts.[7] Cardiac dysrhythmias are *seldom* primary events but occur secondary to an abnormal quality of blood delivered to the myocardium and conduction system. Abnormalities may include electrolyte imbalance (especially potassium and calcium), hypoxia (which is the usual case during pediatric arrests), hypercapnia, acidosis, and alterations in temperature (both hyperthermia and hypothermia). Drug-related problems may also induce cardiac dysrhythmias in the pediatric population, e.g., digoxin toxicity, excessive beta adrenergic blocking agent or catecholamine use, and ingestion of toxins (both accidental or intentional).

The pediatric patients in whom cardiac dysrhythmias are a special risk include those children who arrive at the emergency department following surgical repair of congenital heart defects. Surgical injury can alter impulse initiation and conduction around the site of the surgical repair. Bradycardias may occur after cardiac surgery involving the atria, e.g., Senning or Mustard procedures for transposition of the great arteries, atrial septal defect repair, or endocardial cushion defect repair. Ventricular dysrhythmias may be present in the pediatric patient with ischemic or hypertrophied ventricles, e.g., those with aortic stenosis or tetralogy of Fallot, those with postright ventriculotomy, those who were older at the time of cardiac surgery, and especially in pediatric patients with residual intracardiac defects.[8]

Cardiac dysrhythmias may also be the first indication that a problem exists. Such is the case in acquired heart disease, e.g., myocarditis and myocardiopathy.

RHYTHM ASSESSMENT

The normal pediatric (as well as adult) cardiac rhythm depends upon repetitive impulse initiation at a single site in the heart, the sinoatrial (SA) node, and orderly sequence of propagation and repolarization. Tremendous electrocardiographic (ECG) changes occur during cardiac system maturation. It is imperative that nurses consider these normal age-related changes when assessing the pediatric rhythm strip (Table 14–1). In addition, nurses must also consider the patient's activity level, medication history, and possible positive cardiac history.

When assessing the rhythm strip a systematic approach is essential so that nothing is overlooked. Assessment includes the heart rate and rhythm, P wave, P : QRS relationship, PR interval, QRS duration, ST segment, T wave, QTc interval, and U wave. To apply the following parameters a standardized lead II rhythm strip should be used, i.e., paper speed at 25 mm/second and a 1-mv stimulus equals a 10 mm stylus deflection.

Heart Rate

The heart rate gradually increases during the first week to month of life, then gradually decreases throughout childhood (Table 14–1). Sinus tachycardia and sinus bradycardia are defined as heart rates above and below the child's norm for age. Individual heart rates should reflect the patient's cardiac output requirement, e.g., a sinus tachycardia of 200 is an expected finding in a febrile, hypovolemic, or crying 1-month-old, whereas sinus bradycardia of 90 is expected in the afebrile, normovolemic, sleeping infant. Incongruent findings are abnormal and necessitate further nursing assessment.

The inherent rates of other pacemaker sites within the heart are, as with the adult, slower than that of the sinus node but also have age-dependent faster rates. These accessory pacemaker sites (atrial, junctional, and ventricular) are capable of producing faster escape and accelerated

rhythms than seen in the adult population. Pediatric ectopic rhythms cannot be defined on the basis of heart rate alone.

Cardiac Rhythm

The cardiac rhythm should be fairly regular. Sinus arrhythmia is common and is considered normal because of the parasympathetic dominance experienced in this population. Significant sinus arrhythmia, i.e., doubling of the R to R interval with expiration, can frequently be observed in the pediatric patient with increased intrathoracic or intracerebral pressures.

P Wave

The P wave should be evaluated for configuration, amplitude, duration, and consistency. In pediatrics the P wave duration is less than 0.08 second and 2.5 mm in height (0.06 second and 3 mm in the neonate). The P wave should be gently rounded and should always be consistent in configuration. Right and left atrial hypertrophy can be easily assessed from a standardized lead II rhythm strip. Right atrial hypertrophy may be present when the P wave is consistently taller than the norms, while left atrial hypertrophy may be present when the P wave duration is consistently wider than the norms.

P : QRS Relationship

The P : QRS relationship is always 1 : 1. Sinus node discharge produces atrial depolarization, the P wave, then ventricular depolarization, the QRS complex. Any P wave occurring after a T wave should be followed by a QRS complex. If this is not the case the nurse should suspect second- or third-degree heart block.

PR Interval

The PR interval varies according to the patient's age and heart rate (Table 14–1). Ten percent of normal children have first-

TABLE 14–1. PEDIATRIC ECG NORMS

Age	Heart Rate[a]		P Wave		Maximum PR Interval[a]	QRS Duration[d]	QTc Interval[d]
	Mean[b]	Range[b]	Height[c]	Duration[d]	Heart Rate[b] – Interval[d]		
0–24 hr	119	94–145	<3.0	<0.06	94–145<0.11	0.04–0.05	<0.49
1–7 days	133	100–175	<3.0	<0.06	Same as 0–24 hr	0.04–0.05	<0.49
8–30 days	163	115–190	<3.0	<0.06	Same as 0–24 hr	0.04–0.05	<0.49
1–3 mo	154	124–190	<2.5	<0.08	91–110<0.14 111–130<0.13 131–150<0.12 >150<0.11	0.04–0.05	<0.49
3–6 mo	140	111–179	<2.5	<0.08	Same as 1–3 mo	0.04–0.05	<0.49
6–9 mo	140	112–177	<2.5	<0.08	Same as 1–3 mo	0.04–0.05	<0.425
9–12 mo	140	112–177	<2.5	<0.08	91–110<0.15 111–150<0.14 >150<0.10	0.05–0.06	<0.425
1–3 yr	126	98–163	<2.5	<0.08	Same as 9–12 mo	0.05–0.06	<0.425
3–5 yr	98	65–132	<2.5	<0.08	65–132<0.16	0.06–0.08	<0.425
5–8 yr	96	70–115	<2.5	<0.08	<90<0.18 >90<0.16	0.06–0.08	<0.425
8–12 yr	79	55–107	<2.5	<0.08	Same as 5–8 yr	0.08–0.10	<0.425
12–16 yr	75	55–102	<2.5	<0.08	Same as 5–8 yr	0.08–0.10	<0.425

[a]C.H. Cole (Ed.). *The Johns Hopkins Hospital: The Harriet Lane Handbook* (10th ed.). Chicago: Year Book, 1984.
[b]Per minute.
[c]In millimeters.
[d]In seconds.

degree heart block.[9] Prolonged PR intervals may also result from ectopic atrial rhythms, digoxin effect, fever, myocarditis, and some congenital heart lesions, such as an endocardial cushion defect, Ebstein's anomaly of the tricuspid valve, and L-transposition of the great arteries. Short PR intervals (less than 0.08 second to 3 years of age, 0.10 second from 3 to 16 years of age, and 0.12 in children more than 16 years of age)[10] may be present with junctional rhythms, Wolff-Parkinson-White syndrome, and tricuspid atresia.

QRS Duration

The QRS duration, correlating with ventricular mass, can be as short as 0.04 second in the premature infant, less than 0.06 second in infants, and 0.08 second in children (Fig. 14–5). Anything wider *than the child's normal* QRS duration is associated with aberrant conduction, which may occur secondary to bundle branch blocks and premature ectopic contractions.

ST Segment

The ST segment is assessed from the j point, which is identified as the junction of the QRS complex and ST segment. The ST segment may deviate 1 mm from the baseline and be considered normal. The ST segment is abnormal if it is horizontal to or slopes downward from the j point. Digoxin "effect" commonly produces deviation of the ST segment opposite to that of the QRS complex, e.g., elevation with negative QRS complexes and depression with positive QRS complexes. Other deviations are common to those seen in the adult population, e.g., elevation with inflammation or depression with ventricular strain or ischemia.

T Wave

The T wave should be directed along the same plane as the QRS complex, e.g., positive when the QRS complex is positive and negative when the QRS complex is negative. Deviations may be due to primary repolarization abnormalities, such as myocarditis, or may be secondary to depolarization abnormalities, such as premature ventricular contractions.

QT Interval

The QT interval varies according to heart rate, so a QTc, a QT interval corrected for heart rate, should always be calculated in the pediatric patient. The QTc is calculated by dividing the square root of the R to R

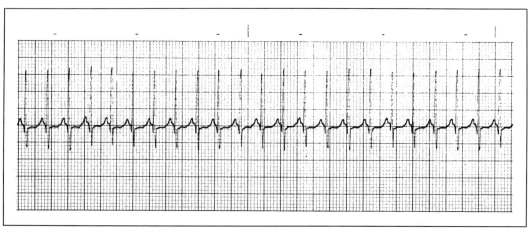

Figure 14–5. Sinus tachycardia in a 2-week-old; note normal QRS duration: 0.04 second.

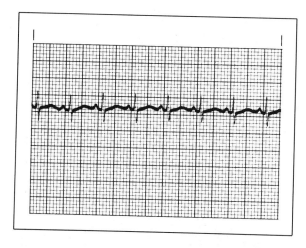

Figure 14–6. Calculation of the QTc. The R-R interval measures 0.40 second; its square root is 0.632. The QT interval measures 0.28 second. The calculated QTc is 0.443. *(Reproduced with permission from M.A.Q. Curley. Pediatric Cardiac Dysrhythmias. Bowie, Md.: Brady Communications, 1985, p. 158.)*

interval into the measured QT interval (Fig. 14–6). The normal should not exceed 0.49 second up to 6 months of age and 0.425 thereafter. Calcium levels alter the QTc interval. Short QTc intervals occur in patients on digoxin. Prolonged QTc intervals occur in patients on quinidine and in those with genetically inherited prolonged QT interval syndrome.[11]

U Waves

Occasionally U waves may be present. Current hypotheses concerning the genesis of these waves include delayed repolarization of the terminal Purkinje's network. Their clinical significance has yet to be determined.

CLINICAL ASSESSMENT

Whenever dysrhythmias are noted in the pediatric age group it is imperative that nurses first assess their hemodynamic effect. These effects or symptoms can be easily understood by noting that to maintain blood pressure when the cardiac output fails, the systemic vascular resistance must increase appropriately. (Blood pressure is equal to the cardiac output times the systemic vascular resistance.) The compensatory peripheral vasoconstriction will produce cool dusky extremities; pallor or mottled skin; increased core with decreased surface temperatures and signs of decreased organ perfusion, e.g., decreased urine output (less than 1 cc/kg/hour or 2 cc/kg/hour in the neonate); decreased level of consciousness; and lethargy. Increased systemic vascular resistance also produces poor capillary refill, which is the quickest and best indicator of cardiac output. Note that the blood pressure will be temporarily maintained even when the cardiac output is significantly decreased. Astute nursing assessment and rapid appropriate intervention is required to improve cardiac output before compensatory mechanisms fail.

REALIZING THE POTENTIAL OF THE LEAD II RHYTHM STRIP

The standardized pediatric lead II rhythm strip can be used as a rapid assessment tool to assist in the detection of electrolyte imbalance, toxic tricyclic overdose, and digoxin toxicity. Intracranial hypertension will also produce many ECG changes, such as tall or notched T waves, U waves, short then prolonged QTc intervals. These alterations are ominous in that they may occur prior to neurologic deterioration and occurrence of lethal ventricular dysrhythmias.[12] Dysrhythmias pose a significant risk in the cerebral hypertensive patient because a rhythm disturbance may alter the mean arterial pressure and thus compromise cerebral perfusion pressure. (Cerebral perfusion pressure is a product of the mean arterial pressure minus the intracranial pressure.)

Electrolyte Imbalance

Whereas serum potassium and calcium levels may be misleading, the rhythm strip graphically represents the ionic movement of these two cations across excitable cardiac cell membranes. Thus the rhythm strip is a useful tool in the assessment of total body potassium and calcium concentration. Hyperkalemia will initially produce tent-shaped T waves, then progress to wide QRS durations, increased PR intervals, broad P waves, atrial arrest, and eventually a sine-wave pattern representing QRS complex and T wave fusion (Fig. 14–7). Hypokalemia will produce depressed ST segments, flattened T waves, and U waves. Hypercalcemia produces a short QTc, while the opposite is true with hypocalcemia.

Tricyclic Overdose

The rhythm strip may also provide more information about the pharmacologic effects of a medication at the receptor level than serum concentrations provide. Prolonged QRS durations (Figs. 14–8 and 14–9) can serve as a guide to immediately predict the incidence of significant complications to tricyclic overdose, i.e., seizures, ventricular dysrhythmias, and death, faster and better than toxic drug levels.[13] The posttricyclic ingestion patient presenting to the emergency department with a prolonged QRS interval should be admitted to an intensive care unit.

Digoxin

Therapeutic digoxin levels are difficult to interpret in infants due to the wide therapeutic range observed in this population. Infants require higher doses of digoxin per kilogram of body weight, and individual levels may be considered toxic if assessed by adult standards. Peak serum digoxin levels of 0.8 to 2.2 ng/ml are considered normal, but 3.5 ng or higher may be required in select infants before therapeutic effects are evident.

Inconclusive level assessment necessitates an accurate lead II rhythm assessment. Digoxin "effect" reflects the normal

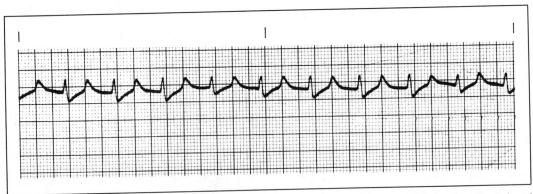

Figure 14–7. Hyperkalemic sine-wave pattern in a 3-year-old; serum potassium was 10.0 mmol/L. *(Reproduced with permission from M.A.Q. Curley. Pediatric Cardiac Dysrhythmias. Bowie, Md.: Brady Communications, 1985, p. 153.)*

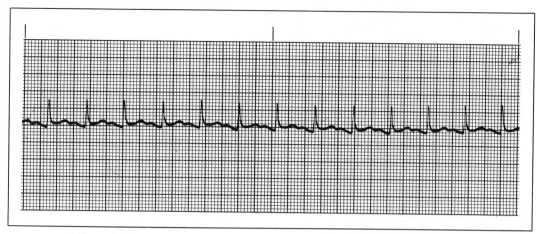

Figure 14–8. Ten hours posttricyclic overdose; note QRS duration: 0.08 second.

ECG changes produced by this drug and are not related to dose, therapeutic range, or toxicity. These changes are minor bradycardia, minor first-degree heart block, short QTc interval, and ST segment deviation opposite to that of the QRS complex. Digoxin toxicity can be identified as significant sinus bradycardia, ectopic atrial activity, junctional tachycardia, AV blocks, and premature ventricular contractions. Any dysrhythmia not present before the digoxin was started may be related to digoxin toxicity (Figs. 14–10, 14–11, 14–12, and 14–13).

Digoxin effect and toxicity are related to potassium ion concentration. Potassium and digoxin compete for myocardial cell-binding sites. Thus increased serum potassium decreases digoxin's effect, while a decreased serum potassium increases the potential for digoxin toxicity. Premature infants and children with renal dysfunction have a decreased rate of digoxin excretion, so they are at increased risk for digoxin toxicity.

Prior to the administration of digoxin to the pediatric patient, the nurse should obtain a lead II rhythm strip and assess for

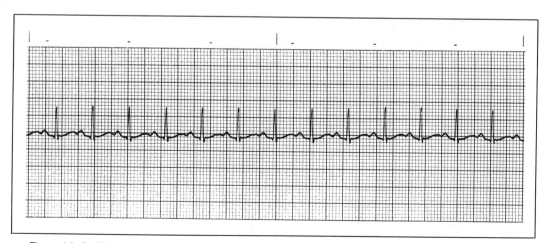

Figure 14–9. Eight hours after rhythm strip in Figure 14–8 was obtained; QRS duration: 0.04 second.

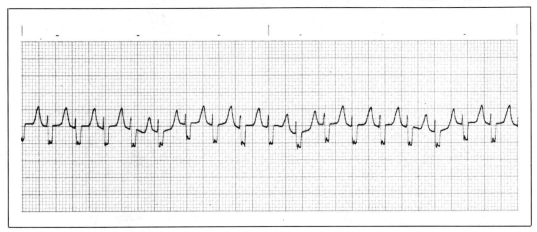

Figure 14–10. Digoxin toxicity in a 7-month-old: junctional tachycardia. *(Reproduced with permission from M.A.Q. Curley. Pediatric Cardiac Dysrhythmias. Bowie, Md.: Brady Communications, 1985, p. 161.)*

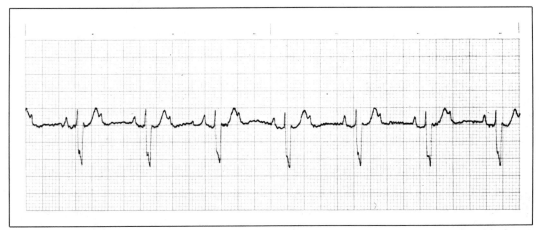

Figure 14–11. Digoxin toxicity in a 7-month-old: 2 : 1 type II AV block. *(Reproduced with permission from M.A.Q. Curley. Pediatric Cardiac Dysrhythmias. Bowie, Md.: Brady Communications, 1985, p. 137.)*

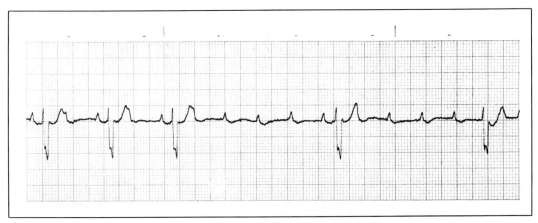

Figure 14–12. Digoxin toxicity in a 7-month-old: 2 : 1 type II AV block to third-degree heart block. *(Reproduced with permission from M.A.Q. Curley. Pediatric Cardiac Dysrhythmias. Bowie, Md.: Brady Communications, 1985, p. 138.)*

262

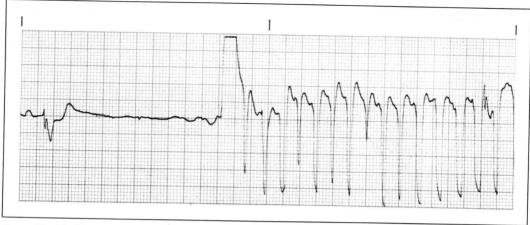

Figure 14–13. Digoxin toxicity in a 7-month-old: ventricular tachycardia. *(Reproduced with permission from M.A.Q. Curley. Pediatric Cardiac Dysrhythmias. Bowie, Md.: Brady Communications, 1985, p. 122.)*

the presence of digoxin effect and toxicity. The rhythm strip along with a notation concerning the heart rate and especially cardiac rhythm should be posted in the patient's record for future reference.

SPECIFIC PEDIATRIC DYSRHYTHMIAS

Supraventricular Tachycardia

Supraventricular tachycardia (SVT) is the most common tachydysrhythmia seen in pediatrics.[14] SVT occurs most often in males under 4 months of age with structurally normal hearts. Occasionally associated congenital heart defects such as Ebstein's anomaly, L-transposition of the great arteries, or tricuspid atresia are identified.

Etiology and Pathophysiology. The etiology of SVT is thought to be the result of increased automaticity of a single focus above the bundle of His or a reentry mechanism. The first is uncommon, having a gradual onset and end, and is frequently noted to be interspersed with sinus tachycardia. The reentry mechanism is thought to be the most common cause of SVT in

pediatrics. In this situation the rapid ventricular rates are perpetuated over a reentry circuit consisting of two functionally distinct pathways or limbs (Fig. 14–14). Both limbs have different repolarization times and allow bidirectional (normal antegrade or retrograde) impulse travel.

SVT is initiated by a premature supraventricular contraction (PSVC) that cannot conduct through one of the limbs (A) because it is still in a refractory period from a previous contraction, but the impulse is able to conduct slowly in a normal antegrade fashion through the other limb (B). By the time the slow antegrade conduction is complete through pathway B, pathway A has had time to complete repolarization, so it is ready to accept an impulse. The *same* impulse is then conducted in a retrograde fashion along pathway A *and* also down to the ventricles, causing ventricular depolarization. When the impulse completes retrograde travel through pathway A, pathway B is again ready to accept another impulse, so the process repeats itself and the reentry circuit is established. Note that this process requires unidirectional block and perfect reciprocal timing of the refractory periods of both limbs.

Intranodal or extranodal reentry cir-

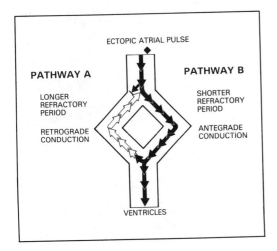

ECTOPIC ATRIAL PULSE

PATHWAY A

LONGER
REFRACTORY
PERIOD

RETROGRADE
CONDUCTION

PATHWAY B

SHORTER
REFRACTORY
PERIOD

ANTEGRADE
CONDUCTION

VENTRICLES

Figure 14–14. Schematic representation of the reentry mechanism. *(Reproduced with permission from M.A.Q. Curley. Pediatric Cardiac Dysrhythmias. Bowie, Md.: Brady Communications, 1985, p. 84.)*

cuits can be established. Intranodal reentry frequently occurs within the AV node, as it contains a dense network of fibers that can facilitate alternate pathway conduction. Extranodal reentry occurs when an active accessory pathway outside the AV node exists, such as in Wolff-Parkinson-White syndrome.

It should be noted that although tachycardia usually increases cardiac output, this mechanism is effective only to a certain point. Excessive tachycardia (SVT) shortens the rapid ventricular filling time that occurs during diastole and thus compromises stroke volume and cardiac output (Fig. 14–15). Excessive tachycardia will also limit diastolic coronary artery filling, thus compromising myocardial perfusion at a time of increased need.

History. Clinical presentation of a patient with SVT depends upon the ventricular

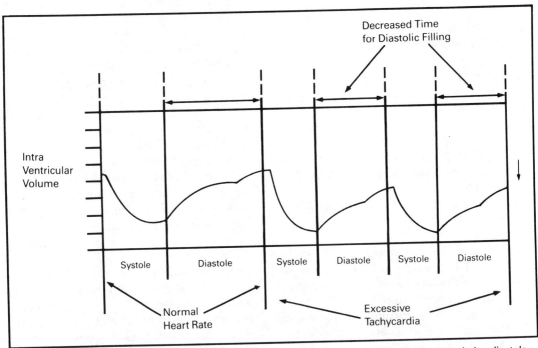

Decreased Time
for Diastolic Filling

Intra
Ventricular
Volume

Systole   Diastole   Systole   Diastole   Systole   Diastole

Normal
Heart Rate

Excessive
Tachycardia

Figure 14–15. Excessive tachycardia shortens the rapid ventricular filling phase/time that occurs during diastole. This mechanism limits stroke volume.

rate, duration, and the underlying condition of the patient's myocardium. SVT is considered a medical emergency in infants under 1 year of age because if the rapid ventricular rates, 260 to 320, are allowed to continue for more than 24 hours, the infant will develop congestive heart failure and then cardiogenic shock. Nursing history usually contains parent's descriptions of poor feeding, pale skin color, and irritable, then lethargic infant behavior. SVT is better tolerated in the older child whose ventricular rates are much slower, approximately 160. Older children may come to the emergency department complaining of chest pain, feeling "sick," palpitations, or abdominal pain with or without vomiting. Children with concurrent congenital heart disease exhibit a decreased hemodynamic tolerance to SVT. These children decompensate rapidly and arrive in severe congestive heart failure or cardiogenic shock.

Assessment. In addition to the nursing history, definitive electrophysiologic criteria (Fig. 14–16) for SVT includes an abrupt onset, which is why SVT is occasionally labeled paroxysmal atrial tachycardia (PAT). The rhythm is monotonously regular, as each QRS complex is an exact replication of the previous. The P waves usually cannot be identified because they are either located on top of the preceding T wave or buried in the previous QRS complex. If visualized the P waves will be different from the patient's normal. If measured the PR interval will be longer than the child's normal. Most often there is 1 to 1 conduction to the ventricles. The QRS complexes are usually normal, but occasionally a rate-related aberrancy, most often RBBB, may be present. Aberrant QRS complexes may also be present when bypass tracts, congenital heart disease, or surgical RBBB is present. In these cases the wide QRS SVT may resemble ventricular tachycardia. ST segment depression, indicating myocardial ischemia, is a frequent finding during SVT or after conversion to normal sinus rhythm.

Physical assessment findings are consistent with those of congestive heart failure and cardiogenic shock.

Management. The treatment goal centers around what is known about the mechanism of this dysrhythmia, e.g., it is known that SVT most frequently is initiated by a

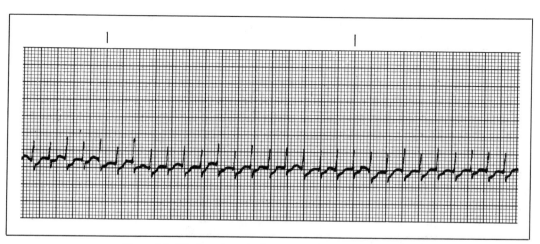

Figure 14–16. Supraventricular tachycardia in a 2-week-old.

PSVC and maintains itself through a reentry mechanism involving the AV node. The treatment goal would then be to break the reentry circuit by interrupting the reciprocating refractory periods of the reentry limbs. Prior to any medical treatment nursing must obtain a high-quality cardiac tracing and an adequate intravenous line and must have ready full resuscitation drugs and defibrillator.

Vagal maneuvers, which induce a negative dromotropic effect through the AV node, are usually attempted first, as they are the least invasive. As anticipated, the vagal maneuvers will induce an all-or-none response with SVT (while only slowing a sinus tachycardia). Vagal maneuvers include unilateral carotid massage, gag reflex induction, rectal stimulation, and ocular pressure. The latter is avoided in the neonate, as it may precipitate retinal detachment. The diving or mammalian reflex has gained popularity due to its effectiveness.[15] The diving reflex is present at birth and produces strong vagal stimulation and sympathetic withdrawal. To induce the diving reflex an ice-cold, wet face cloth, 4C to 5C, is placed abruptly on the infant's face for approximately 6 to 7 seconds, or the older child's face (over 8 years of age)

is immersed in an ice-cold water bath (Figs. 14–17 and 14–18). As anticipated, nurses must instruct, coach, and support the older child to help him or her accomplish this maneuver with as little fear as possible.

Drug therapy for SVT includes verapamil and digoxin. Verapamil has been found to be very effective in the treatment of SVT and will convert 90 percent of the cases within minutes.[16] Verapamil slows both antegrade and retrograde conduction through the AV node by prolonging its effective refractory period. It breaks the reentry circuit by interrupting the reciprocating refractory periods of the reentry limbs. Verapamil is administered very slowly, over 1 minute. Onset is rapid, at 3 to 5 minutes after administration. Because of its negative inotropic effects, verapamil is not the drug of choice if congestive heart failure is present. Side effects are rare but include AV block, extreme bradycardia, hypotension (due to its smooth muscle relaxant effect), and asystole. These side effects occur more frequently with concomitant beta blocker therapy and in the infant under 1 year of age. Treatment of the side effects includes calcium chloride, atropine, and isupril administration.

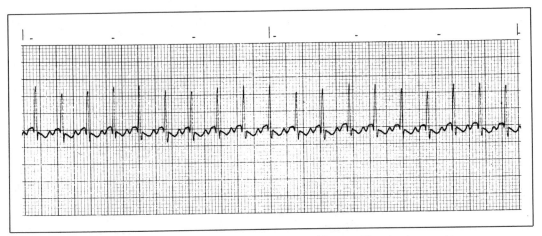

Figure 14–17. Supraventricular tachycardia in a 10-year-old; note slower rate.

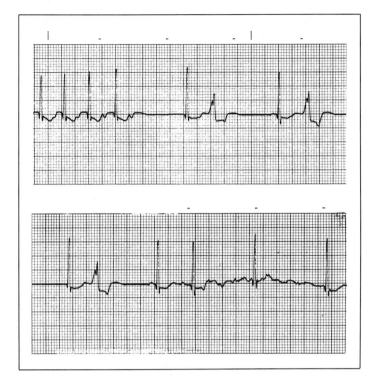

Figure 14-18. Supraventricular tachycardia to ventricular bigeminy to atrial fibrillation then normal sinus rhythm in the same 10-year-old; induced by the diving reflex.

Digoxin is also very effective in the medical management of SVT, but this drug may take up to 10 hours to be effective. Digoxin's vagotonic action directly affects the conductivity and refractoriness of the AV node. One may administer digoxin, wait a few hours, then retry vagal maneuvers.

Cardioversion is the treatment of choice if altered hemodynamic stability or congestive heart failure is present. Mild anesthesia with valium or pentothal is necessary prior to this procedure. The largest paddle size that provides the best chest wall contact should be used. The dose is 0.2 to 1.0 joules/kg. The *lowest possible* joules must be used if the patient is on digoxin because this procedure may induce irreversible cardiac arrest.[17]

Psychosocial Support and Parent Education. SVT can be very frightening to a

child and his or her family. All require nursing support and information congruent with their cognitive development. Patients arriving at the emergency department in SVT are admitted to a monitored pediatric unit for further study. Patient and family teaching includes use of the cardiac monitor with specific information about the alarm system. Parents are not socialized to the hospital environment and consider all alarms worrisome. Families need to know that until the patient is stabilized on medication, recurrences of SVT are common.

Infants usually remain on digoxin for at least 1 year postconversion to normal sinus rhythm. After that time the drug can usually be discontinued without recurrence of SVT. Parents of infants will be able to rest more comfortably at night with the information regarding the 24-hour time element of SVT progression to cardiogenic shock. Older children are assessed on an individual basis. They usually do not require long-term pharmacologic therapy but are taught vagal maneuvers to control their symptoms.

Wolff-Parkinson-White Syndrome

Etiology and Pathophysiology. Normally the atria and the ventricles are separated by a fibrous structure called the trigone, which prevents supraventricular impulses from being conducted to the ventricles except through the AV node and bundle of His. In Wolff-Parkinson-White syndrome (WPW) additional muscle links, capable of impulse conduction, penetrate the trigone connecting the atria to the ventricles. Infants with WPW usually arrive at the emergency department in SVT. Twenty-two percent of infants with SVT have bypass tracts.[18] The activity through bypass fibers is enhanced by the infant's predominant parasympathetic activity. With maturation of sympathetic innervation, these bypass fibers frequently become quiescent, so one can then expect the episodes of SVT to decrease in the first year of life or to disappear spontaneously by the second year. The incidence of WPW is again greater in males at a 3 : 2 ratio, and there is also a greater incidence of WPW in children with congenital heart defects, i.e., Ebstein's anomaly, L-transposition, and familial cardiomyopathy.

Electrophysiologic studies have identified various bypass tracts such as Kent, James, and Mahaim fibers.[19] The atrioventricular bypass tracts, or Kent bundles, are the most common. They appear along the free wall and septal regions of both left and right ventricles. They present electrophysiologically as a short PR interval, indicating AV node bypass; a delta wave, indicating preexcitation or premature activation of the ventricular myocardium; and abnormal QRS due to the delta wave. The delta wave (Fig. 14–19) can be identified as a slurred upstroke of the QRS complex that prolongs the QRS duration, therefore resembling an interventicular conduction delay. The AV nodal bypass tracts, or James fibers, associated with Lown-Ganong-Levine syndrome, connect the atrium to the bundle of His. Their course is perinodal or intranodal, and they produce a short PR interval and normal QRS complex. The nodoventricular bypass tract (connecting the AV node to ventricles) and fasciculoventricular bypass tract (connecting the bundle of His to ventricles) are Mahaim fibers. They are uncommon and produce a normal PR interval, a small Delta wave, and thus an abnormal QRS complex.

WPW's SVT is of two types: an antegrade or retrograde impulse that travels through the AV node. Normally the accessory pathway has a longer refractory period, so the PSVC will first conduct normally through the AV node, then in a retrograde fashion through the accessory pathway producing a normal QRS configuration. This is referred to as orthodromic reentry. Occasionally the PSVC will first conduct through the accessory pathway, then back up in a retrograde fashion through the AV node, producing an abnormal QRS configuration. This is referred to as antidromic reentry. This type is more serious because of the loss of the protective filtering mechanism of the AV node.

History. Clinical presentation to the emergency department is the same as for SVT.

Assessment. Defining electrophysiologic criteria for WPW SVT includes an abrupt onset and end and rapid regular rhythm. The P waves usually cannot be identified but are different from the patient's normal. The PR interval will be longer than the patient's normal with orthodromic reentry and shorter than the patient's nor-

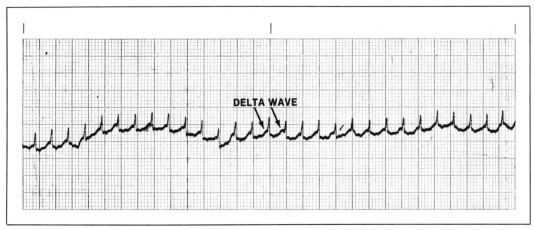

Figure 14–19. Supraventricular tachycardia associated with Wolff-Parkinson-White syndrome; note delta waves. *(Reproduced with permission from M.A.Q. Curley. Pediatric Cardiac Dysrhythmias. Bowie, Md.: Brady Communications, 1985, p. 87.)*

mal with antidromic reentry. Most often there is 1 to 1 conduction to the ventricles. The QRS complexes are normal with orthodromic reentry and widened by delta waves with antidromic reentry. SVT occurring secondary to antidromic WPW may resemble ventricular tachycardia. ST segment depression, indicating myocardial ischemia, may also be present.

Physical assessment findings are consistent with those of congestive heart failure and cardiogenic shock.

After conversion to normal sinus rhythm, sinus impulse conduction to the ventricles may alternate between the AV node and the accessory pathway. This is usually first identified by nurses who observe normal cycles (with normal PR intervals and QRS complexes) interspersed with abnormal cycles of short PR intervals and wide QRS complexes. When observed it is documented by a lead II rhythm strip and is brought to the attention of the physician.

Management. Treatment includes pharmacologic ablation of either limb, so it is the same for SVT except for a few precau-

tions. Digoxin and verapamil are used cautiously if bypass tracts are suspected because while increasing the AV node refractory period they may also decrease the refractoriness of the bypass tracts, thus enhancing conduction to the ventricles. If the patient were to therefore develop atrial flutter or fibrillation with antidromic reentry, all impulses will conduct down to the ventricles, causing ventricular flutter or fibrillation. This effect is uncommon in infants but poses a significant risk in the older child and adolescent.[20]

Propranolol is useful in WPW because it decreases conduction velocity through the AV node. Propranolol also decreases the automaticity of ectopic atrial pacemaker sites and thus decreases the frequency of PSVCs. Side effects include high-degree AV block, bradycardia, asystole, and hypotension. Treatment of these side effects includes isuprel. Propranolol may be used alone or in combination with quinidine, which prolongs the refractory period of the bypass tract. Other drugs that prolong the refractory period of bypass tracts include procainamide and amiodarone.

Psychosocial Support and Parent Education. Psychosocial support and education are fundamentally the same as for SVT. Patients are admitted to a monitored pediatric unit for further study, and reoccurrences of WPW SVT are common. Patients with WPW usually remain on antidysrhythmic therapy longer than 1 year.

Ventricular Dysrhythmias

Etiology and Pathophysiology. Most premature ventricular contractions (PVCs) in pediatrics are benign, yet fear accompanies them because of their ominous nature in the adult population. Idiopathic PVCs with uniform fixed coupling, constant interval from the last normal QRS to the premature QRS, are common in adolescents. PVCs without fixed coupling, multiform PVCs, bigeminy, or couplets in the asymptomatic pediatric patient with a normal heart also may be idiopathic, but consultation with a pediatric cardiologist is warranted.

Table 14–2 provides a summary of the pathogenesis of PVCs in the pediatric population. Severe metabolic or electrolyte imbalance is the most frequent cause of PVCs in the pediatric population.

Management. Treatment depends upon the severity of the ventricular dysrhythmia, as evidenced by an altered hemodynamic effect. Concern for whether PVCs will initiate an unstable ventricular tachydysrhythmia may be warranted in the following cases[21]:

1. Structural heart disease is present. This is related to areas of potential slow conduction or unidirectional block, which can sustain a ventricular tachydysrhythmia.
2. Variable or short coupling intervals are present, especially in the child with significant structural heart disease. The R-on-T phenomena is rare in the pediatric patient with a normal heart.
3. Multiform PVCs are present.
4. The child has prolonged QT interval syndrome. A prolonged QT interval represents prolongation of a vulnerable period in the cardiac cycle, thus the patient is more susceptible to malignant ventricular dysrhythmias and sudden death.[22]
5. A family history of lethal dysrhythmias is present.
6. The PVCs increase with exercise. The opposite is also true, i.e., no treatment is indicated if the dysrhythmias decrease with exercise. Increases may be secondary to endogenous catecholamine release or subendocardial ischemia.
7. A possible history of related dysrhythmia side effects is present, i.e., syncope, idiopathic seizures.

TABLE 14–2. ETIOLOGY OF PREMATURE VENTRICULAR CONTRACTIONS IN THE PEDIATRIC POPULATION

Severe metabolic or electrolyte imbalance: hypoxia, acidosis, hypoglycemia, hyperkalemia/hypokalemia, hypercalcemia/hypocalcemia	Pediatric coronary artery disease: Kawasaki disease, anomalous origin of the left coronary artery
Cardiac manipulation: central line insertion	Mitral valve prolapse
Congenital heart disease: postventriculotomy, residual lesions	Prolonged QT interval syndromes
Cardiomyopathy and myocarditis: idiopathic hypertrophic subaortic stenosis (IHSS)	Toxic drug levels: digoxin, quinidine, sympathomimetics, phenothiazines, tricyclics
	Nervous system induced
	Cardiac tumors
	No identifiable cause

Acute treatment always takes place concurrently with acid-base and fluid-electrolyte correction. Correction of these disturbances may alone convert the ventricular dysrhythmia. Use of antidysrhythmic medications in pediatrics still involves a great deal of empiricism. Lidocaine is effective in 85 percent of the cases, so it is the first drug of choice. The dose of 1.0 mg/kg is administered by intravenous push. Lidocaine is rapid acting but is of short duration, so a repeat bolus is necessary every 3 to 5 minutes until the nurse prepares an intravenous drip. To prepare the infusion, 120 mg of lidocaine is added to 5 percent dextrose in water to make a total volume of 100 cc. This solution is infused at a rate of 1 to 2.5 cc/kg/hr and delivers 20 to 50 μg/kg/min. Therapeutic levels are not clear in the developing heart, so it is difficult to extrapolate adult values to pediatrics. Lidocaine is totally metabolized in the liver, so liver function studies should be followed carefully.

Procainamide is the second drug of choice but is used with caution, as severe peripheral vasodilatation, and thus profound hypotension, can occur. The negative inotropic effects of procainamide are more significant in patients with an already depressed myocardium. This drug may also enhance or induce AV block. Nurses should follow the PR, QRS, and QT intervals, as they should not increase more than 25 percent over pretreatment values.

Bretylium can be used when lidocaine and procainamide are found to be ineffective. Side effects include severe hypotension. Bretylium should not be used if digoxin-related dysrhythmias are suspected because it may enhance them.

Other drugs include propranolol (effective in children with prolonged QT interval syndrome, mitral valve prolapse, obstructive cardiomyopathy), phenytoin (effective in the digoxin toxic or postoperative cardiac surgical patient with residual hemodynamic effects), and amiodarone (new in pediatrics but seemingly effective in patients with ventricular tumors and cardiomyopathies).

Supraventricular Tachycardia versus Ventricular Tachycardia

Ventricular tachycardia may exceed 250 beats per minute in the infant, thus it may be difficult to differentiate supraventricular tachycardia from ventricular tachycardia (VT). Ventricular tachycardia usually produces an irregular rhythm with varied beat-to-beat QRS configurations that are different from the normal supraventricular-originated beat. Supraventricular tachycardia, as noted previously, will be monotonously regular. Unlike the adult, rate-related SVT aberrancy is uncommon in pediatrics. Factors that favor SVT aberrancy include RBBB, presence of bypass tracts (WPW), preceding ectopic atrial activity, and no compensatory pause. The nurse may also scan previous rhythm strips, if available, looking for obvious premature supraventricular or ventricular beats, as the rhythm may be of the same configuration. Fusion complexes, those that resemble both a supraventricular and ventricular beat, frequently appear at the onset or end of the run of ventricular tachycardia. The presence of associated P waves is only present with SVT. This observation can be facilitated by changing the lead system. Lastly, the hyperkalemic sine-wave pattern should also be considered when assessing a pediatric accelerated ventricular rhythm.

Pediatric Arrest-related Dysrhythmias

Unlike the adult population, asystole and bradydysrhythmias account for 90 percent of all pediatric cardiac-arrest dyrhythmias, whereas ventricular dysrhythmias only account for the remaining 10 percent.[23] Ventricular dysrhythmias are observed more frequently in patients with congenital heart disease, in those who experience prolonged resuscitation attempts, in those who are beyond the neonatal period, and in patients who weigh more than 2.23 kg.[24] The nurse should be cognizant of the fact that pediatric arrest dysrhythmias most often occur secondary to hypoxia, acidosis, and electrolyte disturbance, so primary correction is of utmost importance. Table 14–3 provides a review of the most common dysrhythmias observed during pediatric arrests and includes appropriate treatment modalities.

Defibrillation. The basic procedure for defibrillation in pediatrics is the same as in the adult. The defibrillation dose is 2 joules/

TABLE 14–3. PEDIATRIC ARREST-RELATED DYSRHYTHMIAS

Dysrhythmia	Treatment/Comments[a]
Asystole Idioventricular rhythm	Atropine, bicarbonate Epinephrine, Isuprel (IVR)
Bradycardia	Atropine/Isuprel, bicarbonate, epinephrine
Second-degree heart block	Atropine (type I); Isuprel/pacemaker (type II)
Third-degree heart block	Pacemaker If unavailable: atropine, Isuprel, bicarbonate, epinephrine
PVCs	Lidocaine, procainamide bretylium, propranolol, phenytoin, amiodarone
Ventricular tachycardia	Cardioversion at 0.2 to 1.0 joules/kg, lidocaine, bretylium
Ventricular fibrillation	Defibrillation at 2 joules/kg, repeat doubling joules Consider bicarbonate, epinephrine lidocaine, bretylium

[a]Primary treatment *always* includes the ABCs (airway, breathing, circulation) of cardiopulmonary resuscitation and correction of hypoxemia, acidosis, hypoglycemia, potassium and calcium imbalance, hypothermia, and vagal stimulation.

kg, which may be doubled after first reassessing the need for additional hypoxia and acidosis correction. Epinephrine may be used to convert fine ventricular fibrillation (VF) to a coarser form that is easier to defibrillate. Bretylium has been found to be effective in treating both VT and VF, which are refractory to conventional therapy, i.e., lidocaine and repeated countershocks. Defibrillators capable of measuring the amount of delivered joules are essential in pediatrics because of the small doses used. More than usual precautions are necessary to prevent arcing of the electrical current over the small pediatric patient's chest wall, i.e., avoid cross paddle and conduction medium contact. Paddle size and digoxin precautions have been discussed previously.

Psychosocial Support and Parent Education. Much parental and patient fear is associated with any cardiac dysfunction. Parents and children need information and support. Parents' baseline knowledge is frequently oriented to adult coronary artery disease, so they may fear sudden death from a ''heart attack.'' The nurse can be instrumental in providing appropriate reassurance and easily comprehended information to child and family. A parent teaching booklet that specifically addresses pediatric cardiac dysrhythmias is available from the American Heart Association.[25] This teaching aid contains illustrations that can be used in part to facilitate individualized family instruction.

NOTES

1. D.P. Southall, P.G.B. Johnson, J.M. Richards, & E.A. Shinebourne. Study of heart rate and rhythm in normal school children. *British Heart Journal* 42(1979):234.
2. D.P. Southall, J. Richards, P. Mitchell, D.J. Brown, J.G.B. Johnston, E.A. Shine-

bourne. Study of cardiac rhythm in healthy newborn infants. *British Heart Journal* 43(1980):14–20.

3. A. Garson. Pediatric dysrhythmias: Distinguishing those that require intervention. *Consultant* November 1984, 99–126.

4. A. Zaritsky, & B. Chernow. Medical progress: Use of catecholamines in pediatrics. *Journal of Pediatrics* 105, no. 3(1984):341–350.

5. Ibid., pp. 341–350.

6. J.H. Moller, & W.A. Neal. *Heart Disease in Infancy.* New York: Appleton-Century-Crofts, 1981.

7. M. Slota, L. Beerman, & G. Sanchez. Pediatric electrocardiography overview. *Heart & Lung* 11, no. 1(1982):69–82.

8. E. Krongrad. Postoperative arrhythmias in patients with congenital heart disease. *Chest* 85, no. 1(1984):107–113.

9. L. Chameides. Reading a child's ECG. *Emergency Medicine* 16, no. 2(1984):78–111.

10. M.K. Park, & W.G. Guntheroth. *How to Read Pediatric ECGs.* Chicago: Year Book, 1981, p. 36.

11. B.M. Barnes. Romano-Ward syndrome. *Critical Care Nurse* 3, no. 4(1983):22–24.

12. L.J. Zegeer. Systemic cardiovascular effects of intracranial disorders: Implications for nursing care. *Journal of Neurosurgical Nursing* 16, no. 3(1984):161–167.

13. M.T. Boehnert, & F.H. Lovejoy. Value of the QRS duration versus the serum drug level after an acute overdose of tricyclic antidepressants. *New England Journal of Medicine* 313, no. 8(1985):474–478.

14. A. Garson, P.C. Gillette, & D.G. McNamara. Supraventricular tachycardia in children: Clinical features, response to treatment, and long-term follow-up in 217 patients. *Journal of Pediatrics* 98, no. 6(1981):875–882.

15. R.L. van der Horst, & A.R. Hastreiter. Initiation of the diving reflex in neonates with supraventricular tachycardia. *Heart & Lung* 9, no. 3(1980):518–520.

16. E. Shahar, Z. Barzilay, & M. Frand. Verapamil in the treatment of paroxysmal supraventricular tachycardia in infants and children. *Journal of Pediatrics* 98, no. 2(1981):323–325.

17. L. Chameides, R. Melker, J.R. Raye, D. To-dres, & P.H. Viles. Guidelines for defibrillation in infants and children. In K.M. McIntyre, & A.J. Lewis (Eds.), *Textbook of Advanced Cardiac Life Support.* Dallas: American Heart Association's Office of Communications, 1983, pp. 266–267.

18. Garson, Gillette, & McNamara, Supraventricular tachycardia in children, pp. 875–882.

19. W.M. Gersony, & A.J. Hordof. Cardiac arrhythmias. In J.D. Dickerman, & J.F. Lucey (Eds.), *Smith's—The Critically Ill Child: Diagnosis and Medical Management.* Philadelphia: W.B. Saunders, 1985, pp. 242–286.

20. Chameides, Reading a child's ECG, pp. 78–111.

21. Gersony, & Hordof, Cardiac arrhythmias, pp. 242–286.

22. Barns, Romano-Ward syndrome, pp. 22–24.

23. American Heart Association. Standards and guidelines in resuscitation and emergency cardiac care: Pediatric advanced life support. *JAMA* 255, no. 21(1986):2961–2969.

24. C.K. Walsh, & E. Krongrad. Terminal cardiac activity in pediatric patients. *American Journal of Cardiology* 51(1983):557–561.

25. American Heart Association. *Abnormalities of Heart Rhythm: A Guide for Parents.* Publication No. 50-058-A/11-83-75M. Dallas: American Heart Association's Office of Communications, 1983.

BIBLIOGRAPHY

American Heart Association. *Abnormalities of Heart Rhythm: A Guide for Parents.* Publication No. 50-058-A/11-83-75M. Dallas: American Heart Association's Office of Communications, 1983.

American Heart Association. Standards and guidelines in resuscitation and emergency cardiac care: Pediatric advanced life support. *JAMA* 255, no. 21(1986):2961–2969.

Barnes, B.M. Romano-Ward syndrome. *Critical Care Nurse* 3, no. 4(1983):22–24.

Boehnert M.T., & Lovejoy, F.H. Value of the QRS duration versus the serum drug level after an acute overdose of tricyclic antidepressants. *New England Journal of Medicine* 313, no. 8(1985):474–478.

Chameides, L. Reading a child's ECG. *Emergency Medicine* 16, no. 2(1984):78–111.

Chameides, L., Melker, R., Raye, J.R., et al. Guidelines for defibrillation in infants and children. In McIntyre, K.M., & Lewis, A.J. (Eds.), *Textbook of Advanced Cardiac Life Support*. Dallas: American Heart Association's Office of Communications, 1983, pp. 266–267.

Curley, M.A.Q. *Pediatric Cardiac Dysrhythmias*. Bowie, Md.: Brady Communications, 1985.

Garson, A. The six most common acute cardiac dysrhythmias in children. *Applied Cardiology* 12, no. 5(1984):16–21.

Garson, A. Pediatric dysrhythmias: Distinguishing those that require intervention. *Consultant* November 1984, 99–126.

Garson, A., Gillette P.C., & McNamara, D.G. Supraventricular tachycardia in children: Clinical features, response to treatment, and long-term follow-up in 217 patients. *Journal of Pediatrics* 98, no. 6(1981): 875–882.

Gersony, W.M., & Hordof, A.J. Cardiac arrhythmias. In Dickerman, J.D., & Lucey, J.F. (Eds.), *Smith's—The Critically Ill Child: Diagnosis and Medical Management*. Philadelphia: W.B. Saunders, 1985, pp. 242–286.

Gillette, P.C. Advances in the diagnosis and treatment of tachydysrhythmias in children. *American Heart Journal* 102, no. 1(1981):111–119.

Johnson, D.L. Pediatric arrhythmias: A nursing approach. *Dimensions of Critical Care Nursing* 2, no. 3(1983):147–157.

Krongrad, E. Postoperative arrhythmias in patients with congenital heart disease. *Chest* 85, no. 1(1984):107–113.

Levin, D.L., Morriss, F.C., & Moore, G.C. *A Practical Guide to Pediatric Intensive Care* (2nd ed.). St. Louis: Mosby, 1984.

Moller, J.H., Neal, W.A. *Heart Disease in Infancy*. New York: Appleton-Century-Crofts, 1981.

Park, M.K., & Guntheroth, W.G. *How to Read Pediatric ECGs*. Chicago: Year Book, 1981.

Plauth, W.H. Kawasaki disease. *Critical Care Quarterly* 8, no. 3(1985):39–47.

Shahar, E., Barzilay, Z., & Frand, M. Verapamil in the treatment of paroxysmal supraventricular tachycardia in infants and children. *Journal of Pediatrics* 98, no. 2(1981):323–325.

Slota, M., Beerman L., & Sanchez, G. Pediatric electrocardiography overview. *Heart & Lung* 11, no. 1(1982):69–82.

Southall, D.P., Johnson, P.G.B., Richards, J.M., & Shinebourne, E.A. Study of heart rate and rhythm in normal school children. *British Heart Journal* 42(1979):234.

Southall, D.P., Richards, J., Mitchell, P. et al. Study of cardiac rhythm in healthy newborn infants. *British Heart Journal* 43(1980):14–20.

van der Horst, R.L., & Hastreiter, A.R. Initiation of the diving reflex in neonates with supraventricular tachycardia. *Heart & Lung* 9, no. 3(1980):518–520.

Walsh, C.K., & Krongrad, E. Terminal cardiac activity in pediatric patients. *American Journal of Cardiology* 51(1983):557–561.

Webster, H. Hemodynamic monitoring in children. In Daily, E.K., & Schroeder, J.S. (Eds.), *Techniques in Bedside Hemodynamic Monitoring*. St. Louis: Mosby, 1985.

Zegeer, L.J. Systemic cardiovascular effects of intracranial disorders: Implications for nursing care. *Journal of Neurosurgical Nursing* 16, no. 3(1984):161–167.

Zaritsky, A., & Chernow, B. Medical progress: Use of catecholamines in pediatrics. *Journal of Pediatrics* 105, no. 3(1984):341–350.

EMERGENCY DEPARTMENT CARE GUIDE FOR THE CHILD WITH A DYSRHYTHMIA

Nursing Diagnosis	Interventions	Evaluation
Alteration in cardiac output: decreased, related to dysrhythmia	Continually assess and support airway, breathing, and circulation Assess skin color and temperature Obtain ECG Insert intravenous line Administer medications as ordered Prepare child and equipment for defibrillation	Vital signs remain stable Child's skin is pink and warm Child's heart rhythm returns to normal sinus rhythm
Alteration in tissue perfusion: cardiopulmonary, related to dysrhythmia	Continually assess and support airway, breathing, and circulation Perform cardiopulmonary resuscitation if cardiac arrest occurs Assess capillary refill time Administer medications as ordered Obtain arterial blood gas samples Continually monitor serum electrolytes	Vital signs remain stable Child's heart rhythm returns to normal sinus rhythm Capillary refill is adequate Arterial blood gas values remain normal Child's serum electrolytes remain within normal limits
Alteration in urinary elimination pattern: decreased output related to decreased circulation	Carefully monitor urinary output Insert Foley catheter Carefully monitor fluid intake	Urinary output remains normal (> 1 ml/kg/hr)
Fear related to hospital procedures and strange environment	Carefully explain all procedures and equipment to child Allow parents to remain with child once child's condition has stabilized	Child appears relaxed Child engages in appropriate play activities
Knowledge deficit (parental) related to child's cardiac condition	Explain procedures to parents Continually inform parents of child's condition Explain the etiology of dysrhythmias to parent Instruct parents on the discharge care of child, or prepare parents for hospital admission	Parents demonstrate an understanding of procedures and child's condition Parents demonstrate an understanding of the cause of child's dysrhythmias Parents demonstrate knowledge in the home care of their child

15 | Cardiac Emergencies

Ruth A. Fisk
Susan J. Kelley

To suggest that one or two clues can establish a diagnosis would be unwise; however, if the history and physical assessment of a child reveal known congenital heart disease, a recent cardiac surgical procedure, presence of pleuritic chest pain, or a pericardial friction rub, the emergency department nurse should consider these findings to be strongly suggestive of a cardiac component in the child's present illness.

Endocarditis

Infective endocarditis (also called bacterial endocarditis) is an infection of the endocardium, or lining of the heart, which may invade the valves and conduction system as well. It is uncommon in the general pediatric population and when encountered occurs almost exclusively in those with congenital or acquired heart disease. Of those affected, approximately 80 percent have congenital defects, 15 percent acquired heart disease, and the remainder no heart disease.[1] Precipitating events may be cardiovascular or other major surgery, invasive diagnostic or dental procedures, or focal infections elsewhere in the body. Mortality, although decreasing, is still significant (15 to 20 percent)[2] and is higher in children less than 10 years of age and in individuals of any age infected with *Staphylococcus aureus*.[3]

Etiology and Pathophysiology. The infectious process begins with the introduction of bacteria into the blood stream. All individuals, with or without congenital heart disease, are subject to at least transient bacteremia secondary to the most mundane activities, such as tooth brushing or chewing candy. In the vast majority of cases the body's own immune system destroys the bacteria before any harm is done. Since only a small percentage of those with congenital heart disease (9.7 to 13 percent)[4] ever develop endocarditis, it may be speculated that those so affected have a fundamental deficiency in their immune system. Those with defects in which turbulent or high-velocity blood flow can cause changes in the endocardium, such as tetralogy of Fallot or ventricular septal defect, or those with prosthetic materials within the heart, have been shown to be at greatest risk.

Once established in the endocardium, the microorganisms multiply and may form vegetations on valve surfaces or invade the conduction system. Fragments of vegetative material may eventually break off and create systemic or pulmonary emboli, depending upon the location of the infected area; sequelae may thus include neurologic deficits, hematuria, dyspnea, and other localized phenomena.

History. Early signs and symptoms may be subtle and nonspecific. The child (endocarditis is extremely rare in infants) may have a history of recurrent low grade fevers, malaise, anorexia, and fatigue. Clinical presentation may be obscured by oral antibiotics that have been prescribed for a suspected lesser infection. Such partial treatment may delay identification of the causative organism and consequent prescription of appropriate antibiotics. In more advanced cases high fever with shaking chills, a change in the cardiac examination, splenomegaly, and evidence of emboli may be present. If the child arrives with symptoms of infective endocarditis and acute cardiac changes, such as new aortic insufficiency, heart block, or congestive heart failure, he or she should be considered acutely ill, and immediate surgical intervention to replace the infected valve may be required. In this acute stage hemodynamic changes can occur rapidly, and the child must be closely monitored while treatment decisions are made.

Careful history taking should include the child's cardiac diagnosis and identification of possible predisposing events or focal infections, as well as any antibiotic recently prescribed. Information should be gathered regarding onset of present symptoms and daily patterns of temperature fluctuation; changes in behavior or other symptoms attributable to embolic phenomena must be noted.

Assessment. Nursing assessment should include a complete set of vital signs and auscultation of the heart with notation of any irregularities in rhythm; the presence, location, and quality of murmur(s) should be documented, with special attention to the early diastolic murmur of aortic insufficiency, best heard at the left midsternal border. The child must be evaluated for signs and symptoms of congestive heart failure (tachypnea, retractions, grunting or nasal flaring, tachycardia, diaphoresis, hepatomegaly, jugular venous pressure visible more than 3 cm above the clavicle, and facial or pedal edema). Splenomeg-

aly may be present. Examination of the skin may reveal evidence of emboli, as may funduscopic examination. Neurologic screening should be done to determine if any deficits exist.

Laboratory Data. Blood cultures must be drawn from these children even in the absence of classical clinical findings. At least two, and preferably three, sets of cultures must be drawn before any treatment is initiated. Other blood tests are of little definitive diagnostic value. Urine should be checked for the presence of hematuria, and urine and sputum cultures must be sent to rule out potential sites of localized infection. An electrocardiogram (ECG) may reveal a prolonged PR interval or varying degrees of heart block. Echocardiography should be performed to assess the competence of the valves and also to determine if vegetations can be visualized within the heart.

Two or more positive blood cultures without an extracardiac source of infection are considered diagnostic of infectious endocarditis in the pediatric population. In those with congenital heart disease and persistent fever without an identified extracardiac source, a presumptive diagnosis of endocarditis may be made in the absence of positive blood cultures, especially if a change in murmur, microscopic hematuria, or signs of embolic events are noted.

Management. If necessary, the child's airway, breathing, and circulation (ABCs) are supported. The nurse should prepare the child and family for the necessity of serial blood cultures, explain their purpose, and support the family through the drawing of the first set. If the child is acutely ill or is in significant congestive heart failure, an intravenous line will need to be inserted for medication administration at this time as well.

A cardiologist should be called for

consultation, as he or she may be able to speed the diagnosis with information gained from specialized procedures, such as the echocardiogram mentioned above. If the evaluation has revealed acute cardiac changes, the child's condition may warrant evaluation by a cardiac surgeon as well.

Medications may be indicated for management of congestive heart failure; digoxin (Lanoxin), for its inotropic and negative chronotropic effect, and furosemide (Lasix), for vigorous diuresis, are drugs of choice. Both may be given orally or, for more rapid action, intravenously. Close monitoring of the child's condition is necessary after administration both to evaluate the effectiveness and possible side effects of these medications (see section on CHF) and to keep abreast of any alterations in hemodynamic status secondary to the infectious process.

It is preferable, whenever possible, to delay the initiation of antibiotic therapy until the causative organism has been identified so that the antibiotics to which the organism is most sensitive can be selected. If the child's condition mandates treatment before the results of cultures are available, initial parenteral therapy with triple antibiotics should be instituted, based upon the high probability that the offending organism is either *Staphylococcus aureus* or *Streptococcus viridans*, the two bacteria isolated in fully two thirds of the documented cases of endocarditis. Oxacillin sodium, ampicillin, and gentamicin will ordinarily be chosen for broad coverage, and first doses may be given in the emergency department. The nurse must be aware of appropriate dosages, scheduling, and dilutions to maintain optimal blood levels and to minimize infusion problems (Table 15–1).

Whether the child goes to surgery or not, a diagnosis of infective endocarditis implies 4 to 6 weeks of intravenous antibiotic therapy. Parent teaching in the emergency department should include general information about bacterial endocarditis, its possible causes, and signs and symptoms that the parents should be familiar with, as well as preparation for the long-term treatment. If the parents have not already been instructed about antibiotic prophylaxsis by their cardiologist, the rationale for coverage of children at risk can be outlined (Table 15–2), and a printed sheet with current recommendations for physicians and dentists may be given to them.

Any child suspected of having bacterial endocarditis should be admitted to the hospital for further observation and assessment while awaiting the results of the blood cultures. If all cultures prove to be negative and other findings are not suggestive of endocarditis, the child will be discharged, with close follow-up scheduled. If cultures are positive or therapy has already been instituted due to the acuity of illness, the antibiotics will continue for 6 weeks, with possible changes in dosage or agent based upon culture and sensitivities, serum antibiotic levels, bactericidal levels, and clinical progress. The option now exists, with the establishment of home health care agencies staffed by nurses experienced in intravenous therapy, for very stable patients to receive several weeks of the total therapy at home. This service, and the use of heparin locks, can substantially reduce both the cost and the boredom associated with long-term inpatient antibiotic therapy. Patients requiring surgical intervention and those with a less stable course are usually obligated to remain in the hospital for the duration of treatment.

Pericardial Disease

The major manifestations of pericardial disease are (1) pericarditis, an inflammatory or infectious process characterized by fibrin deposition on the pericardium; (2) effusion, the accumulation of a greater-

TABLE 15-1. ANTIBIOTICS USED TO MANAGE INFECTIVE ENDOCARDITIS

Antibiotic	Dose/kg/day	Minimum IV Dilution	Rate of Infusion	Nursing Implications
Ampicillin	200–400 mg/kg/ day divided every 4–6 hr	50 mg/ml (infants)	10–20 min	Observe for skin rash
Cephalothin (Keflin)	100 mg/kg/day in children older than 1 year divided every 8 hr	50 mg/ml	15–20 min	Observe for neph- rotoxicity, leuko- penia, thrombo- cytopenia, and an increase in serum SGOT and SGPT
Gentamicin	1–3 mg/kg/day di- vided every 8 hr up to 6 mg/kg/ day	1 mg/ml	30 min–2 hr	Observe for oto- toxicity (en- hanced by Lasix); increase in BUN, bilirubin, and creatinine levels; may de- crease serum calcium; peak serum level 8– 20 µg/ml
Penicillin G potas- sium	100,000– 150,000 U/kg/ day	Total of 10–15 ml of fluid	15–20 min	Monitor electro- lytes, renal, and hematopoietic systems
Methicillin	100–200 mg/kg/ day divided every 6 hr	50 mg/ml	10–20 min	Monitor for renal and hepatic function during long-term ther- apy; incompati- ble with any other drug
Oxacillin sodium	50–100 mg di- vided every 6 hr	50 mg/ml (infant); 100 mg/ml (child)	10–20 min	Monitor renal, liver, and hema- topoietic sys- tems
Vancomycin	40 mg/kg divided every 6 hr	2.5–5 mg/ml	30–60 min (new- born); 60 min (child)	Nephrotoxic and ototoxic; may cause diarrhea and foul-smelling stools; will cause necrosis and sloughing with extravasa- tion; toxic con- centration greater than 80– 100 µg/ml

Abbreviations: IV = intravenous; SGOT = serum glutamic-oxaloacetic transaminase; SGPT = serum glutamic-pyruvic trans- aminase; BUN = blood urea nitrogen.
From D. Dance, & M. Yates. Nursing Assessment and care of children with complications of congenital heart disease. Heart & Lung 14, no. 3(May 1985):211.

TABLE 15-2. RECOMMENDED ANTIBIOTIC REGIMEN FOR ENDOCARDITIS PROPHYLAXIS

	Dental/Respiratory	Genitourinary/Gastrointestinal
Standard regimen Most congenital heart defects,[a] acquired valvar dysfunction, mitral valve prolapse	PO: > 27 kg—Penicillin VK 1 g 1 hr before procedure, 1 g 6 hr later < 27 kg—Penicillin VK 1 g 1 hr before procedure, 500 mg 6 hr later IM or IV: Aqueous penicillin G 2 million U (children 50,000 U/kg) 30-60 min before procedure, 1 million U (children 25,000/kg) 6 hr later	PO: Amoxicillin 3 g (children 50 mg/kg) 1 hr before procedure, 1.5 g (children 25 mg/kg) 6 hr later[b,d] IM or IV: Ampicillin 2 g (children 50 mg/kg) *plus* gentamycin 1.5 mg/kg (children 2 mg/kg) 30 minutes before procedure. May be repeated 8 hr later
Special regimen High-risk patients— *all* individuals with prosthetic valves, those with surgically created systemic-pulmonary shunts	IM or IV: Ampicillin 1-2 g (children 50 mg/kg) *plus* gentamycin 1.5 mg/kg (children 2 mg/kg) 30 min before procedure, 1 g *oral* Penicillin VK (or previous parenteral combination) 6 hr later	IM or IV: As above
Penicillin-allergic patients	PO: Erythromycin 1 g (children 20 mg/kg) 1 hr before procedure 500 mg (children 10 mg/kg) 6 hr later[b] IV[c]: Vancomycin 1 g (children 20 mg/kg) slowly over 1 hr, starting 1 hr before procedure	IV: Vancomycin 1 g (children 20 mg/kg) slowly over 1 hr *plus* gentamycin 1.5 mg/kg (children 2 mg/kg) 1 hr before procedure. May be repeated 8 to 12 hr later

Abbreviations: PO = orally; IM = intramuscularly; IV = intravenously.
[a] Prophylaxis not recommended for isolated ASD secundum, ASD secundum repaired without a patch ≥ 6 months ago, PDA divided and ligated ≥ 6 months ago.
[b] Children's dosages figured in mg/kg should not exceed maximum adult doses.
[c] For high-risk patients allergic to penicillin.
[d] For minor or repetitive procedures (i.e., bladder catheterization, liver biopsy).
Adapted from S. Shulman, D. Amkren, A. Bisno, et al.[5]

than-normal volume of fluid in the pericardial space; and (3) fibrous scarring of the pericardial tissue, creating a restrictive pericardium. (Figure 15-1 illustrates the anatomic relationship of the pericardial tissues.) Although these processes are often sequential, each can occur in the absence of others; most children, however, are affected by the first two. Precipitating factors or events may be focal or systemic infection, neoplastic disease, or injury or surgical incision of the pericardium. Of particular concern in this disease entity is the frequent necessity of addressing both the implications of an infectious process and the hemodynamic consequences of effusion or a restrictive pericardium, i.e., an increasing pericardial pressure and, ultimately, cardiac tamponade. Bacterial or purulent pericarditis and tamponade of any etiology both constitute medical emergencies and require immediate intervention.

Table 15-3 summarizes information on the four types of pericardial disease discussed below.

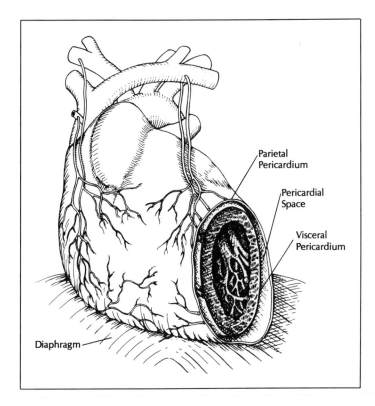

Figure 15-1. The clinical manifestations of pericardial disease are influenced by the anatomic relationships of the pericardial tissues. Effusion of blood or fluid into the pericardial space may lead to tamponade. *(Reproduced with permission from E.W. Hancock. Pericardial disease—Differential diagnosis and management. Hospital Practice April 1983, p. 102.)*

Parietal Pericardium

Pericardial Space

Visceral Pericardium

Diaphragm

Bacterial or Pyogenic Pericarditis. Bacterial pericarditis in children may be the result of either direct spread of the organism from the lungs to the pericardium, as with *Streptococcus pneumoniae* or *Hemophilus influenzae,* or hematogenous spread from a remote site of infection, as is commonly the case with *Straphylococcus aureus.* With bacterial invasion of the pericardium, the volume of pericardial fluid may increase rapidly, due to an influx of fluid containing leukocytes. The chest pain associated with pericarditis is created by friction between the pericardium and the adjacent pleura; the pain is aggravated by changes in position that increase friction or by such activities as swallowing, coughing, or deep breathing. Identification of the causative organism may be accomplished through culture of the pericardial fluid, which may be grossly purulent when withdrawn; in cases of hematogenous transmission, blood culture will also be positive.

The child with bacterial pericarditis will present a clinical picture similar to that associated with many acute infectious processes; high fever, tachycardia, and tachypnea with nasal flaring are often seen, especially in young children. The presence of chest pain and a pericardial friction rub are common and strongly suggestive of pericarditis.

Idiopathic or Viral Pericarditis. Idiopathic or viral pericarditis has a less clearly defined etiology; although isolation of a viral source has been documented in less than 20 percent[6] of these patients, no alternative etiology has been definitely established. An upper respiratory tract infection often precedes the onset of presenting symp-

TABLE 15-3. AN OVERVIEW OF PERICARDIAL DISEASE

	Bacterial	Viral/Idiopathic	Tuberculous	Postpericardotomy Syndrome
Source of pathogen or precipitating event	Recent respiratory infection, remote focal infection, bacteremia	Recent upper respiratory infection, viral syndrome or unknown	Tubercular lymph nodes or remote encapsulation	Opening of pericardium 7-21 days previously; probable autoimmune response
Onset	Acute	Acute	Gradual	Acute
Signs, symptoms	High fever, tachycardia, pleuritic chest pain, pericardial rub	Low-grade fever, pleuritic chest pain, pericardial rub	Cough, dyspnea, orthopnea, pleuritic chest pain, night sweats, weight loss	Low-grade fever, malaise, possible pleuritic chest pain
Incidence	Seen more frequently in children than adults	In both children and adults	Rare in this country, 25% of cases children	Very rare in infants less than 2 yrs old. Affects 25%-30% of older children and adults undergoing pericardotomy
Laboratory findings	Increased WBC, positive blood cultures in 40%-80% of cases, organism cultured from pericardial fluid	WBC normal, increased lymphocytes, occasional viral organism or malignant process identified from pericardial fluid.	Positive PPD, organism identified in pericardial fluid	Increased WBC and erythrocyte sedimentation rate. High anti-heart antibody titre, sterile pericardial fluid
Other studies	Chest x-ray—enlarged cardiac silhouette	Chest x-ray—enlarged cardiac silhouette if effusion present	Chest x-ray—enlarged cardiac silhouette	Chest x-ray—enlarged cardiac silhouette if effusion present, frequently pleural effusions
	ECG—diffuse ST segment, T wave abnormalities	ECG—as in bacterial	ECG—as in bacterial	ECG—as in bacterial
Pericardiocentesis	Diagnostic	Diagnostic *only* if effusion present, therapeutic if tamponade	Diagnostic, therapeutic if tamponade	Therapeutic if tamponade
Incidence of tamponade	Occasional	Rare	Frequent	Rare
	High-dose IV antibiotics 4-6 wk; surgical drainage of pericardial fluid	Symptomatic: bed rest, salicylates, use of steroids controversial, analgesia	Aggressive chemotherapy with streptomycin, INH and anti-TB drugs	Symptomatic: bed rest, use of steroids controversial, analgesia

TABLE 15-3. *(Continued)*

	Bacterial	Viral/Idiopathic	Tuberculous	Postpericardotomy Syndrome
Additional information	Causative organisms in majority of cases: *Staphylococcus aureus, Streptococcus pneumoniae, H. influenzae*	Viral source isolated in approx. 20% of cases; duration 2–3 wk with occasional recurrence	Constrictive pericarditis a common sequela	Self-limited duration 2–3 wk, with infrequent late recurrence

toms. Inflammatory changes in the pericardium occur as they do in bacterial pericarditis, but the course of this disease process is, by comparison, relatively benign and self-limiting.

These children, upon arrival in the emergency department, will usually appear less acutely ill than those with bacterial pericarditis. Low-grade fever (38C) is common, as are mild chest pain and pericardial rub. The children do not appear to be septic. Further symptomatology is directly related to the size of the pericardial effusion, if present (refer to the section on tamponade), or to the occasional presence of pleural effusion, which may cause some respiratory distress, manifested by tachypnea, substernal retractions, or shortness of breath.

Tuberculous Pericarditis. The incidence of tuberculous pericarditis has declined with the incidence of tuberculosis itself; it is now rarely seen, although 25 percent[7] of those cases identified are in the pediatric age group. The organism is usually spread directly from the lymph nodes and is most often seen in individuals with advanced miliary tuberculosis. Pericarditis may rarely occur as the first manifestation of the disease, without evidence of parenchymal lung involvement.

Presentation of these children is more consistent with that of tuberculosis than of other forms of pericarditis. Common signs and symptoms are cough, dyspnea, orthopnea, chest pain, and a history of night sweats and weight loss. Infrequently encountered, and indicative of a more acute disease process, are fever, tachycardia, and pericardial rub; indications of rapidly increasing pericardial effusion may be present in this instance (see the section on tamponade). Analysis of pericardial fluid will establish the diagnosis.

Postpericardotomy Syndrome. This syndrome consists of a febrile illness with pericardial and pleural reaction and effusion occurring 7 to 21 days after wide incision and opening of the pericardium. Infants less than 2 years of age are rarely affected; in the older pediatric population the incidence is 25 to 30 percent of those undergoing pericardotomy.[8] Although a viral etiology has been suggested, it appears more likely to be an autoimmune reaction. Recent studies noted that antiheart antibodies were present in the majority of those exhibiting clinical evidence of the syndrome. Involvement is usually limited to one episode that resolves in 2 to 3 weeks. Recurrences may occasionally appear months or years later.

Within the postoperative time frame indicated, children will usually present with low-grade fever, malaise, and irritability. Chest pain may be present, as may an intermittent pericardial rub. Most children appear only moderately uncomfortable, although a few may be acutely ill, with high fever and evidence of tamponade.

Tamponade

The possibility of pericardial effusion exists in all types of pericarditis. With the exception of bacterial infection, when the purulent pericardial fluid must be drained to combat the infectious process, management of pericardial effusion will usually be conservative, with pericardiocentesis for therapeutic purposes performed only if the volume of fluid threatens to compromise cardiac function. In most instances a small to moderate effusion will resolve spontaneously. When fluid accumulates so rapidly, however, that the compensatory mechanisms of reabsorption and pericardial distensibility cannot keep pace, cardiac tamponade may occur. With the acute increase in volume in the pericardial space, intrapericardial pressure rises, interfering with diastolic filling of the heart and causing decreased cardiac output with subsequent fall in blood pressure. This may result from bleeding into the pericardial space secondary to surgery or trauma as well as from pericarditis and constitutes an acute medical emergency. Signs and symptoms of tamponade, in addition to those of the precipitating process or event, are tachycardia, distant or muffled heart sounds, falling blood pressure with a narrowing pulse pressure, distended neck veins (reflective of rising central venous pressure), and pulsus paradoxus greater than 10 mm Hg (during inspiration, fluid in the pericardium compresses the heart further, causing a sharp drop in cardiac output). Pericardiocentesis must be performed on an emergency basis to restore normal cardiac output.

History. The history should begin with a description of the onset and intensity of signs and symptoms prior to arrival in the emergency department and should continue with a review of past illnesses and surgical procedures. Any recent infections, viral syndromes, flu-like illnesses, cardiac or other surgeries, or injuries should be explored; any medications prescribed should be noted. A history of tuberculosis or tuberculosis-like symptoms, such as daily temperature spikes, night sweats, or weight loss in the child or family members should be noted.

Assessment. If the initial impression of the child suggests an acute illness, the history, assessment, and beginning interventions may, of necessity, be simultaneous. Baseline vital signs should be obtained and noted. Respiratory status must be assessed for presence of cough, dyspnea, retractions, flaring, locally diminished breath sounds, and a preference for the upright position. Cardiovascular assessment will include auscultation for quality of heart sounds and presence of the to and fro sound of a pericardial friction rub at the left sternal border. The patient should be examined for signs of elevated central venous pressure, e.g., full or pulsating neck veins when in an upright position and paradoxical pulse. The latter can be evaluated by using a sphygmomanometer and observing any fluctuation in the patient's arterial pressure with respiration. A drop of more than 10 mm Hg with inspiration constitutes paradox. If the initial blood pressure was low, it should be rechecked frequently to determine if it is continuing to fall and if the pulse pressure is narrowing. The abdomen should be palpated for the presence of hepatosplenomegaly. If the child is in pain, he or she should be asked to describe or point to its location, to describe what it feels like, and to explain what makes it feel better (or worse). If the child's condition is deteriorating and symptoms suggestive of tamponade are present, preparations for pericardiocentesis must be made.

Laboratory Data. Table 15–3 provides a summary of relevant laboratory and diagnostic findings. In general, the most useful bloods to obtain are a white blood cell (WBC) count with differential, erythrocyte sedimentation rate (ESR), and at least two sets of blood cultures when indicated. Cultures of sputum, urine, and wound or local infection sites, if present, should be sent to identify pathogens; viral cultures may be sent if suggested by the clinical picture. A PPD should be planted if there is any suspicion of tubercular involvement.

Chest x-ray will often reveal cardiomegaly or an enlarged cardiac silhouette with normal pulmonary vascular markings, and a diffuse ST segment elevation with T wave abnormalities may be noted on the ECG. Echocardiography is currently the most convenient and accurate method of detecting and evaluating pericardial effusion. Computerized tomography (CT) may be useful to determine size and location of effusions in difficult diagnostic situations.

Pericardial tap for diagnostic purposes may be done in all types of pericarditis (except postpericardotomy syndrome) if there is evidence of a sizeable effusion. Culture and analysis of pericardial fluid will provide a definitive diagnosis of either bacterial or tubercular pericarditis and may identify a viral agent.

Differential diagnosis will be made ultimately on the basis of these cultures, although clinical presentation and history will often be highly suggestive of one category or another before culture results are available. The proximity in time to cardiac surgery will be virtually diagnostic of postpericardotomy syndrome, although careful attention to physical examination and other findings is warranted to differentiate this syndrome from congestive heart failure.

Management. As the child with pericardial disease may be extremely frightened and uncomfortable due to chest pain, a first priority, if he or she is stable, is to make the child as relaxed and comfortable as possible. Often the pain will be relieved by sitting up, so this position should be maintained whenever practical.

The child and parents should be prepared for the upcoming diagnostic procedures. In many institutions pericardiocentesis in the pediatric patient will be performed by a cardiothoracic surgeon in the catheterization laboratory under fluoroscopy or in the intensive care unit where sophisticated monitoring capabilities are available. In an acute situation this may not be possible; the nurse in the emergency department may find himself or herself assisting with this procedure. Table 15–4 summarizes the procedures involved in a pericardiocentesis.

A cardiologist should promptly be called for consultation, as his or her expertise in echocardiography and electrocardiography will facilitate diagnosis and provide information as to the volume of pericardial fluid present.

Any child who is suspected of having pericardial disease will be admitted to the hospital (or transferred to a medical center, if appropriate facilities are not available locally). If, after assessment and evaluation by the nurse and cardiologist, there is a suggestion of impending tamponade, the nurse should alert the appropriate inpatient unit and expedite the admission process.

It is essential that the nurse monitor and document trends in the child's hemodynamic status. Another priority is preparation of the child for admission with information appropriate to his or her

TABLE 15–4. A SUMMARY OF PERICARDIOCENTESIS

Goal

Rapid relief of increased intrapericardial pressure

Possible Complications

Myocardial puncture

Pneumothorax secondary to lung penetration

Ventricular fibrillation

Procedure

The child is placed in a semi-Fowler's position and is connected to a cardiac monitor. The epigastrium is cleansed and draped with sterile towels. Local anesthetic (1% lidocaine) is given intracutaneously to the left of the xiphoid process, and a No. 20 gauge needle is inserted, aimed at the left shoulder. The appearance of fluid in the needle or evidence of a PVC on the monitor is an indication to advance no further. If the fluid is grossly bloody, the needle should be withdrawn slightly.

Once properly placed, the initial needle is removed and is replaced by a No. 14 intracath needle through which intracath tubing is inserted into the pericardium. Fluid may be withdrawn into a syringe or drained into a collection device. The tubing may be left in place for further drainage. Rapid improvement in hemodynamic status will often be evident after removal of a relatively small volume of fluid. Samples of the pericardial fluid should be sent for viral and tuberculosis cultures as well as for bacterial cultures and sensitivites.

Nursing Interventions

Prepare the child for the procedure

Have the defibrillator at hand

Support the child physically and emotionally through the procedure

Monitor his or her overall condition during the procedure while others concentrate on specific tasks; document changes in status

Ensure that a CXR is done after the procedure to check for pneumothroax or hemothorax and changes in the cardiac silhouette

Arrange for transfer to the appropriate inpatient unit for observation or further treatment

---

developmental level and current emotional status.

The majority of nursing interventions beyond the initial diagnostic period will take place in the inpatient setting. The hospital course of the child diagnosed with bacterial pericarditis will include at least 4 to 6 weeks of high-dose intravenous antibiotic therapy directed at the causative organism and surgical drainage of the pericardium. Antibiotics will not be discontinued until the child is afebrile and has a normal WBC. As with the treatment of bacterial endocarditis, completion of the final weeks of antibiotic therapy at home is currently a possibility in carefully selected patients.

The child with viral or idiopathic pericarditis will receive symptomatic treatment: bed rest, salicylates, and, occasionally, steroids. The use of steroids is controversial at present: some report dramatic improvement with their administration, while others cite a rebound phenomenon after discontinuation. Newer nonsteroid anti-inflammatory agents may be equally effective with fewer side effects.

Vigorous treatment of the child with tuberculous pericarditis is indicated. The chemotherapeutic regimen currently recommended combines streptomycin, which diffuses into the pericardial space, INH or para-aminosalicylic acid, and an antitubercular drug such as rifampin.

The child with postpericardotomy syndrome will be treated similarly to those with viral pericarditis: bed rest, analgesia, and possibly steroids. In this population studies indicate a prompt response in clinical signs and a drop in heart reactive antibody with the use of steroids.

If pericardial effusion recurs to the point of causing symptoms in any of these children, serial pericardiocenteses or insertion of a chest tube may be indicated. In isolated instances when control of effusions cannot be accomplished medically, surgical creation of a pericardial window that allows continuous drainage of fluid may be necessary.

Hypoxemia/Hypercyanosis

Some children with decreased pulmonary blood flow secondary to congenital heart disease, primarily those with tetralogy of Fallot, are subject to intense hypoxic episodes. These episodes, also referred to as "cyanotic spells," "Tet spells," or "hyperpneic episodes," may range from manifestation of mild, transient duskiness and irritability to prolonged periods of deep cyanosis, convulsions, unresponsiveness, or even death. Mild episodes are often not recognized as such by parents, but children manifesting more pronounced symptoms are usually brought for emergency attention.

Etiology and Pathophysiology. Cyanotic spells are due to acute insufficiency of pulmonary blood flow, increased right-to-left intracardiac shunting, and systemic hypoxemia. It has long been suggested that these episodes are caused by infundibular spasm, further reducing an already limited blood flow from the right ventricle to the pulmonary circulation. Other explanations include changes in systemic resistance and venous return, alteration in sensitivity of the respiratory center, or marked changes in heart rate. Another hypothesis is that spells are triggered or maintained by hyperpnea. Most of the episodes occur early in the day, shortly after the child has awakened, and are associated with crying, defecating, or feeding, activities that increase oxygen demands and may stimulate hyperpnea. In normal children hyperpnea leads to increased cardiac output from both ventricles and ultimately causes an increase in effective filling pressure of the right ventricle. In tetralogy of Fallot, however, since the pulmonary stenosis is a fixed resistance to flow, pulmonary blood flow does not increase, and cardiac output is increased only with increased right-to-left shunting. The resultant arterial hypoxemia further stimulates respiration, and a vicious cycle is established.

History. A history of previously diagnosed heart disease, prior surgery, or use of medications should be elicited. The episode or spell will often have resolved upon arrival in the emergency department, leaving the child fatigued but no more cyanotic than is usual for him or her. If the child is still markedly cyanotic, he or she will usually be irritable, inconsolable, and hyperpneic as opposed to tachypneic or lethargic.

Assessment. The presence of deep cyanosis; rapid, deep respirations; and a known diagnosis of cyanotic congenital heart disease suggest the diagnosis immediately. The pulmonary ejection murmur of tetralogy of Fallot, normally best heard at the second left intercostal space, may be reduced in intensity or absent entirely at this time. Arterial blood gases are uniformly low during such a spell, but blood drawing, as an additional source of stress, should initially be avoided in favor of prompt intervention.

Management. Table 15–5 summarizes the management of cyanotic spells in the emergency department. Therapeutic measures consist of morphine sulfate 0.1 mg/kg given subcutaneously, oxygen by hood or face mask at 5 to 8 L/minute, and placement of the child in a knee-chest position; these almost always afford relief within minutes. Morphine is thought to

TABLE 15–5. NURSING INTERVENTIONS FOR CYANOTIC SPELLS

Administer *morphine sulfate* 0.1 mg/kg subcutaneously

Administer O_2 at 5–8 L/min

Place child in *knee-chest* position.

break the hyperpneic cycle by acting on the respiratory center; it may also relax the infundibulum. The effect of oxygen administration may not be dramatic in the presence of a fixed limitation of pulmonary blood flow, but any increase in saturation is desirable. Whether the knee-chest position acts to decrease or increase the return of desaturated venous blood to the heart is unclear. Proponents of both theories agree that the net result is increased arterial oxygenation. Intravenous hydration may be given if the child is volume depleted. If he or she does not respond to the initial measures, propranolol 0.1 mg/kg intravenously may be effective. If not, in the most severe and protracted spells intubation and ventilation may be necessary.

Reassurance of the parents should be ongoing while interventions are carried out. An explanation of what is planned and the anticipated outcomes can help parents cope with this frightening experience. Allowing the parents to remain within sight of their child or to hold the child in the knee-chest position if practical may be of great therapeutic value to all concerned, since minimizing stress for the child is a primary concern. When the child's condition has stabilized, a more complete history can be obtained. This may often reveal that he or she is at least moderately cyanotic at rest, that he or she squats or lies down after exertion, and that similar, less severe episodes have occurred in the past. Once "spells" have begun to occur, they usually increase in both frequency and severity.

A cardiology consultation should be promptly arranged so that plans for overall management can be made. Occurrence of a cyanotic spell sufficiently severe to bring a child to the emergency department is currently considered an indication for surgical intervention within the immediate future. Those rare children requiring intubation will proceed to the operating room as soon as is feasible. If for any reason surgery is to be postponed for more than a few days, the child may be started on propranolol 0.5 to 2.0 mg/kg orally in four divided doses. As a beta blocker this medication acts to counter sympathetic stimulation that promotes the cycle described above.

Even in the absence of cyanotic spells, primary surgical correction of tetralogy of Fallot is now routinely done within the first 6 months of life, avoiding not only occurrence of these stressful episodes but also the limitations and sequelae of unrepaired cyanotic heart disease.

Congestive Heart Failure

Congestive heart failure (CHF) is a clinical syndrome in which the heart is unable to maintain a level of tissue perfusion adequate to meet metabolic needs. In childhood these needs also include growth and development.[9] The majority of pediatric patients developing CHF are under 1 year of age.

Etiology. The primary cause of CHF in the pediatric population is congenital heart disease. Acquired heart conditions in which CHF may develop includes myocarditis, cardiomyopathy, pericardial disease, rheumatic heart disease, cor pulmonale, and endocarditis. Other causes of CHF include hypoglycemia, acute hemorrhage, sepsis, electrolyte imbalances, or ingestion of a cardiac drug such as digoxin. The etiologic considerations for CHF are summarized in Table 15–6.

Pathophysiology. The distinction between left-sided and right-sided heart failure is less obvious in the newborn or young infant than it is in the older child or adult.[10] Clinically it is unusual to observe solely right-sided or left-sided heart failure, since each side of the heart is dependent on the adequate performance of the other. In

TABLE 15–6. ETIOLOGIC CONSIDERATIONS FOR CONGESTIVE HEART FAILURE

Congenital Heart Disease	Acquired Heart Disease	Endocrine/Metabolic	Other
1. Pressure overload: Ventricular outflow obstruction (e.g., aortic stenosis; severe coarctation) Left ventricular inflow obstruction (e.g., cor triatriatum) 2. Volume overload: Left-to-right shunts (e.g., ventricular septal defect) Anomalous pulmonary venous return Valvar regurgitation (e.g., aortic insufficiency) Arteriovenous fistulas 3. Other structural disease Anomalous coronary artery Traumatic injury 4. Rhythm disturbance Supraventricular tachycardia Complete heart block 5. Postoperative heart disease Malfunctioning prosthetic valve	1. Myocarditis: Viral infections Kawasaki syndrome Collegen vascular disease 2. Cardiomyopathy Chronic anemia (e.g., thalassemia major) Storage diseases 3. Pericardial disease 4. Rheumatic heart disease 5. Cor pulmonale Acute (e.g., upper airway obstruction) Cystic fibrosis Neuropathies 6. Endocarditis	1. Hypoglycemia 2. Chronic anemia or acute blood loss 3. Sepsis 4. Calcium or magnesium disorders 5. Electrolyte disturbances	1. Ingestions Cardiac toxins (e.g., digitalis) Arrhythmogenics (e.g., tricyclic antidepressants)

Reproduced with permission from M.H. Gewitz, & V.L. Vetter. Congestive heart failure. In G. Fleisher, & S. Ludwig (Eds.), Textbook of Pediatric Emergency Medicine. Baltimore: Williams & Wilkins, 1983, p. 291.

right-sided heart failure the right ventricle pumps an inadequate amount of blood into the pulmonary artery. This results in less blood being oxygenated by the lungs and an increased pressure in the right atrium and systemic circulation. In left-sided heart failure the left ventricle pumps an inadequate amount of blood into the systemic circulation, resulting in increased pressure in the left atrium and pulmonary veins.

History. A thorough history is critical in any infant or child suspected of CHF. Eliciting a history of a preexisting cardiac disease or hematologic disorder is obviously important. A history of any respiratory difficulties should also be sought. This information should include any changes in respiratory rate and regularity and presence of cough. Fatigue, especially during feedings, poor weight gain, persistent vomiting, and a decrease in voiding are other important symptoms that should be elicited from the parents. Also, parents should be carefully questioned regarding the presence of any edema, such as facial or periorbital edema. Infants and young children may have sacral edema. Male infants may present with a history of scrotal edema.

Assessment. Immediate evaluation of the airway, breathing, and circulation (ABCs) in patients with CHF is critical. The airway should be examined for patency. Since infants are obligate nose breathers, patency of the nasal passages should be maintained. Endotracheal intubation may be indicated in severely compromised patients.

A thorough respiratory assessment should be performed. Any difficulty in respirations should be noted. The lungs should be carefully auscultated for movement of air and presence of wheezes, rhonchi, and crepitant rales. Crepitant rales are often present in the early stages of CHF and wheezing is often present in later stages. The respiratory rate should be carefully monitored. Tachypnea is often the first indicator of CHF. The respiratory rate is often 60 to 100 breaths per minute. Breathing is often rapid and shallow. These respiratory symptoms are the result of pulmonary venous engorgement and interstitial edema. In later stages, dyspnea, manifested by retractions, is often present. Changes in circulation may be manifested with tachycardia, with a heart rate of 150 to 200 beats per minute at rest. A cardiac monitor should be used to monitor heart rate and rhythm. A gallop rhythm is often noted in infants with CHF. A third heart sound in the presence of tachycardia may be an early finding in left-sided failure.[11]

Presence of pallor or cyanosis should be noted. Peripheral circulation should be carefully assessed. Peripheral pulses are usually weak and should be carefully monitored. Peripheral edema may be present. Facial edema, usually periorbital, is often found, as well as sacral and scrotal edema. Edema of the lower extremities, although less common in the pediatric than adult patient with CHF, should be noted. Diaphoresis with cool, moist extremities may be found, reflecting peripheral vasoconstriction secondary to catecholamine release and the need to maintain blood pressure in the face of reduced cardiac output.

Hepatomegaly often accompanies CHF. The liver is often 3 to 5 cm below the costal margin and has a round, blunted edge.[12] Inadequate growth and undernutrition often accompany the infant or child with CHF. This may be related to increased caloric expenditure and feeding difficulties.

The child's neurologic status should be continually assessed. Depending on the severity of the CHF, the patient's level of consciousness may be affected and should therefore be carefully monitored. The infant or child may also appear lethargic, restless, or irritable.

Laboratory Data. The chest x-ray in CHF shows an increased cardiothoracic ratio and pulmonary congestion. Plural effusions are common.

An electrocardiogram (ECG) should be obtained. The ECG is a nonspecific indicator of cardiac decompensation. The ECG may help establish an etiology for CHF secondary to cardiac arrhythmia or myocardial ischemia.[13]

Complete blood count, arterial blood gases, serum electrolytes and osmolarity, and urinalysis should be obtained. The blood gas analysis may indicate metabolic acidosis due to prolonged tissue hypoperfusion. Electrolyte imbalances may include hyponatremia and hypochloremia. The hematocrit may be lowered based on dilutional factors. Additionally, in infants with CHF, serum glucose and calcium should be monitored, since deficiencies in either may be responsible in large measure for the impaired cardiac function.[14]

Management. The primary goals of therapy are improved cardiac function and reduction of the work load of the heart. Table 15–7 provides a summary of the priorities of nursing care of the patient with CHF. Improved cardiac function is achieved through restoration of a more effective contractile force with use of a digitalis preparation. Digoxin, as opposed to

digitoxin, is used in pediatrics almost exclusively. Digoxin has a more rapid onset and decreased risk of toxicity as the result of a much shorter half-life. Digitalis preparations increase the force of contraction, decrease the heart rate, and indirectly enhance diuresis by increased renal perfusion. During digitalization it is important to closely monitor the child by ECG for arrhythmias, followed by continuous cardiac monitoring, even during transfer to the ICU.

Reducing the work load of the heart involves reduction of the volume of fluid with which the heart is confronted. Volume reduction can usually be accomplished with a rapid action diuretic such as furosemide if blood pressure and renal function are reasonably normal. Electrolyte imbalances, particularly potassium and chloride losses, must be carefully monitored during diuretic therapy. Hypokalemia may precipitate or enhance digitalis toxicity. Based on the patient's serum level, potassium replacement of 1 to 4 mEq per kg should be given to maintain serum potassium levels of 3.5 to 4.5 mEq/L. An indwelling urinary catheter should be inserted prior to the administration of the diuretic. Urinary output and fluid intake must be judiciously monitored. Fluid restriction may be required in the acute states of CHF. Blood products in the form of packed cells may be administered if the child is severely anemic. In situations of severely compromised cardiac output, isoproterenol (Isuprel) or dopamine, may be administered.[15]

Other interventions to decrease the cardiac demand include decreasing physical activity; using the semi-Fowler's position to reduce respiratory efforts; administration of supplemental cool-humidified oxygen, and administration of a medication to sedate an agitated or uncomfortable child. Morphine sulfate, 0.05 to 0.1 mg/kg is often used for this purpose.

TABLE 15–7. PRIORITIES IN THE NURSING MANAGEMENT OF CHF

Support of airway, breathing, circulation
Oxygen therapy
Place child in semi-Fowler's position
Medication administration (digitalis, lasix, analgesic)
Cardiac monitoring
Fluid and electrolyte balance
Psychosocial support

The nurse must continually evaluate the infant or child in CHF in terms of heart rate, respiratory status, cardiac rhythm, circulation, hepatomegaly, and fluid and electrolyte balance. Patients who arrive in the emergency department in CHF should be stabilized and then transferred to a pediatric intensive care unit or cardiac unit, if one is available.

Psychosocial Support and Parent Education. The patient with CHF and family members will need a tremendous amount of support while in the emergency department. The infant or child who is experiencing difficulty breathing is often agitated by the resultant air hunger. The examination and procedures are often frightening and may result in an increase in both heart and respiratory rates. To decrease anxiety, all procedures should be carefully explained to the patient and family members.

The infant or child's parents are usually very frightened by the rapid deterioration that may take place. Parents need to be reassured that everything possible is being done. They should be allowed to remain at the bedside of their infant or child as much as possible to provide support and reassurance. The child and parents will also need to be prepared for the child's admission to the hospital.

Anaphylaxis

Anaphylaxis, or anaphylactic shock, is an acute systemic reaction that results from extreme allergy or hypersensitivity to an antigen. Anaphylaxis is a life-threatening emergency that requires immediate intervention. Anaphylactic reactions occur immediately after exposure to the offending antigen and usually only after repeated exposure to the particular antigen over a period of time. The most common causes of anaphylaxis in children are insect stings, parenteral administration of penicillin, hyposensitization antigens, or iodinated contrast media used in radiography procedures.

Penicillin and penicillin derivatives are probably the most common cause of anaphylactic reactions. The reaction often occurs in individuals with no previous history of sensitivity. The reaction to an insect sting may be local or systemic. The insects usually involved are bees, hornets, yellow jackets, or wasps. The reactions that occur are against the venom from the insect. Foods, particularly in older children, have been known to cause anaphylaxis. The foods most often implicated are nuts, peanuts, shellfish, eggs, milk, and berries. Drugs other than penicillin may lead to anaphylaxis. Such drugs include salicylates, cephalosporins, sulfonamides, tetracyclines, streptomycin, morphine, and codeine.

Pathophysiology. Anaphylactic shock is the systemic manifestation of an immediate hypersensitivity reaction that necessitates formation of reaginic antibodies that are usually of the IgE class. Antigens interact with antibodies on the surfaces of mast cells and basophils, which then release certain chemical mediators, such as SRS-A, histamine, and bradykinin. In turn these mediators have profound effects on the pulmonary and vascular systems, resulting in bronchospasm, increased vascular permeability, and laryngeal edema. These physiologic changes produce a variety of respiratory, cutaneous, and vascular signs and symptoms that can be precursors to shock.[16] Circulatory collapse and sudden death may ensue unless appropriate lifesaving interventions are implemented immediately.

History. A careful history is necessary to identify the causative agent. Since these reactions are the result of an immediate hypersensitivity reaction, the history should focus on the period of time immediately before the reaction began. The time of exposure to the causative agent and the time of onset of symptoms are important to elicit. Determine if the child or parents initiated any intervention prior to arrival in the emergency department. A careful history of any past allergic reactions should be elicited.

Assessment. The priorities of emergency management of the child in anaphylactic shock are summarized in Table 15–8. A rapid assessment of the airway, breathing, and circulation (ABCs) is essential. Vital signs, especially blood pressure, must be continually monitored. Cardiac monitoring is important, since arrhythmias often occur. Skin color, temperature, and presence of urticaria should be assessed.

The clinical manifestations of anaphylaxis are usually immediate in onset and include urticaria, pruritis, laryngeal edema with stridor or hoarseness, and bronchospasm with bilateral wheezing. Any patient who demonstrates stridor on inspiration or difficulty speaking has significant laryngeal edema. The gastrointestinal response may involve severe abdominal cramping and diarrhea. Massive histamine release increases vascular permeability and causes loss of vascular tone, resulting in hypotension and shock.

TABLE 15–8. PRIORITIES IN THE EMERGENCY MANAGEMENT OF THE CHILD IN ANAPHYLACTIC SHOCK

Establish and maintain airway, breathing, and circulation (ABCs)
Administrer high-flow oxygen
Carefully monitor vital signs
Administer epinephrine
Apply tourniquet proximal to site of insect sting or drug injection
Administer intravenous fluids
Assess for cardiac arrthythmias
Provide emotional support to child and family members

Management. The first priorities of intervention are to support the ABCs. Patency of the airway must be maintained. Oxygen should be administered early on. Equipment for intubation and tracheostomy should be readily available. Epinephrine (1 : 1000) 0.01 ml/kg to a maximum dose of 0.4 ml should be administered intravenously or subcutaneously. This may produce an immediate dramatic response. The dose may be repeated every 20 minutes for a maximum of three injections. Epinephrine often causes tachycardia and heart palpatations, which can be very frightening to the child. The child will need to be reassured that this is normal and will soon subside. Parents should also be informed that any changes in the child's behavior such as hyperactivity are related to the administration of epinephrine.

If the precipitant has been either an insect sting or a drug injection, a tourniquet should be applied proximal to the injection site to impede further systemic absorption of the antigen. One half of the calculated systemic dose of epinephrine should be injected intradermally around the antigen injection site to retard the development of anaphylaxis.[17]

Intravenous therapy should be initiated as soon as possible with either normal saline or Ringer's lactate. Aminophylline, 6 mg/kg intravenously may be administered over 20 minutes to manage bronchospasm. Vasopressor agents are occasionally indicated. Metaraminol, 0.4 mg/kg by slow intravenous infusion, is often given until systolic blood pressure rises to at least 80 mm Hg. Antihistamines, such as diphenhydramine, 1 to 2 mg/kg intravenously, may be given to manage the urticarial components of anaphylaxis.[18]

Children who have experienced airway obstruction or significant hypotension are usually admitted to the hospital for further treatment and close observation.

Psychosocial Support and Parent Education. Anaphylaxis or any severe allergic reaction is an extremely frightening experience for the child and parents. The onset of symptoms is abrupt and severe. The parents often feel helpless and fear that the child may die prior to medical intervention. The parents should be allowed to remain with the child as long as possible in the emergency department providing they are not interfering with lifesaving interventions. Both the child and parents need a tremendous amount of support and reassurance that everything possible is being done.

The child and parents need to be taught how to best avoid the causative agent. Parents should be instructed to obtain a Medic-Alert card and bracelet for their child that contains the appropriate information about the child's allergy. In some cases the parents will be given a prescription for an anaphylaxis kit and will need careful instructions in its use.

NOTES

1. M.H. Gerwitz, & V.L. Vetter. Cardiac emergencies. In G. Fleisher, & S. Ludwig (Eds.), *Textbook of Pediatric Emergency Medicine*. Baltimore: Williams & Wilkins, 1983, p. 321.
2. Ibid., p. 323.
3. C. Johnson, & K.H. Rhodes. Pediatric endocarditis. *Mayo Clinic Proceedings* 57 (1982):86.
4. Ibid., pp. 86–87.
5. S. Shulman, D. Amkren, A. Bisno, et al. Prevention of bacterial endocarditis—A statement for health professionals by the Committee on Rheumatic Fever and Infective Endocarditis of the Council on Cardiovascular Disease in the Young. *Circulation* December 1984, pp. 1123–1127.
6. G. Noren, E. Kaplan, & N. Staley. Infectious inflammatory disease of the pericardium and pericardial space. In F. Adams, & G. Emmanoulides (Eds.), *Heart Disease in Infants, Children, and Adolescents* (3rd ed.). Baltimore: Williams & Wilkins, 1983, p. 590.
7. Ibid., p. 589.
8. M.A. Engle. Postpericardotomy syndrome. In A. Forrest, & G. Emmanoulides (Eds.), *Heart Disease in Infants, Children, and Adolescents* (3rd ed.). Baltimore: Williams & Wilkins, 1983, p. 589.
9. M.H. Gewitz, & V.L. Vetter. Congestive heart failure. In G. Fleisher, & S. Ludwig (Eds.), *Textbook of Pediatric Emergency Medicine*. Baltimore: Williams & Wilkins, 1983, p. 290.
10. H.L. Chernoff, & M.B. Kreidber. Congestive heart failure. In R.M. Reece (Ed.), *Manual of Emergency Pediatrics* (3rd ed.). Philadelphia: W.B. Saunders, 1984, p. 66.
11. Chernoff, & Kreidber, Congestive heart failure, p. 68.
12. Ibid., p. 66.
13. Gewitz, & Vetter, Congestive heart failure, p. 295.
14. Ibid.
15. Ibid., p. 298.
16. A. Harmond, & D. Harmond. Anaphylaxis: Sudden death at any time. *Nursing '80* 10(1980):43.
17. I.K. Rosner. Anaphylaxis. In R.M. Reece, (Ed.), *Manual of Emergency Pediatrics* (3rd ed.). Philadelphia: W.B. Saunders, 1984, p. 13.
18. Ibid.

BIBLIOGRAPHY

Endocarditis

Chernoff, H.L., & Kreidberg, M.B. Infective endocarditis. In Reece, R.M. (Ed.), Manual of Emergency Pediatrics (3rd ed.). Philadelphia: W.B. Saunders, 1984, pp. 501–505.

Dance, D., & Yates, M. Nursing assessment and care of children with complications of congenital heart disease. *Heart and Lung* 14, no. 3(1985):209–212.

Hazinski, M.F. Critical care of the pediatric cardiovascular patient. *Nursing Clinics of North America* 310(1984):1495–1499.

Hook, E.W. The war against endocarditis. *Emergency Medicine* 14, no. 18(1982):28–32.

Johnson, C., & Rhodes, K.H. Pediatric endocarditis. *Mayo Clinic Proceedings* 57(1982):86–94.

Kaplan, E., & Shulman, S. Endocarditis. In Forrest, A., & Emanoulides, G. (Eds.), *Heart Disease in Infants, Children, and Adolescents* (3rd ed.). Baltimore: Williams & Wilkins, 1983, pp. 565–574.

Mead, R.H. et al. Infective endocarditis: Timely intervention depends on prompt recognition. *Consultant* 24, no. 4(1984):109–111, 113.

Newburger, J.W. Cardiac disorders. In Graef, J., & Cone, T. (Eds.), *Manual of Pediatric Therapeutics* (3rd ed.). Boston: Little, Brown, 1985, pp. 252–255.

Rubin, D., & Friedland, G. Infections and the febrile patient. In May, H. (Ed.), *Emergency Medicine*. New York: Wiley, 1984.

Shulman, S., Akmren, D., Bisno, A., et al. Prevention of bacterial endocarditis—A statement for health professionals by the Committee on Rheumatic Fever and Infective Endocarditis of the Council on Cardiovascular Disease in the Young. *Circulation* December 1984:1123–1127.

Pericardial Disease

Brundage, B., & Chomka, E. Clinical applications of cardiac CT imaging. *Modern Concepts of Cardiovascular Disease* 54, no. 8(1985):39–43.

Conner, R.D. Acute pericarditis and the EKG. *Critical Care Nursing* 3, no. 5(1983):40–42.

Engle, M.A. Postpericardotomy syndrome. In Forrest, A., & Emmanoulides, G. (Eds.), *Heart Disease in Infants, Children, and Adolescents* (3rd ed.). Baltimore:Williams & Wilkins, 1983, pp. 749–752.

Hancock, W.E. Pericardial disease—Differential diagnosis and management. *Hospital Practice* 18, no. 4(1983):101–107, 111–112.

Moncada, R., Baker, M., Salinas, M., et al. Diagnostic role of computerized tomography in pericardial heart disease: Congenital defects, thickening neoplasms and effusions. *American Heart Journal* 103(1982):263–282.

Newburger, J.W. Cardiac disorders. In Graef, J., & Cone, T. (Eds.), *Manual of Pediatric Therapeutics* (3rd ed.). Boston: Little, Brown, 1985, pp. 252–255.

Noren, G., Kaplan, E., & Staley, N. Infectious inflammatory disease of the pericardium and pericardial space. In Adams, F., & Emmanoulides, G. (Eds.), *Heart Disease in Infants, Children, and Adolescents* (3rd ed.). Baltimore: Williams and Wilkins, 1983, pp. 585–591.

Sanders, J. Pericardiocentesis. In May, H. (Ed.), *Emergency Medical Procedures*. New York: Wiley, 1984, pp. 127–132.

Wise, P., & O'Rourke, P.P. Acute care. In May, H. (Ed.), *Emergency Medical Procedures*. New York: Wiley, 1984, p. 57.

Hypoxemia/Hypercyanosis

Fought, S., & Throwe, A. *Psychosocial Nursing Care of the Emergency Patient*. New York: Wiley, 1984.

Gevins, L., & Ricks, J. Assessment of clinical manifestations of cyanotic and acyanotic heart disease in infants and children. *Heart and Lung* 14, no. 3(1985):200–204.

M.H. Gewitz, & V.L. Vetter. Cardiac emergencies. In Fleisher, G., & Ludwig, S. (Eds.), *Textbook of Pediatric Emergency Medicine*. Baltimore: Williams & Wilkins, 1983, pp. 321–327.

Guntheroth, W., Kawabori, I., & Baum, D. Tetralogy of Fallot. In Forrest, A., & Emmanoulides, G. (Eds.), *Heart Disease in Infants, Children, and Adolescents* (3rd ed.). Baltimore: Williams & Wilkins, 1983, pp. 215–227.

Hazinski, M.F. Congenital heart disease Part II: Cyanotic and aortic obstructive heart lesions. *Life Support Nursing* October 1982, 7–12.

Congestive Heart Failure

Chernoff, H.L., & Kreidber, M.B. Congestive heart failure. In Reece, R.M. (Ed.), *Manual of Emergency Pediatrics* (3rd ed.). Philadelphia: W.B. Saunders, 1984, pp. 66–72.

Dillion, T.R., Jones, G.G., Meyer, R.A., et al. Vasodilator therapy for congestive heart failure. *Journal of Pediatrics* 96(1980):623.

Furgal, C.L. Pediatric cardiology: Stressors, reactions, interventions. *Issues in Comprehensive Pediatric Nursing* 5(1981):21–31.

Gewitz, M.H., & Vetter, V.L. Congestive heart failure. In Fleisher, G., & Ludwig, S. (Eds.), *Textbook of Pediatric Emergency Medicine*. Baltimore: Williams & Wilkins, 1983, pp. 290–299.

Hazinski, M.F. Critical care of the pediatric cardiovascular patient. *Nursing Clinics of North America* 16(December 1981):671–698.

Huntington, J. Congestive heart failure. In Oakes, A.R. (Ed.), *Critical Care Nursing of Children and Adolescents*. Philadelphia: W.B. Saunders, 1981, pp. 139–143.

Modrcin, M.A., & Schott, J. An update of congestive heart failure in infants. *Issues in Comprehensive Pediatric Nursing* 3(1979):6–22.

Smith, K.M. Recognizing cardiac failure in neonates. *American Journal of Maternal Child Nursing* 4(1979):98–100.

Whaley, L.F., & Wong, D.L. Congestive heart failure. In *Nursing Care of Infants and Children*, 2nd ed. St. Louis: Mosby, 1983, pp. 1319–1328.

27(1980):525.

Grodin, M., & Crone, R. Shock in the pediatric patient. *Pediatric Clinics of North America* 26(1979):821.

Guthrie, M. (Ed.). *Shock.* New York: Churchill Livingstone, 1982.

Harmond, A., & Harmond, D. Anaphylaxis: Sudden death at any time. *Nursing '80* 10(1980):40–43.

Morse, T.S. Shock in infants and children. In Pierog, J.E., & Pierog, L.J. (Eds.), *Pediatric Critical Illness: Assessment and Care*. Rockville, Md.: Aspen 1983, pp. 181–186.

Perkin, R., & Levin, D. Shock in the pediatric patient. *Journal of Pediatrics* 101(1982):319.

Rosner, I.K. Anaphylaxis. In Reece, R.M. (Ed.), *Manual of Emergency Pediatrics*, 3rd ed. Philadelphia: W.B. Saunders, 1984, pp. 12–14.

Sheehy, S.B., & Barber, J. Anaphylactic shock. In *Emergency Nursing: Principles and Practice* (2nd ed.). St. Louis: Mosby, 1985, p. 248.

Anaphylaxis

Cohen, S. Nursing care of patients in shock. *American Journal of Nursing* 82(1982):943–964.

Crone, R.K. Acute circulatory failure in children. *Pediatric Clinics of North America*

EMERGENCY DEPARTMENT CARE GUIDE FOR THE CHILD WITH A CARDIAC EMERGENCY

Nursing Diagnosis	Interventions	Evaluation
Alteration in cardiac output: decreased, related to cardiac emergency	Continually monitor vital signs; Implement electrocardiac monitoring; Insert intravenous line; Administer cardiac medications as ordered; Carefully assess capillary refill, skin color, and skin warmth	Vital signs remain stable; Child's cardiac rhythm is normal; Child's cardiac output increases, as evidenced by increased blood pressure; Capillary refill, skin color, and temperature are normal
Fluid volume excess related to fluid retention	Restrict fluid intake; Carefully monitor and record intake and output; Administer diuretics as ordered	Fluid intake is restricted; Urinary output increases
Alteration in cardiopulmonary tissue perfusion related to decreased cardiac output	Administer cardiac medications as ordered; Monitor vital signs carefully; Administer humidified oxygen; Assess child's skin color and warmth	Vital signs are stable; Child's skin color and warmth return to normal

Nursing Diagnosis	Interventions	Evaluation
Impaired gas exchange related to cardiac emergency	Administer humidified oxygen Obtain arterial blood gases Prepare for endotracheal intubation if necessary	Arterial blood gases return to normal
Activity intolerance related to cardiac emergency	Enforce strict bedrest Provide activities for child that require no exertion of energy, such as having parent read to child	Child cooperates in bed rest
Fear related to emergency department environment and painful procedures	Carefully explain all procedures to child Encourage parents to remain at child's bedside	Child demonstrates an understanding of procedures Child remains calm and cooperative
Knowledge deficit related to cardiac disorder	Carefully explain all procedures and treatments to child and parents Provide information related to the etiology and pathophysiology of child's cardiac condition	Child and parents verbalize an understanding of child's cardiac disorder and necessary treatments

16 | Hematologic Emergencies

Susan J. Kelley

Sickle Cell Disease

Sickle cell disease is an autosomal recessive hereditary disorder characterized by the presence of an abnormal type of hemoglobin (hemoglobin S) in the red blood cell. Hemoglobin S may be manifested as active sickle cell disease or as the sickle cell trait. Approximately one out of every 500 black American children have sickle cell disease, while 8 to 10 percent have sickle cell trait.[1] Sickle cell disease is found predominantly in people from Africa, the Mediterranean, the Near East, and parts of India.

Individuals with sickle cell trait usually are not as severely affected as those with sickle cell disease. Those with sickle cell trait, however, may be affected by decreased ability to tolerate extreme physical activity. These individuals are often unable to withstand atmospheric conditions of low oxygen and may have difficulty with pregnancy.

The prognosis for children with sickle cell disease is grave, although recent advances have been made in treatment of sickle cell disease. Death may occur in childhood or young adulthood. Infection is the leading cause of death in children under 3 years with sickle cell disease.[2] In the older child or young adult death is usually the result of the long-term effects of repeated infarcts and complications.

Etiology and Pathophysiology. The basic defect in sickle cell disease is the substitution of valine for glutamic acid in the sixth position of the beta polypeptide chain of the hemoglobin molecule. This structural change facilitates the sickling phenomenon. In the presence of deoxygenation, a stacking of sickle hemoglobin molecules occurs, and the cell assumes an irregular shape. The abnormally shaped cells increase blood viscosity, which results in stasis and sludging of the cells and further deoxygenation. This leads to further sickling, eventual occlusion of small vessels, and tissue ischemia with infarction and necrosis.[3]

Sickle Cell Crisis. Episodes of sickling with localized or generalized pain, profound anemia, debilitation, and weakness are referred to as sickle cell crisis. The sickling phenomenon takes place when the oxygen tension in the blood is lowered. This may be precipitated by infection, dehydration, exposure to cold, and physical or emotional stress.

There are three primary types of sickle cell crises: vaso-occlusive, aplastic, and sequestration. Vaso-occlusive crisis is the most common. It is caused by intravascular sickling, stasis, and occlusion of the vessels. The most common sites for a vaso-occlusive crisis include the bones, mesenteric vessels, liver, spleen, brain, lungs, and penis.[4]

A careful history may reveal a recent infection, physical exertion, exposure to cold, or emotional stress. In some instances no precipitating event is identified. The pain is usually intense in the organ where vascular occlusion is occurring. These children may complain of painful and swollen joints, severe abdominal pain, back pain, as well as severe headache. The hemoglobin and hematocrit values may be unchanged or slightly elevated due to hemoconcentration.

Aplastic crisis often occurs in association with an upper respiratory infection, gastroenteritis, or viral syndrome. In an aplastic crisis erythropoiesis ceases or drastically decreases while hemolysis continues. This can result in a life-threatening anemia. The hemoglobin will be low compared to the patient's baseline hemoglobin count, and no reticulocytosis is seen.[5]

In the more uncommon and rapidly fatal sequestration crisis, the blood pools in the spleen and other visceral organs, resulting in severe anemia and hypovolemic shock. The child may initially appear pale and lethargic, with left-sided abdominal pain, a rapidly enlarging spleen, chills, fever, and jaundice. Hypovolemic shock rapidly ensues, and death can occur.

History. The patient with sickle cell disease may arrive at the emergency department in any of a variety of physical states. The undiagnosed infant may have a history of frequent infections, failure to thrive, jaundice, or anemia. Manifestation of sickle cell disease rarely occurs before the age of 6 months due to the presence of fetal hemoglobin. Between the ages of 6 months and 2 years, dactylitis (hand-foot syndrome) is commonly observed in the child with sickle cell anemia. It is characterized by soft tissue swelling and tenderness over the affected appendages. Older children may have a history of joint pain, frequent infection, abdominal pain, headache, nausea, and vomiting. The diagnosis of sickle cell disease should be considered in any black child with a history of unex-

plained joint pain or swelling, pneumonia, meningitis, sepsis, neurologic abnormality, splenomegaly, or anemia.

A family history of sickle cell disease or trait should be carefully elicited. It is important to identify any medications or analgesics taken on a regular basis or within the past 24 hours. A history of any past hospitalizations or surgery, such as a splenectomy, should be noted. Patients with sickle cell disease often have G6PD, which is discussed in a later section in this chapter.

Laboratory Data. Blood sickling tests such as the Sickledex test and sickle cell slide prep test are used to screen for the presence of hemoglobin S. If the screening test is positive, a stained blood smear or hemoglobin electrophoresis is used to diagnose sickle cell disease.

Hematologic values in sickle cell disease are outlined in Table 16–1. In addition to a complete blood count with differential and reticulocyte count, it is necessary to obtain serum electrolytes, liver function tests, arterial blood gases, urine culture, urinalysis, and blood cultures. Chest, abdominal, and joint x-rays should be obtained if indicated. An electrocardiogram (ECG) should also be obtained. Biventricular hypertrophy is common in this population. Cor pulmonale may result from recurrent pulmonary infarcts.

Assessment. Nursing assessment includes an initial evaluation of airway,

TABLE 16–1. HEMATOLOGIC VALUES IN SICKLE CELL DISEASE

	Normal Values	Sickle Cell Disease
Hemoglobin (g/dl)	12	5.5–9.5
Hematocrit (%)	36	17–29
Reticulocytes (%)	1.5	5–25
WBC count (mm³)	7,500	12,000–35,000

breathing, and circulation (ABCs). The vital signs, including temperature, should be continually monitored, with special attention to any signs of hypovolemic shock. Location, type, and intensity of pain should be assessed.

Painful or swollen joints should be examined for redness, degree of warmth, and range of motion. Sickling in the mesenteric vessels may cause a complaint of abdominal pain. There may be tenderness upon palpation, guarding, and rebound. The liver and spleen may be enlarged. Before the age of 10 the spleen in children with sickle cell anemia may become completely infarcted, often referred to as autosplenectomy. This loss of splenic function makes these children susceptible to life-threatening infections.[6]

Hydration status should be assessed and fluid intake and output carefully recorded. Respiratory status should be assessed, since these children are susceptible to bacterial pneumonias. Any sign of cyanosis should be noted. Scleral icterus is typically present in children with sickle cell disease, but any increase should be noted. Parents may be helpful in observing any increase in scleral icterus. A neurologic assessment should be conducted, since a central nervous system infarction can occur with severe sequelae.

Management. Impairment of circulation and oxygenation should be treated with administration of oxygen, hydration, and restoration of circulatory volume. Increased hydration by mouth or intravenous route is critical. Fluids should be administered at 1.5 to 2.0 times maintenance. Dehydration causes decreased blood volume, sludging, increased blood viscosity, and further sickling.

Administration of packed red blood cells may be indicated during aplastic or hyperhemolytic crises at a rate of 5 to 10 ml/kg over 3 to 4 hours. Close observation for signs of blood incompatibility is important. Raising the hemoglobin to high levels diminishes bone marrow production of additional sickle cells and dilutes the existing sickle cells with normal transfused erythrocytes.

The moderate to severe pain experienced by the child in sickle cell crisis usually requires administration of a narcotic analgesic such as demerol or morphine. Antipyretics should be administered to febrile patients, as fever will accelerate dehydration. The use of aspirin should be avoided if the patient also has G6PD. A cooling blanket may be needed. The child should be placed on bed rest with the head of the bed elevated.

The potential for infection is markedly increased in this population. Patients with sickle cell disease should be isolated from other infectious children in the emergency department. Bacterial infection is the leading cause of death in children with sickle cell disease. Pneumococcus is the common pathogen responsible for complications such as meningitis, septicemia, and pneumonia. Salmonella is the organism largely responsible for osteomyelitis in these children.

Psychosocial Support and Parent Education. The child in sickle cell crisis and family members are often fearful and require extensive emotional support while in the emergency department. Children in sickle cell crisis fear painful procedures and repeat hospitalizations. Some children may express feelings of anger and frustration while in the emergency department.

In some cases the patient has known family members or friends who have died during a sickle cell crisis. The child therefore needs a tremendous amount of reassurance from a calm, sensitive, nurse. Younger children are fearful of separation from their parents and of painful procedures such as venipunctures and intramuscular injections. Parents should be permitted to remain close to their child while in the emergency department to alleviate the child's fears and anxiety. Children should be provided with age-appropriate toys that will serve as a source of distraction to their pain while in the emergency department.

Children with sickle cell disease and their parents have many learning needs. Parents should be instructed to protect their child from excessive cold, dampness, and exposure to infections and to seek prompt medical attention for all injuries and illnesses. Minor pain crises may be managed at home with analgesics, rest, and hydration. The emergency department nurse should see to it that the family seeks not only episodic care during a crisis but is also closely followed at a sickle cell disease treatment center or hematology clinic where the child can benefit from comprehensive, preventive, supportive, and educational measures.

Families can receive further information from any of the following agencies:

National Sickle Disease Program
National Institutes of Health
Sickle Cell Disease Branch
Room 4 a-27, Bldg. 31
Bethesda, MD 20014

National Association for Sickle
  Cell Disease, Inc.
945 S. Western Ave.
Suite 206
Los Angeles, CA 90006

and from the Sickle Cell Medical Advisory Committee, American Sickle Cell Anemia Association, Cleveland, OH.

Hemophilia

Hemophilia refers to a group of inherited coagulation disorders in which there is a deficiency of one of the blood clotting factors. It affects males almost exclusively but is carried by females. The three most common forms of the disease are classic hemophilia (hemophilia A or factor VIII deficiency), Christmas disease (hemophilia B or factor IX deficiency), and von Willebrand's disease. Classic hemophilia accounts for 75 percent of the hemophiliac population.

The prognosis varies greatly and can be predicted from the level of factor-coagulant activity. Patients with hemophilia are generally categorized into three groups, based on the severity of the factor deficiency. Severe hemophiliacs include those with less than 1 percent of the normal amount of factor involved. These children may bleed spontaneously or from mild injury. Those with moderate hemophilia have 1 to 5 percent of the normal amount of factor. This group does not usually bleed spontaneously but will bleed with only minimal trauma. Mild hemophiliacs have levels of 5 to 25 percent of the normal amount of factor, and significant trauma is needed to cause bleeding. These patients may be asymptomatic for years until serious injury or surgery ocurs. Although very low factor VIII coagulant activity is associated with severe bleeding in von Willebrand's disease, the relationship between laboratory findings and clinical course is less predictable than in other forms of hemophilia. The severity of von Willebrand's disease is judged on an individual basis, depending on the child's bleeding history.[7]

Hemophiliacs from any of these three categories may seek emergency care. The classification of inherited bleeding disorders is very important in assessing these patients in the emergency department. For example, after mild head trauma the patient with severe hemophilia is at greater risk of developing intracranial bleeding than the patient with mild hemophilia. In a patient with mild hemophilia and extensive hemorrhage, severe trauma has probably occurred, and injury to internal organs should be suspected.[8]

History. Children with hemophilia may have a history of traumatic or spontaneous bleeding. Prolonged bleeding may occur internally or externally. Subcutaneous and intramuscular hemorrhage, as well as hemarthrosis, or bleeding into the joints, especially the ankles, knees, and elbows, are common. Prolonged bleeding may occur after circumcision or tooth extraction. Bleeding into the airway, neck, or chest is serious because of the potential of occluding the airway or respiratory tract. Bleeding into the central nervous system is often fatal. A history of head trauma is therefore very significant. Hematuria and epistaxis may also result from spontaneous bleeding. A careful history of previous bleeding episodes and hospitalizations is important. A family history of hemophilia should be obtained.

Assessment. Vital signs should be carefully monitored with close attention to heart rate and blood pressure. Tachycardia and hypotension may indicate impending shock. Careful assessment of the cardiovascular, respiratory, central nervous, musculoskeletal, and gastrointestinal systems is important. Emergency personnel should be alert to any unexplained or difficult-to-control bleeding in a previously undiagnosed patient.

Hemophilic patients with a history of headache, vomiting, altered mental status, or seizures may be experiencing an intracranial bleed. Paralysis, weakness, and asymmetric neurologic findings may signify a spinal cord hematoma.

Laboratory Data. The following laboratory data should be obtained: complete blood count with hematocrit, blood coagulation studies, urinalysis, and x-rays as indicated by history and physical findings. A computerized tomography (CT) scan is indicated with a history of head trauma.

Management. Emergency management is aimed at controlling bleeding, replacing volume, administering the missing coagulation factor, and providing comfort. The type and amount of factor replacement depends on the factor deficiency and location and severity of hemorrhage. Fresh frozen plasma may be administered in the emergency department if the missing factor is not readily available. Table 16–2 describes the factor levels for bleeding episodes, and Table 16–3 describes the therapeutic concentrates for factor replacement.

If hemarthosis is present, the joint should be immobilized. Analgesics may be necessary until the swelling subsides. Aspirin should never be used, since its inhibitory effect on the platelet function may further aggravate the clotting disorder. Application of a cold pack to the affected joint may decrease pain and swelling. Arthrocentesis may be performed by the physician to remove blood from the joint to allow early mobilization and to increase range of motion. Aspiration of a joint is a very frightening procedure for children, and the nurse may need to restrain the child during this procedure while providing reassurance and emotional support.

Muscle bleeding is usually superficial and easily controlled with a single dose of replacement therapy. When extensive hemorrhage does occur, it is most commonly found in the retroperitoneal area and thighs. Bed rest and administration of an analgesic will be necessary.[9]

Subcutaneous bleeding may occur but is rarely dangerous and rarely requires therapy. A subcutaneous bleed in the neck, however, may cause compression of the airway. Any bleeding in the neck muscles should be carefully monitored, and equipment to maintain a patent airway

TABLE 16-2. FACTOR LEVELS FOR BLEEDING EPISODES IN PATIENTS WITH HEMOPHILIA

Site of Bleeding	Factor Level (%) Desired	Comments
Common joint	20–40	Phone follow-up at 24 and 48 hr
Joint (hip or groin)	40	Repeat transfusion in 24–48 hr
Soft tissue or muscle	20–40	No therapy if small and not enlarging; transfuse if enlarging
Muscle (calf or forearm)	30–40	Admit if impending or actual anterior compartment syndrome; surgical consultation
Muscle: deep (thigh, hip, or ilipsoas)	40–60	May require admission; transfusion, then another at 24 hr, then as needed
Neck or throat	50–80	Admit; consider airway mangement
Mouth, lip, tongue, or dental work	40	Aminocaproic acid (Amicar)
Laceration	40	Transfuse until wound is healed; if sutured, continue transfusion until 24 hr after suture removal
Hematuria		Mild to moderate; prednisone, rest, hydration
	40	Severe; transfuse to 40% plus prednisone, rest, hydration
Gastrointestinal	60–80	Admit
Head trauma (no evidence of central nervous system bleeding)	50	Very close follow-up
Head trauma (probable or definite central nervous system bleeding, headache, vomiting, neurologic signs)	100	Admit; investigate (CT scan, etc.); maintain peak and trough factor levels at 100% and 50%, respectively, for 14 days if documented central nervous system bleeding
Surgery	80–100	At time of surgery, maintain peak and trough factor levels at 60% and 30%, respectively, for 1 wk postoperatively; add aminocaproic acid for mouth surgery

The minimum hemostatic level for factors VIII and IX is 10%–20%.
Reproduced with permission from R.A. Yanofsky. Hematologic disorders, Hemophilia. In R.M. Barkin, & P. Rosen, (Eds.), Emergency Pediatrics. St. Louis: Mosby, 1984, p. 563.

should be readily available, since airway obstruction could be sudden. Likewise, any bleeding in the oral cavity should be carefully monitored.[10] Aminocaproic acid (Amicar) is given orally in conjunction with replacement therapy for any mouth, lip, or tongue bleeding.

Because of the numerous blood product transfusions that children with hemophilia receive, they are at an increased risk of developing acquired immune deficiency syndrome (AIDS). All bodily secretions and blood specimens should therefore be handled with the appropriate precautions.

The majority of children with hemophilia will be treated and discharged home. Those with head trauma, retropharyngeal bleeding, or gastrointestinal bleeding will usually be admitted for observation and further intervention.

TABLE 16-3. THERAPEUTIC CONCENTRATES USED FOR FACTOR REPLACEMENT

Product	Available Forms	Coagulation Factors	Average Units/Bag or Unit	Half-life (hours)	Comments
Cryoprecipitate		VIII	60–125 (average: 100)	12	Use for mild hemophilia and those <5 yr: less hepatitis risk; inconvenient
Factor VIII	Hemofil Humafac Koate Profilate	VIII	280–300	12	Convenient; hepatitis risk; expensive
Factor IX	Konyne Proplex	IX II, VII, X	400–600	24	Convenient; hepatitis risk; useful for factor VIII inhibitor

Reproduced with permission from R.A. Yanofsky. Hematologic disorders, hemophillia. In R.M. Barkin, & P. Rosen (Eds.). Emergency Pediatrics. St. Louis: Mosby, 1984, p. 556.

Psychosocial Support and Parent Education. The child and parents are usually frightened by the bleeding episode and seek much reassurance and support from nursing personnel. All procedures and treatments should be carefully explained to the child and parents. The parents should be encouraged to remain at the child's bedside during the emergency department visit. Age-appropriate toys or reading materials should be provided to the child to keep the child calm and resting.

The parents of a child with hemophilia should be referred to a parent support group. The National Hemophilia Foundation has more than 50 chapters across the country to help families with financial, emotional, and medical needs.

Parents of hemophiliacs also have many learning needs. Prevention of injury is very important. The nurse needs to teach the parents how to protect the child from injury without becoming overprotective. Exercise should be encouraged to build strong muscles to help protect the joints from injury. All contact sports, however, should be avoided. A referral to a visiting nurse may be indicated to help the parents plan a safe home environment according to the child's developmental level.

Idiopathic Thrombocytopenic Purpura

Idiopathic thrombocytopenic purpura (ITP) is caused by a pronounced reduction in circulating platelets, causing purpura, or bleeding into the tissues. It is the most frequently encountered platelet disorder of childhood. ITP is usually an acute, self-limited disease but can also be chronic, with numerous remissions. Serious bleeding is rare, occurring in only 2 to 4 percent of cases.[11] Most cases resolve within 6 months.

Etiology and Pathophysiology. The thrombocytopenia is caused by an antiplatelet antibody produced in the spleen. It is associated with a spectrum of viral illnesses, including measles, rubella, mumps, chicken pox, infectious mononucleosis, and the common cold. Other causes include systemic lupus erythematosus, transfusions, and drug sensitivities. Possible complications, although rare, include intracranial hemorrhage, gastrointestinal bleeding, and hematuria.[12]

History. The acute form of ITP is preceded by a viral infection in 50 percent of cases. It can last anywhere from 3 weeks to several months. The chronic form of the ITP is more indolent in its early stages but may recur over the years. Both forms are characterized by abrupt onset of petechiae and ecchymoses over boney prominences; bleeding from the gastrointestinal tract, mouth, or gums; or epistaxis. Twenty percent of patients with ITP may have a mildly enlarged spleen. Acute leukemia should be considered when children present with purpura.[13]

Laboratory Data. The platelet count is usually reduced to below 50,000 platelets/mm^3 (normal platelet count is 150,000 to 400,000/mm^3). If the count falls below 20,000 platelets/mm^3 the patient is at great risk for hemorrhage. The tourniquet test, bleeding time, and clot reaction will be abnormal. Coagulation studies will be normal. A bone marrow aspiration is usually performed to confirm the diagnosis and to rule out aplastic anemia or leukemia.

Assessment. The skin should be carefully examined. The lesions in ITP are minute red hemorrhages ranging in size from 0.5 to 3.0 or 4.0 mm and are flat. They often occur in association with petechiae. Bleeding should be noted from the mucous membranes of the mouth and nose.[14] Hematuria and bloody stools may occur. The child with ITP who has sustained head trauma should be carefully evaluated for signs of increased intracranial pressure.

Management. Emergency management focuses on controlling bleeding and preventing hemorrhage. The patient must be continually evaluated for shock and signs of increased intracranial bleeding. Transfusion with packed red blood cells may be necessary. Platelet transfusions may be administered during acute bleeding. Survival of the transfused platelets, however, is brief. Steroids are administered in severe or chronic cases. The effects of steroid therapy are usually apparent in 48–72 hours. Splenectomy is reserved for

children with thrombocytopenia that persists past 6 months or in the event of a life-threatening hemorrhage. Patients with platelet counts of less than 50,000 platelets/mm^3 should be admitted for evaluation and close monitoring.

Psychosocial Support and Parent Education. In the initial phase of assessment, parents often fear that their child has a life-threatening illness, such as leukemia. They are also greatly disturbed by the changes in the appearance of their child caused by the purpura and petechiae. Parents and child need a great deal of emotional support and reassurance while in the emergency department.

If the child is discharged home, the parents need to be instructed to observe for any abnormalities. Accident prevention should be stressed, and the child should be instructed not to play any contact sports or rough games. The use of aspirin and aspirin products should be avoided. If steroids are prescribed the parents should be instructed in their administration with special emphasis on not abruptly discontinuing them. The side effects of steroids, such as facial edema, weight gain, and increased appetite, should be explained.

Disseminated Intravascular Coagulation

Disseminated intravascular coagulation (DIC) is an acquired disorder of hemostasis that occurs with the activation of clotting mechanisms leading to a depression of clotting factors and intravascular formation of fibrin. DIC is manifested by diffuse hemorrhage and thrombosis.

Pathophysiology. DIC is not a primary disease but rather is a secondary disorder that complicates a pathologic process such as hypovolemic shock; septic shock; viral, bacterial, rickettsial, or parasitic infections; multiple trauma; burns; respiratory distress syndrome; neoplasms; leukemia; intrauterine infections; severe birth asphyxia; snake bites; and heat stroke.[15]

DIC occurs when the first stage of the coagulation process is abnormally stimulated. Thrombin is generated in larger amounts than can be neutralized by the body, with rapid conversion of fibrinogen to fibrin with aggregation and destruction of platelets. In the second stage the fibrinolytic mechanism is activated, causing extensive destruction of clotting factors. The child is then susceptible to uncontrollable hemorrhage and damage and hemolysis of red blood cells.

History. A history may reveal one of the secondary disorders described above. Careful attention should be given to the details of a history of bacterial or viral illness. DIC most often is associated with bacterial septic shock.

Assessment. The child with DIC may present with petechiae, purpura, excessive bleeding from a venipuncture site, hypotension, acrocyanosis, ischemic necrosis of the skin and subcutaneous tissues, and dysfunction of organs from infarction and ischemia. Thrombosis in a blood vessel serving the central nervous system may cause changes in level of consciousness. Hematuria may indicate renal system involvement.

Laboratory Data. Hematologic abnormalities include anemia, prolonged prothrombin time, prolonged partial thromboplastin time, prolonged thrombin time, decreased platelet count, decreased fibrinogen, decreased factors V and VIII, and distortion of red blood cell morphology. Blood and urine cultures, complete blood count, and arterial blood gases should also be obtained.

Management. Initial attention should be directed toward stabilizing the patient,

and treatment involves correcting the underlying cause, supportive measures, and administration of heparin to inhibit thrombin formation. Heparin is given intravenously 50 units/kg, followed 4 hours later by 10 to 15 units/kg/hour by constant intravenous infusion. Vitamin K should be administered intravenously. Fresh whole blood or packed red blood cells are administered if there is significant hemorrhage.[16]

Platelets and fresh frozen plasma may be administered to replace lost plasma components. Humidified 40 percent oxygen should be administered. Vital signs and temperature should be carefully monitored. Cardiac monitoring should be implemented. Continued assessment of neurologic, respiratory, and circulatory status is imperative during stabilization in the emergency department and subsequent transfer to an intensive care unit. The emergency department nurse should protect the child from any unnecessary bleeding episodes. The child's energy should be conserved in the emergency department by bedrest.

Psychosocial Support and Parent Education. Parents are often frightened by the complication of DIC to an already stressful illness or injury in their child. Parents need to be informed of the child's progress and prepared for the child's admission to the intensive care unit. Parents should be allowed to spend as much time as possible at the child's bedside while in the emergency department.

NOTES

1. C. Kneut. Sickle cell anemia. *Issues in Comprehensive Pediatric Nursing* 4(1980):19.
2. L. McMahon. Sickle cell disease. In R.M. Reece (Ed.), *Manual of Emergency Pediatrics* (3rd ed.). Philadelphia: W.B. Saunders, 1984, p. 311.
3. P.E. Green, & L.M. Bloomquist. The hemopoietic system. In G.M. Scipien (Ed.), *Com-*

prehensive Pediatric Nursing New York: Mc-Graw Hill, 1979, p. 724.

4. McMahon, Sickle cell disease, p. 309.
5. Kneut, Sickle cell anemia, p. 24.
6. McMahon, Sickle cell disease, p. 310.
7. J.W. Bender, & A.R. Cohen. Hematotologic emergencies. In G. Fleisher, & S. Ludwig (Eds.), *Textbook of Pediatric Emergency Medicine.* Baltimore: Williams & Wilkins, 1983, p. 480.
8. Ibid., pp. 480–481.
9. Ibid., p. 481.
10. Ibid., p. 482.
11. R.M. Barkin, & P. Rosen. Idiopathic thrombocytopenic purpura. In *Emergency Pediatrics.* St. Louis: Mosby, p. 478.
12. Ibid., p. 566.
13. Ibid.
14. M.E. Osband. Bleeding disorders. In R.M. Reece (Ed.), *Manual of Emergency Pediatrics* (3rd ed.). Philadelphia: W.B. Saunders, 1984, p. 29.
15. Barkin, & Rosen, *Emergency Pediatrics*, p. 558.
16. Ibid., pp. 559–560.

BIBLIOGRAPHY

Sickle Cell Disease

Bender, J.W., & Cohen, A.R. Sickle hemoglobin disorders. In Fleisher, G., & Ludwig, S. (Eds.), *Textbook of Pediatric Emergency Medicine.* Baltimore: Williams & Wilkins, 1983, pp. 467–473.
Eoff, M.J. Sickle cell disease. In Mott, S., Fazekas, N.F., & James, S.R. (Eds.), *Nursing Care of Children and Families.* Menlo Park, Calif.: Addison-Wesley, 1985, pp. 1233–1238.
Gibbons, P.T. Transfusion therapy in sickle cell disease. *Nursing Clinics of North America* 18(1983):201–206.
Giller, R.H. Sickle cell disease. In Barkin, R.B., & Rosen, P. (Eds.), *Emergency Pediatrics.* St. Louis: Mosby, 1984, pp. 569–574.
Goodwin, M., & Baysinger, M. Understanding antisickling agents and the sickling process. *Nursing Clinics of North America* 18(1983):207–214.
Green, P.E., & Bloomquist, L.M. The hemopoietic system. In G.M. Scipien (Ed.), *Com-prehensive Pediatric Nursing* (2nd ed.). New York: McGraw-Hill, 1979, pp. 724–727.
Kneut, C. Sickle cell anemia. *Issues in Comprehensive Pediatric Nursing* 4(1980):19–27.
McMahon, L. Sickle cell disease. In Reece, R.M. (Ed.), *Manual of Emergency Pediatrics* (3rd ed.). Philadelphia: W.B. Saunders, 1984, pp. 308–312.
Rooks, Y., & Pack, B. A profile of sickle cell disease. *Nursing Clinics of North America* 18(1983):131–138.
Stoeppel, A. Care of the child with a hematopoietic disorder. In Oakes, E.A. (Ed.), *Critical Care Nursing of Children and Adolescents.* Philadelphia: W.B. Saunders, 1981, pp. 266–268.
Sullivan, D. The crises of sickle cells. *Emergency Medicine* 13(1981):28–43.
Walters, I. The complications of sickle cell disease. *Nursing Clinics of North America* 18(1983):139–184.
Williams, S., Earles, A.N., & Pack, B. Psychological considerations in sickle cell disease. *Nursing Clinics of North America* 18(1983):215–230.

Hemophilia

Bender, J.W., & Cohen, A.R. Disorders of coagulation. In Fleisher, G., & Ludwig, S. (Eds.), *Textbook of Pediatric Emergency Medicine.* Baltimore: Williams & Wilkins, 1983, pp. 480–486.
Buchanan, G.R. Hemophilia. *Pediatric Clinics of North America* 27(May 1980):309–326.
Budassi, S.A., & Barber, J.M. Hemophilia. In *Emergency Nursing: Principles and Practice.* St. Louis: Mosby, 1981, p. 513.
Cohen, S.A. (Ed.). Hemophilia factors VIII and IX. In *Pediatric Emergency Management: Guidelines for Rapid Diagnosis and Management.* Bowie, Md.: Robert Brady, 1982, p. 205.
Dressler, D. Understanding and treating hemophilia. *Nursing '80* 10(1980):72–73.
Eoff, M.J. Hemophilia. In Mott, S.R., Fazek, N.F., & James, S.R. (Eds.), *Nursing Care of Children and Families.* Menlo Park, Calif.: Addison-Wesley, 1985, pp. 1240–1249.
Green, P.E., & Bloomquist, L.M. Hemophilia. In Scipien, G.M. (Ed.), *Comprehensive Pediatric Nursing* (2nd ed.). New York: McGraw-Hill, 1979, pp. 727–730.
Whaley, L.F., & Wong, D.L. Hemophilia. In *Nursing Care of Infants and Children* (2nd ed.). St. Louis: Mosby, 1983, pp. 1361–1366.

Yanofsky, R.A. Hemophilia. In Barkin, R., & Rosen, P. (Eds.), *Emergency Pediatrics*. St. Louis: Mosby, 1981, pp. 562–566.

Idiopathic Thrombocytopenic Purpura

Bender, J.W., & Cohen, A.R. Idiopathic thrombocytopenic purpura (ITP). In Fleisher, G., & Ludwig, S. (Eds.), *Textbook of Pediatric Emergency Medicine*. Baltimore: Williams & Wilkins, 1984, pp. 478–479.

Green, P.E., & Bloomquist, L.M. Idiopathic thrombocytopenic purpura. In Scipien, G.M. (Ed.), *Comprehensive Pediatric Nursing* (2nd ed.). New York: McGraw-Hill, 1979, pp. 739–740.

Lightsey, A.L. Thrombocytopenia in children. *Pediatric Clinics of North America* 27(1980):293–308.

Osband, M.E. Bleeding disorders. In Reece, R.M. (Ed.), *Manual of Emergency Pediatrics* (3rd ed.). Philadelphia: W.B. Saunders, 1984, pp. 28–32.

Whaley, L.F., & Wong, D.L. Idiopathic thrombocytopenic purpura. In *Nursing Care of Infants and Children* (2nd ed.). St. Louis:

Mosby, 1983, pp. 1366–1367.

Disseminated Intravascular Coagulation

Cohen, S.A. (Ed.) Disseminated intravascular coagulation. In *Pediatric Emergency Management*. Bowie, Md.: Brady, 1982, p. 206.

Lanros, N.E. Disseminated intravascular coagulation. In *Assessment and Intervention in Emergency Nursing* (2nd ed.). Bowie, Md.: Brady, 1983, pp. 291–292.

McMahon, L. Disseminated intravascular coagulation. In Reece, R.M. (Ed.), *Manual of Emergency Pediatrics* (2nd ed.). Philadelphia: W.B. Saunders, 1978, pp. 105–106.

O'Brien, B.S., & Woods, S. The paradox of DIC. *American Journal of Nursing* 78(1978): 1878–1880.

Stoeppel, A. Disseminated intravascular coagulation. In Oakes, A.R. (Ed.), *Critical Care Nursing of Children and Adolescents*. Philadelphia: W.B. Saunders, 1981, pp. 263–264.

Whaley, L.F., & Wong, D.L. Disseminated intravascular coagulation. In *Nursing Care of Infants and Children* (2nd ed.). St. Louis: Mosby, 1983, pp. 1367–1368.

EMERGENCY DEPARTMENT CARE GUIDE FOR THE CHILD WITH A HEMATOLOGIC EMERGENCY

Nursing Diagnosis	Interventions	Evaluation
Alteration in tissue perfusion related to hematologic emergency, i.e., bleeding disorder or sickle cell crisis	Administer humidified oxygen Administer intravenous fluids or blood products Carefully monitor vital signs Control bleeding with external pressure	Skin color is normal Capillary refill is adequate (<3 seconds)
Impaired gas exchange related to decreased oxygen-carrying capacity of blood	Administer humidified oxygen Administer blood products Assess arterial blood gases Assess hemoglobin and hematocrit values Continually assess vital signs	Arterial blood gases are within normal range Hemoglobin and hematocrit return to normal Vital signs are normal
Potential for infection related to chronic illness	Assess child's body temperature	Child's temperature remains normal

Nursing Diagnosis	Interventions	Evaluation
	Prevent exposure to infectious diseases in the emergency department	Child is not exposed to infectious agents
Alteration in comfort: pain related to sickle cell disease and vaso-occlusive crisis	Administer analgesic as indicated Immobilize any joint that is painful and swollen	Child describes a decrease in pain
Activity intolerance related to chronic illness, i.e., hemophilia or sickle cell disease	Decrease level of activity while in emergency department Discuss child's toleration of physical activity with parents	Child rests while in emergency department Parents demonstrate an understanding of child's capacity for strenuous activity

17 | Respiratory Emergencies

Anne Phelan

Conditions that alter the normal breathing patterns of a child of any age are stressful to both child and parents. This factor must be considered when providing emergency nursing care to any child with an acute respiratory impairment. Nursing intervention must be directed toward normalizing air exchange, minimizing respiratory effort, providing adequate hydration, and easing anxiety. As is the case with children of all ages, careful attention must be paid to giving parents and children adequate, understandable explanations of all procedures, treatments, and signs of improvement throughout the emergency department visit.

ASSESSMENT OF THE RESPIRATORY SYSTEM

When a child first arrives in the emergency department with any respiratory problem, a rapid but thorough assessment to determine the nature and severity of the problem must be performed. It is best to develop an organized, systematic approach to assessment, including the four steps of observation, palpation, percussion, and auscultation. Keep in mind that with young children the best results will be obtained by performing the least intrusive procedures first. Refer to Figure 17–1 for a review of the anatomy of the respiratory system.

Observation. Although observation is the simplest assessment tool, it gives the nurse a high yield of information about the possible origins and severity of respiratory difficulty. The child's bare chest is inspected for structural abnormalities, symmetry of movement during both inspiration and expiration, and use of accessory muscles. Careful documentation is made of the location and severity of retractions; the intercostals, the areas above the manubrium and clavicles and below the xyphoid process, are most common (Fig. 17–2). Any movement of the head in association with respiratory effort indicates severe distress. Paradoxical or diaphragmatic (abdominal) breathing is normal in infancy.[1,2]

Palpation. In addition to its use in the detection of abnormal growths, palpation is used in instances of known or suspected trauma to detect the presence of bony abnormalities, areas of tenderness, and swelling. Crepitant swelling most often indicates the free air of a subcutaneous emphysema or pneumomediastinum. The trachea should also be palpated for the deviation from midline associated with unilateral pneumothorax. Tactile fremitus may be elicited by placing the whole hand over various thoracic sites to detect abnormalities in sound transmission during the cries of the infant and during light conversation with the older child. Abnormalities in sound transmission may indicate atelectasis or consolidation in that area.[3]

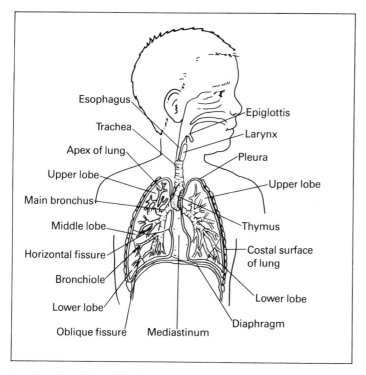

Esophagus
Epiglottis
Trachea
Larynx
Apex of lung
Pleura
Upper lobe
Upper lobe
Main bronchus
Middle lobe
Thymus
Horizontal fissure
Costal surface of lung
Bronchiole
Lower lobe
Lower lobe
Diaphragm
Oblique fissure   Mediastinum

Figure 17-1. Respiratory system.

Percussion. Percussion may be performed on infants by tapping with a single finger. The normal percussion note is hyperresonant over all lung fields. Any variations, excluding the sternal area, connote possi-ble lobar consolidation, intrathoracic mass, or presence of pleural fluid.[4]

Auscultation. The bell or small diaphragm of a stethoscope is used to listen for nor-

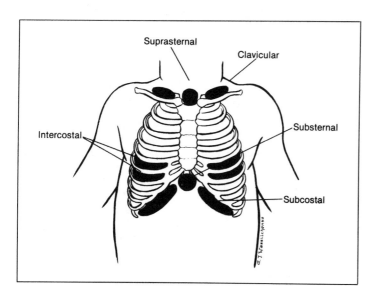

Suprasternal
Clavicular
Intercostal
Substernal
Subcostal

Figure 17-2. Location of retractions. *(Reproduced by permission from L.F. Whaley, & D.L. Wong. Nursing Care of Infants and Children (3rd ed.). St. Louis: Mosby, 1987.)*

mal bronchovesicular breathing. Any adventitious breath sounds must be localized and documented. Infants and small children normally have irregular rate and depth of respiration necessitating a full minute of auscultation during a quiet time to obtain an accurate respiratory rate.

Management. The signs and symptoms of respiratory distress are summarized in Table 17–1.

The child presenting with a respiratory problem should be considered emergent if any of the following are present, either alone or in combination:

- Asymmetric movement of the chest wall during the respiratory cycle
- Crepitant swelling
- Dullness of the percussion note
- Retractions or nasal flaring
- Adventitious breath sounds, i.e., rales (high pitch crackles), rhonchi (coarse rattles), wheezes (inspiratory or expiratory, not cleared by coughing), stridor, or decreased air movement.

RESPIRATORY DISORDERS

Some common disease entities affecting the respiratory system must be dealt with in an individual manner. The following emergent respiratory problems have specific presenting symptomatology and must be readily identified by the emergency department nurse to institute prompt and appropriate intervention.

Bronchiolitis

Bronchiolitis is an acute, self-limiting, viral inflammatory process involving the bronchioles and alveoli. It occurs more often in boys than in girls and is most frequently seen in winter and spring. Bronchiolitis affects infants under 18 months of age, with a rare incidence after the second year of life. The case mortality rate is 1 to 5 percent.[5]

Etiology and Pathophysiology. The most common causative organism is the respiratory syncytial virus (RSV). Other viruses

TABLE 17–1. SIGNS AND SYMPTOMS OF RESPIRATORY DISTRESS

Clinical Feature	Infants	Children
Respiratory rate	Newborn: 60 respirations/min 1–12 mo: 40 respirations/min	1–4 yr: 32 respirations/min 5–18 yr: 28 respirations/min 10–14 yr: 24 respirations/min
Respiratory observations	Nasal flaring Substernal retracting Seesaw abdominal breathing Subcostal retracting	Nasal flaring Substernal retracting Supraclavicular retracting Intercostal or subcostal retractions
Breath sounds	Expiratory grunt Inspiratory stridor Inspiratory or expiratory wheezes Diminished breath sounds	Expiratory grunt Inspiratory stridor Inspiratory or expiratory wheezes Diminished breath sounds
Color	Palor, circumoral or general cyanosis, mottled, dusky	Palor, cyanosis, dusky
Behavior	Irritability Lethargy Refusal to drink fluids Weak cry	Irritability Lethargy Refusal to eat or drink

have also been implicated in bronchiolitis such as influenza, parainfluenza, rhinovirus, adenovirus, and *Mycoplasma pneumoniae.*

The viral agent settles in the mucosal lining of the bronchioles, causing the cells of the lining to slough. During this process the bronchial mucosa become edematous and secrete copious amounts of mucus, which adds to the debris of dead cells, causing irregular patterns of obstruction and plugging. The irregularity of obstruction leads to air trapping, making it difficult for the child to exhale completely, hence the picture of hyperinflation seen on x-ray. The wheezing, heard clinically, is caused by air attempting to flow through these partially obstructed passages. Air trapping distal to the point of obstruction causes abnormal ventilation or perfusion at the alveolar level, leading to hypoxemia. Hypercapnia is actually a late sign and may indicate that respiratory failure is likely to occur.[6,7]

History. The typical clinical picture is of an infant who presents with dyspnea, a rapid respiraroty rate, varying degrees of cyanosis, wheezing, and decreased tolerance for food and drink. There is usually a history of a "cold" for a few days prior to the onset of dyspnea. There may be a family history of allergies or asthma as well as prior history of a bronchiolitic episode in the infant. Fever may be present but will usually be low grade.

Careful history taking will elicit the point at which dyspnea began. Since the critical period of bronchiolitis usually occurs during the first 24 to 72 hours after its onset, this information becomes important in predicting the course. An infant who exhibits cyanosis, areas of decreased air flow, and tiredness on day 1 should be considered to be far more critical than a child with moderate wheezing who is tolerating

oral fluids on day 3. Obtaining a history of the infant's normal feeding pattern in comparison to the present as well as a history of any decrease in urination or onset of diarrhea is important in assessing the hydration status of the infant. Poor tolerance of oral feedings, including refusal to eat or drink and choking spells, indicates significant respiratory distress.

Assessment. Assessment of the infant with bronchiolitis must always include a full set of vital signs. Tachycardia may indicate impending failure, so the child with an apical pulse rate approaching 200 should be carefully observed. The respiratory rate, usually 50 to 80 per minute, is most valuable when taken for a full minute when the infant is at rest. Observe the bare chest for the increased anteroposterior diameter or barrel chest associated with hyperinflation. Also, cautiously document the location and severity of any nasal flaring or retractions observed, as these may change over short periods of time. Infants with bronchiolitis typically have retractions in the intercostal and substernal areas. Deep retractions involving several sets of accessory muscles are more worrisome.

Restlessness should be viewed as a sign of hypoxemia, while cyanosis, pallor, and lethargy may herald respiratory failure.[8] Palpation for tactile fremitus should be performed in a gentle manner. Any areas of decreased sound transmission usually indicate areas of consolidation or atelectasis and provide the nurse with a valuable clue as to where areas of decreased air movement will be heard on auscultation. Dullness of the percussion note in any area other than sternal would also indicate fluid buildup or consolidation.

Auscultation of the chest of an infant with bronchiolitis should be performed with careful attention to the quality and character of the wheezing as well as comparisons of the quality of sounds from one area of the lung to another. An infant with loud, moist wheezing and good air movement throughout is far less worrisome than the infant with dry crackles and decreased air flow in sections of lung fields.

Assessment procedures should be performed frequently and should be carefully documented to provide a basis for evaluating improvement or worsening of the condition. Upon arrival in the emergency department and completion of the initial assessment, the child should be brought to an acute care area where nursing observations can be made continuously.

Laboratory Data. The posteroanterior and lateral views of the chest radiograph usually show hyperinflation, with peribronchial cuffing and flattened diaphragms indicative of the air trapping of bronchiolitis. In addition to the complete blood count, a throat or nasopharyngeal culture should be obtained in an effort to isolate the causative viral agent. Arterial blood gas determinations of PaO_2 under 60 or $PaCO_2$ over 45 indicate respiratory compromise.[9]

Management. The disease entity most commonly thought of in conjunction with bronchiolitis is asthma. The differences between the child with bronchiolitis and the child with asthma are summarized in Table 17-2. In an effort to rule out reactive airway disease, a trial dose of epinephrine (1 : 1000—.01 cc/kg) should be given. Epinephrine is contraindicated in children with tachycardia. The infant should then be observed carefully for any signs of improvement for the next 15 to 20 minutes. Since epinephrine has no effect in true bronchiolitis, if no improvement is seen after the first injection, a second dose should not be given. The next major cause of wheezing in infancy is the aspiration of a foreign body. A suggestive history accompanied by more localized wheezing should indicate the need for a lateral radiograph of the neck and chest to detect an opaque foreign body. If suspicion of a foreign body remains high in the absence of radiopaque findings, fluoroscopy may be necessary to localize the object.

Since bronchiolitis is a self-limiting, viral illness, antibiotics are of little or no use, and therapy is largely supportive. The use of a mist tent in the emergency department should be encouraged, as it serves

TABLE 17-2. DIFFERENTIATION OF BRONCHIOLITIS AND ASTHMA

Clinical Features	Bronchiolitis	Asthma
Etiology	Viral	Allergic or infectious
Occurrence	12 mo or younger	Over 1 yr of age
Respirations	Wheezing, expiratory or inspiratory	Wheezing, expiratory or inspiratory
	Shallow	Shallow
	Tachypnea	Tachypnea
	Retractions	Retractions
Chest films	Hyperinflation ± scattered infiltrate	Hyperinflation
Response to beta-adrenergic drugs or theophylline	None	Reversal of bronchospasm

the dual purpose of providing the desired oxygen concentration, 30 to 40 percent, and a moist environment to prevent fluid loss due to increased respiratory rate and to liquefy secretions. Some symptomatic relief may be noted within 30 minutes. Observation of the infant during feeding will give the nurse a valid impression of the baby's current ability to tolerate oral hydration. Refusal to drink fluids or choking usually indicate the need for intravenous hydration and hospital admission.

The child may be treated as an outpatient only if (1) the respiratory rate is below 60; (2) hydration status is adequate and the infant is tolerating oral fluids; (3) the parents own or have access to a cool mist vaporizer or have an adequate supply of hot water for showers to provide humidification; (4) cyanosis is absent and the Pa_{CO_2} remains near normal levels (35 to 45 mm Hg); (5) parent or caretaker feels comfortable caring for the baby at home; (6) the child is over 3 months of age.

Parent Education. Once the decision is made to discharge the infant from the emergency department, care must be taken to advise the parents of all signs of increased respiratory distress as well as comfort measures. Parents should be told to expect rapid improvement about 3 days after the breathing trouble began but that the child may not be completely well for about 2 weeks. Refer to Appendix A for instructions to parents of a child with bronchiolitis.

Asthma

Asthma may be best described as recurrent reactive airway disease. It is characterized by constriction of bronchiole smooth muscle, mucosal edema, and increased mucous production as well as its reversal in response to beta-stimulating drugs. It is estimated that 5 to 10 percent of all American children are asthmatic. Asthma is seen more frequently in male children than in female children.[10]

Etiology and Pathophysiology. When the asthmatic child is exposed to allergens, respiratory infections, emotional trauma, exercise, or the inhalation of an irritating substance, the smooth muscles of the bronchioles react by constricting. The narrower air passages result in decreased ability to move air out of the lungs and the first feelings of tightness. This is shortly followed by excessive mucous production, which, if left unchecked, eventually leads to edema of the lining of the bronchioles and further obstruction to air flow and gas exchanges. Generally speaking the longer an asthmatic attack is allowed to progress without intervention, the more medication will be required to reverse the process.[11]

The typical asthmatic child will arrive in the emergency department wheezing audibly, with some nasal flaring and shoulder lifting on inspiration. Suprasternal, intercostal, and substernal retractions may also be present. The child may be pale or may exhibit some cyanosis. He or she also may have difficulty talking.

History. The history of an asthmatic child will usually reveal other evidence of atopic problems such as eczema and hay fever. The family history usually shows other members who are asthmatic. The emergency department nurse's history for a previously diagnosed asthmatic should include time of onset of the present episode of wheezing, cough, and dyspnea; medications taken prior to arrival with times of each dose; and presence of a recognized trigger for the attack (i.e., exposure to a known allergen, upper respiratory infection, prolonged exercise, weather change). Noting the time since the last attack or admission is also helpful.

Assessment. The vital signs of an asthmatic child will initially show dyspnea and tachycardia, which should gradually resolve with therapy. Vital signs should be obtained and recorded frequently and always prior to the administration of each medication. This, along with the intermittent auscultation of the chest, provides a valuable indication of therapeutic effectiveness.

The blood pressure of an older asthmatic child may exhibit a phenomenon called pulsus paradoxus. Pulsus paradoxus may be described as the fluctuation of arterial pressure with the respiratory cycle. When in severe respiratory distress, the arterial pressure may rise with expiration and fall with inspiration. The emergency department nurse can measure this by stopping the fall of mercury at the point of the first systolic sound and observing for variations of the mercury level during the respiratory cycle. If the difference in arterial pressure during the respiratory cycle is equivalent to 30 mm Hg, the patient is said to have a pulsus of 30. Pulsus paradoxus will disappear as intrathoracic pressures resolve.

Observe the child's chest bare for the presence, location, and depth of retractions. The presence of nasal flaring, shoulder lifting, and cyanosis should be carefully documented.

Auscultation of the chest over all lung fields will yield a wealth of information. The characteristic wheezing may vary in intensity from loud musical wheeze with other coarse sounds present to the tight squeaking wheeze usually indicative of markedly decreased air movement through the narrowed bronchioles. Auscultation should always be performed comparing the same site on both sides alternately with an ear toward detecting any inequality of breath sounds indicative of decreased air flow. Due to the asthmatic child's difficulty with expelling air, auscultation should include a timed value for the inspiration to expiration ratio. Initially the expiratory phase may be quite prolonged.

The supraclavicular and intercostal areas should be palpated for the crepitant swelling indicative of a pneumomediastinum or interstitial emphysema. The trachea should also be palpated for any deviation from midline associated with a unilateral pneumothorax.

It is important to remember that wheezing does not always mean asthma, and an asthmatic attack may be present when wheezing is not. An asthmatic attack may also manifest itself by a persistent cough, usually occurring in spells, or the feeling of tightness associated with decreased air flow. The child with no personal or family history of asthma should therefore be assessed for the possibility of an aspirated foreign body, pulmonary edema, or, in infants, a tracheoesophageal fistula. Conversely, the child with a known history of asthma who presents with dyspnea, a tight feeling, or a spasmotic cough in the absence of wheezing should be given a trial dose of epinephrine and should be observed carefully for response.[12,13]

Laboratory Data. In the presence of fever a complete blood count should be drawn prior to the administration of any medications; epinephrine most notably affects the results by dramatically raising the white blood cell count. A child who is on prophylactic or maintenance medications and who is suspected of needing dosage adjustment should have a serum level drawn before therapy begins, with careful notation of how many hours have elapsed since ingestion of the medication.

Arterial blood gas determinations may be made periodically during the course of therapy, although this invasive and painful procedure is usually reserved for severe attacks that are not responding well.

The chest radiograph of an asthmatic during an attack will usually show hyperinflation and gas trapping; areas of consolidation or atelectasis may also be present. The chest radiograph in Figure 17–3 shows subcutaneous emphysema and pneumomediastinum during a severe asthma attack.

Ideally the child's pulmonary functions should be measured directly on initial presentation in the emergency department and periodically throughout treatment through the use of a peak flow meter. The FEV_1 (forced expiratory volume at 1 second) value together with arterial blood gas results provide the best possible indication of bronchiole smooth-muscle relaxation and improved gas exchange.

Management. The first therapeutic consideration is to increase the child's oxygen consumption by administering O_2 in a 40 percent concentration in a manner comfortable for the child. After the initial assessment of the child's vital signs and degree of respiratory distress are documented, the medication regimen begins. Table 17–3 summarizes the medications used in the management of the asthmatic child in the emergency department.

Typically two to three doses of aqueous epinephrine are administered at 15-to-20-minute intervals followed by the inhalation of either Bronkosol, Alupent, or Isuprel if the breath sounds do not clear. If signs of cardiac irritation (increased blood pressure, sinus tachycardia, or tachyarrhythmias) develop after administration of epinephrine, lower doses of this drug or an alternate sympathomimetic with more pure beta$_2$ stimulation such as terbutaline, may be subsequently administered. For the same reasons Bronkosol would be the drug of choice over Isuprel for this patient.[14]

Fluids should be offered frequently as

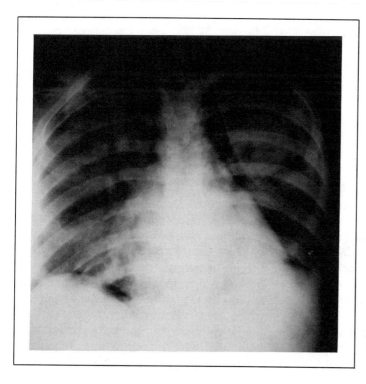

Figure 17–3. A 14-year-old with intractable asthma with subcutaneous emphysema and pneumomediastinum. *(Photo courtesy of Richard De-Nise, MD, and the Pediatric Radiology Department of Boston City Hospital.)*

TABLE 17-3. DRUGS USED IN THE MANAGEMENT OF ACUTE ASTHMA

Drug	Dose and Route	Frequency	Nursing Implications
Aqueous epinephrine 1:1000 (Adrenalin)	0.01 ml/kg to a maximum of 0.4 cc/dose, subcutaneously	Every 20 min to a maximum of 3 doses	Assess vital signs prior to each dose. May cause cardiac irritation, hypertension, tachyarrhythmias, nausea and vomiting, diaphoresis, and headache; may cause necrosis at injection site
Terbutaline sulfate injection (Brethine, Bricanyl)	0.01 mg/kg subcutaneously	Every 30 min to a maximum of 2 doses	Not yet approved by FDA for children under 12 years; causes less cardiac irritability. Monitor blood pressure carefully. Be alert for decrease in diastolic pressure
Isoproterenol (Isuprel)	0.25 ml in 2.5 ml normal saline	Every 4 hr	Close cardiac monitoring is necessary. Observe patient carefully for signs of cardiac irritation
Aminophylline (Anhydrous theophylline)	5–6 mg/kg intravenously administered slowly over 30 min or constant infusion at 0.9–1.1 mg/kg/hr	Every 6 hr	Cardiac monitor should be used. Observe carefully for tachyarrhythmias. Monitor vital signs every 10 minutes. Do not administer simultaneously with epinephrine
Methylprednisolone (Solu-Medrol)	1–2 mg/kg intravenous bolus	Every 6 hr	Incompatible with aminophylline and Ringer's lactate; given to reduce the the mucosal edema associated with a prolonged or severe attack
Bronkosol (Isoetharine)	0.25–0.5 cc, diluted with 2.5 ml normal saline to a nebulizer	Every 2–4 hr	May cause tachycardia, headache, and nausea
Epinephrine (Sus-Phrine) (1:200)	0.005 ml/kg up to 0.2 ml, subcutaneously	Every 8–12 hr	A long-acting epinephrine; given to child who has stopped wheezing prior to discharge home

soon as the child feels comfortable taking them to liquefy and to mobilize secretions. Albuterol (Ventolin) is a new and very effective sympathomimetic drug that is available in a metered-dose inhaler for home use. Children sent home with inhalers should be cautioned against overuse because of the risk of tachyarrhythmias associated with inhaler abuse.

When wheezing and dyspnea persist after inhalation therapy and chest physical therapy, an intravenous line should be started. A bolus of aminophylline is administered 3- to-7-mg/kg intravenously over 20 to 30 minutes, with the dose depending on the estimated serum theophylline level that is determined from peak and trough action of the last administered dose. Cardiac monitoring by oscilloscope should be maintained from the beginning of the bolus administration for the earliest possible detection of the tachyarrhythmias associated with aminophylline. When the asthmatic attack has been present for a protracted period of time or when the child continues to manifest signs of air hunger after the above regimen, the administration of steroids by intravenous infusion should be considered, and the patient is said to be in status asthmaticus.[15]

Admission should be considered when (1) the child fails to respond to the epinephrine and inhalation treatments; (2) tachypnea, retractions, or cyanosis continue in the absence of wheezing; (3) a viral illness with vomiting as a symptom is present and the child is unable to tolerate oral medications; (4) the child has made frequent recent visits to the emergency department, i.e., three visits/week; or (5) parental exhaustion or apprehension exist to such a degree that the provision of adequate home care is questionable.

If the wheezing has subsided, the child may be given Sus-phrine, a long-acting form of epinephrine, 0.005 cc/kg, subcutaneously to a maximum dose of 0.2 cc.

Parent Education. Parents of asthmatic children need much ongoing support and teaching. Instruction for the parents of the child with asthma are listed in Appendix A.

Croup

Croup (laryngotracheobronchitis) is a viral inflammatory process of the subglottic area including the trachea and bronchi. Croup occurs most frequently in infants and children between 6 months and 3 years of age, affects more boys than girls, and may be recurrent. It is most frequently seen in late fall and late spring.

Etiology and Pathophysiology. The most common viral agent isolated in croup is the parainfluenza type 1. Rhinoviruses, parainfluenza type 2 and 3, RSV, measles, and influenza A are also viral etiologic considerations. Bacterial superinfection, although rare, may be caused by pneumococcus or *Hemophilus influenzae*.

Pathophysiology. The inflammatory process of viral croup produces edema of the trachea and bronchi. The edematous airways secrete tenacious mucus, which, along with sloughing of ciliated epithelial lining, leads to problematic secretion removal that interferes with gas exchange at the alveolar level[16] (Fig. 17–4).

History. The history will most likely reveal an upper respiratory infection for several days followed by the onset of the characteristic hoarse, barking cough. It is important to elicit whether the child has had a prior history of croup and what the parents' impressions or apprehensions about the disease are. A history of a fever and of medications taken should also be determined.

Assessment. Nursing assessment should focus on the child's cardiorespiratory status, hydration, anxiety or fatigue level, and parental anxiety. Observe the child's face for the classic open-mouth gulp breathing, amount of drooling, expressions of anxiety, and cyanosis or pallor in the areas around the mouth, nose or ears. The presence and depth of chest wall retractions should be carefully noted and the quality of stridor listened to. The frequency and quality of the cough must be recorded as well as frequent vital signs. Remember that exhaustion and decreased retractions plus decreased air movement plus increased pulse indicate impending respiratory arrest.[17] Auscultation of all lung fields should be performed frequently to ascertain the amount of actual air movement and prolongation of the inspiratory phase. The importance of frequent assessments and meticulous documentation cannot be overemphasized because just as rapid improvement may be

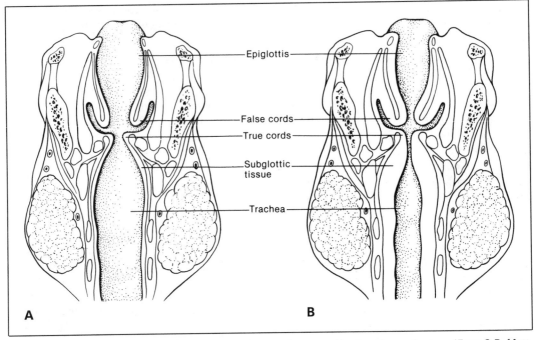

Figure 17–4. (A) Normal larynx. **(B)** Obstruction and narrowing caused by the edema of croup. *(From S.R. Mott, N.F. Fazekas, & S.R. James. Nursing Care of Children and Families. Menlo Park, Calif.: Addison-Wesley, 1985, p. 1131.)*

noted in a humidified environment, rapid deterioration is also a possibility.

The presenting symptomatology will vary in severity according to the degree of inflammation and the amount of exhaustion experienced by the child. In cases of mild croup the child may appear comfortable, will have a hoarse cough on occasion, and stridor may only be heard on auscultation or may be audible when the child is upset. With more severe cases air hunger is evident, inspiratory stridor is audible at rest, cough is more intense and frequent, retractions are visible, notably in the suprasternal area, and substernal depression may be present. In cases of moderate to severe croup the child may appear frightened and restless and may exhibit tachycardia and tachypnea, which are characteristic of hypoxia. Cyanosis, hypercapnea, and acidosis are late signs and may be an

indication for artificial airway support. The increased respiratory effort, air hunger, and inability to take in calories lead to exhaustion, which may seem to relieve the stridor but which should be viewed as a sign of impending respiratory arrest.[18]

Clinical grading of croup divides children with croup into three classifications based on observable data. These classifications are as follows:

- Grade I: quiet at rest, barking cough and stridor occur when disturbed or agitated.
- Grade II: the child has stridor and some retraction of the sternum when quiet.
- Grade III: profound stridor, deep sternal retraction, restlessness, cyanosis.

Grade III is indicative of severe disease and these children require aggressive airway management. Similarly, a clinical scoring system exists which rates the amount of stridor and depth of sternal retraction with grades of 1 to 3 to indicate a mild, moderate or severe clinical state.

The differential diagnosis most often associated with croup is epiglottitis. Epiglottitis differs from croup in that epiglottitis has a rapid onset of symptoms and is bacterial in etiology. In addition, the child's fever is high, he or she drools excessively, is unable to tolerate fluids by mouth, and refuses to lie down. The major differences between croup and epiglottitis are summarized in Table 17–4. The suspected diagnosis of epiglottitis is always an indicator for immediate and expert intubation under anesthesia. All diagnostic procedures, including x-rays, should be postponed until a patent airway is assured. Laryngotracheal foreign body aspiration and measles may also produce croup-like symptoms.

Laboratory Data. It is advisable to keep intrusive procedures to a minimum, as crying and fear increase the work of breathing. In cases of croup many physicians will forego the visualization of the epiglottis in favor of the anteroposterior and lateral neck and chest films as the primary diagnostic tool. The radiograph in Figure 17–5 demonstrates the characteristic ''steeple sign'' and narrowing of tracheal diameter seen in the radiographs of children with croup. Any attempt to visualize the epiglottis may cause severe laryngospasm, necessitating immediate intubation or tracheoostomy. The complete blood count may reveal a moderately elevated white blood cell count. Baseline determinations of arterial blood gases should be made in the emergency department.

Management. The nursing interventions in croup are focused on relieving anxiety and reducing air hunger. Cool-mist tent

TABLE 17–4. DIFFERENTIATION OF CROUP AND EPIGLOTTITIS

Clinical Features	Croup	Epiglottitis
Etiology	Viral agent—usually one of the parainfluenza type	Bacterial agent—usually *Hemophilus influenzae* type B
Occurrence	Seasonal—late fall and late spring, age 6 mo to 3 yr; more often in boys; may recur	Not seasonal; seen in boys and girls aged 2–7 yr with equal frequency
Respirations	Inspiratory stridor; varying degrees of substernal retractions may involve suprasternal notch; inspiratory phase usually prolonged	Inspiratory stridor; deep substernal retractions; unable to manage oral secretions (drooling is constant)
Assessment findings	History reveals a few days of upper respiratory infection with slow progression to hoarse barking cough; may have low-grade fever; will accept oral fluids	Sudden onset of high fever (102F–105F); rapid development of hoarse barking cough; drooling; refusal to lie down. These symptoms usually heighten over 2–4 hr after onset, and intervention must be immediate
Chest films	Laryngotracheal narrowing is the hallmark ''steeple sign''	Inflamed epiglottis causing partial airway obstruction
Response to antibiotic therapy	None	Once a patent airway is established, intravenous ampicillin and chloramphenicol should be started as second priority

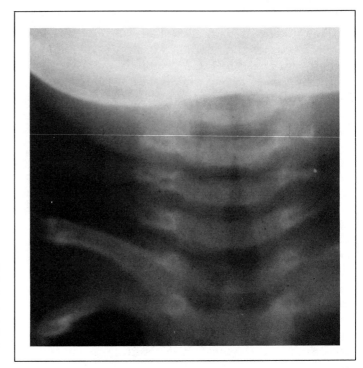

Figure 17–5. A 3-year-old male with tracheobronchitis (croup). Note the airway ''steeple sign'' and the narrowing of the tracheal diameter. *(Photo courtesy of Richard DeNise, MD, and the Pediatric Radiology Department of Boston City Hospital.)*

therapy should be begun in the emergency department. Most procedures can be performed in the tent. Racemic epinephrine may be administered by nebulizer or in a dose of 0.5 cc of a 2¼ percent solution in 3.5 cc of normal saline or distilled water. The use of racemic epinephrine is usually reserved for severe, or Grade III, cases of croup. Racemic epinephrine has been noted to reduce mucosal edema and laryngospasm. Children receiving this therapy may experience profound relief with hourly administrations but should be observed carefully for a rebound worsening of their condition. The rebound effect is thought to be due to actual clinical deterioration rather than effects of the drug. A one fourth percent phenylephrine solution may be used as an alternate therapy.[19]

Antibiotics are of little use in uncomplicated cases of croup. Sedation should

be avoided because restlessness is used as an indicator of the degree of hypoxia, although arterial blood gases are the most reliable indicator. The patient may want to lie down, but keeping the head of the bed slightly elevated is advisable.

The decision for hospital admission rests on the degree of respiratory distress, the ability to maintain adequate hydration, the child's ability to rest, and the degree of parental apprehension.

Parent Education. If the child's croup is judged to be mild and the parents feel comfortable caring for the child at home, the parents should be given careful instructions for home care. These instructions should include comfort measures aimed at easing the child's respiratory effort and a list of observable signs of increased respiratory distress. Refer to Appendix A for instructions to parents of a child with croup.

Epiglottitis

Epiglottitis, or supraglottic laryngitis, is the most emergent type of acute airway obstruction of childhood. This disease produces rapid-onset inflammatory edema of the epiglottis and supraglottic structures. Epiglottitis occurs throughout the year, is seen in boys and girls with equal frequency, and usually affects 2- to 7-year-olds.

When the child with epiglottitis arrives in the emergency department, an aura of heightened anxiety usually surrounds him or her. The anxiety on the part of the child and parent usually stems from the fact that the child appeared well until just about 2 to 4 hours prior to arrival. The child will probably be febrile, will drool excessively, will exhibit signs of air hunger (open-mouthed gulping respirations, tachypnea, stridor, retractions, and a prolonged inspiratory phase), will refuse or choke on oral fluids, and will refuse to lie down.

Etiology and Pathophysiology. Epiglottitis is bacterial in origin. *Hemophilus influenzae* type B is by far the most common organism involved, with an occasional streptococcal, pneumococcal, and staphylococcal incidence.

Following the colonization of the *H. influenzae*, onset of symptomatology and clinical course is rapid. Significant supraglottic edema is evident within 2 hours of onset (Fig. 17–6). This is followed by increased mucosal secretion that may lead to secondary bronchopneumonia, atelectasis, pulmonary edema, or pleural effusion. This, in turn, interferes with gas exchange at the alveolar level. The difficulty in inspiring air past inflamed supraglottic structures causes inspiratory stridor, air hunger, retractions, tachypnea, and anxiety. Due to the fulminant nature of this bacterial infection, fever is usually present. As the clinical hypoxia progresses, cyanosis will become apparent.[20]

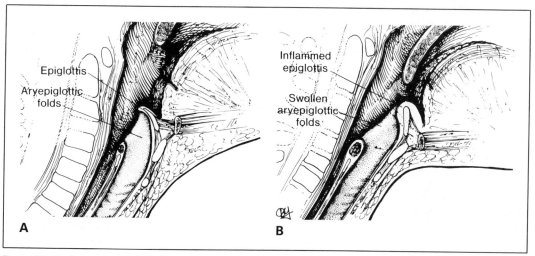

Figure 17-6. Appearance of the lateral neck region in the normal child **(A)** and the child with epiglottitis **(B)**. *(From G.R. Fleisher, & S. Ludwig (Eds.). Textbook of Pediatric Emergency Medicine. Baltimore: Williams & Wilkins, 1983. Used by permission.)*

History. The history of the child with epi-glottitis typically reveals a child who appeared well until 2 to 4 hours prior to arrival in the emergency department. The parent will usually describe a rapid onset of fever, inability to eat or drink, drooling or choking, and difficulty breathing.

Assessment. Nursing assessment must be detailed and rapid, but invasive or disturbing techniques should be avoided. If the child is quiet while sitting in the parent's lap, leave him or her there. The child's excessive crying or attempts to make the child lie down may lead to severe laryngospasm and airway obstruction.

The most valuable assessment tools with this child are observation and auscultation. After the baseline vital signs have been obtained, the nurse should observe and carefully document the signs of air hunger. Such observations include the presence and extent of stridor relative to the respiratory cycle; any timed prolongation of the inspiratory phase; presence and depth of chest-wall muscle retractions; presence and location of cyanosis; and degree of tachypnea and tachycardia. Such observations must be made continually to provide early detection of any changes.

Croup is the condition most closely resembling epiglottitis. Differentiation should occur rapidly in light of the rapidity of onset and fulminant course. Aspiration of a foreign object lodged in the upper airway and asthma may also be diagnostic considerations.

Laboratory Data. Although determinations of arterial blood gases, complete blood count with differential, sedimentation rate, and blood culture may be helpful indicators of the need for supportive therapies, the performance of these blood tests should be deferred until the artificial airway has been established. Likewise, the visualization of the cherry-red epiglottis,

radiographic studies, and the insertion of an intravenous line should also be delayed until a patent airway is assured.

The arterial blood gas will usually show some degree of hypoxemia, while the results of the complete blood count usually show an elevation of the leukocyte count indicative of a bacteriologic infectious process. Cultures will usually be positive for *H. influenzae* type B. Radiographic studies usually reveal a marked increase in the size of the epiglottis as well as some edema of the supraglottic structures. Some increases in lung fluid may be evident in the chest films. The radiograph in Figure 17–7 illustrates a swollen epiglottis that is almost completely obstructing the airway.

Management. Nursing intervention must take place swiftly while at the same time a concerted effort is made to explain the procedures and treatments to the child and parents. The primary focus is to maintain a patent airway. Efforts must be directed toward keeping the child calm and comfortable. If the child is quiet while sitting on the parent's lap, allow him or her to remain there during the brief history and physical examination.

As soon as epiglottitis is suspected, the nurse must gather all of the equipment necessary to perform a tracheostomy and intubation. It is imperative that the anesthesiologist, otorhinolaryngologist, or pediatrician who is prepared to perform tracheostomy or intubation have the appropriate equipment at hand at all times and that the child is never left unattended.

Ideally the establishment of an artificial airway should occur rapidly and in a controlled environment, such as the operating room. The child should be carried to the operating room in an upright position, preferably by the parent.

Hospital admission is always necessary in cases of known or suspected epiglottitis. Intravenous fluid maintenance

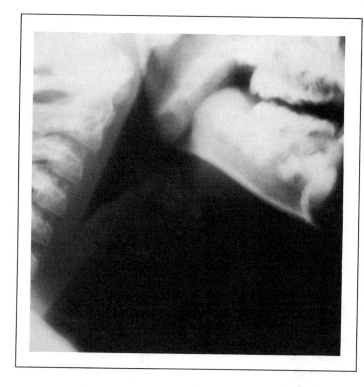

Figure 17–7. A 5-year-old male with epiglottitis. Note the swollen epiglottis almost completely obstructing the airway. *(Photo courtesy of Richard DeNise, MD, and the Pediatric Radiology Department of Boston City Hospital.)*

will be necessary until oral fluids are easily tolerated postextubation. This is also the route of preference for the administration of antibiotics. Ampicillin (100 to 250 mg/kg/day) is the drug of choice to combat *H. influenzae*, but there are strains of this organism known to be ampicillin resistant. Dual coverage with a drug such as chloramphenicol (50 to 100 mg/kg/day) is usually desirable until the culture and sensitivity results are available.[21] The initial doses should be administered as soon as possible in the emergency department. The child must also be maintained in a humid, oxygen-enriched environment, such as that provided with a mist tent. Epiglottitis seldom recurs in the same child.

Pneumonia

Pneumonia may be best defined as an acute inflammation of the lungs, which may be caused by a variety of agents including bacteria and viruses as well as fungi and other agents. Pneumonia is one of the most common infections of the lower respiratory tract in children.

Etiology and Pathophysiology. A variety of organisms causes pneumonia in children. Respiratory viruses are most common. The bacterial organisms most frequently associated with pneumonia in children are *Streptococcus pneumoniae* in all age children and *H. influenzae*. In the preschool age child *Streptococcus pyogenes*, *Staphylococcus aureus*, *Pseudomonas aeruginosa*, *Klebsiella pneumoniae*, *Escherichia coli*, and *Mycobacterium tuberculosis* are also known to cause pneumonia.[22]

The viral agents that have been identified as caustive in childhood pneumonia include RSV, enteroviruses, adenoviruses, influenza, varicella, rubeola, and reoviruses. Also implicated are *Mycoplasma pneumoniae*, chlamydia, Q fever, and protozoa as well as several types of fungi. Pneumonia may also manifest itself after aspiration syndromes.[23]

Causative agents of pneumonia in children may vary with the age of the child or area of infiltration on radiograph. Segmental or lobar pneumonias are usually caused by *Streptococcus pneumoniae* and may be associated with an empyema. Staphylococcus pneumonia occurs in young infants, is less common, and is usually associated with empyema, pneumonoceles, and a high mortality rate. *H. influenzae* pneumonia is a frequent occurrence in children under 2 years old and is usually associated with a pleural effusion. Klebsiella pneumonia has a fulminant course and is seen in young infants or children with chronic pulmonary problems. Bronchopneumonias may be mixed viral and bacterial in etiology. Mycoplasma pneumonia is usually seen in older children and adolescents. Chlamydia pneumonia is usually found in infants from birth to 3 months of age, and occurs as a sequelae of vaginal delivery by an infected mother and conjunctivitis in the infant.[24]

History. The child with pneumonia will have a differing clinical picture according to his or her age, the causative organism, and the duration of evident symptomatology. The young infant often has a history of fever and dyspnea that may have been preceded by symptoms of a "cold," i.e., stuffy or runny nose, crankiness, and cough. There are also some generalized symptoms associated with pneumonia in an infant, which include poor feeding, vomiting, or diarrhea. An extensive or fulminant pneumonia should be suspected when an infant has tachypnea, high fever, circumoral cyanosis, nasal flaring, retractions, and the hallmark "expiratory grunt." Adventitious breath sounds are not always present in infants with pneumonia.

The older child with pneumonia often has fever, chills, cough (may be productive), headache, stomach pain, and chest pain that is not necessarily localized to the area of infection. Tachypnea, tachycardia, dyspnea, retractions, and circumoral pallor or cyanosis may also be present.

A careful tracing of the onset of symptoms, beginning when the child last appeared well and continuing to the present, should be obtained and recorded. The progression of symptomatology over time may be an important factor in determining the possible causative agent. In the young infant a history of conjunctivitis or maternal vaginitis around the time of delivery should be carefully documented. The history of any prior hypersensitivity to antibiotics in this child should be carefully elicited. Carefully document the history or presence of any related symptomatology, i.e., vomiting, headache, chest or abdominal pain, and lethargy.

Assessment. The infant should be assessed in terms of the quality of respirations (tachypnea with minimal distress versus slower respirations); presence, location and depth of retractions; presence of a cough; presence and location of cyanosis (including assessment of capillary filling in distal portions of limbs); nasal flaring; and presence of expiratory grunting. Document the location of any adventitious or decreased breath sounds as well as the quality of the infant's cry. Some assessment of the infant's ability to tolerate oral fluids should be made to determine the infant's ability to maintain adequate hydration.

The older child may exhibit increased vocal tactile fremitus, a dull percussion note over the affected area, and rales on auscultation. Careful documentation must also be made with regard to the child's respiratory effort as a baseline to assess improvement versus deterioration of condition. Such assessment should include presence, location, and depth of retractions; presence and location of cyanosis; and degree of lethargy.

The child who arrives in the emergency department with a primary episode of wheezing and dyspnea should be suspected of having pneumonia as a precipitating factor. The aspiration of a foreign body must also be considered a possibility.

Laboratory Data. Blood studies on a child with suspected pneumonia should include an arterial blood gas, complete blood count, and blood culture. A cold agglutinin should also be drawn on an older child or adolescent with pneumonia. Sputum for culture and sensitivity should be obtained as well as a smear for microscopic examination in the emergency department. The sputum smear is the most immediate determinant of appropriate antimicrobial therapy.

The anteroposterior and lateral chest x-rays will be most helpful in confirming the diagnosis of pneumonia as well as identifying areas of involvement. Figure 17–8 contains a radiograph of a 2-month-old with left upper-lobe pneumonia.

Management. Treatment will vary according to the age of the child and the suspected causative agent. Infants less than 6 months of age with pneumonia should be treated with double intravenous antibiotics in dosages appropriate to treat either gram-positive or gram-negative sepsis.

Children from infancy to 6 years of age usually contract viral pneumonia. If

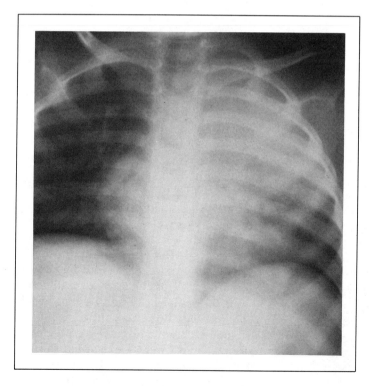

Figure 17–8. A 2-month-old female with consolidation of lingula and left uppler lobe. Diagnosis: LUL pneumonia. *(Photo courtesy of Richard DeNise, MD, and the Pediatric Radiology Department of Boston City Hospital.)*

the white blood cell count is sufficiently elevated (above 20,000), however, *Streptococcus pneumoniae* or *H. influenzae* should be suspected as the causative agent in this age group. Intravenous ampicillin may be administered to children who have severe pneumonia or refuse fluids. Children who appear well and are drinking adequate volumes of fluid may be treated with oral amoxicillin, 40 mg/kg/day, in three divided doses.

In addition to viral and bacterial etiology in school-aged children and adolescents, *Mycoplasma pneumoniae* should be considered. The antibiotic therapy of choice, therefore, in this age group is erythromycin, 40 mg/kg/day to a maximum of 250 mg every six hours. Erythromycin is also the drug of choice to combat chlamydia and bronchopneumonias. Bear in mind that antibiotic therapy can be changed or discontinued when the sputum and blood culture and sensitivity results become available.

In addition to the antibiotic regimen, other measures are essential to the comfort and recovery of any age child with pneumonia. Adequate hydration must be maintained through the administration of fluids by mouth or intravenously. A variety of electrolytes may be required with intravenous fluid therapy, and their use must be monitored according to serum levels. Humidification of inspired air is desirable whether or not oxygen therapy is in use. Oxygen concentrations higher than environmental concentrations should be administered when arterial blood gases or the clinical picture indicates the necessity. Chest physical therapy and postural drainage are essential measures to dislodge and remove accumulated secretions. This technique must be carefully taught to parents when the child is to be treated as an outpatient.

Hospital admission is recommended when (1) the degree of respiratory distress is significant; (2) the child is unable to tolerate fluids or medications by mouth (due to degree of respiratory distress or the presence of vomiting); (3) the infant is under six months of age; (4) underlying pathology is present. Refer to Appendix A for instructions to parents on the care of a child with pneumonia.

Pertussis

Pertussis or "whooping cough" is an acute bacterial infection of the respiratory tract. It most commonly affects infants (under 1 year of age) who are without immunity. The incidence in adolescents, however, has increased recently. Although vaccination with diphtheria-pertussis-tetanus (DPT) has contributed to the marked decrease in the frequency of this disease, several thousand cases occur yearly in the United States.[25]

Etiology and Pathophysiology. Pertussis is caused by *Bordetella pertussis*, which primarily affects the bronchi and bronchioles. It is spread by droplet nuclei and can be cultured from the nasopharynx early in the process.

There are three well-defined stages of pertussis. The initial catarrhal stage resembles a simple upper respiratory tract infection lasting 1 to 2 weeks. The child begins with rhinorrhea, sneezing, and a cough that usually occurs at night. Over the initial stage the child slowly worsens, developing a low-grade fever and a cough during the day as well.[26]

The paroxysmal phase is marked by the onset of prolonged coughing spasms that end with the hallmark inspiratory whoop. The effort expended by the child in these spasmodic coughing episodes is such that vomiting, sweating, neck vein distention, confusion, and convulsions may occur in the aftermath. During this phase mucus becomes thick and tenacious and may cause obstructive emphysema or atelectasis through plugging. In very young infants choking spells may be observed instead of the whoop. It should be remembered that the coughing spasms are exacerbated by the inhalation of irritants, by excitement, or by sudden changes in activity or temperature.[27]

The convalescent phase lasts approximately 2 weeks. During this time the severity of the paroxysms decreases, while the interval between spasms gradually increases until resolved.[28]

If the child arrives in the emergency department during the first phase of pertussis, the diagnosis will probably be missed. Pertussis is usually indistinguishable from the common cold until the paroxysmal stage. The child in this stage will have fever, hypoxia, and the classic cough. The child may also exhibit evidence of hemorrhages from the neck up, otitis media, pneumonia, atelectasis, vomiting, and the sudden appearance of hernias as a result of exertion during coughing.

History. The history of the child with pertussis typically reveals the progression of the symptoms of an upper respiratory tract infection with gradual worsening of the cough until the onset of the spasms with inspiratory whoop.

Assessment. Since excitement and crying tend to worsen the coughing paroxysms, care should be taken to keep the child as calm as possible. Observe the child for cyanosis prior to, during, and following paroxysm. Note the depth of substernal retraction during the inspiratory whoop. Time the frequency and length of the coughing spasms. Auscultation should be performed during a quiet time with careful attention to the detection of pneumonia, air trapping, or the diminished breath sounds over an area of atelectasis.

Other types of respiratory infections may mimic pertussis. These include RSV,

influenza, adenoviruses, and chlamydial infections. The possibility of an inhaled bronchial foreign body must also be considered.

Laboratory Data. In the early stages a nasopharyngeal swab culture will usually grow *Bordetella pertussis*. In later stages a sputum culture must be obtained from deeper suctioning to isolate the organism. The complete blood count may show a leukocytosis.

Management. Although strict isolation is difficult to achieve in an emergency department, it is necessary and should be started there. All persons in the room should wear masks, and gowns and gloves should be worn when handling the child or his or her secretions. Isolation needs only to be maintained until the brief (5- to 10-day) course of antibiotics is completed. The antibiotic of choice for pertussis is erythromycin, 50 mg/kg/day for 7 to 10 days. Antibiotic therapy is effective in the decontamination of secretions but cannot be relied upon to shorten the course of the disease. Intravenous antibiotic therapy may be initiated in the emergency department. Preliminary studies show that salbutamol may be helpful in reducing the effort of paroxysms in pertussis. But since results are largely inconclusive as yet and since dosage is uncertain, its use is usually reserved for the most severe cases.

Humidified oxygen should be on hand at all times for administration during and after coughing episodes. Gentle, deep suctioning will also be necessary to remove thick secretions. Ongoing assessment and documentation of the child's condition should be made. These include the frequency, duration, and sequelae of paroxysms as well as observations of color changes during these events.

Hospital admission is usually recommended for children with pertussis. Arrangements must be made to treat exposed persons. Exposed children under 7 years of age who have had a primary series of pertussis vaccine should receive a booster of pertussis vaccine, preferably as DPT vaccine, as well as the erythromycin prophylaxis. Older children and other adults who have been exposed and who have not received pertussis vaccine should also be provided prophylaxis with erythromycin.[29]

Upper Respiratory Tract Infections

The uncomplicated common cold is a mild, self-limiting, upper respiratory tract infection characterized by inflammation of the lining of the upper respiratory passages. Children under 4 years old contract approximately eight colds per year. Colds tend to be seasonal, with peaks in early fall, midwinter, and spring. Colds are seen more frequently in boys under 3 years old, but over that age girls are more frequently affected.

The child with an upper respiratory tract infection may be febrile and will usually have rhinorrhea, loss of appetite, cough, sore throat, headache without meningismus, earache, and general malaise. Infants and young children may have dyspnea due to clogged nasal passages, and nasal breathing may predominate. Childen may also have concurrent vomiting and diarrhea.

Etiology and Pathophysiology. The simple upper respiratory tract infection has a viral etiology. Numerous types of viruses can cause a cold, but the rhinovirus is the most frequent agent. The upper respiratory infection is contracted through contact with the airborne droplets of an infected person. Prolonged exposure increases a person's chances of contracting a cold.

Symptoms usually develop within 2 days after exposure. The mucosal swelling causes pharyngeal irritation and hypersecretion of the nasal passages. The systemic effects that may accompany a cold include listlessness, headache, excessive tearing and redness of the conjuctiva and sclera, low-grade fever, and body aches.

History. The nursing history begins at the point when the child last appeared well. The appearance, duration, and any apparent resolution of symptoms should be recorded. It is helpful to elicit comfort measures that have been used at home and their degree of success. Documentation of other ill family members will also be helpful.

Assessment. The physical assessment of the child with a cold must include documentation of upper respiratory tract symptoms as well as examination for the possible complications of superinfection. The pliability of the neck must be checked for the presence of meningismus, the ears examined carefully for otitis media, the pharynx visualized for erythema or exudate, and the lungs auscultated for differentiation between the coarse nasal-referred sounds and the adventitious sounds indicative of pneumonia. The chest of the infant should be observed for retractions.

The differential diagnosis for upper respiratory tract infections is lengthy. It includes allergic conditions, infectious mononucleosis, otitis media, streptococcal pharyngitis, pneumonia, bronchitis, bronchiolitis, sinusitis, influenza, pertussis, foreign body aspiration, and pulmonary edema associated with congestive heart failure and tuberculosis.

Laboratory Data. A complete blood count may be helpful in differentiating a viral cold from a bacterial infection. A throat culture should be obtained when the pharynx is erythematous or the tonsils are infected. An anteroposterior and lateral chest film will be helpful when the breath sounds are questionable. Infants under 2 months of age who are febrile and irritable may require a blood culture and lumbar puncture to rule out septicemia and viral or bacterial meningitis. A mono spot test may be desirable for older children.

Management. Children with uncomplicated, viral, upper respiratory tract infections do not require hospital admission. Emphasis is placed on teaching the parents to provide supportive care to their child. It is essential to explain that antibiotic treatment has no effect on a cold and may indeed be harmful due to the developing strains of resistant bacteria. There are, however, medications that may provide symptomatic relief. These include Tylenol for fever reduction and pain relief, antihistamines, decongestants, and expectorants. Cough suppressants should be used with caution in children if at all. A cool mist vaporizer may help liquify and drain secretions. For infants and very young children who are unable to blow their noses, the use of normal saline nose drops and nasal bulb suctioning must be carefully taught to the parents. Increased fluid intake is necessary to replace water loss and to liquefy secretions. Rest is the natural response to the listless feeling, and it is not uncommon for children to take longer and more frequent naps.

Pneumothorax

Pneumothorax is best described as a collection of air in the pleural space due to rupture of alveoli on the surface of the pleura, resulting in partial collapse of one or both lungs.[30]

Mild cases of unilateral or bilateral pneumothorax may be asymptomatic and will remain undetected unless specifically examined for. More extensive pneumothoraces will be painful and will cause tachypnea and dyspnea. The older child may complain of being unable to take a deep breath.

Etiology and Pathophysiology. Pneumothoraces may occur secondary to bronchial obstruction, trauma, atelectasis, or ruptured abscesses. The leakage of small amounts of air unilaterally or bilaterally may be asymptomatic. By contrast, large amounts of displaced air prevents full expansion of the lung on the side(s) involved. This causes tachypnea, dyspnea, grunting, hypoxia, and cyanosis. Contrary to most respiratory problems that cause retractions of the chest wall musculature, pneumothorax may cause bulging of these muscles, especially the intercostals over the affected area. Unilateral tension pneumothorax causes a mediastinal shift that pushes the heart toward the affected side.[31,32]

Pneumomediastinum differs from pneumothorax in the location of trapped extrapleural air. The free air of a pneumomediastinum is located between the lungs, around the heart anteriorly or posteriorly. This condition may manifest itself with dyspnea, crepitant swelling in the supraclavicular area and neck vein distention, and distant heart sounds. Breath sounds may appear normal.

History. A history of events leading to the current problem should be obtained as well as a subjective description of symptoms. A prior history of a pneumothorax increases the likelihood that this is a recurrence of the problem. It is important to note whether there was a sudden onset of symptoms or whether progressive respiratory illness has preceded the problem. A history of trauma to the chest should be elicited.

Assessment. Observe the chest for symmetry of movement during inspiration and expiration, presence of retractions or bulging neck vein engorgement, and change in coloring. Palpate the neck and chest for crepitant swellings. Palpate the trachea for any deviation from midline. Auscultate the chest for heart and lung sounds. Bear in mind that with pneumothorax the breath sounds seem distant or diminished over affected areas, and the location of heart sounds may have shifted. Conversely, with pneumomediastinum the breath sounds are usually normal, while heart sounds are muffled or distant. The percussion note over affected areas will be hyperresonant.

Laboratory Data. An arterial blood gas will provide a baseline estimation of the degree of interference with gas exchange. The child who is symptomatic of a pneumothorax should never be sent to radiology unaccompanied. Rather, anteroposterior and lateral films may be obtained in the emergency department prior to intervention. Figure 17–9 is a chest radiograph of a 15-year-old with a spontaneous left-sided pneumothorax.

Management. Bedrest and the administration of humidified 100 percent oxygen are the only treatments necessary for partial, mildy symptomatic pneumothorax or pneumomediastinum.

Tension pneumothorax or unilateral pneumothorax resulting in the near total collapse of a lung, however, is a life-threatening emergency requiring immediate intervention. The child may be placed in a sitting or supine position while a large bore needle or catheter is introduced between the second and third ribs on the anterolateral portion of the chest for immediate relief. Equipment should be available to insert a chest tube into this location as soon as possible. The chest tube must be attached at all times to a closed-seal drainage apparatus with the air fluid level clearly marked. Symptoms will be relieved as the lung reexpands.

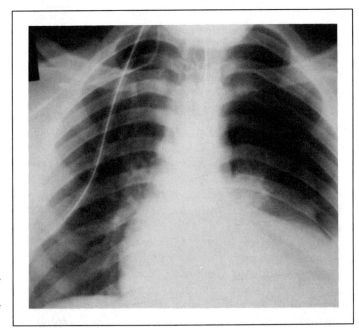

Figure 17–9. A 15-year-old with a left pneumothorax. This was a spontaneous event. *(Photo courtesy of Richard DeNise, MD, and the Department of Pediatric Radiology of Boston City Hospital.)*

Admission is recommended for any child who is symptomatic of a pneumothorax. Children who are asymptomatic and have evidence of small pneumothoraces may be followed on an outpatient basis.

Foreign Body Aspiration

Aspiration of a foreign body occurs when material is inhaled and becomes lodged in the lower respiratory tract. This phenomenon is usually seen in children 4 years of age and under and occurs more often in boys than girls.

Etiology and Pathophysiology. By far the most common agent involved in foreign body aspiration is food material. Nuts are most frequently implicated; sunflower seeds, beans, popcorn, peelings, hot dogs, and inorganic objects have also been identified. In the period immediately following the aspiration there is usually an episode of choking, coughing, gagging, or wheezing. Then symptoms may subside for days, weeks, or months without recurrence unless the object becomes dislodged and moves. This cessation of symptoms occurs as the lining of the respiratory tract adapts to the presence of foreign material. Disturbance of ventilation distal to the foreign body, however, continues over time. Although aspiration of organic foreign bodies is by far more common than inorganic, the identification of organic materials on x-ray is more difficult due to their radiolucency.

Bronchial foreign body aspiration is far more common. The usual site of lodging is the right mainstem bronchi, with the left mainstem the second most frequent site. The signs of bronchial aspiration include cough, dyspnea, reduced air entry, fever, wheezing, rales, and cyanosis. The most common radiographic finding is obstructive emphysema, although as time goes on a secondary pneumonia or atelectasis distal to the location of the foreign body may be seen. If the foreign body goes undetected for a period of weeks to months, the child may experience recurrent pneumonias.[33]

Laryngotracheal foreign body aspirations are rarer than bronchial aspirations and are usually more difficult to detect. The chest x-ray on inspiration and expiration may appear normal, necessitating a fluoroscopic examination for detection. Fluoroscopic examination may also yield normal findings, placing the emphasis on the history and clinical picture. The signs of a laryngotracheal foreign body include dyspnea, cough, stridor, and cyanosis.[34]

When the child arrives in the emergency department in the immediate period following bronchial aspiration of a foreign body, the child may exhibit paroxysmal coughing, dyspnea, wheezing, rales, and cyanosis. Over time the wheezing and rales may persist, with fever intermittently making differentiation between aspiration, asthma, and pneumonia more difficult.

History. In all cases of inhaled foreign bodies the history of an observed aspiration or choking spell is the single most important diagnostic tool. In cases where the child has exhibited periods of intermittent wheezing, stridor, dyspnea, or cyanosis over time, the nurse must exact a meticulous history of events leading to the primary episode. The parent may recall witnessing the aspiration or the immediate sequelae, then negating its importance in light of the temporary resolution of symptoms.

Assessment. Since the emphasis of detection of an inhaled foreign body is usually placed on the history and clinical picture rather than on radiologic or laboratory tests, careful attention must be paid to documentation of physical findings. Observe the child for respiratory effort and presence of cyanosis, pallor, or retractions. Palpate the trachea for any deviation from midline associated with mediastinal shifting in cases where lobar collapse secondary to obstruction exists.

Auscultation must be performed with careful attention to minute details. The presence of adventitious or decreased breath sounds must be noted with detailed description of their exact location and intensity. The most frequent complications of aspiration of foreign bodies are pneumonia, atelectasis, bronchiectasis, and pneumothorax.

Any infant or toddler who arrives in the emergency department with a clinical picture resembling asthma, bronchitis, pneumonia, or croup must be assessed in terms of an aspirated foreign body. The history of the respiratory problem should be elicited carefully for any correlation with an aspiration. As previously discussed, this may involve retracing events as far back as a few months.

Laboratory Data. In cases of moderate to severe respiratory impairment, an arterial blood gas should be obtained. When the child presents with symptomatology suggestive of pneumonia, a complete blood count and blood cultures will be helpful.

Although the chest films, as previously mentioned, may be inconclusive, every attempt should be made to obtain high-quality anteroposterior and lateral views of the chest during inspiration and expiration. The chest radiograph in Figure 17–10 is an example of the findings of a nonopaque foreign body in the right mainstem bronchus. Figure 17–11 contains a radiograph of a 7-month-old infant with a foreign body in the hypopharynx.

Fluoroscopy may be necessary to determine the location of a bronchial foreign body, but children with laryngotracheal foreign bodies may also have normal fluoroscopic examinations. A lung scan may be needed to localize the object in such cases.

Management. The child who has aspirated a foreign body that completely occludes the airway is an acute emergency. This child will probably be in cardiorespiratory arrest by the time he or she reaches the emergency department. The history of such an aspiration necessitates immediate delivery of a series of back blows and chest thrusts in an attempt to remove the object.[35] If these measures fail to restore a patent airway, an immediate tracheostomy must be performed to open the airway before cardiopulmonary resuscitation can be effective.

Hospital admission is always recommended in cases of suspected foreign body aspiration due to its potential for mortality. Attempts to dislodge and remove laryngotracheal or bronchial foreign bodies should be reserved for a controlled environment such as the operating room. They are usually removed under anesthesia with laryngoscopy, tracheoscopy, or bronchoscopy. Emergency attempts at removal may result in mere relocation of the object and further respiratory compromise.

Emergency department treatment is focused on supportive measures for more effective respiration. Humidified oxygen is desirable when any cyanosis is present or when wheezing or stridor are significant. An intravenous line should be established for administration of fluids and medications. Antibiotics are necessary with pneumonia and at times are used prophylactically prior to removal of the foreign body. Steroids may be helpful in reducing edema prior to removal of the foreign body and postremoval. Bear in mind that as is true with esophageal foreign bodies, after the removal of a single foreign body the child must be assessed for the presence of another foreign body.

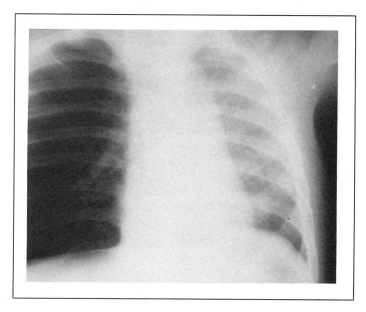

Figure 17–10. The evidence of a nonopaque foreign body in the right mainstem bronchus includes hyperventilation of right lung, hypoventilation of left lung, and shift of the mediastinum to the left. *(Photo courtesy of Richard DeNise, MD, and the Pediatric Radiology Department of Boston City Hospital.)*

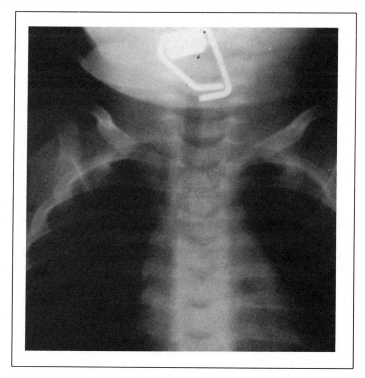

Figure 17–11. A 7-month-old found lying on the floor gasping and coughing. Diagnosis: clothespin in the hypopharynx. *(Photo courtesy of Richard DeNise, MD, and the Pediatric Radiology Department of Boston City Hospital.)*

Carbon Monoxide Poisoning

Carbon monoxide poisoning is a toxic condition produced when carbon monoxide gas is inhaled, usually in a fire, from car exhaust fumes or coal burning in a closed space.

The clinical picture will differ according to the extent of toxicity and symptoms may be generalized in children, making diagnosis in the absence of known exposure very difficult. At the lower spectrum of toxicity, nausea, vomiting, headache, dizziness, or blurred vision may be present. One should anticipate a carboxyhemoglobin in the 20 to 40 percent range when the child is tired and irritable and has muscle weakness, nausea or vomiting, and palpitations. Children with carboxyhemoglobin levels above 40 percent, if conscious, will be ataxic and will manifest central nervous system damage that may progress to coma and death.[36]

Etiology and Pathophysiology. Carbon monoxide is a colorless, odorless gas that, when inhaled, combines with hemoglobin at a rate 240 times faster than oxygen. The normal arterial carboxyhemoglobin level ranges from 1 to 10 percent and may run as high as 15 percent in smokers. Once inhaled carbon monoxide is rapidly absorbed into the hemoglobin molecule and interferes with oxygenation of all body tissues. With prolonged exposure and high carboxyhemoglobin levels, acidosis is profound. Irritability, confusion, and ataxia may progress to coma and death. Generally speaking, the central nervous system damage incurred is permanent.[37]

History. The history of a known or possible exposure to carbon monoxide gas (fire, car exhaust, or coal) provides the emergency department nurse with the best possible indication for the immediate intervention necessary. When the clinical index of suspicion is high, the parents should be questioned closely for a relevant history. Time of onset of symptoms and their progression must be carefully noted.

Assessment. A brief but thorough assessment should be performed, including baseline determinations of vital signs, observations of coloring, respiratory pattern and effort, nausea or vomiting, and manifestations of central nervous system alterations.

The differential diagnosis for carbon monoxide poisoning includes the inhalation of other noxious gases, drug ingestion, diabetes, hypoglycemia, and other conditions that have toxic appearances.

Laboratory Data. An arterial blood gas with carboxyhemoglobin level is mandatory and should be repeated frequently as treatment ensues. Chest radiographs may be helpful in providing baseline data that later aids in detecting complications, but radiographs should be deferred until adequate treatment has been provided.

Management. The primary treatment modality remains the administration of 100 percent oxygen, which should be initiated immediately in any case of suspected carbon monoxide poisoning. In children with evidence of central nervous system impairment, elective intubation will ensure adequate ventilation with 100 percent oxygen. In severe cases with carboxyhemoglobin levels above 60 percent, a hyperbaric oxygen chamber may be used to reduce the carboxyhemoglobin level quickly.[38] Intravenous maintenance fluids should be administered with caution to avoid cerebral edema. Efforts should be directed toward minimizing the body's oxygen requirements by keeping the child quiet and cool. In some cases acidosis may need to be corrected by administration of intravenous sodium bicarbonate.

Children with known or suspected inhalation of carbon monoxide should always be admitted for close observation and oxygen therapy. Initial carboxyhemoglobin levels may be misleading in that tissues continue to release the carbon monoxide molecules stored for up to 7 days. Pulmonary complications occur in 15 to 20 percent of patients with significant burns and are frequently seen in the victims of fires in the absence of surface burns.[39]

Smoke Inhalation

Smoke inhalation can be described as the breathing in of particles and gases, often the products of combustion, that produce some degree of damage to the structures of the airway.

Children exposed to fires or explosions should be treated as if smoke inhalation has occurred until proven otherwise. A high index of suspicion for smoke inhalation is present when there are burns of the head, neck, or chest; singed facial or nasal hairs; soot in the nasal secretions, oral mucosa, or sputum; edema of the oropharynx or trachea; a history that the exposure took place in a closed environment; a history of lapse of consciousness during the fire; extensive dermal burns; or a history of prior pulmonary or cardiac problems.[40,41]

The structures of the upper airways may suffer actual burns. These result in edema of the oropharynx and trachea, which have the potential to obstruct the airway. Early intubation to ensure a patent airway is critical for these children. Similarly, severe burns of the chest may limit the expansion needed for adequate ventilation. These children may require escharotomies in the emergency department as a life-saving measure.[42]

Etiology and Pathophysiology. The extent of damage to the bronchial lining and smaller tributaries is difficult to assess im-

mediately upon the child's arrival at the emergency department. Indeed the chest films may show minimal or no apparent abnormalities in the first 48 hours. The damage caused by smoke inhalation begins with the destruction of the ciliated epithelium and mucosal edema. The gaseous products of combustion may extend their damage to structures of the lower respiratory tract, affecting the lining of the bronchioles and alveoli. The linings of the trachea and bronchi may actually become necrotic. When the child comes to the emergency department with auscultatory abnormalities such as stridor, wheezing, or rhonchi, assume that major inhalation injury has occurred.[43]

The appearance of the child who has suffered smoke inhalation varies widely with degree of injury. A note of caution: the child who arrives in an alert state with an effective cough and adequate air movement does not necessarily preclude serious respiratory damage. These children should be dealt with as if insult has occurred until an adequate history, physical findings, and laboratory data have proven otherwise. To err on the side of safety may very well minimize delayed complications.

History. Obtaining a meaningful and reliable history when a child arrives after a fire is often a difficult task owing to the possible injuries to persons who witnessed the event. One person from the emergency department team should be designated to gather whatever facts are available while immediate intervention is begun with the child. The odor of smoke will usually pervade the area around the child.

Assessment. The most reliable criteria for intervention in the child with known or suspected smoke inhalation will be determined from the physical findings. Observe the face and neck for color, edema, or blistering indicative of a dermal burn. Inspect the nares for hair singeing or mucosal edema and the presence of soot. Carefully inspect the mouth and pharynx for blisters, color of mucosa, evidence of edema, and presence of soot. Look at the bare chest for evidence of burns, and assess for adequate excursion of the chest through a few deep breaths. Palpate the buccal cavity for degree of dryness. Palpate the trachea gently for any evidence of edema. Auscultation of the lung sounds may yield the normal bronchovesticular breath sounds on initial presentation, and indeed breath sounds may remain normal for up to 2 days postinjury. The presence of adventitious breath sounds upon presentation in the emergency department signifies that moderate to extensive insult has occurred. Ongoing assessment of the child's vital signs with frequent temperatures is essential.

Due to the fact that carbon monoxide is a byproduct of the combustion of several common materials such as polyvinylchloride (in synthetic rubber) and polystyrene (in foam cushions), the level of toxicity should be assessed.

Laboratory Data. Baseline determination of arterial blood gases, pH, and carboxyhemoglobin level should be obtained immediately upon arrival. Because the results may reflect near-normal values initially, it is important to repeat them periodically throughout treatment. Baseline chest films should also be obtained but should be deferred until the patient is stable. Xenon lung scanning or fiberoptic bronchoscopy may be desirable tools to evaluate the extent of lung tissue damage.

Management. As soon as the initial arterial blood gases have been drawn, oxygen therapy with 100 percent oxygen should be initiated. In the presence of laryngeal edema, hypoxemia, copious secretions, or clearly audible stridor, nasotracheal or endotracheal intubation should be per-

formed to ensure airway maintenance and the delivery of appropriate oxygen concentrations. When wheezing or stridor are present, intravenous administrations of bronchodilators or steroids may be desirable. Steroids, however, should not be given when the child has burns of the skin. Intravenous fluids should be administered in amounts determined by the extent of the dermal burn. In the absence of dermal burns, intravenous rates should be adjusted to provide maintenance fluids for body weight.

All children with smoke inhalation injuries should be admitted for careful observation owing to the likelihood of delayed onset of complications. The child and family members are often very frightened by the fire and will need much support and reassurance while in the emergency department.

Drowning and Near Drowning

Drowning may be defined as death resulting from submersion asphyxia anytime within 24 hours of the submersion. *Secondary drowning* refers to death resulting from the complications of the submersion more than 24 hours after the episode. *Immersion syndrome* results in sudden death secondary to the "diving reflex," in which extremely cold water enters the nasopharynx, vagally inducing cardiac arrest.[44]

It is estimated that greater than 6000 deaths per year in the United States are the result of drowning. There is a peak incidence in 10- to 19-year-olds, although 40 percent of victims are under 4 years old. Drowning incidents typically involve children who are inadequately attended in or near swimming pools, bathtubs, lakes, hot tubs, and other bodies of water, even those as small as a bucket. The increased risk in adolescents, especially males, is usually attributed to overestimation of ability. The use of alcohol or drugs, trauma, and seizure disorders may also be risk factors. Most incidents of drowning and near drowning occur in close proximity to the victim's home.[45,46]

Pathophysiology. A variety of factors, either alone or in combination, contribute to injury and death after a submersion injury. "Dry drowning" accounts for approximately 10 percent of all fatalities from submersion in which no fluid is aspirated. The remaining 90 percent of near-drowning victims either inhale or swallow large amounts of water and then vomit and aspirate during the initial period of panic, struggle, and breath holding.[47,48]

In theory there should be a difference between salt-water and fresh-water near drowning with respect to clinical findings. Salt-water aspiration should cause intravascular fluid to be drawn into the alveoli, leading to hypovolemia and hemoconcentration with resultant higher levels of serum electrolytes. Similarly, fresh-water aspiration should produce a rapid osmosis of fluid from the alveoli into the intravascular spaces, causing hemodilution and lower serum electrolyte levels. These changes, however, are seldom noted in patients who survive long enough to reach the emergency department because these victims have aspirated less than the estimated 11 ml/kg necessary to cause serum electrolyte imbalances, except in very hypertonic waters such as the Dead Sea.[49]

Asphyxia and the resultant degree of hypoxia are the common causes of tissue injury and death in submersion incidents. Hypoxia is the result of increased intrapulmonary shunting caused by loss of surfactant. Surfactant is rendered inert by fresh water and is diluted by salt water, causing alveolar collapse and areas of atelectasis. The loss of surfactant leads to pulmonary edema and intrapulmonary shunting, which are further aggravated by the inhalation of debris (gastric material, mud, algae, and sewage) that combines to produce a higher degree of hypoxia.[50,51] This may be observed immediately or may have a delayed onset of up to 72 hours after the episode.

As a result of hypoxemia, severe metabolic acidosis and hypercarbia develop, which may lead to central nervous system ischemia, encephalopathy, and seizures. The mechanism of injury must be considered to protect the victim who may have suffered head or neck trauma in addition to the submersion injury. Further insult to the central nervous system may result from fluid resuscitation, which may cause increased intracranial pressure.[52,53]

Immediately upon rescue, most near-drowning victims will have a "death-like" appearance. Children, with the possible exception of those submerged in hot tubs or heated baths, will also suffer some degree of hypothermia. There is evidence that submersion incidents that occur in cold water have higher survival rates than those that occur in warm water. This phenomenon is thought to be due to the peripheral vasoconstriction caused by exposure to cold; thereby blood flow to the periphery is shunted to the brain and heart.[54]

The body's ability to survive a cold-water submersion greatly depends on length of exposure, insulation, and the body's ability to balance heat production with heat loss. One of the ways the body produces heat is through exercise. In very cold water, however, exercise may cause more rapid heat loss by constantly stirring the cold water around the body. Exercise also produces exhaustion and leads to more rapid loss of consciousness. The body loses heat 25 percent more rapidly in cold water than cold air due to conduction differences. A factor that reduces heat loss is insulation either from heavy clothing or body fat.[55]

The sequence of events during sustained hypothermia is believed to progress from shivering to confusion and disorientation to amnesia and cardiac arrhythmias. At this point shivering is replaced by muscle rigidity, and the victim is semiconscious. When the victim becomes unconscious, the pupils dilate and deep tendon reflexes are absent. When hypothermia is sustained, the arrhythmias progress to ventricular fibrillation, then asystole.[56]

Assessment. Assessment factors to consider include the mechanism of injury. If the circumstances suggest a possibility of head or neck trauma, C-spine immobilization must be maintained until the integrity of the C spine has been confirmed by x-rays. If the history reveals that the near drowning occurred during deep sea diving, barotrauma and the need for slow decompression must be considered. For information about decompression chambers, call the Diver's Alert Network, (919) 684-2948; for emergencies call (919) 684-8111.[57]

Assessment of the child on arrival in the emergency department must include the status of the airway and breathing, cardiac rate, rhythm and effective circulation, body temperature (using the hypothermia probe), and mental status. After a submersion accident a child may arrive in the emergency department with a wide range of symptomatology, progressing from alertness and apparent recovery to cardiorespiratory arrest. As one might suspect, those children who arrive unconscious with fixed dilated pupils in sustained cardiorespiratory arrest, despite rapid and competent prehospital care, have the greatest chance of poor outcomes.[58]

Management. The death-like appearance of most children on initial rescue results from apnea, cyanosis or profound pallor, extreme peripheral vasoconstriction, and myocardial depression. Because high percentages of children survive, the child victim should receive skilled vigorous resus-

citative efforts. As in other situations of pediatric arrests, the first drug is oxygen, which is delivered at the highest possible concentration (100 percent) to minimize the danger of progressive hypoxemia, resultant acidosis, and myocardial and central nervous system insult.[59] Table 17-5 summarizes the medications that may be indicated in cases of near downing.

The initial focus of management is aimed at correction of hypoxemia and metabolic acidosis. The initial arterial blood gas determinations guide the effectiveness of oxygen therapy and the need for correction of acidosis with sodium bicarbonate. The formula for correction[60] is

$$\text{mEq NaHco}_3 = \frac{\text{BD} \times \text{BW} \times 0.6}{2}$$

with BD being base deficit and BW being body weight in kilograms. Subsequent arterial blood gases will document effectiveness of therapy and will monitor progress.

All child victims should be monitored for cardiac rate, rhythm, blood pressure, respiratory effort, and auscultation of breath sounds. Children with persistent respiratory distress, hypoxemia, and pulmonary edema may require intubation and ventilation with positive and expiratory pressure (PEEP) or continuous positive airway pressure (CPAP). If arterial oxygen levels remain inadequate, intermittent mandatory ventilation (IMV) may be necessary.[61,62]

When the child's blood pressure has reached an adequate and stable level, intravenous fluids should be limited to one-half maintenance, and diuretic therapy should be initiated. This may improve oxygenation in lungs with decreased surfactant and compliance while maintaining renal function. Children who remain comatose after a submersion incident often have signs of increased intracranial pressure. Subarachnoid bolts or intraventricu-

TABLE 17-5. MEDICATIONS FOR NEAR DROWNING VICTIMS

Indications	Medications	Dose/Comments
Increased intracranial pressure	O_2 hyperventilation	Maintain $PaCO_2$ at 25-30 mm Hg
	Furosemide (Lasix)	1-3 mg/kg/dose; repeat every 2-6 hr as indicated
	Mannitol	0.5 g/kg/dose; repeat every 3-4 hr; may have rebound effect
	Dexamethasone (Decadron)	0.25 mg/kg/dose every 6 hr; use is controversial
	Pentobarbital (Nembutal)	Maximum dose 50 mg/kg/24 hr. Barbiturate use is reserved for significant cerebral edema and only when bolt or other means is established to monitor and maintain intracerebral pressure ≤15 mm Hg and cerebral perfusion pressure ≥50 mm Hg
Hypoxic seizures	Diazepam (Valium)	0.2-0.3 mg/kg/dose; repeat every 2-5 min

Adapted from A.E. Thompson. Environmental emergencies. In G. Fleisher, & S. Ludwig (Eds.), Textbook of Pediatric Emergency Medicine. Baltimore: Williams & Wilkins, 1983, pp. 582-587.

lar catheters are frequently inserted to measure and to monitor pressures and effectiveness of therapy.

Rewarming the child to a minimum core temperature of at least 30C is essential prior to pronouncement of death and cessation of resuscitation efforts. Techniques for rewarming children include the use of heat lamps directed to the trunk, warmed blankets, warmed intravenous fluids, and gastric or rectal lavage with warmed fluids.

All children with a history of a near-drowning incident should be admitted for observation. Children who appear to be asymptomatic require monitoring and observation for a minimum of 12 to 24 hours to assess the delayed onset of symptoms of secondary near drowning. Admission to intensive care should be considered for any child who required even brief periods of resuscitation.

Laboratory Data. Laboratory studies include baseline determinations of the complete blood count, coagulation studies, serum electrolytes, arterial blood gases (ABGs), and a chest x-ray. The need for

additional studies, such as skull and neck films, medication levels, toxic screens, and serum alcohol (ethanol alchohol, ETOH) levels, will be determined by the history of possible precipitating factors.

Psychosocial Support and Parent Education. Prevention may be the single most effective method of reducing morbidity and mortality rates from submersion accidents. All pools should be properly enclosed to limit access to unsupervised children. Adults must be diligent in their supervision of children, especially infants and toddlers, around water, including the bathtub. Swimming and water safety should be taught to children at early ages. Rules forbidding alcohol and illicit drug use near swimming areas and hot tubs should be strictly enforced.

One of the most important and sometimes difficult roles for nurses in the emergency department is supporting the family of the near-drowning victim. It is important to keep the family updated on the child's progress during resuscitation. The child's parents should be informed that everything possible is being done for their child. Parents should be prepared for poor outcomes when indicated. A nonjudgmental approach is important, since family members may already be experiencing guilt, depending on the circumstances surrounding the accident.

NOTES

1. R.A. Hoekelman. The pediatric physical exam. In B. Bates (Ed.), *A Guide to Physical Examination* (2nd ed.). Philadelphia: Lippincott, 1979, p. 346.
2. M.A. Visich. Knowing what you hear: A guide to assessing breath and heart sounds. *Nursing '81* 2, no. 11(1981):66–71.
3. Hoekelman, *A Guide to Physical Examination,* p. 346.
4. Ibid.
5. R.M. Reece. Bronchiolitis. In R.M. Reece (Ed.), *Manual of Emergency Pediatrics* (3rd ed.). Philadelphia: W.B. Saunders, 1984, p. 416.
6. H. Levinson, E. Tabachnik, & C.J.L. Newth. Wheezing in infancy, croup and epiglottitis. In L. Gluck (Ed.), *Current Problems in Pediatrics.* Chicago, Year Book, 12, no. 3(January 1982):12–13.
7. R. Simkins. The crisis of bronchiolitis. *American Journal of Nursing* 81, no. 3(March 1981):514–515.
8. G. Scipien, M.U. Barnard, M.A. Chard, et al. *Comprehensive Pediatric Nursing* (2nd ed.). New York: McGraw-Hill 1979, pp. 603–604.
9. Levinson, Tabachnik, & Newth, Wheezing in infancy, croup and epiglottitis, p. 213.
10. Scipien, Barnard, & Chard, *Comprehensive Pediatric Nursing,* p. 616.
11. I.K. Roser. Asthma: Status asthmaticus and respiratory failure. In R.M. Reece (Ed.), *Manual of Emergency Pediatrics* (2nd ed.). Philadelphia: W.B. Saunders, 1978.
12. Levinson, Tabachnik, & Newth, Wheezing in infancy, croup and epiglottitis, p. 14.
13. Roser, Asthma: Status asthmaticus and respiratory failure, p. 24.
14. C.H. Fanta, T.H. Rossing, & E.R. McFad-den. Emergency room treatment of asthma. *American Journal of Medicine* 72(March, 1982):420.
15. L.H. Kiriloff, & S.C. Tibbals. Drugs for asthma, a complete guide. *American Journal of Nursing* 83, no. 1(January 1983):66–67.
16. Levinson, Tabachnik, & Newth, Wheezing in infancy, croup and epiglottitis, p. 40.
17. R. Simkins. Croup and epiglottitis. *American Journal of Nursing* 81, no. 3(March 1981):519–520.
18. Levinson, Tabachnik, & Newth, Wheezing in infancy, croup and epiglottitis, p. 41.
19. M.P. Fried. Controversies in the management of supraglottitis and croup. *Pediatric Clinics of North America* 26, no. 4(November 1979):939.
20. Levinson, Tabachnik, & Newth, Wheezing in infancy, croup and epiglottitis, p. 43.
21. N. Huang, D. Schidlow, & J. Palmer. Antibiotics in pediatric respiratory disease. *Clinics in Chest Medicine* 1, no. 3(September 1980):390.
22. J.O. Klein. Pneumonia. In R.M. Reece (Ed.), *Manual of Emergency Pediatrics* (3rd ed.). Philadelphia: W.B. Saunders, 1984, pp. 521–523.
23. Ibid.
24. Ibid.
25. G. Fleisher (Ed.). Pertussis. In *Textbook of Pediatric Emergency Medicine.* Baltimore: Williams & Wilkins, 1983, p. 386.
26. J.O. Klein. Pertussis. In R.M. Reece (Ed.), *Manual of Emergency Pediatrics* (3rd ed.). Philadelphia: W.B. Saunders, 1984, pp. 666–667.
27. Ibid.
28. Ibid.
29. Ibid.
30. J.W. Chamberlain. Pneumothorax. In R.M. Reece (Ed.), *Manual of Emergency Pediatrics* (3rd ed.). Philadelphia: W.B. Saunders, 1984, pp. 214–215.
31. Ibid.
32. J.P. Hall, & V.D. Jackson. Adult respiratory medical emergencies. *Nursing Clinics of North America* 16, no. 1(March 1981):81.
33. M. Pinney. Foreign body aspiration. *American Journal of Nursing* 81, no. 3(March 1981):511–512.
34. Ibid.

35. J. Greesher, & H.C. Mofeson. Emergency treatment of the choking child. *Pediatrics* 70, no. 1(July 1982):110–111.
36. J. Brandeburg. Inhalation injury: Carbon monoxide poisoning. *American Journal of Nursing* January 1980, pp. 98–100.
37. Ibid.
38. M.A. McGuigan. Carbon monoxide. In R.M. Reece (Ed.), *Manual of Emergency Pediatrics* (3rd ed.). Philadelphia: W.B. Saunders, 1984, pp. 230–232.
39. I.K. Rosner. Smoke inhalation and burns of the respiratory system. In R.M. Reece (Ed.), *Manual of Emergency Pediatrics* (3rd ed.). Philadelphia: W.B. Saunders, 1984, pp. 312–314.
40. Ibid.
41. J.F. Burke. The sequence of events following smoke inhalation. *Journal of Trauma* 21, no. 8(August 1981):721–722.
42. J.A. Surveyor. Smoke inhalation injuries. *Heart and Lung* 9, no. 5(September-October 1980):825.
43. Ibid., pp. 827–828.
44. D.L. Levin. Neardrowning. *Critical Care Medicine* 8, no. 10(October 1980):590.
45. A.E. Thompson. Environmental emergencies. In G. Fleisher, & S. Ludwig (Eds.), *Textbook of Pediatric Emergency Medicine*. Baltimore: Williams & Wilkins, 1983, pp. 582–587.
46. L. Whaley, & D. Wong. *Nursing Care of Infants and Children*. St. Louis: Mosby, 1983, p. 1209.
47. D.L. Levin. Neardrowning. *Critical Care Medicine* 8, no. 10(October 1980):591.
48. T.G. Martin. Neardrowning and cold water immersion. *Annals of Emergency Medicine* 13, no. 4(April 1984):263.
49. Levin, Neardrowning, p. 591.
50. Ibid.
51. Martin, Neardrowning and cold water immersion, p. 264.
52. Levin, Neardrowning, p. 593.
53. Thompson, Environmental emergencies, p. 582.
54. Whaley, & Wong, *Nursing Care of Infants and Children*, p. 1209.
55. Martin, Neardrowning and cold water immersion, p. 265.
56. Ibid., p. 267.
57. R.M. Barkin, & P. Rosen (Eds.). *Emergency Pediatrics*. St. Louis: Mosby, 1984, p. 242.
58. Levin, Neardrowning. p. 594.
59. Thompson, Environmental emergencies, p. 583.
60. Ibid., p. 584.
61. Martin, Neardrowning and cold water immersion, p. 270.
62. Thompson, Environmental emergencies, p. 584.

BIBLIOGRAPHY

Respiratory Assessment

Block, G.J., Nolan, J.W., & Dempsey, M.K. *Health Assessment for Professional Nursing, A Developmental Approach* (2nd ed.). New York: Appleton-Century-Crofts, 1986.
Ferhold, J.D.L. *Clinical Assessment of Children: A Comprehensive Approach to Primary Pediatric Care.* Philadelphia: Lippincott, 1980.
Hoekelman, Robert A. In Bates, B. (Ed.), *A Guide to Physical Examination* (2nd ed.). Philadelphia: Lippincott, 1979.
Malasanos, L. et al. *Health Assessment.* St. Louis: Mosby, 1981.
Thompson, J., & Bowers, A. *Clinical Manual of Health Assessment.* St. Louis: Mosby, 1980.
Visich, M.A. Knowing what you hear: A guide to assessing breath and heart sounds. *Nursing 81* 2, no. 11(1981):64–72.
Whaley, L.F., & Wong, D.L. *Nursing Care of Infants and Children* (2nd ed.). St. Louis: Mosby, 1983.

Bronchiolitis

Alexander, M., & Brown, M. *Pediatric History Taking and Physical Diagnosis for Nurses* (2nd ed.). New York: McGraw-Hill, 1979.
Beasley, J.M., et al. Continuous positive airway pressure in bronchiolitis. *British Medical Journal of Clinical Research* 283, no. 6305(December 5, 1981).
Colditz, P.B., et al. Apnea and bronchiolitis due to RSV. *Australian Pediatric Journal* 18, no. 1(March 1982).
Levinson, H., et al. Wheezing in infancy, croup and epiglottitis. *Current Problems in Pediatrics* 12, no. 3(1982):22–25.

Mortola, J.P., et al. Dynamics of breathing in infants. *Journal of Applied Physiology* 52, no. 5(May 1982).

Reece, R.M. Bronchiolitis. In Reece, R.M. (Ed.), *Manual of Emergency Pediatrics* (3rd ed.). Philadelphia: W.B. Saunders, 1984, p. 517.

Scipien, G., Barnard, M.U., Chard, M.A., et al. *Comprehensive Pediatric Nursing* (2nd ed.). New York: McGraw-Hill, 1979.

Simkins, R. The crisis of bronchiolitis. *American Journal of Nursing* 81, no. 3(March 1981):514–515.

Whaley, L., & Wong, D. *Nursing Care of Infants and Children* (2nd ed.). St. Louis: Mosby, 1983.

Wieczorek, R., & Natapoff, J. *A Conceptual Approach to the Nursing of Children: Health Care from Birth through Adolescence.* Philadelphia: Lippincott, 1981.

Asthma

Arnold, A.G., Lane, D.J., & Zapata, E. The speed of onset and severity of acute severe asthma. *British Journal for Diseases of the Chest* 76(1982):157–163.

Bottenfield, M.D., & Cohen, S.N. Theraputics in the pediatric emergency room. *Pediatric Clinics of North America* 26, no. 4(November 1979):867–872.

Fanta, C.H., Rossing, T.H., & McFadden, E.R. Emergency room treatment of asthma. *American Journal of Medicine* 72(March 1982):416–422.

George, R.B. Some recent advances in the management of asthma. *Archives of Internal Medicine* 142(May 1982):933–935.

Kiriloff, L.H., & Tibbals, S.C. Drugs for asthma, a complete guide. *American Journal of Nursing* 83, no. 1(January 1983):66–67.

Levinson, H. Wheezing in infancy, croup and epiglottitis. *Current Problems in Pediatrics* 12, no. 3(1982):10–22.

Milner, A.D. Childhood asthma: Treatment and severity. *British Medical Journal* 285, no. 6336(July 1982):155–156.

Picone, F. Asthma: Status asthmaticus and respiratory failure. In Reece, R.M. (Ed.), *Manual of Emergency Pediatrics* (2nd ed.). Philadelphia: W.B. Saunders, 1978.

Scipien, G., Barnard, M.U., Chard, M.A., et al. *Comprehensive Pediatric Nursing* (2nd ed.). New York: McGraw-Hill, 1979, pp. 616–621.

Simkins, R. Asthma: Reactive airways disease. *American Journal of Nursing* 81, no. 3(March 1981):522–524.

Vermeir, P. Combined use of theophylline and beta agonists in asthma. *European Journal of Respiratory Diseases* 63(1982):372–375.

Wabschall, J.M. Nursing management of children during a mild to moderate asthma attack. *Journal of Emergency Nursing* 12(1986): 134–141.

Webber, J.E., & Bryant, M.K. Over-the-counter bronchodilators. *Nursing 80* 10(January 1980).

Whaley, L., & Wong, D. *Nursing Care of Infants and Children* (2nd ed.). St. Louis: Mosby, 1983.

Croup

Barker, G.A. Current management of croup and epiglottitis. *Pediatric Clinics of North America* 26, no. 573(1979).

Cherry, J.D. The treatment of croup: Continued controversy due to failure of recognition of historic, ecologic, etiologic and clinical perspectives. *Journal of Pediatrics* 94, no. 194(1979):352–354.

Corkey, C.W.B., Barker, G.A., Edmonds, J.F., et al. Radiographic tracheal diameter measurements in acute infectious croup. *Critical Care Medicine* 9, no. 587(1981):587–590.

Davison, F.W. Acute laryngeal obstruction in children. *Journal of the American Medical Association* 171, no. 1301(1979).

Fried, M.P. Controversies in the management of supraglottitis and croup. *Pediatric Clinics of North America* 26, no. 4(November 1979):931–941.

Fried, M.P. Supraglottitis and croup. In Reece, R.M. (Ed.), *Manual of Emergency Pediatrics* (3rd ed.). Philadelphia: W.B. Saunders, 1984, pp. 329–337.

Leipzig, B., Oski, F.A., Cummings, C.W., et al. A prospective randomized study to determine the efficacy of steroids in treatment of croup. *Journal of Pediatrics* 94(1979):194–196.

Levinson, H., Tabachnik, E., Newth, C.J.L. Wheezing in infancy, croup and epiglottitis. *Current Problems in Pediatrics* 12, no. 3(1982): 38–43.

Simkins, R. Croup and epiglottitis. *American Journal of Nursing* 81, no. 3(March 1981):519–520.

Whaley, L., & Wong, D. *Nursing Care of Infants*

and Children (2nd ed.). St. Louis: Mosby, 1983.

Zullinger, J.J., Schuller, D.E., Beach, T.P., et al., Assessment of intubation in croup and epiglottitis. *Annals of Otorhinolaryngology*, 91(1982):403–406.

Epiglottitis

Barker, G.A. Current management of croup and epiglottitis. *Pediatric Clinics of North America* 26, no. 573(1979).

Costigan, D.C., & Newth, C. Respiratory status of children with epiglottitis with and without artificial airway. *American Journal of Diseases of Children* 137(February 1983).

Davison, F.W. Acute laryngeal obstruction in children. *Journal of the American Medical Association* 171, no. 1301(1979).

Huang, N.N., Schidlow, D.V., & Palmer, J.J. Antibiotics in pediatric respiratory diseases. *Clinics in Chest Medicine* 1, no. 3(September 1980):385–399.

Levinson, H., Tabachnik, E., & Newth, C.J.L. Wheezing in infancy, croup and epiglottitis. *Current Problems in Pediatrics* 12, no. 3(1982): 38–43.

Reece, R.M. Bronchiolitis. In Reece, R.M. (Ed.), *Manual of Emergency Pediatrics* (3rd ed.). Philadelphia: W.B. Saunders, 1984, p. 333.

Scipien, G., Barnard, M.U., Chard, M.A., et al. *Comprehensive Pediatric Nursing* (2nd ed.). New York: McGraw-Hill, 1979.

Simkins, R. Croup and epiglottitis. *American Journal of Nursing* 81, no. 3(March 1981):519–520.

Whaley, L., & Wong, D. *Nursing Care of Infants and Children* (2nd ed.). St. Louis: Mosby, 1983.

Zullinger, J.J., Schuller, D.E., Beach, T.P., et al. Assessment of intubation in croup and epiglottitis. *Annals of Otorhinolaryngology*, 91(1982):403–406.

Pneumonia

Causes of primary pneumonia. *Lancet* 2(November 28, 1981).

Hall, J.P., & Jackson, V.D. Adult respiratory medical emergencies. *Nursing Clinics of North America* 1b, no. 1(March 1981):75–83.

Huang, N.N., Schidlow, D.V., & Palmer, J.J. Antibiotics in pediatric respiratory diseases.

Clinics in Chest Medicine 1, no. 3(September 1980):385–399.

Klein, J.O. Pneumonia. In Reece, R.M. (Ed.), *Manual of Emergency Pediatrics* (3rd ed.). Philadelphia: W.B. Saunders, 1984, pp. 521–523.

Levinson, H., Tabachnik, E., & Newth, C.J.L. Wheezing in infancy, croup and epiglottitis. *Current Problems in Pediatrics* 12, no. 3(1982):11–12.

Pinney, M. Pneumonia. *American Journal of Nursing* 81, no. 3(March 1981):517–518.

Whaley, L., & Wong, D. *Nursing Care of Infants and Children* (2nd ed.). St. Louis: Mosby, 1983.

White, R.J., Blainey, A.D., & Harrison, K.J. Causes of pneumonia presenting to a district general hospital. *Thorax* 36(1981):566–570.

Wieczorek, R., & Natapoff, J. *A Conceptual Approach to the Nursing of Children: Health Care from Birth through Adolescence.* Philadelphia: Lippincott, 1981.

Pertussis

Craine, E.F., & Gershel, J.C. (Eds.) Pertussis. In *A Clinical Manual of Emergency Pediatrics.* Norwalk, Conn.: Appleton-Century-Crofts, 1986, pp. 313–315.

Fleisher, G. (Ed.) Pertussis. In *Textbook of Pediatric Emergency Medicine.* Baltimore: Williams & Wilkins, 1983, p. 386.

Huang, N. Antibiotics in pediatric respiratory diseases. *Clinics in Chest Medicine* 1, no. 3(September 1980):390.

Klein, J.O. Pertussis. In Reece, R.M. (Ed.), *Manual of Emergency Pediatrics* (3rd ed.). Philadelphia: W.B. Saunders, 1984, pp. 666–667.

Peltola, H., & Michelsson, K. Efficacy of salbutamol in treatment of infant pertussis demonstrated by sound spectrum analysis. *Lancet* (February 6, 1982):310–313.

Scipien, G., Barnard, M.U., Chard, M.A., et al. *Comprehensive Pediatric Nursing* (2nd ed.). New York: McGraw-Hill, 1979, pp. 606–609.

Whaley, L., & Wong, D. *Nursing Care of Infants and Children* (2nd ed.). St. Louis: Mosby, 1983.

Wieczorek, R., & Natapoff, J. *A Conceptual Approach to the Nursing of Children: Health Care from Birth through Adolescence.* Philadelphia: Lippincott, 1981.

Upper Respiratory Tract Infections

Hutchinson, R. The common cold primer. *Nursing 79* 9, no. 3(March 1979):57–61.

Reece, R.M. Chronic cough. In Reece, R.M. (Ed.), *Manual of Emergency Pediatrics* (3rd ed.). Philadelphia: W.B. Saunders, 1984, pp. 394–396.

Teele, D.W. Upper respiratory infection (common cold). In Reece, R.M. (Ed.), *Manual of Emergency Pediatrics* (3rd ed.). Philadelphia: W.B. Saunders, 1984, p. 516.

Whaley, L., & Wong, D. *Nursing Care of Infants and Children* (2nd ed.). St. Louis: Mosby, 1983.

Wieczorek, R., & Natapoff, J. *A Conceptual Approach to the Nursing of Children: Health Care from Birth through Adolescence.* Philadelphia: Lippincott, 1981.

Pneumothorax

A stab at pneumothorax. *Emergency Medicine* 13, no. 3(February 15, 1981):109–110.

Bevelaqua, F.A., & Conrado, A. Management of spontaneous pneumothorax with small lumen catheter manual aspiration. *Chest* 81, no. 6(June 1982):693–694.

Chamberlain, J.W. Pneumothorax. In Reece, R.M. (Ed.), *Manual of Emergency Pediatrics* (3rd ed.). Philadelphia: W.B. Saunders, 1984, pp. 214–215.

Cohen, S. How to work with chest tubes. *American Journal of Nursing* (April 1980):685–706.

Hall, J.P., & Jackson, V.D. Adult respiratory medical emergencies. *Nursing Clinics of North America* 16, no. 1(March 1981):75–83.

The shapes of pneumomediastinum. *Emergency Medicine* 14, no. 8(April 30, 1982):75–83.

Schuster, M.J. Pneumomediastinum as a cause of dysphagia and pseudodysphagia. *Annals of Emergency Medicine* 10, no. 12(December 1981):648–651.

Yamazaki, S., Ogawa, J., Shohzu, A., & Suzuki Y. Pulmonary blood flow to rapidly reexpand lung in spontaneous pneumothorax. *Chest* 81, no. 1(January 1982):118–120.

Foreign Bodies in the Respiratory Tract

Blazer, S., Naveh, Y., & Friedman, A. Foreign body in the airway, a review of 200 cases. *American Journal of Diseases of Children* 134(January 1980):60–71.

Greesher, J., & Mofeson, H.C. Emergency treatment of the choking child. *Pediatrics* 70, no. 1(July 1982):110–112.

Levinson, H., Tabachnik, E., & Newth, C.J.L. Wheezing in infancy, croup and epiglottitis. *Current Problems in Pediatrics* 12, no. 3(January 1982):28–31.

Pinney, M. Foreign body aspiration. *American Journal of Nursing* 81, no. 3(March 1981):511–512.

Simon, D.J. Coins in the esophagus: Two for the price of one. *Annals of Emergency Medicine* 10, no. 9(September 1981):489–491.

Whaley, L., & Wong, D. *Nursing Care of Infants and Children* (2nd ed.). St. Louis: Mosby, 1983.

Wieczorek, R., & Natapoff, J. *A Conceptual Approach to the Nursing of Children: Health Care from Birth through Adolescence.* Philadelphia: Lippincott, 1981.

Carbon Monoxide

Brandeburg, J. Inhalation injury: Carbon monoxide poisoning. *American Journal of Nursing* (January 1980):98–100.

Crain, E.F., & Gershel, J.C. Inhalation injury. In *A Clinical Manual of Emergency Pediatrics.* Norwalk, Conn.: Appleton-Century-Crofts, 1986, pp. 161–167.

Hall, J.P., & Jackson, V.D. Adult respiratory medical emergencies. *Nursing Clinics of North America* 16, no. 1(March 1, 1981):75–83.

Mcguigan, M.A. Carbon monoxide. In Reece, R.M. (Ed.), *Manual of Emergency Pediatrics* (3rd ed.). Philadelphia: W.B. Saunders, 1984, pp. 230–232.

Strohl, K.P., Feldman, N.T., Saunders, N.A., & O'Connor, N. Carbon monoxide poisoning in fire victims: A reappraisal of prognosis. *Journal of Trauma* 20, no. 1(January 1980):78–80.

Surveyer, J.A. Smoke inhalation injuries. *Heart and Lung* 9, no. 5(September-October 1980): 825–832.

Whaley, L., & Wong, D. *Nursing Care of Infants and Children* (2nd ed.). St. Louis: Mosby, 1983.

Wieczorek, R., & Natapoff, J. *A Conceptual Approach to the Nursing of Children: Health Care from Birth through Adolescence.* Philadelphia: Lippincott, 1981.

Smoke Inhalation

Burke, J.F. The sequence of events following smoke inhalation. *Journal of Trauma* 21, no. 8(August 1981):721–722.

Gaston, S.F., & Schumann, L.L. Inhalation injuries: Smoke inhalation. *American Journal of Nursing* (January 1980):94–97.

Hall, J.P., & Jackson, V.D. Adult respiratory medical emergencies. *Nursing Clinics of North America* 16, no. 1(March 1, 1981):75–83.

Head, J.M. Inhalation injury in burns. *American Journal of Surgery* 139, no. 4(1980):508–512.

Horovitz, J.H. Diagnostic tools for use in smoke inhalation. *Journal of Trauma* 21, no. 8(August 1981):717–719.

Moylan, J.A. Inhalation injury. *Journal of Trauma* 21, no. 8(August 1981):720–723.

Surveyer, J.A. Smoke inhalation injuries. *Heart and Lung* 9, no. 5(September-October 1980): 825–832.

Ward, P.A. The role of the complement system in smoke inhalation. *Journal of Trauma* 21, no. 8(August 1981):722–723.

Near Drowning

Barkin, R.M., & Rosen, P. (Eds.). *Emergency Pediatrics.* St. Louis: Mosby, 1984.

Levin, D.L. Neardrowning. *Critical Care Medicine* 8, no. 10(October 1980):590–595.

Martin, T.G. Neardrowning and cold water immersion. *Annals of Emergency Medicine* 13, no. 4(April 1984):263–270.

Thompson, A.E. Environmental emergencies. In Fleisher, G., & Ludwig, S. (Eds.), *Textbook of Pediatric Emergency Medicine,* Baltimore: Williams & Wilkins, 1983, pp. 582–587.

Whaley, L., & Wong, D. *Nursing Care of Infants and Children.* St. Louis: Mosby, 1983.

EMERGENCY DEPARTMENT CARE GUIDE FOR THE CHILD IN RESPIRATORY DISTRESS

Nursing Diagnosis	Interventions	Evaluation
Ineffective airway clearance related to increased mucus in airway	Assess and clear airway Suction upper airway as needed Insert oropharyngeal airway Prepare for endotracheal intubation if necessary	Airway remains patent
Ineffective breathing pattern related to respiratory infection or obstruction	Carefully auscultate breaths Observe chest movements for symmetry Continually monitor vital signs Provide humidified oxygen via face mask Position child in semi-Fowler's position to facilitate respiratory efforts	Breath sounds remain clear Child's respiratory rate is normal Vital signs are stable Child tolerates use of facial mask with oxygen
Impaired gas exchange related to inadequate oxygenation	Administer humidified oxygen by face mask Monitor arterial blood gases Administer medications (i.e., antibiotics or antiasthmatics as ordered) Provide bed rest to reduce oxygen requirements Observe for duskiness or cyanosis	Arterial blood gas values are normal Child responds to medications Child's respiratory rate and skin color return to normal

(Continued)

Nursing Diagnosis	Interventions	Evaluation
Potential fluid volume deficit related to insufficient intake and increased metabolic needs	Encourage oral intake of clear fluids as tolerated Administer intravenous fluids as ordered Carefully measure and record fluid intake and output Obtain urine-specific gravity Obtain serum electrolyte values	Fluid intake is sufficient to meet increased needs Urinary output is adequate (>1 ml/kg/hr) Urine-specific gravity is normal Serum electrolyte values are within normal range
Hyperthermia related to infection	Continually monitor child's body temperature Administer antipyretics Administer antibiotics as ordered	Child's body temperature returns to normal
Potential for infection of others related to communicable disease	Enforce strict respiratory precautions in emergency department Isolate child with respiratory infection from other patients in emergency department Administer initial doses of antibiotics as soon as possible	Emergency department staff and other patients are protected from exposure to infectious organism Antibiotics are administered as soon as possible
Alteration in comfort related to respiratory distress and fatigue	Provide emotional support to child Encourage bed rest and decreased activities Provide age-appropriate activities to distract child from discomfort Provide humidified oxygen Encourage parents to remain at child's bedside	Child breathes without discomfort Child rests in bed and engages in activities that do not require physical exertion
Knowledge deficit related to respiratory illness	Carefully explain nature and cause of child's respiratory condition to child and parents Carefully explain all procedures and treatments Prepare parents and child for child's discharge home or admission to hospital	Child and parents demonstrate understanding of respiratory condition and all procedures and treatments Child and parents demonstrate knowledge of home care or reasons for hospital admission and hospital policies

18

Gastrointestinal Emergencies

Arlene M. Sperhac

Gastrointestinal emergencies make up one of the largest categories of diseases in the pediatric population. As emergency department nurses we must be prepared to deal with the physical and psychosocial needs of these children and their parents.

When children have abdominal discomfort they are usually terribly frightened. Past admonitions to not eat certain types of foods or to refrain from doing things that might make them ill can create guilt feelings in children about the activities that they feel precipitated the event. Thus children may be even more anxious than is usually expected. A calm, reassuring, supportive approach is needed by the nurse.

If possible the parents should be allowed to remain with the child when the assessment is done. In a frightening, strange environment it is helpful for the children to see their familiar, trusted family members as much as possible.

Privacy should be maintained when assessing the abdomen. To the school-aged child or young adolescent with a rapidly changing body, modesty can be a major concern. In addition, sights and sounds that are familiar to emergency department personnel can seem ominous to children and should be explained if children cannot be shielded from them.

Not only the child but the family as well needs to be kept informed about what will be occurring. With the young child the assurance that nurses give to the parents by keeping them up to date is usually transmitted to the child. Well-informed parents convey an attitude that is rational and that may convey their trust in the emergency department staff. The staff's realistic assessment of the child's condition, as critical as it may be, is often less frightening than the parents' own perceptions of the situation; therefore the family should be kept as informed as possible.

The nurse's manner and his or her attention to comfort measures are important in gaining the confidence of the child. For example, warming hands and stethoscope before placing them on a tender abdomen and the general responsiveness to the needs of the child and the family can do much to assuage the child's fear. The frightened child in pain and his or her family must feel confident in the emergency department staff.

History. In children with gastrointestinal diseases, a complete and careful history almost always points to the correct diagnosis.[1] Questions that deal with the duration and onset of the problem, recent infections, medication, new foods, weight loss and associated symptoms, and level of activity should be asked. Both prenatal and perinatal events, a complete dietary history, and a history of allergy or gastrointestinal disease in other family members should be sought.

When obtaining the history of a child with a gastrointestinal dysfunction, age is probably the most important factor. In the child less than 2 years of age the parents interpret the "cries" as abdominal pain. The 2- to 5-year-old can point a finger to the exact location. In older children the history is more reliable and the symptoms better described.

For each age group different disease entities must be considered.[2] Figure 18-1 provides a review of the anatomy of the gastrointestinal tract in the child. In the infant with an acute abdomen, a gastroin-

tinal malformation, an incarcerated hernia, or a torsion of the testis or of the ovarian pedicle should be considered. In the preschool child the acute abdomen is frequently related to infections or to an inflammatory process rather than to a mechanical obstruction.

In addition to age, sex needs to be considered, since some entities are more frequently encountered in males than in females. Growth parameters also need to be noted.

In most cases the history will be obtained from the parents, but the children should also be questioned for validation and clarification, if possible. Close attention should be paid to the events preceding the problem, since a significant num-

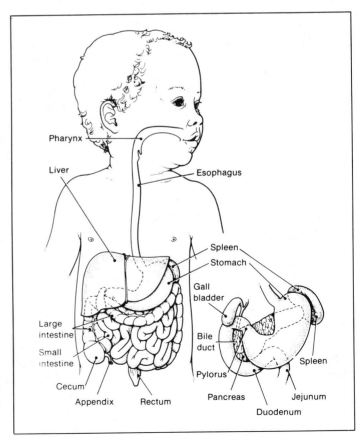

Figure 18-1. Anatomy of the gastrointestinal tract. *(From G.M. Scipien, M.U. Barnard, M.A. Chard, et al. (Eds.). Comprehensive Pediatric Nursing (2nd ed.). New York: McGraw-Hill, 1979, p. 746.)*

ber of children admitted to the hospital with acute abdominal pain recover spontaneously because the pain can, in some cases, be attributed to a degree of emotional maladjustment.[3]

Clinical Presentation. Children suffering from acute disease of an intra-abdominal organ can have pain, bleeding, jaundice, or some combination thereof. Other signs and symptoms may prove to be valuable aids in arriving at the correct diagnosis or in determining a course of management. For example, nausea and vomiting are often reflex phenomena and may not be related to the physiologic process, but these symptoms give important information and need to be noted. Pain, bleeding, and jaundice, however, are the three main complaints of children with gastrointestinal dysfunction.

Pain is the most useful of all subjective data.[4] A precise characterization of pain accurately differentiates inflammations from nongangrenous mechanical obstructions. An instantaneous onset or the sudden worsening of pain usually indicates an origin from a vascular accident or rupture of some hollow viscus, i.e., a surgical condition. "Colicky" or intermittent pain usually develops when there has been an anatomic obstruction to the lumen of a peristaltic hollow conduit. Information regarding the onset, situation, nature, persistence, and radiation of the pain should be sought. Wilson[5] suggests the use of computer analysis in assessing pain, since clinical impressions can be corrected by precise mathematical analysis.

Bleeding usually causes a mildly inflammatory, painless reaction. Hemorrhage into the lumen of the gastrointestinal tract is the single most impressive finding. If the bleeding is internal, acute anemia or hypovolemic shock may be the presenting feature.

Jaundice is usually associated with diseases of the liver or biliary duct system. Jaundice is more common in infancy than at any other time in life and may be normal. Hepatic diseases in older children frequently appear in a similar manner.

Abdominal and pelvic injuries present special problems of diagnosis, since the extent of the trauma is often not immediately apparent. An accurate history and a careful record of all relevant information regarding the nature of the trauma sustained needs to be made as an aid to diagnosis.

Pain with Gastrointestinal Emergencies

Inflammatory Conditions. Inflammatory disease within the peritoneal cavity is generally characterized by unremitting abdominal pain. Sudden onset of pain or the rapid worsening of symptoms usually indicates hollow viscus perforation. Gradual intensification of pain is associated with commonly encountered inflammatory conditions.

Location of the pain should be noted. Foregut diseases (stomach and duodenum) give symptoms that are epigastric in location; midgut problems (small bowel and right and transverse colons) generally are referred to the periumbilical region; hindgut inflammations (descending and sigmoid colons) are referred to the intraumbilical and suprapubic areas.[6]

In the younger age group localization of pain is usually inaccurate, since the child invariably points to the umbilical region irrespective of the site of the disease. Vague periumbilical pain in the older child, except in early appendicitis, is usually of little significance. Pain localized to one of the abdominal quadrants, however, suggests local organic disease.[7]

Local abdominal tenderness confirms the existence of peritoneal irritation. With an anxious child with a low pain threshold, reaction to direct palpation can give little information. In adults and older children rebound tenderness identifies the site of maximal irritation with much greater accuracy. In young children, however, rebound tenderness is a sign with limited clinical value, and no attempt to elicit it should be made.[8]

Muscle spasm, also called guarding, is involuntary whenever the inflammatory process is intense, is located beneath the area palpated, and is maintained as a continuous muscular contraction. If the guarding is voluntary, a warm hand in contact with the abdominal wall for several minutes will permit the examiner to distinguish between these two forms of muscle spasm.

Alimentary Tract Obstructions. The pain described with alimentary tract obstructions is characteristically intermittent, since it is associated with the major peristaltic wave. Younger children frequently cannot communicate this verbally, but watching for intermittent facial grimacing or abdominal guarding may provide this information. Older children, upon specific questioning, may describe the pain as dull and cramping, rising slowly in a crescendo pattern and reaching a maximum that lasts about 30 seconds. Since in older children the major peristaltic wave in the small bowel occurs every 2 to 3 minutes, and in the colon every 15 to 20 minutes, this feature can be used to localize the site of the obstruction.[9] Episodic pain is associated with intestinal peristalsis.

Since bowel sounds occur with peristalsis, cramping abdominal pain coexisting with high-pitched, rushing, continuous bowel sounds, which are sounds characteristic of intestinal obstruction, is the foundation on which the diagnosis of mechanical obstruction can be made. There is a temporal relationship between the abdominal pain and the peristaltic wave.

Uncomplicated alimentary tract obstruction rarely results in anything other than mild tenderness to palpation. More severe tenderness usually indicates peritonitis. This is an important sign in a child with an obstruction, since it means that a perforation has occurred or that a gangrenous bowel is present. A bowel necrosis necessitates prompt surgical intervention.

Other findings that may be helpful in diagnosis of alimentary tract obstruction include abdominal distention and a history of irregular bowel function. Abdominal distention is frequently felt to be characteristic of obstruction. The absence of distention, however, does not obviate the presence of an obstruction, since a high obstruction is not associated with abdominal distention. In lesions proximal to the upper jejunum, protracted and projectile vomiting can alleviate distention. As the obstruction progresses distally, vomiting becomes less prominent and more characteristic (such as the feculent vomitus of ileal contents), while abdominal distention becomes more prominent.

Irregular bowel function can be a feature of alimentary tract obstruction. If there is complete obstruction passage of feces would not occur. Bowel content distal to the obstruction, however, would be evacuated. Likewise, the presence or absence of feces in the rectum on digital examination does not indicate the presence of an obstruction. Obstruction and continued fecal passage can coexist only in high-grade incomplete or partial intestinal obstruction.[10]

Diagnosis

A combination of a complete history and a careful examination is essential in the diagnosis of inflammatory conditions and alimentary tract obstructions. The examination should include inspection of the fully exposed abdomen, palpation, auscultation, and a rectal or pelvic examination.

The most important part, however, is a complete and detailed history. With information from the history and the physical examination, decisions regarding laboratory and radiographic studies can be made.

In inflammatory conditions routine laboratory tests include a complete blood count and a urinalysis. A rapid measurement of red cell mass (hematocrit or hemoglobin) is extremely useful, since it gives evidence of an established anemia, provides an estimate of the severity of dehydration, and serves as a baseline when hemorrhage is the immediate problem. The white blood cell (WBC) count with differential generally reflects the intensity of the inflammatory process. Extreme leukocytosis (greater than 25,000 WBC/mm^3) and leukopenia (less than 5,000 WBC/mm^3) are noted in cases of profound sepsis or even septic shock. The urinalysis is important in detecting the presence of a urinary tract infection, which may coexist or may be responsible for the patient's symptoms. Pyuria and bacilluria are the findings in such cases. Other abnormal findings of diagnostic value are the hematuria associated with renal trauma, renal stones, or a tumor; glycosuria in the diabetic (who may present in ketoacidosis with abdominal pain as the prominent symptom); and bile in the urine of children with liver or biliary tract disease.

Blood chemistries are valuable in assessing the presence and severity of preexisting disease states as well as the magnitude of derangements caused by the acute peritoneal inflammation itself. The standard blood chemistries are serum electrolytes, blood urea nitrogen, and blood glucose.

Fiberoptic endoscopy has simplified the analysis of gastrointestinal problems. This is done before any barium studies.

A diagnosis of alimentary tract obstruction is usually obvious from the history and physical examination. No characteristic changes of obstruction are reflected by examination of the blood, except perhaps some degree of nonspecific dehydration. A WBC evaluation that is markedly elevated may be of benefit in cases in which impending or actual necrosis or inflammatory bowel disease is suspected. Since these suspicions have implications for management, radiographic studies to further aid in the confirmation of a diagnosis are done.

Radiographic studies are the most valuable diagnostic aids in inflammatory conditions and alimentary tract obstructions. Plain films of the supine abdomen will give evidence of solid organ location, size, and contour; bowel patterns in relation to displacement, distention, distribution of intraluminal gas, and abnormal masses; free intra-abdominal gas; and the presence and approximate quantity of peritoneal fluid. An upright chest film can reveal subdiaphragmatic free gas; pneumonia, which can be the cause of the abdominal symptoms; and previously unrecognized cardiopulmonary pathology. Radiographic studies may also aid in confirmation of child abuse.[11]

Contrast studies are often required, since they furnish information about the size and location and adjacent viscera. Air insufflation of the stomach, upper gastrointestinal series, barium enemas, and intravenous pyelograms are also sometimes used.

INFLAMMATORY CONDITIONS

Appendicitis

Appendicitis is the inflammation of the vermiform appendix, or blind sac at the end of the cecum. It is the most common reason for abdominal surgery during childhood, with the incidence increasing after the first year of life. While rare in children under 2 years of age, it is associated with increased complications and mortality in this age group. Appendicitis in early childhood is characterized by a low incidence (1 percent), an overwhelming male predominance (8 : 1), a short history, and rapid progress of the disease.[12]

In the adolescent population, however, the male to female ratio is closer to 1 : 1, and the progress of the disease is somewhat less rapid.[13]

It is usually an acute condition that, when undiagnosed, progresses to perforation and peritonitis. The estimated total incidence of appendicitis in the United States is 200,000 cases per year with 2000 deaths.[14]

Etiology. While the exact cause of appendicitis is poorly understood, obstruction seems to be a primary factor in the pathogenesis. The obstruction may be secondary to inflammatory changes from blood-borne or enteric infections or may be mechanical from parasitic infestation, a fecalith, a foreign body, or stenosis. Decreased fiber and residue content in the diet may also play a role as a factor in obstruction.

The progression of appendicitis in children has been described.[15] Acute obstruction is followed by inflammation, since the local defense mechanisms are impaired sufficiently to allow invasion by the bacterial organisms in their lumen. The initially inflamed and then infected appendix may then progress to perforation and peritonitis. Young children have a thinner appendiceal wall, hence progression is much more rapid. In addition, the younger child has an omentum that is not fully developed and is less efficient in walling off the inflammation, sealing perforated viscera, and confining an intraperitoneal disease process. The close proximity of abdominal and pelvic organs further favors the spread of peritonitis to other structures.

Clinical Presentation. Classically, the most common signs and symptoms of appendicitis are abdominal pain, which begins as generalized and shifts to the right lower quadrant, localized abdominal tenderness, and fever. The most intense site of pain may be McBurney's point, which is approximately 3.75 cm above the anterior superior iliac crest along a straight line drawn from the umbilicus. Other important signs include rebound tenderness, hypoactive or absent bowel sounds, anorexia, nausea, and vomiting. Signs of peritonitis include sudden relief from pain after perforation. Then there is a subsequent increase in pain, which is diffuse and is accompanied by guarding of the abdomen, progressive abdominal distention, rapid shallow breathing (since abdominal muscles are not used), pallor, irritability, restlessness, and tachycardia.

About 70 percent of children 5 years of age or younger have a perforation of the appendix when they are first seen in the emergency department. Since they cannot localize the pain or communicate their discomfort, the prodromal manifestations are not appreciated. Abdominal pain, tenderness, temperature elevation, and vomiting, which are the most common findings, are not communicated. Consequently there is a progression from simple to complicated appendicitis with peritonitis, which is more rapid in the child than it is in the adult. Upon arrival at the emergency department, therefore, the young child is frequently very ill, with grunting respirations, a rigid abdomen, an ashen color, and an anxious expression. Active peristalsis can persist for some time with generalized peritonitis. The temperature, after development of peritonitis, is usually elevated to 39.5C or more (103F to 105F).

The initial symptom in the older child is persistent pain that becomes progressively severe. Vomiting, bowel sounds that are not hypoactive, and temperature elevation are also significant signs and symptoms.[16]

It is important to remember, however, that the clinical course of appendicitis varies enormously, and the duration of symptoms has a wide range that is partly independent of the pathologic findings.[17]

History. A history of persistent abdominal pain, insidious or abrupt in onset, accompanied by persistent localized tenderness in the right lower quadrant, involuntary muscle spasm, and rigidity are evidence of localized intraperitoneal irritation. Nausea and vomiting are frequently present, and a low-grade fever is more common than a high fever and chills at the onset of the disease.

Assessment. The clinical presentation of a child in distress with signs of localized peritoneal irritation is significant. It is, however, important to distinguish between voluntary and involuntary muscle spasm, or guarding of the abdomen in children. A young child frequently tenses the abdominal muscles at the sight of a nurse's uniform or with the touch of a cold hand. So a gentle, unhurried approach that helps to reassure the child and allows him or her to relax, will provide more reliable information. In some cases sedation may be ordered to allay apprehension and to eliminate voluntary muscle guarding. Narcotic analgesics should not be given, since they may mask the signs of intraperitoneal inflammation.

Other signs of peritoneal irritation such as rebound tenderness are helpful when elicited. The only sign of an inflamed retrocecal appendix, however, may be deep tenderness, and when the appendix is in the pelvic area, there may be no abdominal findings.

A rectal examination is the final step in the physical examination and further aids assessment. Peristalsis is generally decreased or absent in the presence of intraperitoneal infection, although in the early stages there may be hyperactivity. A positive psoas sign (a drawing up of the legs) is also suggestive of a right lower-quadrant inflammatory lesion.

Laboratory Data. The most important laboratory evaluation is a WBC. The WBC is usually elevated but is seldom higher than 15,000 to 20,000/mm with a preponderance of immature polymorphonuclear cells.[18] Excessively high total leukocyte counts are suggestive of an abscess or peritonitis.[19] In acute appendicitis, neutrophilia supports the diagnosis, and leukocytosis indicates the prognosis. In other words, the ratio of infection appears to increase as the total leukocyte count rises above the upper normal limit, and a decreased neutrophil percentage suggests appendicitis. In some studies, however, patients with appendicitis had a normal WBC.[20]

The WBC should be only a small part of the overall assessment. Priority should be given to the physical findings, and the WBC and neutrophil percentage should be used to support or question these findings.[21]

Other laboratory studies are helpful in differentiating appendicitis from other conditions. In addition, studies such as a urinalysis help to provide an overall assessment of fluid loss. Sedimentation rate, electrolytes, glucose, blood urea nitrogen (BUN), amylase, serum glutamic-oxalo-acetic transaminase (SGOT), and bilirubin should also be ordered.[22]

Radiographs may further aid in the diagnosis of appendicitis. Abdominal films may show an appendiceal fecalith, which, although rare, clearly indicates the diagnosis of appendicitis. In many cases of appendicitis, however, abdominal radiographs are absolutely normal.[23] A barium enema may increase the accuracy of diagnosis in difficult cases.[24] The barium enema may demonstrate nonfilling or partial filling of the appendix when there is appendicitis.[25] The use of a barium enema as an adjunct may be helpful if the findings are positive, but negative findings should not be relied upon to delay surgery in the child with positive peritoneal signs in the right lower quadrant.[26]

Differential Diagnosis. One of the most difficult diagnoses in children is that of acute appendicitis.[27] So many conditions mimic appendicitis and vice versa that frequently many diagnostic tests as well as the detailed history and physical examination are needed. Other diagnostic possibilities when appendicitis is being considered include Crohn's disease, mesenteric adenitis, Meckel's diverticulitis, acute rheumatic fever, diabetes mellitus, regional enteritis, abdominal epilepsy, ovarian lesions, intussusception, acute gastroenteritis, constipation, sickle cell crisis, and infectious mononucleosis. In addition, there can be infection of the urinary tract, which may be ruled out with a urinalysis and an intravenous pyelogram, and pneumonia, in which case a chest x-ray will clarify the diagnosis.

Management. When appendicitis is suspected, the child must be given nothing by mouth. An intravenous infusion of Ringer's lactate solution is frequently ordered in preparation for surgery. The urine concentration (specific gravity) and output per hour are generally used as guides for adequacy of fluid therapy. A nasogastric tube to low suction is also frequently ordered. Vital signs need to be monitored frequently. If the diagnosis of appendicitis is definitive, preoperative antibiotics such as a cephalosporin or ampicillin are ordered. If perforation is believed to have occurred, an aminoglycoside antibiotic such as gentamicin or tobramycin are usually ordered. All efforts are directed toward the delivery of definitive therapy, which in appendici-

tis is surgery. Appendectomy is the only appropriate treatment for acute appendicitis. If there has been appendiceal perforation, antibiotics, transperitoneal drainage, and delayed wound closure is used. Delayed wound closure has been shown to reduce the incidence of wound infection after perforation by 75 percent.[28]

Psychosocial Support and Patient Education. During the preparation time an explanation geared to the age level of the child should be provided. This should be done in a calm, reassuring way. If the parents are available, they should also be kept informed and should be encouraged to help communicate to the child what can be expected. Any question of the possibility of appendicitis should warrant as immediate a hospital admission as if the diagnosis were certain.[29]

Intestinal Parasites

An intestinal parasite is an organism that relies on its host (the child) for nourishment and physical protection and does not reciprocate in kind. The effect of the parasite on the child may be negligible or, if there is a heavy infestation, fatal.

Geographic and ecologic conditions are important in the prevalence of parasitic infections. Sanitary conditions in the community, personal hygiene, and food processing and cooking constitute additional factors that affect the epidemiology of infestations. The parasitic diseases of the intestine are often complicated by poor socioeconomic conditions, poor hygiene, and malnutrition.

There are numerous portals of entry through which the parasite invades the host organism. The most common portal is by mouth, either ingested in food or water or transferred to the mouth from the soil by way of hands or other objects.

Etiology. There are two main groupings of intestinal parasites. The first is intestinal protozoal diseases, which include amebiasis, which is caused by *Entamoeba histolytica*, and giardiasis, which is caused by the *Giardia lamblia*. The second main grouping is the helminthic diseases, which are caused by roundworm infestations and which include ascariasis, pinworm (oxyuriasis), hookworm, trichuriasis, and the tapeworms.

In both of the protozoan diseases, amebiasis and giardiasis, transmission is by way of ingestion of multinucleated cysts through water or through contact with feces. Humans are the main reservoir for amebiasis, and for giardiasis, humans, beavers, rats, mice, and beagle pups are the reservoirs.

The helminthic diseases, or those caused by roundworms that are generally seen, are caused by ingestion of the eggs, which enable the worms to eventually lodge in the intestine or, in the case of hookworm, by skin contact with contaminated soil. Ascariasis occurs when the Ascaris eggs are ingested, as when toys or fingers that have come in contact with fecally contaminated topsoil are placed in the mouth.

Oxyuriasis, or pinworms, is caused by ingested eggs frequently found in contaminated dog feces in soil or sand in children's play areas. Hookworm disease is caused by adult *Ancylostoma duodenale* and *Necator americanus*, which enter the body from the soil through the skin, are carried to the lungs, ascend to the pharynx, and are swallowed, allowing them to reach and lodge in the intestine. Trichuriasis, or whipworm, is caused by ingested eggs in water, food, or dirt.

The tapeworms include *Taenia saginata* (beef), *Taenia solium* (pork), and *Hymenolepis nana*. Both the beef and the pork tapeworm can be spread by contaminated human feces or by the ingestion of the contaminated meat that has not been properly prepared by freezing or by thorough cooking. *H. nana*, or the dwarf tapeworm, which is most common in the United States, are spread by direct patient-to-patient ingestion of eggs.

Clinical Presentation. With amebiasis, the child has diarrhea, fever, and vomiting. There are diarrheal stools that contain blood-streaked mucus, and tenesmus (spasmodic contraction of the anal sphincter with pain) along with abdominal pain and distention are noted. The bowel sounds are hyperactive, and fluid losses can be significant.

The child with giardiasis has diarrhea, a poor weight gain, abdominal distention, and steatorrhea (fatty stools). Some children complain of abdominal cramping.

Ascariasis is seen throughout North America, but few children are symptomatic because the parasite is well adapted to its human host. In some cases the child may complain of colicky abdominal pain and may have vomiting, anorexia, weight loss, and some irritability.

In large numbers, however, a bolus of ascarids can be formed, causing a mechanical obstruction with resultant intestinal spasm and pain. This, however, is rare. In most cases the mother telephones or brings the child to the emergency department stating that a 6-inch pencil-sized roundworm has been passed or vomited.

With oxyuriasis, or pinworm, the main complaint is anal itching, which is most marked at night. There is controversy as to whether pinworms cause abdominal pain.[30,31] Adult worms can migrate into the vagina and even into the fallopian tubes and cause vaginitis and salpingitis in females. In males, meatitis can occur.

The clinical presentation with hookworm varies as to the stage at which the child is seen. Initially the area of skin, which is usually on the feet, where the larvae enter is red and edematous. Cough is prominent during the pulmonary transit, and as the hookworms migrate to the small intestine, epigastric pain, tender-

ness, vomiting, and diarrhea are the complaints. About 6 weeks after entry, blood
loss and anemia are seen. The anemia may
reach such proportions as to cause cardiac
failure.[32]

Children who are heavily infested
with *Trichuris* show diarrhea, tenesmus,
anemia, eosinophilia, weight loss, and abdominal distention. If the tenesmus is severe, rectal prolapse can occur.

With the infestation of the tapeworms
T. saginata and *T. solium* from infested un-
dercooked beef or pork, vague abdominal
pain, nausea, increased appetite, nausea,
and weight loss occur. *H. nana*, the dwarf
tapeworm, in large numbers causes headache, anorexia, intermittent diarrhea, and
abdominal pain.

History. The history is an important diagnostic tool in the assessment of intestinal
parasites. Information should be sought
about the occurrence and progression of
symptoms in the child and in other family
members or close friends. The type and
size of housing, the number of people in
the dwelling, and the available sanitary facilities should also be explored. In cases of
possible beef or pork tapeworm infestation, information on storage and preparation of meats should be obtained.

Assessment. To assess for intestinal parasites, the history of the signs and symptoms the child has exhibited and his or her
living conditions and home environment
also need to be considered. Crowded living conditions, poor sanitation, and inadequate nutrition increase a child's susceptibility to intestinal parasites. Some of these
children also have immunoglobulin deficiencies. To identify a specific organism,
however, the organism needs to be re-
trieved from the child's body. This is usually done by examination of fresh fecal material.

Assessment for the presence of protozoa is done in several ways. To assess for
amebiasis, the rectal mucosa is swabbed,
and the freshly prepared slide is examined
to detect the larval or adult stages of the
parasite. In cases of suspected giardiasis, a
gelatin-weighted capsule on a string,
passed into the small intestine and re-
trieved after 4 hours, has shown the organism adhering to mucus on the string.

When there is infestation by worms,
in most cases, such as in ascariasis, hookworm disease, and tapeworm, the worms
can be easily isolated and identified in the
stool. With pinworms or oxyuriasis, however, fecal examination is a poor method.
The most efficient technique entails placing adhesive cellophane tape on the perianal skin for a few seconds to secure the
organisms, which are then placed on a
slide.

Laboratory Data. In addition to routine
laboratory tests and attempts to isolate and
identify the intestinal parasite, various
other diagnostic tests are done to complete
the assessment, since isolation is not always possible.[33] If amebiasis is suspected,
a sigmoidoscopy is frequently done, which
shows hemorrhage and shallow or deep
discrete ulcerations of the mucosa; if feces
is obtained it is examined immediately for
the active motile amebae. Duodenal aspiration is performed when giardiasis is suspected; the procedure yields the organism
in 90 percent of the cases in which there is
giardiasis. In ascariasis, x-rays may demonstrate the parasite. In hookworm disease the WBC is elevated with an eosinophilia that reaches 15 to 30 percent. In
trichuriasis, a sigmoidoscopy can be done
in which the worms, which look like waving threads, can be seen obliterating the
mucosa.

A positive diagnosis can be made on
obtaining and identifying the organism.
Frequently, however, the child has some
immunoglobulin deficiency that needs to

be assessed. The parasitic infestation also often causes anemia, which needs to be treated.

Management. Interventions in cases of intestinal parasites should not only include treatment of the infestation but prevention of reinfection. Good hygiene and health habits need to be emphasized. The need for careful hand washing before eating or handling food, after using the toilet, and before placing fingers in the mouth should be emphasized to the child. Parents and children need to be cautioned about washing foods that have been in or near the soil, such as raw fruits and vegetables. Children need to be discouraged from biting their nails, scratching the bare anal area, and going without shoes outside the house.

In most cases of pinworm infestation, the entire family is treated with medication (Table 18–1). When other members are treated, the family needs to understand the nature of transmission and that in many cases the medication is repeated in 2 weeks to 1 month to kill organisms that have hatched since the initial treatment. In addition, all underwear and bed linen

needs to be washed in hot water to kill the pinworm eggs that persist.

Most children with intestinal parasites are discharged to their home from the emergency department. It is very important for nurses to assume the responsibility for making sure that the treatment regimen is explained and reinforced and that the parents and children understand how to follow the regimen.

Acute Gastroenteritis
Acute gastroenteritis is an illness in which vomiting or diarrhea predominate. (Mild vomiting and loose stools of slightly increased frequency can accompany most acute illnesses in childhood.) Vomiting involves the loss of gastric contents with loss of bile and pancreatic secretions by reverse peristalsis. Diarrhea involves increased peristalsis and decreased transit time with incomplete absorption and reabsorption of bile, pancreatic secretions, water, and electrolytes.

Etiology. Gastroenteritis can be attributed to a number of specific causes and predisposing factors. Some specific causes of gastroenteritis include an inflammatory

TABLE 18–1. MEDICATIONS FOR SPECIFIC INTESTINAL PARASITE INFESTATION

Parasite	Medication	Dosage
Amebiasis	Metronidazole (Flagyl)	50 mg/day in 3 divided doses for 10 days
Giardiasis	Metronidazole (Flagyl) or Quinacrine (Atabrine)	35–50 mg/kg for 10 days or 6 mg/kg for 5 days
Ascariasis	Pyrantel pamoate (Antiminth) or Mebendazole (Vermax)	10 mg/kg or 100 mg twice daily for 3 days
Pinworm (Oxyuriasis)	Pyrvinium pamoate (Povan)	Single dose of 5 mg/kg
Hookworm	Mebendazole (Vermax)	100 mg twice daily for 3 days
Trichuriasis	Mebendazole (Vermax)	100 mg twice daily for 3 days
	Hexylresorcinol	0.2 percent to rapidly cleanse worms from the colon
Tapeworm (beef)	Niclosamide	500 mg given in a fasting state
Tapeworm (pork)	Quinacrine (Atabrine)	6 mg/kg for 5 days
Hymenolepsis nana	Niclosamide	500 mg given in a fasting state

process of infectious or viral origin. The bacterial or viral organisms that cause gastroenteritis in children are varied. These include the *Shigella, Yersinia, Campylobacter,* and *Salmonella* groups of bacteria, as well as *Staphylococcus aureus* and *Escherichia coli,* which are normal flora but which cause problems under certain circumstances. Pseudomonas, klebsiella, and proteus organisms are occasionally responsible. The main virus responsible for almost 90 percent of all infectious gastroenteritis in children is the rotavirus.[34]

Intestinal parasites can also be responsible for gastroenteritis. A toxic reaction to bacterial exotoxins, or the ingestion of poisons or certain antibiotics, or dietary indiscretions are also causes. Allergy and intolerance to specific foods and episodes of nervous excitement or periods of emotional tension can also be responsible.

Four main factors predispose a child to gastroenteritis. The first two factors are age and state of health. The younger the child and the more impaired his or her health, the more susceptible and more severe the gastroenteritis. Climate is the third factor. Many of the causative organisms are more prevalent in warmer climates. The fourth factor is environment. Crowding, substandard sanitation, and poor facilities for preparation and refrigeration of food all tend to increase the likelihood of gastroenteritis. It has also been found that breast-fed infants are less susceptible and are better protected against reduced intake during gastroenteritis.[35]

Clinical Presentation. The clinical presentation depends on the cause and the intensity of the illness. The child's age and health status are also influences.

The most serious and immediate physiologic disturbances of gastroenteritis are dehydration, acid-base derangements with acidosis, and shock that occurs when dehydration progresses to the point that circulatory status is seriously disturbed. Signs of dehydration include grey, cool skin with poor turgor, dry mucous membranes, little or no tearing or salivation, sunken eyeballs and fontanels, rapid pulse and respirations, decreased urine, and decreased blood pressure. The metabolic acidosis that occurs from the increased bicarbonate losses from diarrhea is compensated for by the respiratory system through rapid deep breathing, which is referred to as Kussmaul's or air hunger respirations. Signs of shock resulting from severe depletion of extracellular fluid volume include tachycardia, decreased blood pressure, cool mottled skin, and dry mucous membranes.

History. Since there are many causes of gastroenteritis, a history is important in diagnosing the cause. The history should include questions on the onset, number, duration, type, and color of the diarrhea or stools, and the vomitus; the amount of fluid intake and the type of fluids that are taken; the diet and any recent medications or new foods that have been introduced; and recent infections. Information regarding weight loss, possible contact with contaminated foods, food allergy, and an estimation of recent urine output is also helpful.

Assessment. The assessment is based on the history, with particular attention being paid to the relative intake and output. The state of consciousness and general appearance of the child should be assessed. Urine output should be measured and a specific gravity obtained. The weight of the child should be compared to the pre-illness weight. Vital signs should be taken and recorded. When counting respirations it should be determined if there is presence of ketone smell on the breath. A fever or signs of shock (decreased blood pressure, increased pulse) necessitates immediate attention, as does severe dehydration and metabolic acidosis. Assessment of mild, moderate, or severe dehydration should be made based on the clinical presentation.

The age of the child provides further clues as to the etiology. In the first year of life in bottle-fed infants, and later in breast-fed infants, E. coli is the usual disease agent. Shigella is most common from ages 2 to 4 years, but the most severe form is apt to occur in children over 5. Salmonella and the viral causes are most prevalent under age 2, although they can appear at any age.

If there are multiple cases of gastroenteritis in a household, the cause is frequently Shigella. A single case in a young child is more likely to be E. coli, a milk allergy, a new food, overfeeding, or starvation.

Laboratory Data. In addition to a complete blood count and a urinalysis, electrolytes, blood urea nitrogen, venous blood gases, and examination of the stool should be done. Many band forms in the differential WBC are indicative of shigellosis. The dehydrated infant will have an increased hematocrit as a result of fluid loss. The specific gravity of the urine, in general, gives good indication of hydration, while the presence of ketones reflect increased ketoacid production as a result of increased fat metabolism due to caloric deprivation. Venous gases, which are obtained without a tourniquet to prevent lactate buildup, reflect the degree of bicarbonate loss, while the P_{CO_2} indicates the degree of compensation. In the measurement of electrolytes, the sodium will indicate if the dehydration is hypotonic, isotonic, or hypertonic. The serum potassium does not necessarily reflect the total body potassium, since cellular concentration is not measured. If there is a question regarding potassium depletion, an electro-

cardiogram (ECG) can be done, which will show flattened T waves.

An elevated blood urea nitrogen will be found in reduced renal circulation but will be falsely low if the child has not ingested protein in the preceding 24 hours.

Examination of the stool is indicated in gastroenteritis. Stool examination with indicator paper for pH and a clinitest tablet will detect stool containing carbohydrates, indicative of disaccharide intolerance. Bulky, fatty stools suggest malabsorption. Examination of the stool for leukocytes is important because no leukocytes are found in normal stools or if the disease producing agent is a virus. Rectal swabs for culture are indicated if a bacterial agent is suspected.

Differential Diagnosis. Occasionally the history may indicate the source and nature of the infection or the possibility of food poisoning, but in most instances the cause can be determined by bacteriologic and virologic studies of the stool, which are definitive.

When the diagnosis is not definite and the illness is severe, other factors need to be considered. In cases of overfeeding or starvation, the dietary history may provide the needed information. There have also been instances of child abuse with the use of laxatives or poisons that have caused gastroenteritis;[36] thus these possibilities may also need to be considered. Other entities in which gastroenteritis is one facet of the illness includes Crohn's disease, ulcerative colitis, immunodeficiencies, carbohydrate and fat malabsorption, intractable diarrhea of infancy, and Hirschsprung's disease.

Management. In most cases of gastroenteritis, pharmacologic agents are not recommended. Antiemetics are rarely effective and tend to alter the level of consciousness. Antidiarrheal agents are also rarely effective and may be harmful; Kaopectate may facilitate bacterial penetration, and the opiates and Lomotil may encourage the proliferation of pathogens.[37]

Mild or moderate gastroenteritis, consisting of vomiting alone or vomiting with diarrhea, can be managed by simple measures when there is an understanding, cooperative parent. Instructions are given regarding diet and signs and symptoms that may indicate a worsening of the condition, which would necessitate another emergency department visit. Initially the child is given nothing by mouth for a period of time, depending on age. For young infants the period of restriction is 2 to 4 hours; for children aged 1 to 5 it is 4 hours; and for older children 6 to 8 hours. This helps slow down the increased intestinal activity and provides a period of rest for the gastrointestinal tract by reducing the number and volume of stools. Clear liquids such as Pedialyte or Lytren for infants and gingerale, cola, Kool-Aid, Jello water, Gatorade, and Popsicles for older children can be given starting with small amounts (1 tablespoon every 15 minutes), to minimize gastric distention. The amounts can be gradually increased and the feedings made less frequent depending on the age of the child. If there is diarrhea with no vomiting, clear liquids in large amounts every 3 to 4 hours should be given, since the lower frequency of feedings reduces activation of the gastrocolic reflex. It is important to emphasize that milk should be withheld for at least a week after symptoms disappear, and for young children a hydrolyzed lactose-free formula should be used instead of milk.[38]

If clear liquids are tolerated, soft foods such as gelatin desserts, soups (not creamed), bananas, applesauce, strained carrots, and toast can be given. The parent should be further instructed that if the child develops signs of complications, such as deep breathing, listlessness, re-

duced urinary output, weight loss, or blood in the stools, the parent should return to the emergency department with the child.

In moderately severe to severe cases, appropriate treatment of the physiologic distrubances is the primary concern. Parenteral fluid therapy, comprehensive evaluation, and hospitalization are warranted. Fluid therapy in the emergency department is directed to restoring circulation rapidly in this resuscitation phase, which lasts approximately 1 to 2 hours. The fluid generally used is 5 percent dextrose in normal saline at 20 to 30 cc/kg/hour and must be closely monitored. In hypertonic dehydration with shock, plasma substitutes, such as a 5 percent albumin solution, are used. Measures to control fever and the administration of oxygen may also be necessary in some cases. The child should be isolated to prevent possible spread to others. Accurate intake and output measurement is important. A urine collector is placed on the child to determine the volume of output and to measure specific gravity.

In cases of mild to moderate diarrhea, if the parent seems to understand the instructions given regarding diet and potential for complications and appears to be cooperative, the child may be discharged home. Detailed instructions in oral dietary therapy, however, need to be given.[39] If there is some question as to the care the child will receive or a question about the severity of his or her condition, especially with an infant, hospitalization is indicated. In cases of moderately severe to severe diarrhea, hospitalization is generally indicated.

Anal Fissure

An anal fissure is a small slit or crack in the anus that extends into the mucocutaneous junction. It is the most common cause of rectal bleeding in infants.

Etiology. The cause is most often a hard, sharp, or bulky stool. It sometimes develops after explosive diarrhea. It may also be caused by overzealous cleansing or by skin conditions such as eczema.

The edges of a fresh fissure are clean and sharp, but if the fissure becomes chronic, the edges thicken and frequently pucker.[40]

Clinical Presentation. Typically there is a small amount of bright red blood in the diaper or bloody streaking of the stool of an otherwise healthy looking child. Significant bleeding is rare. The child cries before or during defecation and may refuse to defecate. The fissure, a small slit, can usually be visualized on external examination.

History. The parents usually give a history of bright red blood-streaked stool and of the child crying during defecation. There may be reported a difference in the diet, which might explain the change in the child's bowel habits.

Assessment. The diagnosis is made by inspection of the anal area, preferably when the child is straining to enable the examiner to better visualize the fissure.

Laboratory Data. The routine complete blood count and urinalysis are usually the only studies ordered. The hematocrit or hemoglobin may indicate some degree of anemia if there has been significant bleeding or if the bleeding has occurred over a period of time.

A diagnosis of anal fissure is relatively straightforward based on the history and visualization of the defect. There should be questioning about diet and stool habits, since constipation may cause this condition and will certainly aggravate it.

Management. Since the acute fissure heals quickly with careful cleansing of the anus, the parents should be shown how to cleanse in a gentle, nonirritating manner using a mild soap with a lot of water and a minimum of friction. The cleansing should be done several times a day and after each defecation.

The local irritation causing the fissure should be lessened or eliminated. The stool can be softened by increasing the sugar content of the formula; some children may need the addition of mineral oil or some other stool softener.

Anal pain and the withholding of stool secondary to it are alleviated by the local application to the fissure of an anesthetic ointment. The child with an anal fissure can be discharged following instructions to the parents on the care of the fissure.

Perirectal Abscess

A perirectal abscess often follows infection of deep perianal fissures or peritonitis. There is a male predominance of 79 to 90 percent.[41] The majority of these patients are less than 3 years of age.[42]

Etiology. The infectious etiology is usually *Staphylococcus aureus* or *E. coli*, both of which are normally found in feces. In 25 percent of the children a primary serious illness with neutropenia or immune deficiency occurs. It is felt that diarrhea or hard stools injure the canal and promote bacterial invasion with obstruction of the anal glands. An abscess develops in the poorly draining duct that may extend through, within, or outside the rectal sphincter to the anus to form fistula-in-ano or that may be perirectal, which may be associated with scrotal or gluteal cellulitis.

Clinical Presentation. The main symptoms are pain and swelling. Defecation is painful, and the child is unable to sit comfortably. The temperature is not very elevated unless the perirectal space is involved. Systemic signs such as fever and leukocytosis reflect the severity of the process.

History. The child under 3 years usually will be irritable. The parents may have noted crying during defecation and an inability to sit comfortably.

Assessment. A painful swelling can be noted over the ischiorectal fossa with redness, heat, induration, and fluctuation. During rectal examination, a mass that is adjacent to the rectum and is fluctuant can be noted.

Laboratory Data. Besides the routine urinalysis and a complete blood count, a barium enema may be ordered. The barium enema will show an extrinsic pressure defect in the rectum.[43]

Differential Diagnosis. A diagnosis of perianal abscess can be made with some degree of certainty based on the relatively clear signs and symptoms. The child, however, should be assessed for a primary illness that may have contributed to the development of a perirectal abscess because of an immune deficiency and neutropenia.

Management. If the abscess is developing, antibiotics are ordered as well as warm soaks to the rectal area, which provide symptomatic relief and which localize the abscess. If the condition is more severe, incision and drainage are recommended.

Since the child is so uncomfortable, medication for pain is ordered, and the child must be handled in such a way that no direct pressure is placed on the anal area.

Because of the degrees of severity of perirectal abscess, the child must be carefully assessed. The child with a fever and leukocytosis is probably in need of hospital admission, while the child with no fever and beginning anal redness and discomfort will be discharged home with instructions to the parents about antibiotic administration and warm soaks to the anal area.

Anal Fistula

Anal fistula is an abnormal connection between the anorectal canal and the perianal skin. It is not a very common condition, occuring in only 25 to 30 percent of children following a perirectal abscess.

Etiology. An acquired fistula is the residual of an abscess and is open to the skin surface. There is frequently a history of one or more incisions into the abscess.

Clinical Presentation. The symptoms of an acquired fistula are those of a painful swelling that recurs intermittently, followed by purulent drainage. When the fistulous tract becomes obstructed, there is redness, swelling, and warmth underlying its opening.

History. The child frequently has a history of incision and drainage of the perirectal abscess or of spontaneous rupture of the abscess. Information should be gained about the occurrences and treatment of perirectal abscesses.

Assessment. An opening into the skin beside the anal orifice can be readily visualized. Purulent or fecal material may be draining from this lesion. A probe can be placed into this perianal opening that can go into the anal crypt or even further into the rectum.

Laboratory Data. The routine laboratory studies, a complete blood count and a urinalysis, may be normal. The WBC will be elevated if there is infection.

Radiologic examination of the colon

with barium or retrograde injection of dye into the fistula will show the communicating tract.

Differential Diagnosis. The presence of an opening beside the anal orifice that allows an introduction of a probe clearly indicates an anal fistula. The child should be further assessed for cellulitis with beta-hemolytic streptococci and furuncles.[44]

Management. There is some controversy over the recommended treatment of anal fistulas. Some investigators believe that conservatism is indicated in the care of fistulas in infants, since it is felt that frequently the fistula will close spontaneously without surgery.

If surgery is needed, simple incision and removal of the fistulous tract with packing of the resultant defect is effective.[45] Gryboski and Walker[46] believe that while in a few cases the tract will remain closed after drainage and constant cleansing of the area, for a complete cure complete excision of the fistula is required. Silverman and Roy[47] also believe that fistulectomy is necessary to prevent recurrences.

If the child is an infant and has no symptoms of infection or inflammation, the parents may be instructed to observe the area and to keep it clean. When a simple incision and drainage have been done, the child may be discharged with instructions to the parents on the use of warm soaks to the area and on antibiotic administration. A child who has a fistula and cellulitis may need hospitalization.

Hiatal Hernia

A hiatal hernia is a congenital herniation through a diaphragmatic defect that allows the cardiac end of the stomach to slide or roll above the diaphragm and back into the abdomen. The muscular ring of the hiatus is not snug and permits the sliding of the cardiac end of the stomach from the thorax to the abdomen. This sliding or rolling through the esophageal hiatus frequently causes inflammation of the distal esophagus because of reflux of gastric contents into the esophagus with subsequent regurgitation. To distinguish it from the adult with a hiatal hernia, some pediatric gastroenterologists use the term ''partial thoracic stomach.''[48]

Etiology. The diaphragm forms between the eighth and tenth weeks of fetal life from four separate embryonic structures that fuse to form the partition separating the thoracic and abdominal cavities. Apertures through which the esophagus and great vessels traverse the diaphragm are normally found. A much larger esophageal aperture results in a hiatal hernia.

Clinical Presentation. The most common symptom is vomiting. It is sometimes so severe that there is loss of calories sufficient to cause weight loss and failure to thrive.

Repeated irritation of the esophageal lining with gastric acid can lead to esophagitis and consequently bleeding. Blood loss causes anemia and is seen as hematemesis or melena. Heartburn is a symptom in older children but may go unrecognized in infants.

Reflux of the stomach contents also predisposes to aspiration and the development of respiratory symptoms, especially pneumonia.

History. A history is an important part of the diagnostic evaluation. Particular attention should be paid to the child's eating habits and the occurrence of symptoms, especially vomiting.

Assessment. Persistent vomiting is the principal complaint. Only occasionally is the onset of vomiting delayed until after a year of age. Vomiting is usually copious and is typically projectile. It occurs most frequently during or shortly after feeding in early infancy, and in late infancy the vomiting occurs at night. Occasional brown staining from the vomit due to blood is a characteristic feature. When questioning the parents it is important to refer to discoloration rather than to the presence of blood, since the brown discoloration of vomitus is frequently not equated with the presence of blood.

Gastric peristalsis may be seen and a "pyloric tumor" may be felt, leading to an incorrect diagnosis of pyloric stenosis. The "tumor" in hiatal hernia, however, tends to be softer.

Arising from loss of nourishment, these infants are hungry and take feedings eagerly. The majority are underweight and may be dehydrated. Constipation is common.

Laboratory Data. Several tests are available to evaluate the presence of a hiatal hernia. The initial test is the barium esophagram in which the reflux of barium from the stomach to the esophagus can be seen by fluoroscopy.

Differential Diagnosis. Since there are other conditions that produce the return of stomach contents into the esophagus, a hiatal hernia must be differentiated from other causes of gastrointestinal reflux. In newborns gastrointestinal reflux is considered normal. Reflux is thought to result from delayed maturation of the lower esophageal neuromuscular function or impaired local hormonal control mechanisms.[49] Other causes of persistent vomiting are feeding problems (especially underfeeding), pyloric stenosis, and urinary tract infections.[50]

Management. Nursing interventions vary greatly depending on the condition of the child and on whether the child can be managed conservatively or surgically.

Conservative management consists of positioning these patients and a modified feeding regimen. These infants are placed in an upright posture at an angle of approximately 40 to 60 degrees to reduce gastrointestinal reflux. This position facilitates clearance of regurgitated gastric juice from the terminal esophagus. This posture should be maintained consistently, particularly at night when gastric contents are neither buffered nor diluted by feedings. Thickened small-volume feedings are also helpful.

Although there is usually a significant reduction in the frequency of vomiting within 2 to 4 weeks of starting treatment, it may take longer. By 6 weeks a normal physiologic barrier to reflux usually develops.[51]

Once symptoms have been controlled for 4 to 6 weeks, therapy can be reduced in intensity. The reduction might consist of the child being removed from the upright posture for a short period of time before the next feeding.

Surgical intervention is selected for those children with severe complications such as respiratory distress, esophagitis, or esophageal stricture. A commonly used surgical procedure is the Nisson fundoplication, which creates a valve mechanism by wrapping the fundus of the stomach around the distal esophagus.

An overall assessment of the infant needs to be made because he or she may range from healthy to critically ill. The infant with mild dehydration and a history of persistent vomiting may only require home care management of positioning and feeding. An infant who is very ill may have major fluid loss, anemia, and aspiration pneumonia from severe persistent vomiting. The fluid, electrolyte, and acid-base imbalances will require the infant's hospitalization for parenteral correction and possible surgical intervention.

ALIMENTARY TRACT OBSTRUCTIONS

Intussusception

Intussusception is the invagination or telescoping of a segment of intestine into itself. The ileocecal region is most commonly involved. It is one of the most frequent causes of intestinal obstruction during infancy with half of the cases occurring in the first year and the other half in the second year of life.[52] The condition is three times more common in males than females.

Etiology. While reasons for intussusception are uncertain, several theories have been suggested.[53] The greater disparity between the size of the ileum and the ileocecal valve in infants is felt to encourage telescoping at this point, where 95 percent of intussusception occurs (Fig. 18–2). In approximately the other 5 percent, enlarged lymph nodes along the gastrointestinal tract that occur with respiratory infections, cystic fibrosis, foreign bodies, gastrointestinal polyps, or Meckel's diverticulum appear to be the recognizable lead points. One study has implicated the human rotavirus as an etiologic agent.[54]

Intussusception causes an interference with the vascular supply as well as an obstruction of the gastrointestinal tract. Interference with lymphatic and venous drainage leads to edema, increased tissue pressure, and capillary and venule engorgement, which form a vicious cycle. With increasing edema and eventual total venous obstruction, tissue pressure rises until arterial flow is stopped, which fosters necrosis. Goblet cells are stimulated to dis-

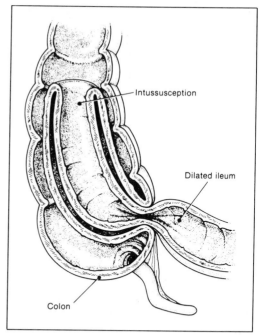

Figure 18–2. Telescoping bowel in the presence of intussusception. *(From G.M. Scipien, M.U. Barnard, M.A. Chard , et al. (Eds.). Comprehensive Pediatric Nursing (2nd ed.). New York: McGraw-Hill, 1979, p. 776.)*

charge mucus, which mixes with the blood to create the "currant jelly" stool.

Clinical Presentation. Generally, intussusception occurs as an acute or subacute illness in previously healthy infants or children. The classical signs and symptoms are intermittent abdominal pain, vomiting, blood and mucus in the stools, and a palpable tumor, a "sausage-shaped mass" in the upper epigastrium, although frequently one or several of these traits are missing. Accompanying features such as an upper respiratory infection, fever, and diarrhea may be misleading and may postpone the diagnosis. Some children have no pain but are pale, listless, and apparently ill. If treatment is not sought, the child becomes acutely ill with fever, prostration, and signs of peritonitis.

History. A detailed history is an important aid in making the diagnosis. The typical history is of a well infant who screams and draws up his knees. Vomiting occurs soon after, and there are bouts of colicky pain at regular intervals. Gradually the child becomes apathetic, and when the diagnosis has been delayed, currant jelly stools are seen.

Assessment. The assessment is based on the history. An unhurried examination should be done during a pain-free interval. To identify the sausage-shaped characteristic mass, it is helpful to stand at the head of the infant and attempt to roll the mass against the under surface of the liver. A rectal examination may allow for direct palpation of the intussusception itself and may reveal the characteristic bloody mucoid discharge.

Laboratory Data. Blood should be obtained for a baseline complete blood count and differential, and a hemoglobin, hematocrit, and type-and-crossmatching should be obtained. With a urinalysis attention should be paid to the specific gravity to assess hydration.

X-rays of the abdomen show a scant amount of gas in the gut and little or no bowel content. Barium enema studies provide the definitive diagnosis of intussusception where the intussusception can be shown.

Differential Diagnosis. Barium enema studies provide visualization of the intussusception. Since other problems, such as polyps or Meckel's diverticulum, may be a causative factor in intussusception, the child needs to be assessed as to the possible cause of the condition.

Management. Initially a nasogastric tube should be inserted and connected to low suction, intravenous fluids should be

started, and antibiotics should be given, since edematous bowel is permeable to bacteria. The treatment of choice is nonsurgical hydrostatic reduction by barium enema.[55]

The diagnostic enema is continued, and the intussusception is observed by fluoroscope until the mass disappears in the ileum and several loops become filled with barium. This can take from a few minutes to a half hour and is successful in 75 percent of cases. Failure of the barium enema to reduce the intussusception is an obvious indication for surgery.

If the intussusception is reduced by barium enema, the child's condition is good, and the parents are reliable and can easily return to the hospital, the child may be sent home after a brief period of observation in the emergency department. If any of these factors are questioned or if the child needs surgical reduction, the child is hospitalized.

Pyloric Stenosis

Pyloric stenosis occurs when there is an obstruction of the pyloric sphincter by hypertrophy of the circular muscle of the pylorus. It is five times more common in males than in females with an incidence of 4 to 5 per 1000 live births.

Etiology. The most popular theory is one of hypertrophy of the circular smooth fibers of the pyloric sphincter secondary to spasm. Narrowing of the canal between the stomach and duodenum occur until, over time, it progresses to a complete obstruction. The muscle is thickened to as much as twice its normal size, and the stomach is dilated (Fig. 18–3).

Clinical Presentation. The full-term infant typically manifests symptoms between the second and sixth weeks of life.[56] The vomiting is at first intermittent, increasing in frequency and severity until it follows

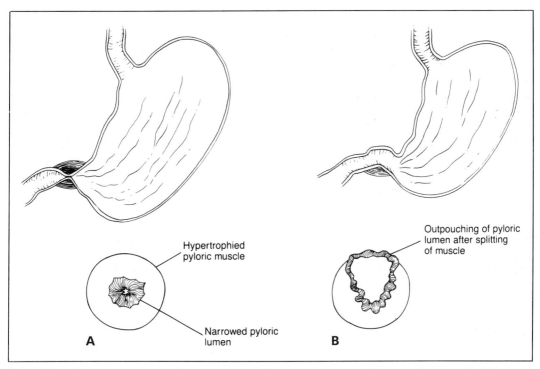

Figure 18–3. Pyloric stenosis. **A.** Obstruction of pyloric lumen by hypertrophied muscle layers. **B.** Release of submucosal layer after pyloromyotomy. *(From S.R. Mott, N.F. Fazekas, & S.R. James (Eds.) Nursing Care of Children and Families. Menlo Park, Calif.: Addison-Wesley, 1985, p. 1329.)*

every feeding and is projectile. The infant is hungry, and a second feeding after a vomiting episode produces vomitus of sour formula or clear gastric content. As less food and water make their way through the pylorus, the number of stools decreases and the urine becomes scanty. Weight loss is light or severe, depending on the duration and severity of symptoms. The upper abdomen is frequently distended, visible peristaltic waves can be seen that move from left to right across the epigastrum, and there is a palpable olive-shaped tumor in the epigastrium, just to the right of the umbilicus.

History. A careful history should be obtained, since the diagnosis can be made with a high degree of accuracy for the patient who has a history of progressive,

nonbilious vomiting that becomes projectile and may be blood tinged.[57]

Assessment. A history of progressive vomiting, failure to gain weight, or weight loss indicates the need for an assessment for pyloric stenosis. Examination reveals a distended upper abdomen and gastric peristaltic waves. An olive-shaped tumor, felt to the right of the umbilicus, is more readily palpable after the infant has vomited. The infant is active, irritable, and eager to feed. Dehydration, loss of skin turgor, fretfulness, and apathy may be present in severe cases of long duration.

Laboratory Data. In addition to the routine laboratory tests, electrolyte studies should be done, because the vomiting leads to metabolic alkalosis and sodium and potassium depletion. An upper gastrointestinal series is usually done, which demonstrates the elongation of the pylorus. Ultrasound demonstration of the thickened ring may aid in diagnosis, but some investigators feel that false-negative examinations are frequent.[58]

Differential Diagnosis. In the gastrointestinal series a study of the esophagus should be done so that a stricture can be ruled out. Benign tumors may lead to symptoms similar to pyloric stenosis, but the age of onset and x-ray findings are different.

Management. Surgical relief of pyloric obstruction by pylorotomy is simple, safe, and effective. Before this can be done, however, the metabolic alkalosis needs to be corrected. An intravenous infusion is started with 0.45 percent normal saline in 5 percent dextrose with potassium added. Intake and output need to be closely monitored. An explanation of the diagnosis and treatment needs to be given to the parents.

In most cases of pyloric stenosis the child will be admitted from the emergency department. Postponement of treatment will only worsen the condition, because the child will continue to vomit.

Foreign Body

A foreign body in the alimentary tract is the result of a child ingesting an article that cannot be digested. Foreign bodies include objects such as coins, marbles, buttons, thumbtacks, and bones. The majority of children with gastrointestinal foreign bodies are 6 months to 4 years of age. In older children the ingestion is usually accidental or is associated with psychiatric abnormalities.

Etiology. When a foreign object is swallowed the common places for it to become lodged are the esophagus and the stom-

ach. As a general rule, any object that can be swallowed and that reaches the stomach will pass through the intestine without difficulty in 90 percent of the cases.

A foreign body that remains in the esophagus needs immediate attention, since it may cause perforation. Foreign bodies are most frequently found in a cricopharyngeal area, which corresponds to the fourth cervical vertebrae. Children who have had surgery for tracheoesophageal fistula are most prone to impaction with partially chewed meat because of narrowing of the lumen and dysmobility of the anastamosed esophagus.

Clinical Presentation. Symptoms of an esophageal foreign body include gagging, attempts at vomiting, retrosternal pain, hypersalivation, and respiratory distress. If left in place, ulceration with bleeding and finally perforation with mediastinitis can occur.

A foreign body lodged in the stomach or intestine may cause abdominal pain. Gastrointestinal bleeding from the irritation may result. Complications of foreign bodies distal to the esophagus include hemorrhage, pressure necrosis, complete obstruction, and perforation with peritonitis.

History. A history is needed to help determine what type of object the child might have swallowed. An approximate estimate of when the ingestion occurred is also very important information, since in the case of foreign bodies trapped in the esophagus perforation and mediastinitis can occur very rapidly after ingestion.

Assessment. The child's symptoms and the history are most important to the assessment. The child with an esophageal foreign body will generally appear in distress, with gagging, attempts at vomiting, hypersalivation, and respiratory distress.

The child with a foreign body lower in the alimentary tract may complain of pain, but if the object has been lodged for a period of time, complications of hemorrhage and peritonitis may occur.

Laboratory Data. The routine laboratory tests are not remarkable unless there are bleeding and mediastinitis or peritonitis, which would be reflected in the hematocrit and the differential.

X-rays of the area are done. If the object is opaque, as, fortunately, coins and many swallowed objects are, they can be readily visualized (Fig. 18–4). If an object is non-opaque an esophagram will determine its size and location. Visualization of the foreign body by radiography provides a definite diagnosis. The child must be watched closely for complications.

Management. In cases of smooth foreign objects in the proximal esophagus, the usual site of occurrence, removal can be accomplished by means of a Foley catheter, which is passed beyond the object, is inflated, and is withdrawn, bringing the foreign body with it.[59] Mouth gag and forceps should be ready for use when the object nears the child's mouth. The procedure is carried out under fluoroscope. With sharp objects or objects lodged in the distal esophagus, removal is done under general anesthesia with an esophagoscope equipped with appropriate forceps.

For foreign bodies that have reached the stomach, conservative management is in order. The progress of the foreign body can be followed by serial roentgenograms. Surgical removal is not considered unless 2 to 3 weeks have gone by without progress. The parents should be instructed to examine all of the child's stools until the object swallowed has been recovered. The child may have a normal diet with extra roughage and should not be given a laxa-

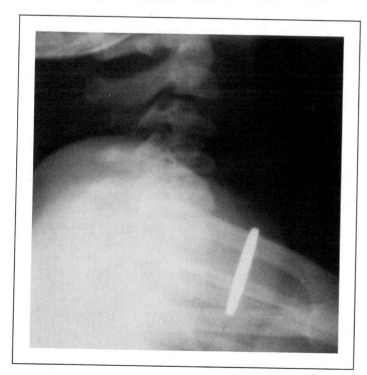

Figure 18–4. Radiograph of lateral view of a coin in the esophagus in a 5-year-old female. *(Radiograph courtesy of Richard DeNise, MD, and the Pediatric Radiology Department, Boston City Hospital.)*

tive. If there is severe abdominal pain, vomiting, or fever, the child should be brought to the emergency department.

If the child had a foreign body in the esophagus that was removed with a catheter and had no complications, discharge is likely. If there is question of trauma and subsequent swelling, hospitalization would be advised. A child requiring general anesthesia for an esophagoscopy would be admitted.

Hospitalization for retrieval of a coin from the stomach may be deferred for 4 weeks but for no more than a few days for removal of an open safety pin caught in the duodenum.

Hirschsprung's Disease

Hirschsprung's disease is a mechanical obstruction caused by inadequate motility in part of the intestine. It is four times more frequent in boys than in girls, and other congenital anomalies accompanying it are unusual.[60]

Etiology. Abnormalities in the pelvic parasympathetic system include the absence of ganglion cells from the distal colon, absence of peristalsis in the affected areas, and partial intestinal obstruction (Fig. 18–5). This condition may be due to anoxia during development, which causes an arrest of the craniocaudal migration of neuroblasts.[61]

Clinical Presentation. Most of the infants are full term, appear normal at birth, and have symptoms within the first few weeks of life that are not always recognized. Only 5 percent of these neonates are known to pass meconium during the first 24 hours. Abdominal distention and bilious vomiting are the usual symptoms. If the disorder is allowed to progress, other signs of intestinal obstruction, such as respiratory distress and shock, develop.

History. A history is generally given of an infant who failed to pass meconium spon-

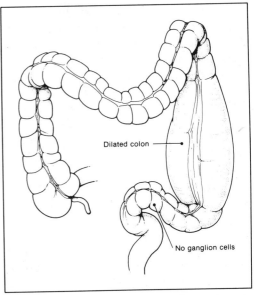

Figure 18–5. The affected bowel in Hirschsprung's disease. *(From G.M. Scipien, M.U. Barnard, M.A. Chard, et al. (Eds.). Comprehensive Pediatric Nursing (2nd ed.). New York: McGraw-Hill, 1979, p. 774.)*

taneously or passed it sparingly. Information on the onset of constipation, the character of stools, and the frequency of bowel movements needs to be obtained. The child does not thrive and has constipation, abdominal distention, and episodes of diarrhea and vomiting.

Assessment. The examination reveals an emaciated and dehydrated infant with a greatly distended abdomen. Dilated small bowel loops are easily visualized and palpated in the abdomen. Fecal impaction in the colon feels like a ropy mass that extends down the left side of the abdomen and across the epigastrum. As the examiner withdraws a finger, a gush of flatus and foul-smelling stool follows.

Laboratory Data. Roentgenographic studies using a barium enema frequently demonstrate the transition zone between the dilated proximal colon (megacolon) and the aganglionic distal segment. The typical megacolon and narrow segment, however, may not develop until 3 to 4 weeks or even months after birth in some children. The definitive method of diagnosis is rectal biopsy done by suction or deep surgical wedge section. Manometric studies that show changes in motor response can also be a helpful diagnostic aid.

Differential Diagnosis. This disease must be distinguished from rectal stenosis and meconium plug syndrome and in older children from physiologic constipation. A definitive diagnosis can be made by rectal biopsy.

Management. Initially there should be correction of fluid and electrolyte deficits with an intravenous infusion. Isotonic enemas may be needed to provide relief from the abdominal distention. A nasogastric tube is inserted. The only definitive treatment is removal of the aganglionic, nonfunctioning segment of bowel. The small infant is usually treated by a colostomy, which is reversed at 8 or more months of age. Surgery, however, is usually postponed until the child is in a good nutritional state; it is not emergency surgery.

Occasionally a child has chronic but not severe symptoms of megacolon, in which case isotonic enemas, stool softeners, and a low residue diet that decrease the bulk of the stool may be ordered. Detailed instructions need to be given to the parents.

Generally the child with Hirschsprung's disease is hospitalized initially to correct fluid and electrolyte levels before surgery can be performed.

Inguinal Hernia

An inguinal hernia is a mass in the inguinal region that contains some part of the abdominal contents. Inguinal hernias account for approximately 80 percent of all hernias and are commoner in males than females. Such hernias are not usually evident until 2 to 3 months of age.

Etiology. An inguinal hernia is derived from persistence of all or part of the processus vaginalis, the tube of peritoneum that precedes the testicle through the inguinal canal into the scrotum during the eighth month of gestation. When the upper portion fails to atrophy, abdominal contents can be forced into it, creating a palpable bulge or mass.

Clinical Presentation. There are no symptoms with an empty hernial sac. The hernia is usually manifested as a painless inguinal swelling that is absent when the child sleeps and that increases in size when there is coughing or straining. Mild external pressure is usually sufficient to bring about reentry of the herniated bowel into the abdominal cavity. When the contents of the hernial sac cannot be reduced, the hernia is said to be incarcerated. Partial or complete obstruction almost invariably follows incarceration. The symptoms of obstruction are tenderness and pain in that area leading to intermittent or continuous crying, nausea, vomiting, and abdominal distention. While inguinal hernias are less frequent in girls, incarceration and obstruction are more frequent in the girls who have them, especially in the first 6 months of life.[62]

History. A good history is of value, since the mass is not always visualized by the examiner. Questions regarding the exact location, when it appeared, aggravating circumstances, and the reducibility of the mass should be asked.

Assessment. Physical findings are often nonexistent, and one is forced to rely on parental observation of the hernia. Careful inspection of both sides of the groin will indicate a small lump beneath a thick layer of adipose tissue. Slight pressure with the fingertips causes reentry of the bowel into the abdominal cavity. Crying causes an increase in the size of the hernia. Because of potential complications of hernia, such as incarceration with intestinal obstruction and possible vascular compromise and bowel necrosis, there is concern about the potential of the processus vaginalis to admit herniated bowel.

Laboratory Data. In addition to the routine laboratory tests, which are not diagnostic in this case, radiographs may be ordered. In uncomplicated inguinal hernia, plain radiographs are of little value, although small bowel obstruction may be seen on plain radiographs with incarceration.[63]

Inguinal herniography can be used to detect children with unilateral inguinal hernia who have a contralateral patent processus vaginalus.

Differential Diagnosis. An inguinal hernia needs to be differentiated from lymph nodes, a hydrocele, an undescended testis, or torsion of the cord. With these conditions an increase in abdominal pressure, such as in crying, does not increase the size of the mass, and the mass is not reducible.

Management. The treatment for hernias is prompt, elective surgical repair. If the hernia is incarcerated, it is best to reduce it immediately before obstruction occurs and the injured tissues recover before surgery is scheduled in 24 to 48 hours.[64] Manipulative reduction with gentle digital pressure can be attempted after sedation of the child with meperidine (1 mg/kg) and by placing him in Trendelenberg's position with an ice bag on the affected side.[65]

Irreducible or strangulated hernias are treated with emergency exploration and herniotomy. In all cases of inguinal hernias, the surgery and follow-up care must be explained to the parents.

The child with an uncomplicated in-guinal hernia can be discharged home with arrangements as to when the elective surgical repair will be done. Preoperative teaching should be done for both child and parents. In the case of an incarcerated or strangulated hernia, the child is admitted and emergency surgery is done.

Umbilical Hernias

A hernia in the umbilical region is a very common defect. It is more common in premature infants and in black infants. A familial incidence is common.

Etiology. An umbilical hernia is caused by incomplete fascial closure of the umbilical ring, although the defect is entirely covered by skin and subcutaneous tissue. As the contents of the cord involute, the hernia becomes apparent.

The size of the umbilical protrusion is variable. The underlying fascial defect can vary from 0.5 cm to 4.0 cm. Herniated small bowel is usually reducible.

History. Information should be gained regarding when the hernia was first noted, if there has been any increase or decrease in its size, and if it is affected by crying, coughing, or vomiting. Because the sight of the hernia is so disconcerting to parents, they need reassurance regarding its innocuous nature.

Assessment. The hernia appears as a fullness in the umbilical region, which increases with crying or straining. It varies in size from that of a fingertip to that of an orange and frequently increases during the first months of life. The sac may contain only omentum, but when herniated bowel occupies it, the sac feels soft and silky, and the hernia is reduced with a gurgling sound. Incarceration and strangulation are very rare but require immediate surgical intervention.

Laboratory Data. In addition to the routine laboratory studies, if there is a large hernia a plain film of the abdomen may be ordered. The protruding hernial sac can be visualized.

Differential Diagnosis. An umbilical hernia can be seen and allows a definite diagnosis. Since it is sometimes a concomitant defect in Down's syndrome, hypothyroidism, and Hurler's syndrome, an additional assessment for these defects may be desirable.

Management. Usually, umbilical hernias close spontaneously during the first year of life and should not be treated. Some investigators advocate taping the hernia, but there is no evidence that it hastens closure of the defect.[66]

Surgery is advisable if the fascial defect still exceeds 1.5 cm at 2 years of age. If the child is having abdominal pain or if the hernia persists until school age, it should be repaired.[67]

Since most umbilical hernias close spontaneously and no treatment is needed, parents need to be reassured of the gradual normal closure and of the low probability of complications (incarceration is 1 in 1500 umbilical hernias).[68]

Most children with umbilical hernias will be discharged home following reassurance of the parents that there is nothing seriously wrong with their child.

BLEEDING

Many lesions may cause bleeding in the gastrointestinal tract. This complication manifests itself by hematemesis and passage of blood in the stool. Depending on the extent of blood loss, signs and symptoms of hypovolemia may be present.

Mixing of blood with acid in the stomach leads to the formation of acid hematin, which is the material responsible for the characteristic tarry or melanotic stools that are frequently seen. Bright red rectal bleeding is usually characteristic of large bowel lesions. Blood on the surface of the stool is characteristic of low rectal or anal bleeding.

Once the child with gastrointestinal bleeding is stabilized with suitable fluids and blood, a complete history should be obtained. Assessment includes a complete physical and diagnostic laboratory tests. The tests frequently done include a gastroduodenal endoscopy, diagnostic angiography, and a gastrointestinal barium study.

With fiberoptic gastroscopy, endoscopy has become increasingly popular for evaluation of gastrointestinal bleeding. This usually does not require general anesthesia and can be done in the emergency department. It permits the identification of the lesion responsible for the hemorrhage in upper gastrointestinal bleeds.

Celiac, superior mesenteric, and inferior mesenteric angiography are useful in the diagnosis of gastrointestinal bleeding. Selection of the artery to be used is based on the clinical impression of the site of the bleeding. Bleeding in excess of 0.5 to 1.0 cc per minute usually can be detected in angiography as extravasation of contrast medium from the bleeding vessel. In cases in which endoscopy is inconclusive, angiography is performed. It is a good method for demonstrating bleeding sites in Meckel's diverticulum, when there are bleeding sites in the small bowel, or in children with variceal bleeding. Barium studies are only occasionally used, because they cannot prove a visualized lesion to be a source of bleeding.

Meckel's Diverticulum
A Meckel's diverticulum results when the omphalomesenteric duct, which connects the ileum to the yolk sac, fails to obliterate. The omphalomesenteric duct normally clo-

ses by the fifth or sixth week of fetal life, but if it persists in all or part of its courses several types of malformations can result. These malformations can be cysts, fistulas, fibrotic cords, or, most commonly, Meckel's diverticulum. It is the most common congenital malformation of the gastrointestinal tract and is present in 1 to 2 percent of the population. The sexes are equally affected, but males have a much higher incidence of complications of the lesion.[69] It is estimated that about 15 percent of the cases develop complications. The majority of symptomatic Meckel's diverticula are seen between 6 months and 2 years of age.[70]

Pathophysiology. Meckel's diverticulum consists of an outpouching of the ileum that may vary in size from a small appendiceal process to a segment of bowel several inches long and wide. It may be connected to the umbilicus by a cord. It is a true diverticulum with a complete wall (Fig. 18–6).

Its mucosal lining may be gastric and ileal, which is most frequent, or colonic and ileal. Sixty percent of clinically significant Meckel's diverticula contain gastric mucosa capable of hydrochloric acid secretion. The acid and pepsin production of the gastric mucosa causes ulceration of the adjacent ileal mucosa with resultant hemorrhage or perforation.

Clinical Presentation. Painless, profuse rectal bleeding is the chief complaint of symptomatic cases in children less than 2 years of age. It is the chief presenting sign in more than half the cases. Severe anemia or shock affects most of these children. The classic description of bleeding from Meckel's diverticulum in older children is the alternate passage of dark and bright blood.

If low intestinal obstruction develops, it is caused by intussusception (telescop-

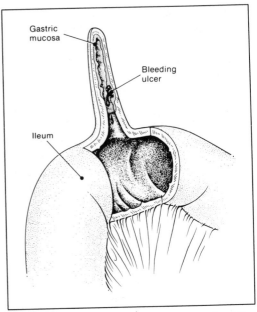

Figure 18–6. This outpouching is an example of the type of abnormality present in Meckel's diverticulum. *(From G.M. Scipien, M.U. Barnard, M.A. Chard, et al. (Eds.). Comprehensive Pediatric Nursing (2nd ed.). New York: McGraw-Hill, 1979, p. 784.)*

ing), by volvulus (twisting) of the small bowel, or by diverticulum about the fibrous remnant of the obliterated omphalomesenteric duct. The diverticulum tends to invert and to cause intussusception more often in infancy than in later life.

If diverticulitis develops, there is fever, leukocytosis, and tenderness and guarding in the right lower quadrant, all of which arouse suspicion of appendicitis. The pain is periumbilical early in the disease but may be to the right of the midline. Acute suppuration may lead to perforation in the infant. With perforation of the diverticulum, there is an increase in temperature and WBC. The abdomen becomes rigid, and bowel sounds decrease or disappear.

History. Diagnosis is usually based on the history. In more than half the cases of Meckel's diverticulum, the child has painless, profuse, rectal bleeding. In some cases there is a history of occasional bouts of bright red blood in the stools and in few instances a history of tarry stools.

Assessment. Since the most frequent manifestation is gastrointestinal bleeding, the child with Meckel's diverticulum is frequently in shock. There is profuse, painless, rectal bleeding.

Laboratory Data. Several diagnostic studies are routinely done if Meckel's diverticulum is suspected. A rectosigmoidoscopy is generally first performed. Blood tests, such as complete blood count and screening tests for bleeding disorders, are done. Abdominal angiography can be beneficial when the individual branch of the superior mesenteric artery leading to the diverticulum can be identified.

An x-ray diagnosis can seldom be made. Very rarely abdominal films following a barium enema show residual barium in the diverticulum.

Diagnostic studies are done to rule out other conditions. Rectosigmoidoscopy and barium enema are usually performed to eliminate other possible diagnoses, such as anal fissure, polyps, and intussusception without Meckel's diverticulum. Blood studies to rule out bleeding disorders are also done.

Management. As with most acute abdominal conditions, the child is to receive nothing by mouth. A nasogastric tube is ordered and should be inserted, secured, and attached to low suction. To correct hypovolemic shock, blood is often started. Intravenous infusions to replace fluid loss are also often needed. All output (urine, nasogastric, and rectal) should be measured and recorded. In the infant with rectal bleeding, the diapers can be weighed and the blood loss estimated. The general rule for measurement is 1 mg = 1 ml. If an

obstructive complication or inflammation is present, intravenous antibiotics may be ordered. In children with severe protracted bleeding, vasopressin intravenously may be ordered.[71]

Cimetidine also may be ordered to stop the bleeding before diverticulectomy is performed.[72] As with all cases of bleeding, vital signs need to be frequently monitored and the child kept on bed rest.

Because the onset is usually rapid and because there is massive bleeding, much psychologic support is needed for both the child and the parents. A calm, reassuring attitude is important for the nurse to maintain.

The child who presents with massive rectal bleeding needs to be made ready for hospitalization.

Esophageal Varices

Esophageal varices are large dilated veins in the submucosal layer of the lower esophageal wall that develop as a result of portal hypertension. This is secondary to obstruction of the portal or splenic venous blood flow. The esophageal varices of portal hypertension are usually in the distal one third of the esophagus.

Etiology. Bleeding from esophageal varices is a direct consequence of increased portal venous pressure and accounts for 5 to 8 percent of all cases of gastrointestinal bleeding in children. Increased resistance to portal flow leads to hemodynamic alterations that redirect the flow of blood away from the liver. As a result there is a reversal of venous blood flow that normally drains into the portal vein and the reopening of preexisting but nonfunctioning collateral circulation. This redirection of blood flow is responsible for the varices.

The causes of portal hypertension are varied. The most common include thrombosis, congenital malformation of the portal or splenic vein, and cirrhosis due to chronic liver disease. Portal vein thrombosis is now recognized as a complication of exchange transfusion and umbilical vein catheterization.

Clinical Presentation. Massive hematemesis is the most frequent symptom. This usually does not occur in the child younger than 5 years of age. The bleeding episodes are often precipitated by a febrile illness. Some investigators suspect that aspirin is responsible rather than the illness. Less frequent symptoms include collateral circulation over the abdomen, ascites and hepatomegaly, and splenomegaly.

History. These children may have an early neonatal history of respiratory distress, omphalitis, or exchange transfusion. There is frequently a history of anemia and growth retardation. There may have been ascites that subsided as a result of recanalization of the thrombosis.

Assessment. Examination of the child may reveal hepatomegaly and splenomegaly. If the liver is very cirrhotic, however, it is not palpable. On the abdomen the caput medusae, a ring of dilated vessels about the umbilicus, may be seen. If ascites is present, the abdomen is dull to percussion and a fluid wave can be elicited. Sigmoidoscopy will reveal internal hemorrhoids or a blue to purple coloration of the rectal mucosa.

If the child is examined after a bleed, the portal system is decompressed and the spleen is no longer palpable. Examination must be repeated after the blood volume has been restored.

Laboratory Data. Routine laboratory tests include a complete blood count, platelet count, and urinalysis. Some additional immediate laboratory studies include tests of liver function and clotting and ceruloplasmin concentration. Endoscopy is performed to visualize the site of the bleeding after the child is stabilized.

Radiologic examination using a thick barium medium can demonstrate varices in up to 80 percent of the cases. Splenoportography, visualization of the portal vein anatomy, is also used.

Differential Diagnosis. The diagnosis of esophageal varices can be made with some certainty based on visualization using endoscopy and radiologic studies. It is frequently difficult to assess the cause of the esophageal varices, however.

Management. Frequently the bleeding has stopped by the time the child reaches the hospital. The care is similar to that of a child with Meckel's diverticulum. Vital signs should be closely monitored, and serial hematocrit determinations should be made. Fresh blood is given to maintain the hematocrit between 30 and 35 percent. Small amounts of oral antacids help to coat the esophagus and to alkalinize any refluxed gastric contents. After the vital signs are stable, endoscopy is performed.

If bleeding persists or recurs after blood replacement, sedation and rest and intermittent doses of intravenous Pitressin are used. If bleeding still persists, a Sengstaken-Blakemore tube is placed in the esophagus and is inflated.

Both the child and the family need a great deal of support, since this often occurs without warning and is a frightening, life-threatening situation. The child is admitted to the hospital for diagnostic workup. The exact cause of the bleed needs to be determined and measures taken to prevent reoccurrence.

JAUNDICE

Jaundice is frequently due to diseases of the liver or biliary duct system. The most common causes of jaundice in the pediatric emergency patient are acute hepatitis and hepatic coma.

Hepatitis

Hepatitis is an inflammation of the liver. It is rapidly emerging as one of the major causes of morbidity in childhood and is a significant cause of mortality.

Etiology. Hepatitis of viral origin is caused by three or four types of virus, hepatitis A virus (HAV, infectious hepatitis) or hepatitis B virus (HBV, serum hepatitis) and one or two types of non-A and non-B viruses. While both produce similar clinical manifestations, they are distinct in their epidemiologic and immunologic characteristics.

Type A mainly affects children under 15 years of age and has an average incubation period of 25 days. The period of communicability is unknown, and the principal route of transmission is the oral-fecal route. Fetal transfer can occur from transplacental blood during the last trimester but is most commonly transmitted during delivery. It is most common in low socioeconomic groups where housing conditions are crowded. Epidemics have been attributed to poor sanitation, with shellfish providing a viral reservoir.

Type B, which affects all age groups, has an incubation period of 6 weeks to 6 months. The period of communicability is variable, and the principal route of transmission is parenteral, although fetal transfer can occur. Certain groups of people who are in contact with blood products or who require blood transfusions are especially at risk for contacting HBV, such as those children with hemophilia or leukemia or those requiring hemodialysis. In adolescents who use illicit parenteral drugs, 50 to 80 percent of acute active or prior HBV infection is found.[73]

In non-A and non-B hepatitis, no antigen or antibody has been identified, but viral particles can be seen in liver cells, and virus-like particles have been found in the circulation of apparently healthy blood donors. Infected serum may transmit the agent in 1 to 5 weeks.

In viral hepatitis pathologic changes occur in the parenchymal cells of the liver. The initial changes involve swelling and degeneration, which are followed by autolysis. This results in impaired bile excretion, elevated transaminase and alkaline phosphatase levels, and decreased albumin synthesis. The disorder is usually self-limiting, with complete regeneration of cells recurring within 2 to 3 months.

Clinical Presentation. The clinical manifestations of viral hepatitis are similar. No distinction can be made in regard to the clinical course except for the incubation period.[74] There is a rapid onset in type A, however, and a slower, more insidious onset in type B. Initially the child has nausea and vomiting, extreme anorexia, easy fatigability, and a slight to moderate fever, all flu-like symptoms. There may be abdominal pain in the epigastrum or upper right quadrant.

Following this period there is evidence of jaundice, which begins with darkening of the urine and light-colored stools and is followed by yellowing of the sclera and skin. As the jaundice worsens the child begins to feel better. The course of rising bilirubin and improved clinical signs is a good prognostic sign. Jaundice and a worsening of symptoms is a poor prognostic sign because most of these children develop fulminant or chronic, active hepatitis.

History. The history includes questioning about the flu-like symptoms of an ill child who is content to stay quiet. The family should be questioned regarding illness of other family members or friends, sanitation practices such as impure drinking water, eating shellfish from contaminated water, recent immunizations or blood transfusions, ingestion of hepatotoxic drugs, parenteral administration of illicit drugs, and sexual contact with someone who uses these drugs.

Assessment. Tender hepatomegaly may be the only important physical finding. The facial expression of the child should be observed as the liver is percussed. At times tenderness is elicited on deep inspiration that permits the liver edge to flip over the examining fingers.

Early in the course of the illness jaundice is not present, and splenomegaly may not be noted. The flu-like symptoms are the only complaints.

Laboratory Data. In the routine tests the complete blood count shows some leukopenia. The urinalysis shows proteinuria and some bilirubinuria early in the disease before jaundice is evident. A liver profile, which shows the severity of the disease, utilizes a screening panel that requires knowledge and understanding of the specificity and selectivity of the individual tests.

Common laboratory tests include sedimentation rate, which is normal with type B but elevated with type A; a serum bilirubin, which is elevated; serum transaminases (SGOT and SGPT), which are elevated; and gamma glutamyl transpeptidose (GGT), which is elevated. No one test is specific for hepatitis. The specific tests for acute viral hepatitis A and B are detection of the hepatitis A antibody (anti-HAV) and the hepatitis surface antigen (HBsAg).

Differential Diagnosis. In children, before a diagnosis of acute hepatitis can be made the following conditions need to be excluded: malformations of the bile duct, sepsis, syphilis, congenital rubella, tox-

oplasmosis, and cystic fibrosis.[75] Hepatitis may also be a manifestation of disseminated viral infections, leptospirosis, or intoxications.[76]

In infants with nonhemolytic jaundice, half will have viral hepatitis, and a quarter will have malformations of the bile duct.

Management. There is no specific treatment for viral hepatitis. Management is based on palliative treatment of symptoms. Good hand washing and proper disposal of waste materials should be used with these patients. An antiemetic drug may be ordered if vomiting is severe. Hemorrhage is a serious early complication of hepatitis and requires immediate blood replacement.

Instructions should be given to the parents regarding home care, as hospitalization is rarely necessary. There is no solid evidence that bed rest, absolute or partial, influences the rate of recovery,[77] therefore the child is allowed to regulate his or her own pace. The child is also allowed to choose the diet, within normal limits. Scrupulous hand washing after toileting and before eating is encouraged, and no drugs should be given unless prescribed because many drugs are excreted by the liver.

In most cases the child with hepatitis is not hospitalized. If the child has had severe vomiting and is dehydrated, hospitalization may be necessary to restore fluid balance.

Hepatic Coma
Hepatic coma is a condition that results from severe liver failure when the blood flow to the liver is decreased and ammonia cannot be detoxified.

Etiology. Hepatic coma occurs when the body's supply of protein, and consequently ammonia, is increased. Central nervous system dysfunction is thought to result from ammonia toxicity. The sources may be food, blood proteins, or the products that result from the breakdown of liver cells in fulminant hepatic necrosis. Other conditions precipitating hepatic coma include fluid and electrolyte imbalance, diuresis, progressive renal failure, and hypoxia. Hepatic necrosis may be drug or poison induced.

Clinical Presentation. The main clinical features are changes in the mental and neuromuscular state. A characteristic odor, fetor hepaticus, similar to the smell of feces, is evident on the breath. Hepatic coma may be divided into four stages:

- Stage I: normal level of consciousness interspersed with reduced mental alertness and periods of hypotonia;
- Stage II: drowsiness, confusion, disorientation, swings in affect and mood;
- Stage III: stupor and coma, fetor hepaticus, decerebrate posturing;
- Stage IV: no response to pain, reflexes disappear, seizures and respiratory arrest.[78]

Mortality is at least 80 percent in children reaching stage IV hepatic coma.[79]

History. Frequently the parent will have noticed behavioral changes. Questions regarding these changes, which might include lethargy and confusion, should be asked. The occurrence of previous liver diseases, such as hepatitis, should be investigated.

Assessment. The clinical features that affect the mental and neuromuscular state are not difficult to recognize. The features begin with confusion and incoordination with tremor, can progress to crying and agitation with roving eyes and muscle twitching, and can further progress to apathy and incontinence ending in coma.

The subtle changes in the respiratory pattern should be noted as an indicator of deepening coma. An increase in the effort of breathing is characterized by deeper inspirations and a more obvious phase of expiration. Fetor hepaticus is the most specific clinical sign of hepatic encephalopathy and occurs in stage III.

Laboratory Data. The specific laboratory tests for hepatic coma include a blood analysis of ammonia concentration, which is significantly elevated; blood urea nitrogen, which is initially low since urea is not formed by the liver and becomes elevated as renal function deteriorates; an elevated blood pH; and electrolyte disturbances. In pre-coma stages, an electroencephalogram, which shows slower brain wave activity, may be a useful diagnostic tool. The specific laboratory tests and history can provide a definite diagnosis of hepatic coma. It may be difficult, however, to identify the cause.

Management. There is no evidence that any treatment so far employed aids the underlying liver disease. Attempts are thus made to reduce the levels of circulating toxins that can benefit the brain. In the previously well child in whom a drug- or poison-induced hepatic necrosis is suspected as the cause, heroic measures are justified. Fluids are started, and there is a correction of deranged clotting factors with fresh frozen plasma. Frequent neurologic assessments and vital signs are performed and recorded. Endotracheal intubation and assisted ventilation may be necessary. Arterial and jugular lines are placed for frequent sampling of blood gases. Antibiotics and steroids may be ordered. Heroic measures can include two-volume blood exchange, peritoneal dialysis, hemodialysis, total body washout with hypothermia, hyperbaric oxygenation, and liver transplantation, among others.[80]

The child with a diagnosis of hepatic coma will be hospitalized.

ABDOMINAL TRAUMA

Abdominal trauma results from injury to the abdominal area caused by some type of force. In children between 5 and 14 years of age, accidental injuries are responsible for over 50 percent of the deaths in boys and for nearly 40 percent of the deaths in girls.[81] Over 90 percent of abdominal injuries in childhood are caused by blunt trauma. The spleen, genitourinary tract, liver, gastrointestinal tract, and pancreas are the organs most commonly involved.

Etiology. Abdominal trauma can be the result of many causes. The trauma may be blunt, such as from a fall, or penetrating. The penetrating wounds may be caused by low velocity objects such as knives or by high velocity objects such as bullets.

The clinical presentation varies according to the extent and severity of the injury. Careful assessment based on a detailed history and physical examination will best clarify the clinical picture.

History. An accurate history is imperative. All information regarding when and how the trauma was sustained should be sought and recorded. The best sources are the child and someone who directly observed the trauma.

Assessment. Observation is most important. The type and extent of trauma may be apparent, such as in a superficial knife wound, or may not be apparent. Whatever the trauma, a baseline should be established as to the amount of pain the child has and how he responds to movement and touch. By palpation, abdominal tenderness is assessed. External signs of injury, including location, depth, and appearance, need to be noted. The abdominal configuration, which may be distended, scaphoid, or show lumbar lordosis, needs to be assessed. Persistent abdominal tenderness is the most consistent sign of an abdominal visceral injury. If there are signs of hypovolemic shock, the diagnosis of ruptured spleen, liver, or kidney is readily apparent. Splenic injury may present with persistent tachycardia or unexplained pallor. The diagnosis of abdominal injury is usually impossible at a single assessment, and close observations and recordings of the changes in a child's condition are as important as initial findings.

Important physical signs of serious injury are shock, pain, abdominal distention, and abdominal rigidity. Respiratory, cardiovascular, and neurologic assessments should be made.

Laboratory Data. A complete blood count and urinalysis are done routinely. Serial hematocrits may be done in cases of overt or suspected bleeding. A serum amylase, which will be elevated, should be done in all cases of suspected visceral injury. If the urinalysis shows hematuria, intravenous pyelography is done. Routine erect and supine x-rays of the abdomen are done. If the child's condition makes an erect view impossible, a lateral decubitus is ordered.[82]

Management. The extent and severity of injuries in abdominal trauma need to be diagnosed. In some cases this is very difficult. If there are respiratory, cardiovascular, and neurologic complications, these need to be addressed initially. (See Chapters 6, 10, and 15 for specific care.) A surgical consult is often routinely made in cases of abdominal trauma as surgery may be necessary. Vital signs are taken at once and frequently thereafter and are recorded. A nasogastric tube is inserted, and the gastric aspirate is tested for bile and blood. Peritoneal lavage may be done if the hematocrit is falling and no source of bleeding is found. An intravenous infusion is begun, and fluids or blood may be started.

Aspiration of peritoneal fluid may be done if there is not a clear reason for a laparotomy. A cannula is inserted, and fluid is aspirated to determine if there is the presence of blood or intestinal contents in the peritoneal cavity.

Frequently surgery is necessary. The child and parents are told what is needed and are reassured that everything possible will be done. Most children with abdominal trauma are hospitalized, since there may be slow, insidious bleeding such as in trauma of the spleen. If the child appears to be doing well and lives within a reasonable distance from the hospital, a decision may be made for discharge with instructions to the parents about the signs and symptoms the child must be observed for and what actions they should take.

NOTES

1. J. Gyrboski, & W.A. Walker. *Gastrointestinal Problems in the Infant* (2nd ed.). Philadelphia: W.B. Saunders, 1983.
2. C.C. Roy, C.L. Morin, & A.M. Weber. Gastrointestinal emergency problems in paediatric practice. *Clinics in Gastroenterology* 10, no. 1(January 1981):225–254.
3. R.B. Crossley. Hospital admissions for abdominal pain in childhood. *Journal of the Royal Society of Medicine* 75, no. 10(October 1982):772–776.
4. G.R. Schwartz, P. Safar, J.H. Stone, P.B. Storey, & D.K. Wagner. *Principles and Practice of Emergency Medicine*, vol. 2. Philadelphia: W.B. Saunders, 1978.
5. D.H. Wilson. The acute abdomen in the accident and emergency department. *The Practitioner* 222(April 1979):480–485.
6. Schwartz, Safar, and Stone, *Principles and Practice of Emergency Medicine*, p. 986.
7. J.A. Black, *Paediatric Emergencies*. London: Butterworths, 1979.
8. Ibid, p. 377.
9. Schwartz, Safar, and Stone, *Principles and Practice of Emergency Medicine*.
10. Ibid., p. 1007.
11. J.J. Buchino. Recognition and management of child abuse by the surgical pathologist. *Archives of Pathology and Laboratory Medicine* 107, no. 4(April 1983):204–205.
12. B. Siegal, E. Hyman, E. Lahat, & U. Oland. Acute appendicitis in early childhood. *Helvetica Paediatrica Acta* 37, no. 3(June 1982):215–219.
13. H.W. Nase, P.J. Kovalcik, & G.H. Cross. The diagnosis of appendicitis. *American Surgeon* 46, no. 9(September 1980):504–507.
14. E.A. Franken. *Gastrointestinal Imaging in Pediatrics* (2nd ed.). Philadelphia: Harper and Row, 1982.
15. N.V. Doraiswamy. Progress of acute appendicitis: A study in children. *British Journal of Surgery* 65, no. 12(December 1978):877–879.
16. Nase, Kovalcik, & Cross, The diagnosis of appendicitis, pp. 504–507.
17. Ibid.
18. V.C. Vaughn, & R.J. Mckay. *Nelson Textbook of Pediatrics*. Philadelphia: W.B. Saunders, 1979, p. 14.
19. N.V. Doraiswamy. Leukocyte counts in the diagnosis and prognosis of acute appendicitis in children. *British Journal of Surgery* 66, no. 11(November 1979):782–784.
20. Nase, Kovalcik, & Cross, The diagnosis of appendicitis, pp. 504–507.
21. R.J. Bower, M.J. Bell, & J.L. Ternberg. Diagnostic value of the white blood count and neutrophil percentage in the evaluation of abdominal pain in children. *Surgery, Gynecology and Obstetrics* 152, no. 4(April 1981):424–426.
22. S.A. Cohen. *Pediatric Emergency Management: Guidelines for Rapid Diagnosis and Therapy*. Bowie, Md.: Robert J. Brady, 1982.

23. Franken, *Gastrointestinal Imaging in Pediatrics*.
24. E.I. Hatch Jr., D. Naffis, & N.W. Chandler. Pitfalls in the use of barium enema in early appendicitis in children. *Journal of Pediatric Surgery* 16, no. 3(June 1981):309–312.
25. Franken, *Gastrointestinal Imaging in Pediatrics*.
26. Hatch, Naffis, & Chandler, Pitfalls in the use of barium enema, pp. 309–312.
27. Roy, Morin, & Weber, Gastrointestinal emergency problems in paediatric practice, pp. 225–254.
28. J.S. Janik, & H.V. Firor. Pediatric appendicitis—a 20 year study of 1,640 children at Cook County (Illinois) Hospital. *Archives of Surgery* 114, no. 6(June 1979):717–719.
29. Schwartz, Safar, & Stone, *Principles and Practice of Emergency Medicine*.
30. A. Silverman, & C. Roy. *Pediatric Clinical Gastroenterology*. St. Louis: Mosby, 1983.
31. Grybosky, & Walker, *Gastrointestinal Problems in the Infant*.
32. Ibid.
33. Ibid.
34. D.A.J. Tyrrell, & A.Z. Kapikan. *Virus Infections of the Gastrointestinal Tract*. New York: Marcel Dekker, 1982.
35. B. Hoyle, M. Yunus, & L.C. Chen. Breast feeding and food intake among children with acute diarrheal disease. *American Journal of Clinical Nutrition* 33, no. 11(November 1980):2365–2371.
36. I. Zahavi, E.A. Shaffer, & D.G. Gall. Child abuse with laxatives. *CMA Journal* 127(September 15, 1982):512–513.
37. H.W. Davis. Acute gastroenteritis and dehydration. *Protocols of Children's Hospital of Pittsburgh*. Unpublished, Children's Hospital of Pittsburgh, 1982.
38. L. Rees, & C.O. Brook. Gradual reintroduction of full-strength milk after acute gastroenteritis in children. *Lancet* 1, no. 8119(April 7, 1979):770–771.
39. D. Pizarro, G. Posada, E. Mohs, M.M. Levine, & D.R. Nalin. Evaluation of oral therapy for infant diarrhea in an emergency room setting: The acute episode as an opportunity for instructing mothers in home treatment. *Bulletin of the World Health Organization* 57, no. 6(1979):983–986.
40. Gryboski, & Walker, *Gastrointestinal Problems in the Infant*.
41. Ibid.
42. Silverman, & Roy, *Pediatric Clinical Gastroenterology*.
43. Ibid.
44. Ibid.
45. Gryboski, & Walker, *Gastrointestinal Problems in the Infant*.
46. Ibid.
47. Silverman, & Roy, *Pediatric Clinical Gastroenterology*.
48. C.M. Anderson, & V. Burke. *Paediatric Gastroenterology*. Oxford, England: Blackwell Scientific, 1975.
49. L.F. Whaley, & D.L. Wong. *Nursing Care of Infants and Children* (2nd ed.). St. Louis: Mosby, 1983.
50. Anderson, & Burke, *Paediatric Gastroenterology*.
51. M. Weissbluth. Gastrointestinal reflux. *Clinical Pediatrics* 20, no. 1(1981):7–14.
52. Silverman, & Roy, *Pediatric Clinical Gastroenterology*.
53. D.K. Wagner. Intussusception. *Emergency Medicine—a Clinical Approach to Challenging Problems*. Philadelphia: F.A. Davis, 1982.
54. Silverman, & Roy, *Pediatric Clinical Gastroenterology*.
55. J.N.H. Du. Ten years experience in the management of intussusception in infants and children by hydrostatic reduction. *Canadian Medical Association Journal* 119(November 4, 1978):1075–1076.
56. Gryboski, & Walker, *Gastrointestinal Problems in the Infant*.
57. Silverman, & Roy, *Pediatric Clinical Gastroenterology*.
58. Franken, *Gastrointestinal Imaging in Pediatrics*.
59. N.R. Fein, Foreign bodies in the esophagus and gastrointestinal tract. In R.M. Reece (Ed.), *Manual of Emergency Pediatrics* (3rd ed.). Philadelphia: W.B. Saunders, 1984, p. 436.
60. Gryboski, & Walker, *Gastrointestional Problems in the Infant*.
61. Franken, *Gastrointestinal Imaging in Pediatrics*.
62. Silverman, & Roy, *Pediatric Clinical Gastroenterology*.

63. Franken, *Gastrointestinal Imaging in Pediatrics.*
64. Ibid.
65. Silverman, & Roy, *Pediatric Clinical Gastroenterology.*
66. Gryboski, & Walker, *Gastrointestinal Problems in the Infant.*
67. Silverman, & Roy, *Pediatric Clinical Gastroenterology.*
68. Ibid.
69. Franken, *Gastrointestinal Imaging in Pediatrics.*
70. Roy, Morin, & Weber, *Gastrointestinal Emergency Problems in Paediatric Practice*, pp. 225–254.
71. Ibid.
72. Silverman, & Roy, *Pediatric Clinical Gastroenterology.*
73. Ibid.
74. Gryboski, & Walker, *Gastrointestinal Problems in the Infant.*
75. Ibid.
76. R. Karasic. Hepatitis. In R.M. Reece (Ed.), *Manual of Emergency Pediatrics* (3rd ed.). Philadelphia: W.B. Saunders, 1984, pp. 488–491.
77. Silverman, & Roy, *Pediatric Clinical Gastroenterology.*
78. Ibid.
79. Ibid.
80. Ibid.
81. Black, *Paediatric Emergencies.*
82. C.M. Illingsworth. *The Diagnosis and Primary Care of Accidents and Emergencies in Children* (2nd ed.). Oxford, England: Blackwell Scientific, 1982.

BIBLIOGRAPHY

Anne, I., & Derom, F. Portal derivation surgery in children—a long term follow-up report. *Acta Chirurgica Belgica* 82, no. 1(January-February 1983):67–71.

Anderson, C.M., & Burke, V. *Paediatric Gastroenterology.* Oxford, England: Blackwell Scientific, 1975.

Bates, B. *A Guide to Physical Examination* (2nd ed.). Philadelphia: Lippincott, 1979.

Black, J.A. *Paediatric Emergencies.* London: Butterworths, 1979.

Block, G.J., Nolan, J.W., & Dempsey, M.K. *Health Assessment for Professional Nursing—A Developmental Approach.* New York: Appleton-Century-Crofts, 1981.

Bower, R.J., Bell, M.J., & Ternberg, J.L. Diagnostic value of the white blood count and neutrophil percentage in the evaluation of abdominal pain in children. *Surgery, Gynecology and Obstetrics* 152, no. 4(April 1981):424–426.

Buchino, J.J. Recognition and management of child abuse by the surgical pathologist. *Archives of Pathology and Laboratory Medicine* 107, no. 4(April 1983):204–205.

Cohen, S.A. *Pediatric Emergency Management: Guidelines for Rapid Diagnosis and Therapy.* Bowie, Md.: Robert J. Brady, 1982.

Crossley, R.B. Hospital admissions for abdominal pain in childhood. *Journal of the Royal Society of Medicine* 75, no. 10(October 1982):772–776.

Davis, H.W. Acute gastroenteritis and dehydration. *Protocols of Children's Hospital of Pittsburgh.* Unpublished, Children's Hospital of Pittsburgh, 1982.

Doraiswamy, N.V. Leukocyte counts in the diagnosis and prognosis of acute appendicitis in children. *British Journal of Surgery* 66, no. 11(November 1979):782–784.

Doraiswamy, N.V. Progress of acute appendicitis: A study in children. *British Journal of Surgery* 65, no. 12(December 1978):877–879.

Du, J.N.H. Ten years experience in the management of intussusception in infants and children by hydrostatic reduction. *Canadian Medical Association Journal* 119, (November 4, 1978):1075–1076.

Dube, S., & Pierog, S. *Immediate Care of the Sick and Injured Child.* St. Louis: Mosby, 1978.

Franken, E.A. *Gastrointestinal Imaging in Pediatrics* (2nd ed.). Philadelphia: Harper and Row, 1982.

Graham, J.M., Pokorny, W.J., & Harberg, F.J. Acute appendicitis in preschool age children. *American Journal of Surgery* 139, no. 2(February 1980):247–250.

Grant, A.K., Skyring, A., & Conn, H.D. *Clinical Diagnosis of Gastrointestinal Disease.* Oxford, England: Blackwell Scientific, 1981.

Gryboski, J., & Walker, W.A. *Gastrointestinal Problems in the Infant* (2nd ed.). Philadelphia: W.B. Saunders, 1983.

Hatch, E.I., Jr., Naffis, D., & Chandler, N.W. Pitfalls in the use of barium enema in early appendicitis in children. *Journal of Pediatric Surgery* 16, no. 3(June 1981):309–312.

Hirschhorn, N. The treatment of acute diarrhea in children—an historical and physiological perspective. *American Journal of Clinical Nutrition* 33, no. 3(March 1980):637–663 (review).

Hoyle, B., Yunus, M., & Chen, L.C. Breast feeding and food intake among children with acute diarrheal disease. *American Journal of Clinical Nutrition* 33, no. 11(November 1980):2365–2371.

Illingsworth, C.M. *The Diagnosis and Primary Care of Accidents and Emergencies in Children* (2nd ed.). Oxford, England: Blackwell Scientific, 1982.

Janik, J.S., & Firor, H.V. Pediatric appendicitis—a 20 year study of 1,640 children at Cook County (Illinois) Hospital. *Archives of Surgery* 114, no. 6(June 1979):717–719.

Joseph, N.H. Ten years' experience in the management of intussusception in infants and children by hydrostatis reduction. *Canadian Medical Association Journal* 119, (November 4, 1978):1075–1076.

Malasnos, L., Barkauskas, V., Moss, M., & Stoltenberg-Allen, K. *Health Assessment* (2nd ed.). St. Louis: Mosby, 1981.

Nase, H.W., Kovalcik, P.J., & Cross, G.H. The diagnosis of appendicitis. *American Surgeon* 46, no. 9(September 1980):504–507.

Pantell, R.H., & Irwin, C.E. Appendectomies during physicians' boycott—analysis of surgical care. *Journal of the American Medical Association* 242, no. 15(October 12, 1979):1627–1630.

Persson, B., Feychting, H., Josephson, S., et al. Rehydration using solutions with and without glucose before emergency abdominal surgery in children. *Acta Anaesthesiologica Scandinavica* 27, no. 1(February 1983):35–38.

Pizarro, D., Posada, G., Mohs, E., et al. Evaluation of oral therapy for infant diarrhea in an emergency room setting: The acute episode as an opportunity for instructing mothers in home treatment. *Bulletin of the World Health Organization* 57, no. 6(1979):983–986.

Pringle, K.C., Reyes, H.M., & Bennett, E.J. Preoperative and postoperative care of the pediatric surgical patient. *Critical Care Medicine* 8, no. 10(October 1980):554–558.

Pullan, C.R., Halse, P.C., & Sims, D.G., et al. Viruses and acute abdominal pain in childhood. *Archives of Disease in Childhood* 54, no. 10(October 1979):780–782.

Reece, R.M. (Ed.). *Reece-Chamberlain Manual of Emergency Pediatrics* (2nd ed.). Philadelphia: W.B. Saunders, 1978.

Rees, L., & Brook, C.O. Gradual reintroduction of full-strength milk after acute gastroenteritis in children. *Lancet* 1, no. 8119(April 7, 1979):770–771.

Roy, C.C., Morin, C.L., & Weber, A.M. Gastrointestinal emergency problems in paediatric practice. *Clinics in Gastroenterology* 10, no. 1(January 1981):225–254.

Rumi, G., Solt, I., Patty, I., & Hamori, A. Interhospital mobile oesophago-gastro-bulboscopy emergency service. *Acta Medica Academiae Scientiarum Hungaricae* 37, no. 3(1980):299–304.

Schwartz, G.R., Safar, P., Stone, J.H., et al. *Principles and Practice of Emergency Medicine*, vol. 2. Philadelphia: W. B. Saunders, 1978.

Siegal, B., Hyman, E., Lahat, E., & Oland, U. Acute appendicitis in early childhood. *Helvetica Paediatrica Acta* 37, no. 3(June 1982):215–219.

Silverman, A., & Roy, C. *Pediatric Clinical Gastroenterology*. St. Louis: Mosby, 1983.

Swadia, N.D., Thakore, A.B., Patel, B.R., & Bhavani, S.S. Unusual form of child abuse presenting as an acute abdomen. *British Journal of Surgery* 68, no. 9(September 1981):668.

Touloukian, R.J., & Krizek, T.J. *Diagnosis and Early Management of Trauma Emergencies: a Manual for the Emergency Service*. Springfield, Ill.: Charles C. Thomas, 1974.

Tyrrell, D.A.J., & Kapikan, A.Z. *Virus Infections of the Gastrointestinal Tract*. New York: Marcel Dekker, 1982.

Wagner, D.K. Intussusception. In *Emergency Medicine—a Clinical Approach to Challenging Problems*. Philadelphia: F.A. Davis, 1982.

Warner, C.G. *Emergency Care—Assessment and Intervention* (3rd ed.). St. Louis: Mosby, 1983.

Whaley, L.F., & Wong, D.L. *Nursing Care of In-*

fants and Children (2nd ed.). St. Louis: Mosby, 1983.

Weissbluth, M. Gastrointestinal reflux. *Clinical Pediatrics* 20, no. 1(1981):7–14.

Wilson, D.H. The acute abdomen in the accident and emergency department. *The Prac-titioner* 222(April 1979):480–485.

Zahavi, I., Shaffer, E.A., & Gall, D.G. Child abuse with laxatives. *CMA Journal* 127(September 15, 1982):512–513.

Zorab, J., & Baskett, P. *Immediate Care.* London: W.B. Saunders, 1977.

EMERGENCY DEPARTMENT CARE GUIDE FOR THE CHILD WITH A GASTROINTESTINAL EMERGENCY

Nursing Diagnosis	Interventions	Evaluation
Alteration in bowel elimination related to gastrointestinal disorder	Assess child's pattern of bowel elimination Continually assess bowel sounds Administer medications as indicated	Child's patterns of bowel elimination return to normal
Potential for infection related to bowel inflammation/obstruction	Assess for signs of localized or systemic infection Administer antibiotics as ordered	Child's infection is adequately treated
Knowledge deficit (parental) of child's condition and treatment	Explain all procedures and treatments to parents Teach parents medication administration and fever control if child is to be discharged home	Parents demonstrate knowledge of child's illness and its treatment
Alteration in gastrointestinal tissue perfusion related to obstruction or inflammation	Carefully monitor vital signs Obtain necessary laboratory specimens Administer medications as ordered Prepare child for surgery Restrict child from oral ingestion	Vital signs remain stable Medications are administered Child is prepared for surgery
Fluid volume deficit related to gastrointestinal disorder	Assess child's hydration status Administer intravenous fluids Carefully measure fluid intake and output	Child remains adequately hydrated Urinary output remains adequate (>1 ml/kg/hr)
Alteration in comfort: pain related to child's gastrointestinal disorder	Assess child's level of pain Administer analgesics as ordered Limit child's level of activity	Child describes a decrease in discomfort

(Continued)

Nursing Diagnosis	Interventions	Evaluation
Fear related to painful procedures and emergency department environment	Carefully explain all procedures to child Allow parents to remain with child as much as possible	Child remains calm and cooperative Child is comforted by parents' presence

19

Endocrine Emergencies

Susan J. Kelley
Carole T. Roberts

Diabetes Mellitus

The hormone insulin is involved in the processes of glucose transport, storage and synthesis of lipids, and protein synthesis. Diabetes mellitus (DM) results from an absolute or functional deficiency of insulin and is thus a disorder of energy metabolism. DM is a common disorder of children and adolescents, affecting one out of every 500 to 800 children under 21 years of age.[1]

DM is classified as type 1 (juvenile onset, insulin dependent) and type II (maturity onset, usually noninsulin dependent). Most children with DM have the type I disorder. The term "maturity" refers to diabetes that exhibits itself during adulthood. In cases where the physiologic characteristics of type II diabetes manifest themselves in a child or adolescent, the term MODY (maturity-onset diabetes of youth) is applied.[2]

Type I and type II have very different manifestations, they differ in genetic composition and medical management.[3] As such it is not possible for a young child's type I diabetes to later convert to the adult type II diabetes; likewise the child's elderly relative's type II diabetes is probably unrelated to the child's type I diabetes.

In DM the primary concern is the cells' ability to obtain glucose from the blood stream. Insulin, natural or synthetic must be available to help in the transport of glucose to the cells. For the child and adolescent, demands for insulin vary greatly, as their physical growth and emotional development change frequently until adulthood. This places the child and adolescent at increased risk for developing an imbalance in insulin/glucose need. They are at increased risk of developing hypoglycemia or hyperglycemia along with their potentially severe ramifications.

Diabetic Ketoacidosis

Diabetic ketoacidosis (DKA) is a physiologic state characterized by hyperglycemia, fluid loss, electrolyte derangements, and acid-base imbalances. In DKA, insulin normally involved in the processes of glucose transport, storage and synthesis of lipids, and synthesis of protein is deficient. As a result glucose and ketones (acids) accumulate within the blood stream. It is the secondary physiologic changes resulting from this initial hyperglycemia and acidosis that threaten the individual's level of consciousness. The diabetic child's increased susceptibility to infection and altered glucose metabolism place him or her at particular risk for developing DKA.

Ketoacidosis may be present in up to 30 percent of newly diagnosed juvenile-onset (type I) diabetics and accounts for 65 percent of all hospital admissions of diabetics under 19 years of age. The mortality rate for children with ketoacidosis is just under 3 percent.[4] DKA, then, is a life-threatening complication of diabetes that demands prompt intervention to achieve a favorable outcome.

Etiology and Pathophysiology. DKA may result from either a situation in which the body's demand for insulin is greater than normal or in which the presence of insulin (natural or synthetic) is lacking. Insulin deficiency can occur in the diabetic patient who is building up resistance to insulin, in a patient who omits his or her insulin dose or fails to take the prescribed dose, or in one who is noncompliant with the dietary plan and increases food intake.[5] Infection is the most common precipitating factor, but trauma, pregnancy, poor diabetic control, certain drugs, emotional stresses such as menstruation, and surgery may also initiate this state.[6]

Hyperglycemia develops primarily from a lack of insulin but may be aided by increased levels of counterregulatory hormones, such as glucagon, cortisol, growth hormone, and catecholamines. Osmotic diuresis occurs as the serum osmolality rises from increasing levels of glucose in the blood. Fluid is pulled from surrounding tissues and is excreted in large quantities. This results in dehydration and electrolyte loss. In the untreated patient hyperosmolality and brain cell dehydration are the main causes of obtundation.[7]

Since insulin deficiency leaves glucose unattainable as a source of energy, protein and fat are broken down to meet the body's demands. Free fatty acids from adipose tissue are released and converted into ketoacids in the liver. These strong acids readily dissociate, producing free hydrogen ions. The result is a metabolic acidosis for which the body tries to compensate by hyperventilation, hence lowering the P_{CO_2} and plasma bicarbonate. The hyperventilation of the child with DKA is referred to as "Kussmaul's" breathing. The characteristic fruity breath of the child with ketoacidosis results from the presence of acetone in the body.

To make matters worse, hepatic glucose production is triggered by this anorexic state, which serves to aggravate the preexisting hyperglycemia. Patients with DKA have a serum glucose in the range of 200 to 300 mg/dl, although significant hyperglycemia of greater than 500 mg/dl is common.[8] Other significant findings include ketonemia at a level greater than 1:2 dilution of the serum, a venous pH less than 7.3, a bicarbonate level less than or equal to 15 mEq/L, a slightly elevated blood urea nitrogen, glycosuria, ketonuria and leukocytosis.[9] The total white blood cell count may be elevated to 18,000 to 20,000/mm in spite of the absence of infection, due to the increase in circulating catecholamines.[10] In DKA, then, there is acidosis with a low serum bicarbonate and pH, the decrease reflecting the severity of the condition.

The primary electrolytes of concern in the patient with DKA are sodium and potassium. Hyponatremia results from increased urinary excretion of sodium. Since serum sodium is calculated relative to both the shifts in water to the extracellular space (Na decreases 1.6 mEq/L per 100 mg/dl rise in glucose) and the increased lipid and protein in the serum, it is important to remember that the true serum sodium value is usually higher than the measured sodium value given by the laboratory report.[11]

On the other hand, although the serum concentration of potassium may be reported as within normal limits, in DKA there is total body potassium deficit. The results may appear normal because serum potassium tends to increase by 0.5 mEq/L for each 0.1 decrease in pH.[12] Potassium is depleted by several mechanisms. (1) Acidosis and extracellular dehydration bring about transcellular shifts of this ion. (2) Protein catabolism secondary to anorexia causes negative nitrogen balance and additional efflux of potassium from cells. (3) Volume depletion causes secondary hyperaldosteronism, which further promotes urinary potassium excretion.[13]

The individual's level of consciousness is affected by the progressive dehydration, hyperosmolality, acidosis, and diminished cerebral oxygen utilization. Electrolyte imbalances increase the risk of cardiac arrest.

History. On admittance to the emergency department children may complain of abdominal pain, nausea, or vomiting. Parents may describe a history of polydipsia, polyuria, nocturia, enuresis, and, with the new onset diabetic, recent weight loss. It is important to determine what precipitated this disruption. The nurse should gather information such as the type and amount of the child's last meal, time and amount of last insulin dose, time and level of recent activities, allergies, recent symptoms of infection, and present developmental or maturational crises. The nurse should also take note of all other medications the child may be taking, since certain medications such as phenobarbital and steroids affect insulin requirements. In cases where the diagnosis of DKA is questionable, it is also helpful to explore the probability of salicylate ingestion.[14] Table 19–1 summarizes the differential diagnosis of DKA.

Laboratory Data. Laboratory data collected in the emergency department serve to assess the degree of metabolic imbalance present in the child. Initial blood tests should include serum glucose, serum electrolytes, complete blood count, osmolality, arterial pH, (ABG), and toxicology screen. Dextrostix may be performed for rapid gross approximation of blood glucose levels. Urine should be sent to the laboratory for culture and sensitivity as well as for measurement of glucose and acetone lev-

TABLE 19–1. DIFFERENTIAL DIAGNOSIS OF DIABETIC KETOACIDOSIS

Metabolic Acidosis	*Polyuria, Nocturia, Abdominal Pain*
Severe gastroenteritis with hypovolemia	Urinary tract infection
Salicylate poisoning	*Hyperglycemia*
Other ingestions	Salicylate poisoning
Ethanol	(hyperglycemia
Methanol	is moderate,
Ethylene glycol	<300 mg/dl)
Phenformin	Hypernatremia
Isoniazid	Stress
Iron	Sepsis
Coma	*Ketonuria*
Hypoglycemia	Fasting states
Sedative hypnotic or narcotic overdose	Gastroenteritis with vomiting
Lactic acidosis	Anorexia of any etiology
Nonketotic hyperosmolar coma	Salicylate poisoning
Central nervous system trauma, infection, bleeding	

Reproduced with permission from E. Crain, & J. Gersher. A Clinical Manual of Emergency Pediatrics. Norwalk, Conn.: Appleton-Century-Crofts, 1986.

els. Blood and urine cultures should be obtained to rule out infection.

Assessment. Assessment of airway, breathing, and circulation (ABCs) are the first priorities of the emergency nurse. These will vary depending upon the level of consciousness of the child. Increased levels of CO_2 in the blood stream have adverse effects on the individual's level of consciousness. The body attempts to compensate for this increase by changing the depth and rate of the individual's respirations. In DKA, then, a child may arrive in the emergency department with characteristic Kussmaul's respirations (deep, rapid, "air hunger" respirations) as the body tries to rid itself of excess CO_2, or the child's respirations may be depressed if the patient is severely acidotic (pH less than 6.90).[15] The odor of the breath should be assessed for the presence of acetone.

Circulatory status is best assessed by measuring the quality and pulse rate, moistness of mucous membranes, blood pressure, and urinary output. The child should be placed on a cardiac monitor and a stat electrocardiogram (ECG) obtained.

Management. Along with securing an open airway and supporting ventilation as necessary, the initial management objective is to restore circulatory volume and to improve perfusion. Pediatric patients should be considered to be 10 percent dehydrated and should be given an initial bolus of 20 cc/kg of normal saline (NS; no glucose or potassium) over 30 minutes.[16] The initial fluid bolus may lead to considerable improvement in serum glucose, osmolality, and pH, so these tests should be repeated every hour, and an ECG obtained before changing the intravenous therapy. The child's blood pressure, pulse and respiratory rates, urine output, and mental status should be assessed frequently.[17] The type of solution used after the initial bolus is based on the results from the laboratory data as well as the results of continued physical assessment of the child. The child's vital signs, neurologic status, urine output, serum osmolality, and sodium, in particular, are evaluated to determine the type of solution that will be used to restore fluid balance. Nursing flow sheets are helpful in organizing all of this data for easy reference.

Potassium may be added to the intravenous solution once the initial bolus has infused, the patient has voided, and it has been determined that the T waves on the ECG are not peaked. Forty milliequivalents of potassium (one half as potassium acetate and one half as potassium phosphate) may be added to each liter of hydrating solution. Patients with severe hypokalemia, however, (potassium less than 3.5 mEq/L) may need as much as 80 mEq/L.[18]

In patients whose serum glucose is greater than 600 mg/dl or in the acidotic patient (pH less than 7.25), a continuous insulin infusion may be started. Special considerations should be taken when infusing insulin. First, since insulin tends to bind to the intravenous tubing, a 50-cc bolus of the insulin solution should be flushed through the tubing to saturate all of the insulin-binding sites prior to connecting the intravenous tubing to the patient. Second, rapid lowering of blood glucose to 250 mg/dl and below may lead to acute cerebral edema. A rapid shift of water from the extracellular fluid to the relatively hyperosmolar brain cells is responsible for producing this cerebral edema. Frequent blood glucose levels should therefore be obtained to ensure that the glucose concentration falls at a linear rate of 75 to 100 mg/dl/hour.[19]

When the serum glucose approaches 250 mg/dl, glucose should be added to the insulin drip to prevent the occurrence of hypoglycemia. This intravenous fluid should contain about one unit of insulin for every 5 g of glucose and should be run at $1\frac{1}{2}$ times the prescribed maintenance rate. This should maintain the glucose level at a steady state. If the serum glucose level should fall too low and the patient remains acidotic, the insulin dose should not be lowered. Instead the concentration of glucose in the intravenous tubing should be increased to D7.5 percent and the rate of the intravenous drip increased to twice the maintenance rate.[20]

Psychosocial Support and Parent Education. For both the child and the family a visit to the emergency department for DKA can be a frightening experience. Younger children may be overwhelmed by the new people and unfamiliarity of the procedures that are taking place. Older children may be overtaken by the fear of what they know to be the possible consequences of DKA. Likewise each family member may feel helpless and fearful during this time of uncertainty.

The circumstances leading to the emergency department visit also play an important role in determining the feelings of the child and family members. If noncompliance was a precipitating factor, the child may feel guilty as well as fearful. Family issues occurring prior to the admission may be intensified as parents search for a cause of the changes in their child. Each parent may feel guilt over the events that are taking place. Keeping the parents informed of the patient's progress and anticipating the parents' need for comfort and privacy are the best means of support.

Education involves informing parents of the precipitating factors to DKA and teaching them to recognize early signs and symptoms of this condition. If the admission results in the diagnosis of a new type I diabetic, the parents will need to receive appropriate education specific to this illness.

Hypoglycemia

Hypoglycemia is defined as serum glucose below 20 mg/dl in the premature or low birth weight infant, below 30 mg/dl in the normal newborn, and below 40 mg/dl in older infants and children. Hypoglycemia in infants and children is most often caused by insulin overdose or decreased glucose intake in the nondiabetic. Other causes of hypoglycemia include decreased absorption secondary to diarrhea, inadequate glycogen reserves, or hyperinsulism. Hypoglycemia can also occur in association with hypothermia, Reye's syndrome, alcohol or salicylate ingestion, sepsis, hypopituitarism, and hypothyroidism. Infants are particularly vulnerable to hypoglycemia. Table 19-2 summarizes the etiologies of hypoglycemia.

Maintaining an adequate supply of serum glucose is critical for all body tissues,

TABLE 19-2. ETIOLOGIES OF HYPOGLYCEMIA

Decreased Glucose	Ingestions
Intake	Alcohol
Fasting	Salicylates
Malnutrition	Oral hypoglycemic
Malabsorption	agents
Hormone Deficiencies	Propranolol
Growth hormone	*Other Etiologies*
Cortisol	Sepsis
Glucagon	Ketotic hypoglycemia
Thyroid hormone	Islet cell adenoma
Liver Disease	
Fulminant hepatitis	
Reye's syndrome	
Glycogenoses	
(type I, III)	
Galactosemia	
Fructosemia	

Reproduced with permission from E. Crain, & J. Gersher. A Clinical Manual of Emergency Pediatrics. Norwalk, Conn.: Appleton-Century-Crofts, 1986.

especially the brain. Prompt recognition of hypoglycemia is important, since the risk of irreversible brain damage is great if the hypoglycemia is prolonged.[21]

History. Since hypoglycemia can occur in association with almost any illness in which there is an associated decrease in glucose intake, a careful history of caloric intake for the past 24 to 48 hours should be obtained in ill infants and children. The parents may give a history of irritability, fatigue, ataxia, seizure activity, or decreased level of consciousness in their child. A careful history of any possible ingestion of alcohol, aspirin products, or hypoglycemic agents should be elicited. In the previously diagnosed diabetic, a careful history of insulin dosages should be obtained.

Assessment. The child's ABCs should be assessed and vital signs carefully monitored. The hypoglycemic infant or child may have tachycardia, tachypnea, tremors, diaphoresis, decreased level of consciousness, and seizure activity. Pupil size and reactivity should be noted.

Laboratory Data. A dextrostix should be obtained immediately in all patients in whom hypoglycemia is suspected for rapid screening, followed by serum laboratory glucose values. Serum insulin levels and liver function tests may also be obtained. Urine should be obtained for glucose and ketones. Serum and urine toxic screens are obtained if the history indicates the possibility of an ingestion.

Management. The patient's ABCs should be supported as a first priority. Glucose, in the form of D25, 0.5 to 1.0 g/kg/dose is administered intravenously. D50 may be given to children over 3 years of age. If the cause of the decreased level of consciousness is hypoglycemia, the patient should respond promptly. Thereafter maintenance may be given through adequate glucose homeostasis and fluid balance by administering 10 to 20 percent glucose in 0.2 NS.[22] When concentrated glucose solutions are administered in peripheral lines, special precautions should be taken to prevent infection at the intravenous site. Most patients with hypoglycemia will be admitted to determine the etiology and to treat the underlying cause.

Psychosocial Support and Parent Education. Parents are often frightened by their child's appearance and behavior while hypoglycemic. The parents therefore will need much support while in the emergency department. All procedures and treatments should be carefully explained. Once the child's condition has been stabilized, the parents should be encouraged to remain with the child. If the child is hospitalized, the procedures for admission and visitation hours should be explained.

Diabetes Insipidus

Diabetes insipidus (DI) is a syndrome characterized by an inability to concentrate urine. DI is caused by a deficiency of antidiuretic hormone. Antidiuretic insufficiency can be caused by a variety of conditions, including tumors, basilar skull fractures, neurosurgical complications, granulomatous diseases, vascular lesions, meningitis, and encephalitis. In approximately 50 percent of cases, however, no obvious primary lesion can be found.[23]

History. Parents may describe the child as being constantly thirsty and voiding large amounts of dilute urine. There may also be a history of irritability, fever of unknown origin, failure to thrive, constipation, and enuresis.

Assessment. The child should be assessed for signs of dehydration, such as sunken eyes, poor skin turgor, and dryness of the mucous membranes. An infant with DI may have a depressed anterior fontanelle.[24] Vital signs should be carefully monitored. Tachycardia and hypotension may also indicate dehydration. Fluid intake and output should be measured and recorded. The child's level of consciousness should be carefully monitored.

Laboratory Data. Urine should be obtained for specific gravity and electrolyte analysis. Serum electrolytes and osmolality values should also be obtained. In cases of DI, serum osmolality is usually elevated (>290 mosm/kg), and serum sodium is elevated or on the high side of the normal range, in the presence of dilute urine.[25]

Management. Rehydration is usually attempted over a 48-hour period. Caution must be taken not to correct the hypernatremia too rapidly, since this may lead to cerebral edema and seizures. Isotonic fluids such as 0.9 NS may be given intravenously at about 20 ml/kg for the first hour, together with vasopressin, 0.1 ml given nasally. After the first 1 to 2 hours the intravenous infusion rate is tapered to about 1½ times maintenance, and 5 percent dextrose in 0.25 NS is substituted.[26]

The child's vital signs and level of consciousness should be continually evaluated during rehydration. In most cases of DI the child will be admitted to the hospital for further evaluation and intervention. The child and parents will need preparation for the child's admission to an inpatient unit.

Acute Adrenal Insufficiency

Acute adrenal insufficiency occurs when the adrenal cortex fails to produce enough cortisol and aldosterone. This can result in a life-threatening emergency. Prompt recognition and treatment are critical.

The most common causes of acute adrenal insufficiency include congenital adrenal hyperplasia, Addison's disease, pituitary deficiency, or brain tumor. The precipitant of a crisis may be infection, fever, trauma, or surgery. Acute adrenal insufficiency has become more common with the widespread use of suppressive doses of corticosteroids in the treatment of such diseases as the nephrotic syndrome, acute lymphoblastic leukemia, status asthmaticus, and others.[27]

History. A careful history may lead to the suspicion of acute adrenal insufficiency. The child may come to the emergency department with a history of fever, weakness, lethargy, anorexia, vomiting, nausea, diarrhea, and adbominal pain. A careful history of past or current medical conditions such as Addison's disease, central nervous system tumor, tuberculosis, or congenital adrenal hyperplasia is important to elicit. A history of recent infection,

trauma, or surgery is also significant. Any medications taken currently or in the past, especially corticosteroids, should be noted.

Assessment. The ABCs should be carefully assessed. Vital signs may reveal hypotension and tachycardia. The patient's skin turgor and mucous membranes should be inspected, since dehydration is often present. The presence of petechiae and purpura indicates overwhelming sepsis. A subtle but valuable clinical finding is increased skin pigmentation on the knees, elbows, and knuckles (areas of friction) and areas of sunlight exposure such as the face and neck. There may also be increased pigmentation in skin creases, oral mucosa, and conjunctiva. These changes are indicative of adrenocorticotropic hormone (ACTH) hypersecretion and suggest primary adrenal insufficiency.[28] The abdomen should be palpated for tenderness and auscultated for bowel sounds.

The child's level of consciousness should be carefully observed. Orientation to person, time, and place should be assessed, since some children with acute adrenal insufficiency may display mental changes or symptoms of psychosis.

Laboratory Data. A serum cortisol level should be obtained as well as a complete blood count with differential and serum electrolytes. The serum cortisol level will be low. Acute adrenal insufficiency causes hyponatremia and hyperkalemia with a decreased sodium/potassium ratio.[29] Hypoglycemia, hemoconcentration, mild metabolic acidosis, variable hypercalcemia, and eosinophilia will also be present. The urine-specific gravity should be obtained.

Management. The ABCs should be supported. An intravenous line should be inserted immediately for rapid replacement of fluid volume and sodium and steroid therapy.

Hydrocortisone, 100 mg, should be administered intravenously and then continued at a dose of 25 to 100 mg every 4 to 6 hours. Alternatively, cortisone acetate, 100 mg, can be given intramuscularly and then 25 to 100 mg repeated every 6 to 12 hours, or dexamethasone, 1 to 4 mg/day, may be administered intravenously.[30]

Intravenous isotonic saline in 5 percent dextrose is administered at 20 ml/kg in the first hour and then at a rate of 1.5 to 2.0 times normal maintenance rate until dehydration has been corrected.[31] Urinary output should be carefully measured. If the patient is unconscious a nasogastric tube should be inserted to prevent vomiting and aspiration. Vital signs should be continually monitored. A cardiac monitor should be used to identify any dysrhythmias. The patient's temperature should be carefully monitored and regulated.

Psychosocial Support and Parent Education. Both the child and the parents may be frightened by the rapid deterioration of the child's condition. All procedures and treatments should be carefully explained. Parents should be encouraged to remain with the child as much as possible while in the emergency department. Both child and parents will need to be prepared for the child's admission to the hospital.

Hyperthyroidism

Hyperthyroidism primarily affects children over 6 years of age, with a peak incidence during adolescence. It appears to affect females more than males. Etiologies of hyperthyroidism include diffuse toxic goiter (Graves' disease), thyroiditis with hyperthyroidism, thyroid adenoma, and exogenous overdosage.[32] Hypothalamic and

pituitary dysfunction are other possible causes. Thyroid storm, or thyroid crisis, is a life-threatening complication of hyperthyroidism that is rarely seen in children.[33] Thyroid storm is caused by a sudden release of thyroid hormone into the circulation.

History. A history may reveal complaints of palpitations, sweating, heat intolerance, weight loss, increased bowel movements, motor hyperactivity with tremor, nervousness, emotional lability, decreased attention span, and poor school performance.[34,35]

Assessment. The neck should be inspected for the presence of a goiter. A characteristic bruit may be heard over the thyroid.[36] Tachycardia and increased systolic blood pressure and widened pulse pressure are common. The skin should be assessed for warmth and diaphoresis. The eyes are usually protruding, with exophthalmos present. Fine tremors of the eyelids, fingers, or tongue may be observed.

Hyperthyroid storm is manifested by acute onset of fever, tachycardia, arrhythmia, decreased level of consciousness, diaphoresis, and gastrointestinal complaints, such as vomiting, abdominal pain, and jaundice.

Laboratory Data. Thyroid function tests are obtained as well as a complete blood count and serum electrolytes. An ECG and chest radiograph are also obtained.

Management

Hyperthyroidism. Oral antithyroid medication, propylthiouracil, 5 to 10 mg/kg/day divided every 8 hours, is prescribed. Patients in a hypermetabolic state are treated with propranolol, 1 to 2 mg/kg/day divided every 6 to 8 hours, by mouth.[37]

Thyroid Storm. If the patient is in thyroid storm, propranolol is given, 0.1 mg/kg/day intravenously. Frequent vital signs and ECG monitoring are important during and after administration. Iodine (Lugol solution, 10 drops three times a day orally) and propylthiouracil (in an initial loading dose of 600 to 1200 mg/day divided every 8 hours) are also administered.[38]

Hyperthermia should be treated with acetaminophen, sponge baths, and, when necessary, cooling blankets.

Dehydration should be treated with intravenous fluid administration. Electrolyte deficits should be replaced. Fluid intake and output should be carefully monitored. Urine-specific gravity should be obtained.

Psychosocial Support and Parent Education. The child and parents may be very frightened by the child's appearance (exophthalmos) and unstable condition and will need much support while in the emergency department. All procedures and treatments should be carefully explained. Parents should be allowed to remain at the child's bedside as much as possible without intervening in lifesaving procedures. Children in thyroid storm will be admitted to the hospital; therefore the child and family will need preparation for admission.

NOTES

1. B. Giordano. The child with altered secretion of insulin. In S.R. Mott, N.F. Fazekas, & S.R. James (Eds.). *Nursing Care of Children and Families*. Menlo Park, Calif.: Addison-Wesley, 1985, p. 1428.
2. Ibid., p. 1429.
3. Ibid.
4. K.R. Lyen, D. Hale, & L. Baker. Endocrine emergencies. In G. Fleisher, & S. Ludwig (Eds.). *Textbook of Pediatric Emergency Medicine*. Baltimore: Williams & Wilkins, 1983, p. 632.
5. C. O'Boyle, D.K. Davis, B.A. Russo, & T.J. Kraf. Disorders of glucose metabolism. In *Emergency Care: The First 24 Hours*. Norwalk, Conn.: Appleton-Century-Crofts, 1985, p. 362.
6. E.F. Crain, & J.C. Gershel, Eds. Diabetic ketoacidosis. In *Clinical Manual of Emergency Pediatrics*. Norwalk, Conn.: Appleton-Century-Crofts, 1986, p. 136.
7. H.I. Hochman. Diabetic ketoacidosis. In R.M. Reece (Ed.), *Manual of Emergency Pediatrics* (3rd ed.). Philadelphia: W.B. Saunders, 1984, p. 101.
8. Crain, & Gershel, Diabetic ketoacidosis, p. 137.
9. Lyen, Hale, & Baker, Endocrine emergencies, p. 635.
10. Crain, & Gershel, Diabetic ketoacidosis, p. 137.
11. Ibid., p. 136.
12. R.M. Barkin, & P. Rosen, Eds. Endocrine disorders. In *Emergency Pediatrics*. St. Louis: Mosby, 1984, p. 500.
13. Lyen, Hale, & Baker, Endocrine emergencies, p. 632.
14. Crain, & Gershel, Diabetic ketoacidosis, p. 138.
15. Ibid., p. 136.
16. Ibid., p. 138.
17. Hochman, Diabetic ketoacidosis, p. 101.
18. Crain, & Gershel, Diabetic ketoacidosis, p. 138.
19. Ibid., p. 139.
20. Ibid., p. 138.
21. Lyen, Hale, & Baker, Endocrine emergencies, p. 639.
22. Hochman, Hypoglycermia, p. 18.
23. Crain, & Gershel, Endocrine emergencies, p. 134.
24. Lyen, Hale, & Baker, Endocrine emergencies, p. 646.
25. Ibid.
26. Ibid.
27. Ibid., p. 640.
28. Crain, & Gershel, Endocrine emergencies, pp. 131–132.
29. Ibid., p. 132.

30. Lyen, Hale, & Baker, Endocrine emergencies, p. 641.
31. Ibid.
32. Crain, & Gershel, Hyperthyroidism, p. 141.
33. Ibid.
34. Ibid.
35. Barkin, & Rosen, Endocrine disorders, p. 504.
36. Crain, & Gershel, Hyperthyroidism, pp. 141–142.
37. Ibid., p. 142.
38. Ibid.

BIBLIOGRAPHY

Barkin, R.M., & Rosen, P. (Eds.). Endocrine disorders. In *Emergency Pediatrics*. St. Louis: Mosby, 1984, pp. 499–503.

Crain, E.F., & Gershel, J.C., Eds. Diabetic ketoacidosis. In *Clinical Manual of Emergency Pediatrics*. Norwalk, Conn.: Appleton-Century-Crofts, 1986, pp. 136–139.

Hochman, H.I. Diabetic ketoacidosis. In Reece, R.M. (Ed.), *Manual of Emergency Pediatrics* (3rd ed.). Philadelphia: W.B. Saunders, 1984, pp. 101–105.

Lyen, K.R., Hale, D., & Baker, L. Endocrine emergencies. In Fleisher, G., & Ludwig, S. (Eds.), *Textbook of Pediatric Emergency Medicine*, Baltimore: Williams & Wilkins, 1983, pp. 632–640.

B. Giordano. The child with altered secretion of insulin. In Mott, S.R., Fazekas, N.F., & James, S.R. (Eds.), *Nursing Care of Children and Families: A Holistic Approach*. Menlo Park, Calif.: Addison-Wesley, 1985, pp. 1428–1440.

O'Boyle, C., Davis, D.K., Russo, B.A., & Kraf, T.J. Disorders of glucose metabolism. In *Emergency Care: The First 24 Hours*. Norwalk, Conn.: Appleton-Century-Crofts, 1985, pp. 351–355.

Sheehy, S.B. Metabolic and endocrine emergencies. *Journal of Emergency Nursing* 11, no. 1(1985):49–52.

Sheehy, S.B., & Barber, J. Metabolic emergencies. In *Emergency Nursing: Principles and Practice* (2nd ed.). St. Louis: Mosby, 1985, pp. 494–509.

EMERGENCY DEPARTMENT CARE GUIDE FOR THE CHILD WITH A DIABETIC EMERGENCY

Nursing Diagnosis	Interventions	Evaluation
Airway clearance: ineffective, related to decreased level of consciousness	Maintain patent airway	Airway remains patent
Ineffective breathing patterns related to decreased level of consciousness	Continually assess and support airway, breathing, and circulation Administer humidified oxygen Monitor arterial blood gases	Respiratory rate is normal Arterial blood gases are normal
Impaired gas exchange related to metabolic acidosis in child in DKA	Assess serum pH, glucose, and electrolytes Administer sodium bicarbonate as indicated Administer normal saline intravenously Monitor arterial blood gases Administer insulin as ordered Carefully monitor vital signs	Metabolic acidosis is corrected; HCO_3 and pH are within normal limits Arterial blood gases are normal Serum glucose returns to normal Serum electrolytes return to normal Vital signs remain normal

Nursing Diagnosis	Interventions	Evaluation
Potential for infection related to hyperglycemia or hypoglycemia	Continually assess serum glucose level Administer insulin or dextrose as ordered Carefully monitor temperature Obtain necessary cultures	Serum glucose level returns to normal Child's body temperature remains normal Cultures identify source of infection
Alteration in patterns of urinary elimination related to endocrine emergency	Assess hydration status Monitor fluid intake and output Monitor serum osmolarity Obtain urine-specific gravity	Child is adequately hydrated, skin turgor is normal, mucus membranes are moist Fluid intake and output are accurately recorded Serum osmolarity and urine-specific gravity are normal
Knowledge deficit related to endocrine disorder	Carefully explain all procedures and treatments to child and parents Explain the cause of the child's illness Provide information that may prevent illness in the future	Child and parents demonstrate an understanding of procedures and treatments Child and parents demonstrate an understanding of cause of child's illness and measures to prevent illness in the future
Potential for cognitive impairment related to altered glucose metabolism	Monitor glucose level frequently Closely monitor child's level of consciousness	Serum glucose level returns to normal Child remains alert and oriented to person, place, and time

Genitourinary and Gynecologic Disorders

Susan J. Kelley

DISORDERS OF THE FEMALE GENITALIA

Gynecologic Examination

The gynecologic examination of the pediatric patient requires sensitivity, patience, and a specialized approach. A careful explanation by the nurse prior to and during the examination is crucial. Younger children may want to be examined in the presence of their mothers. The nurse and physician may choose to examine the child together to avoid having the child go through the examination twice.

The approach to the examination will usually depend on the age of the child. Examination of the external genitalia can usually be accomplished with the younger child on the mother's lap leaning back with the child's legs held apart by the mother in a frog-like position. The older child should be placed on the examination table in the supine position. If old enough the child may choose to assist the examiner by holding her own labia majora apart. This gives the child some sense of control over the examination. The labia minora, introitus, hymen, urethral meatus, and clitoris can then be visualized and inspected for signs of trauma, infection, bleeding, or anatomic abnormality (Fig. 20–1).

The school-aged female should be placed in the knee-chest position to allow visualization of the vagina. This is usually accomplished by asking the child to get up on her hands and knees on the examination table, bringing her knees close to the chest, with the buttocks in the air. She should be instructed to rest her head on her folded arms, facing her mother or the nurse for comfort and support. The child should be instructed to relax her abdominal muscles while the examiner gently separates the labia and buttocks. This will cause the vaginal opening to fall open for visualization with light from an otoscope without a speculum. A vaginal speculum is usually not necessary in the examination of the prepubescent female. Occasionally it is necessary to use a pediatric vaginal speculum or small nasal speculum to examine the vagina. Any discharge, bleeding, hematomas, contusions, or foreign bodies should be noted. After this the child should be returned to the supine position for the collection of specimens.

Vaginal Bleeding Prior to Menarche

Vaginal bleeding can be either a normal event or a sign of disease, and when it is pathologic it can indicate a local genital tract disorder or endocrinologic or hematologic disease. Vaginal bleeding after the first few weeks of life and prior to menar-

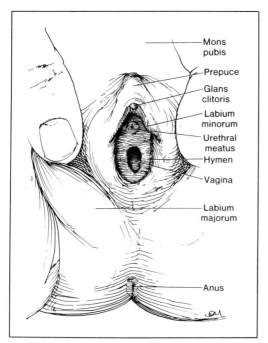

Figure 20-1. Anatomy of the normal female external genitalia. *(From G.R. Fleisher, & S. Ludwig (Eds.). Textbook of Pediatric Emergency Medicine. Baltimore: Williams & Wilkins, 1983, p. 605.)*

che is abnormal.[1] Menarche can occur normally at any age between 9 and 16 years.

Vaginal bleeding in infants and children can be caused by a variety of conditions, including trauma, infection, hormone imbalance, and genital tumors. The possibility of sexual abuse should always be considered in the differential diagnosis. Table 20-1 summarizes possible causes of vaginal bleeding in the prepubescent female.

TABLE 20-1. DIFFERENTIAL DIAGNOSIS IN VAGINAL BLEEDING

Sexual abuse	Pinworms
Trauma	Neonatal hormonal
Foreign body	bleeding
Urethral prolapse	Precocious puberty
Hematuria	Tumor
Rectal bleeding	

Vulvar Bleeding

Trauma to the vulva can include lacerations, hematomas, or ecchymosis. Vaginal or rectal injuries should be considered whenever trauma to the vulva is noted. Urethral prolapse is a common cause of apparent vaginal bleeding in children. Urethral prolapse is identified by the characteristic donut shape, with swollen, dark red, protruding urethral mucosa and central lumen. Often the vaginal orifice is concealed by the prolapse (Fig. 20-2). Most urethral prolapses occur in girls between the ages of 2 and 10 years. Painless vaginal bleeding is often the presenting complaint. The bleeding comes from ischemic mucosa. It may be accompanied by dysuria or urinary frequency. Straight catheterization of the bladder may be performed to confirm patency. If the prolapsed mucosa appears healthy, it may be treated by instructing the parents to use warm compresses or sitz baths for 10 to 14 days. If the prolapsed tissue appears necrotic, surgical intervention may be needed. This

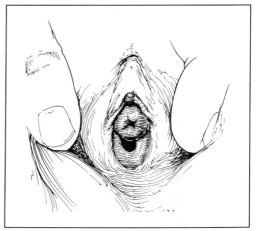

Figure 20-2. The smooth doughnut shape and central lumen are characteristic features of a urethral prolapse, which, if large or swollen, often conceals the vagina below it. *(From G.R. Fleisher, & S. Ludwig (Eds.). Textbook of Pediatric Emergency Medicine. Baltimore: Williams & Wilkins, 1983, p. 611.)*

is often performed within a few days of diagnosis on an elective, outpatient basis.

Another source of vulvar bleeding due to perineal excoriations is rectal *Enterobius vermicularis* infection (pinworms). Pinworms can produce intense itching and scratching, especially at night.

Vaginal Bleeding

Etiology. Vaginal bleeding due to trauma is a potential emergency. A penetrating injury to the vagina can also cause damage to the rectum, bladder, or abdominal viscera. A vaginal laceration may cause only minimal bleeding and may not necessarily reflect the seriousness of the injury.

Assessment. Whenever trauma to the vagina is suspected, the child's abdomen should be carefully evaluated. If intraabdominal injury is present, lower quadrant tenderness may be noted. Surgical consultation is indicated, and the child may need careful examination of the vagina under sedation or anesthesia. Also, whenever trauma to the vagina is suspected, a baseline hemoglobin should be obtained along with a urinalysis to screen for hematuria, which may indicate injury to the urethra or bladder.

Shigella vaginitis can cause vaginal bleeding that is often more noticeable than the associated discharge. A vaginal culture will identify the organism as well as the organism's sensitivity to antibiotics.

Foreign bodies may cause vaginal bleeding. If the foreign body has been in the vagina for more than several days, a foul smelling discharge will usually be present. If the foreign object cannot be easily visualized and removed, it may be necessary to gently irrigate the vaginal cavity with 50 cc of normal saline. If this fails to dislodge and to remove the foreign body, an examination under anesthesia is indicated.

Hormonal Causes of Vaginal Bleeding

There are several hormonal causes of vaginal bleeding in prepubescent females. Vaginal bleeding in the first 3 weeks of life is usually caused by hormonal fluctuations. This is due to exposure to high levels of circulating maternal hormones prior to birth that stimulate growth of the uterine endometrium as well as an increase in breast tissue. Shortly after birth the endometrium sloughs, resulting in a few days of light vaginal bleeding. The bleeding stops spontaneously and requires no treatment.[2] Parents will need a great amount of reassurance that the bleeding is normal and will subside.

Hormonal stimulation that produces vaginal bleeding in an older infant or child may be associated with precocious puberty. The vaginal bleeding may be accompanied by an increase in breast tissue or pubic hair growth. When these occur in children under 8 years of age they should be referred to an endocrinologist for further evaluation.

In cases in which parents give a history of bleeding but no abnormalities or bleeding is noted on examination, a urine and stool specimen should be analyzed for blood. The causes of vaginal bleeding listed in Table 20–1 should also be considered.

Occasionally parents will bring their daughter to the emergency department because she is experiencing her first menstrual period. If the child's age and degree of pubertal development are appropriate, no further evaluation is necessary.[3] The child and family will require teaching regarding the normal menstrual cycle and reassurance.

Vaginal Bleeding After Menarche

A comprehensive history from the adolescent will assist in determining the source of bleeding. A careful history regarding sexual activity, last menstrual cycle, possibility of pregnancy, use of contraceptives, and any previous pregnancies and their outcomes should be ascertained. The patient's mother should be asked if she were exposed to estrogen therapy during pregnancy.

If the patient is pregnant, uterine bleeding during the first 20 weeks indicates either spontaneous abortion or ectopic pregnancy.

A hematocrit, hemoglobin, and pregnancy test should be obtained. A pelvic examination will be performed. If the patient is believed to be pregnant, she should be referred for prenatal care.

Vulvovaginitis

Vulvovaginitis, the most common gynecologic problem in childhood, refers to inflammation of both the vulva and vagina. The vulvovaginitis usually begins with a vulvitis, and the vaginitis then occurs secondarily.

Etiology. Occasionally simple vulvitis may be observed. In these cases the inflammation of the labia may be caused by an infection, trauma, or allergic reaction. Common causes of allergic vulvitis include soaps, bubble bath solutions, and close-fitting synthetic undergarments.

Several factors make children more susceptible to vulvovaginitis. Lack of estrogen in the prepubescent female is responsible for the vaginal lining being thin and dry as well as having a neutral pH. These factors make the prepubescent vagina susceptible to infection. Another factor that contributes to vulvovaginitis in children is poor perineal hygiene, particularly the improper habit of wiping from "back to front" after defecation, resulting in fecal contamination of the genitalia. Also, the labia minora and majora are relatively smaller in the child than in the adult. This results in less protection of the vagina from invasion by microorganisms.[4]

History. The child with vulvovaginitis may give a history of dysuria, vaginal discharge, or pruritus. Parents may have noticed discomfort in the child, manifested by gait disturbance, or rubbing or scratching of the genitalia by the child.

Assessment. Examination of the perineum may reveal erythematous labia major and a slight vaginal discharge or presence of leukorrhea. It is important to note that a white discharge may be noted in the newborn period and that this occurrence is normal and is not due to infection but rather to the result of maternal estrogen in the residual circulation. This condition is self-limited and requires no intervention, except reassurance of the parents. Pubescent females may also experience a mucoid discharge.

The types, causes, clinical presentation, and treatment of nonsexually transmitted vulvovaginitis in children is summarized in Table 20–2.

DISORDERS OF THE MALE GENITALIA

Figure 20–3 provides a review of the anatomy of the male pelvis.

Balanitis

Balanitis, or balanoposthitis, is an inflammation of the glans and foreskin of the penis. It is a cellulitis and has its origin from a break in the penile skin. It may be associated with trauma or poor hygiene. The foreskin may appear crusted, swollen, and reddened. It is often accompanied by deeper rash over the scrotum, pubis, and buttocks. Dysuria is often present.[5]

Management. The area should be carefully cleansed with soap and water and allowed to dry completely. An ointment such as petroleum jelly or bacitracin

TABLE 20-2. VULVOVAGINITIS IN CHILDREN

Type	Cause	Clinical Presentation	Treatment
Mixed, nonspecific bacterial	Poor local hygiene Improper "back to front" wiping technique Transmission of infecting organism from respiratory tract to genital area by contaminated fingers	Red, swollen vulva Vaginal discharge Dysuria Pruritis	Sitz baths Improved local hygiene Antibacterial cream Estrogen cream Triple sulfa cream
Allergic vulvitis	Bubble bath soaps Synthetic, tight-fitting underwear	Red, swollen vulva Pruritis	Identify causative agent and avoid contact Hydrocortisone cream 1% three times daily Instruct parents to use only white, cotton, loose-fitting undergarments for child
Enterobius vermicularis (pinworm)	Pinworms migrate to vagina from rectum	Perivaginal itching Excoriation of vulva from scratching Perianal itching Unexplained irritability at night	Pyrantel pamoate—single dose of 11 mg/kg (to maximum dose of 1 g) orally Treatment of all family members Improve hygiene
Foreign object	Insertion of foreign object into vagina Common objects include wads of toilet paper, beads, stones, coins, hairpins	Profuse, purulent, malodorous vaginal discharge Vaginal bleeding Edema Discomfort Gait disturbance	Removal of foreign object Irrigation of vagina Systemic antibiotic therapy may be necessary

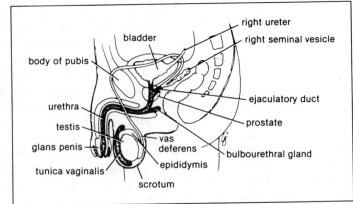

Figure 20-3. Saggittal section of the male pelvis. *(From R.S. Snell. Student's Aid to Gross Anatomy. Norwalk, Conn.: Appleton-Century-Crofts, 1986, p. 430.)*

should be applied sparingly. The child may be placed on ampicillin (50 to 100 mg/kg/24 hours in four divided doses).

If the foreskin produces total obstruction, there may be acute urinary retention. In this event a physician will insert the tip of a mosquito forceps into the orifice of the foreskin to stretch the skin. Any collected pus is removed. Circumcision is performed only after inflammation has subsided.

Parents should be instructed to cleanse and dry the area as well as to change diapers frequently. They may also be instructed to expose the inflamed area to air as much as possible. If there is crusting of the foreskin, warm soaks may be applied three times daily for 20 minutes each time.

Paraphimosis

Paraphimosis is a condition in which the foreskin has been retracted behind the glans and cannot be drawn back into its normal position over the glans. Immediate treatment is necessary, since there is rapidly increasing swelling and potential compromise of circulation to the glans. Poor hygiene and collection of smegma under the foreskin can lead to chronic inflammation.

The child is usually brought to the emergency department with a history of swelling of the glans and an inability to return the foreskin over the glans.

Management. Ice packs should be applied to the penis and a potent analgesic such as morphine or meperidine administered. Manual reduction of the foreskin is then attempted by the physician. If manual reduction fails, a dorsal slit is created to overcome the swelling.[6]

The patient and parents are advised to seek a follow-up appointment with a surgeon to arrange for circumcision once the swelling has subsided and the wound has healed. Proper cleansing of the uncircumcised penis should be taught to the child and parents.

Hernia

Indirect inguinal hernia is the most common surgical condition in childhood. Approximately 50 percent of inguinal hernias occur during infancy, while a majority of the remaining 50 percent occur in children 1 to 5 years of age. Males are affected more often than females. The contents of an inguinal hernial sac is visceral, being intestine in the male and ovary or fallopian tube in the female.

Assessment. Inguinal hernias may appear as uncomplicated masses in the inguinal canal or as surgical emergencies. A hernia is termed incarcerated when its contents cannot be returned to the abdominal cavity. Strangulated hernias occur when the blood supply to the entrapped contents is compromised.

The infant or child with uncomplicated hernia usually has a recent history of fussiness or crying, drawing up of the legs on the abdomen, and swelling of the scrotum. Upon examination the scrotum appears large and gives an impulse on coughing or crying. In cases of incarcerated or strangulated hernia, the scrotal mass will be firm, edematous, painful, and nontranslucent. These are usually not reducible manually.

Management. Manual reduction of inguinal hernias is usually attempted in the emergency department. Prior to reduction, morphine (0.1 mg/kg intramuscularly) is administered. Cold packs should be applied to the groin and the child placed in Trendelenburg's position. The physician will attempt to manually reduce the hernia. If manual reduction is successful the patient is discharged and is referred for elective surgery, since recurrence is very likely. Immediate surgery is indicated if manual reduction is unsuccessful, if incarceration persists for more than 12 hours, or if signs of bowel obstruction are present.

Epididymitis and Orchitis

Epididymitis in males usually occurs by direct extension into the ejaculatory ducts or vas deferens. Epididymitis may be the complication of gonorrhea, urethritis, prostatitis, or instrumentation of the urethra. Orchitis is often preceded by trauma or viral infection, most frequently the mumps.

Both epididymitis and orchitis reveal a history of pain and swelling of the scrotum accompanied by fever. The pain of epididymitis is usually described as dull and aching, whereas with orchitis the pain is more severe and the testes enlarged. Urine cultures should be obtained.

Management. Treatment includes scrotal support, analgesia, sitz baths, and antibiotics, depending upon culture results.

Testicular Torsion

Testicular torsion is caused by twisting of the spermatic cord, leading to venous and arterial obstruction (Fig. 20–4). It is the

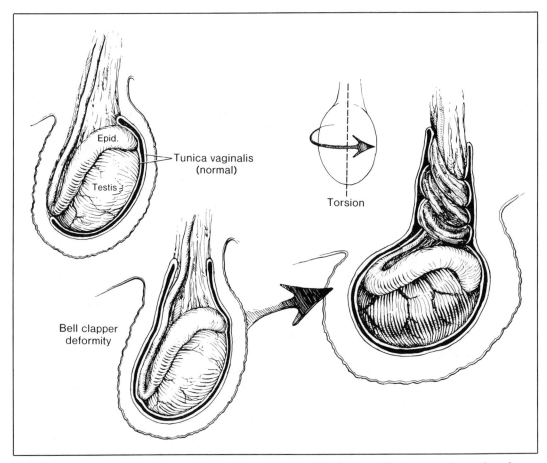

Figure 20–4. Torsion testis. Abnormality of testicular fixation—bell-clapper deformity—permits torsion of spermatic vessels with subsequent infarction of the gonad. Epid. = epididymis. *(From G.R. Fleisher, & S. Ludwig (Eds.). Textbook of Pediatric Emergency Medicine. Baltimore: Williams & Wilkins, 1983, p. 239.)*

leading cause of scrotal swelling and should be suspected in any case of scrotal swelling.

All suspected cases of testicular torsion should be evaluated immediately, since testicular survival depends on the duration of ischemia. At 4 hours there is a 100 percent chance of survival, while chances of survival after 24 hours are 0 percent.[7] Prompt triage is therefore critical, and the urologist or surgeon must be notified immediately.

History. Most often there will be a recent history of trauma to the genitals or strenuous exercise, although testicular torsion can occur at rest or while a patient is asleep. There may have been subacute episodes of scrotal pain prior to the visit to the emergency department. The patient will complain of intermittent or constant pain to the involved testis, groin, or lower abdomen. The patient may also complain of nausea.

Assessment. The involved testis will lie higher in the scrotum, with a horizontal rather than vertical orientation. Scrotal edema is present and does not transilluminate. Doppler examination of the testicles indicates decreased blood flow to the affected testicle. The patient's blood pressure may be elevated due to pain and anxiety. The patient is usually afebrile.

Management. Prompt surgical management is the treatment of choice. The emergency nurse should ensure that the patient takes nothing by mouth while in the emergency department. Often an analgesic will be administered while the patient awaits transport to the operating room.

Psychosocial Support and Parent Education. The emergency nurse should make the patient as comfortable as possible while awaiting evaluation and surgery.

Pain, examination, and surgery to the genitals is embarrassing for the patient and provokes great anxiety. Young children may fear castration. Adolescents may have concerns regarding their future sexuality after surgery. Emotional support and accurate information are therefore extremely important. The patient and family will need to be prepared for the child's admission to the hospital after the surgery.

SEXUALLY TRANSMITTED DISEASES

Sexually transmitted diseases (STD) have become of increased concern and incidence in the pediatric population. The term STD refers to a group of diseases that are usually transmitted from one individual to another during sexual activity. Several STDs, however, can be transmitted from a mother to her fetus or newborn. These congenital infections include herpes simplex virus type II, acquired immune deficiency syndrome (AIDS), gonorrhea, and syphilis. The presence of a STD beyond the newborn period should be considered as acquired through sexual contact and the infant or child regarded as a victim of sexual abuse until proven otherwise. (Refer to Chapter 2 on sexual abuse of children.) Table 20–3 summarizes the STDs most commonly found in the pediatric population and their clinical management.

URINARY TRACT DISEASE

Urinary Tract Infection

Urinary tract infection (UTI) is the second most common form of bacterial infection in children next to upper respiratory tract infections. Between 1 and 2 percent of infants and children have bacteriuria at any given time, and 5 percent of all school-

TABLE 20-3. SEXUALLY TRANSMITTED DISEASES IN CHILDREN

STD	Clinical Presentation	Laboratory Tests	Treatment
Gonorrhea	*Male* Penile discharge Penile swelling Dysuria Pharyngitis Rectal inflammation, discharge *Female* Dsyuria Vaginal discharge Urethral inflammation Lymph gland inflammation Pharyngitis Rectal inflammation, discharge	Pharyngeal, vaginal, penile and rectal cultures plated on Thayer-Martin agar medium Gram-stain smear: may reveal gram-negative diplococci (more reliable in males)	Aqueous procaine penicillin 100,000 U/kg (max. 4.8 million units) intramuscularly along with Probenicid 25 mg/kg (max. dose 1 g) orally *or* Amoxacillin 50 mg/kg (max. 3.5 g) orally (one-time dose) along with Probenicid 25 mg/kg (max. 1 g) *or* If allergic to penicillin: Under 8 years of age—Erythromycin 40 mg/kg/day orally in four divided doses for 7 days Over 8 years of age—Tetracycline 25 mg/kg as initial dose, followed by 40 to 60 mg/kg/day in four divided doses for 7 days
Syphilis	*Primary stage* Chancre may appear on penis, vulva, cervix, rectum, or mouth. Chancre is an ulcer-like sore *Secondary stage* Fever, pharyngitis, generalized rash, lymphadenopathy	Serum VDRL or RPR Dark-field examination of scrapings from genital or mucocutaneous lesion	Benzathine penicillin G 2.4 million units intramuscularly *or* If allergic to penicillin: Under 8 years of age—Erythromycin 500 mg orally four times a day for 15 days Over 8 years of age—Tetracycline 500 mg orally four times a day for 15 days
Herpes simplex virus type II	Multiple painful lesions or vesicles on the vulva, penis, buttocks, and inner thighs Blisters break open after several days, leaving red lesions that eventually form scabs and then heal Acute urinary retention secondary to severe dysuria due to painful lesions Fever and malaise may accompany outbreak	Pap smear reveals multinucleated giant cells and nuclear inclusion bodies Tissue culture necessary to confirm diagnosis	Symptomatic only Sitz baths may give relief If accompanied by severe dysuria, the child may be instructed to urinate in warm bath water Acetaminophen may be given for pain Recurrences are common, and child and parents need to be warned of this

TABLE 20-3. *(Continued)*

STD	Clinical Presentation	Laboratory Tests	Treatment
Trichomoniasis	*Male* Often asymptomatic Mild dysuria Urethral discharge *Female* Vaginal pruritis Vulvar pruritis Yellow, frothy, malodorous vaginal discharge	Fresh smear of discharge will reveal protozoan trichomonial vaginalis	Metronidazole (Flagyl) orally, 35 mg/kg daily in two divided doses for 5 days (max. dose 500 mg daily)
Monilia	*Female* Erythema and edema of vulva Thick, white, cheesey discharge (may occasionally be watery and thin) *Male* May develop balanitis or cutaneous lesions on penis	Microscopic examination of vaginal wall scrapings and vaginal discharge	Nystatin vaginal suppositories twice daily for 7 to 14 days
Condyloma acuminata	Warts on the genitals or rectum	May require biopsy	Local application of Podophylline 20% in tincture of benzoin to affected areas only Must be washed off by parents 2 hours after application

aged females will have a UTI.[8] During infancy males are at increased risk of developing a UTI. This is due to the higher incidence of anatomic defects in males. Following infancy the prevalence rate is much higher for girls than boys. A major reason for this higher incidence in girls past infancy is the short urethra of the female child and the close proximity of the rectum to the urethra. The peak incidence of UTI occurs between 2 and 6 years of age.

Etiology and Pathophysiology. Virtually all UTIs occur by the ascending route. *Escherichia coli* is the most common causative pathogen and is responsible in 70 to 90 percent of cases. Other common pathogens include *Klebsiella pneumoniae, Proteus species, Enterobacter aerogenes, Enterococcus,* and *Staphylococcus epidermidis.*

History and Assessment. Infants and children with UTI often arrive at the emergency department with vague complaints that suggest a variety of clinical entities. The clinical indicators in neonates are more often gastrointestinal than genitourinary in character. Infants with UTI may have jaundice, vomiting, diarrhea, irritability, and a history of poor feeding. Fever may or may not be present. Signs and symptoms of UTI in older children may include abdominal pain, vomiting, dysuria, frequency, and fever. Table 20-4 summa-

TABLE 20–4. CLINICAL MANIFESTATIONS OF URINARY TRACT INFECTIONS

Infants	Children
Fever	Fever
Vomiting	Frequency
Diarrhea	Urgency
Irritability	Dysuria
Jaundice	Enuresis
Poor feeding	Hematuria
Cloudy or malodorous urine	Abdominal pain or discomfort
Failure to thrive or to gain weight normally	

rizes the clinical manifestations of UTIs in infants and children.

Laboratory Data. The diagnosis of UTI is based on the presence of bacteriuria, or organisms in the urine. Proper collection of urine cultures is essential in accurate diag-nosis of UTI. Obtaining uncontaminated urine specimens in infants and children, however, is difficult.

A suprapubic bladder aspiration (Fig. 20–5) performed by the physician is the most effective method of collecting urine in the infant because the urine obtained by this method is generally free of bacterial contaminants. If a suprapubic bladder as-piration is not conducted, a sterile urine collection bag can be applied to the peri-neum after the area has been cleansed. In older children, after proper cleansing a midstream clean-catch urine specimen can be obtained in a sterile receptable by the nurse or mother after the first portion of urine has passed into the toilet.

Catheterization of the urethra to ob-tain a urine specimen should be avoided because of the risk of introduction of bacte-ria during the procedure. A first-morning

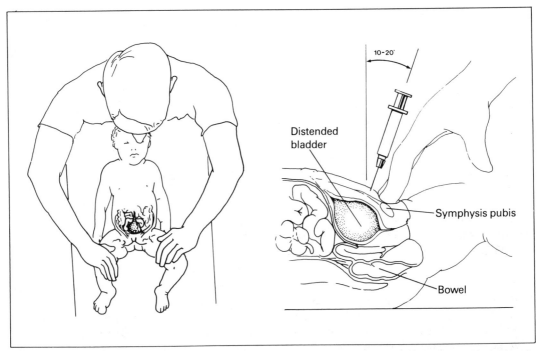

Figure 20–5. Suprapubic bladder aspiration. The infant should be held firmly in a supine position with the legs in a frog-leg position *(left)*. The suprapubic bladder tap is performed by inserting a 22 gauge needle (attached to a 3 ml syringe) into the bladder and aspirating urine as the syringe is gradually withdrawn *(right)*.

void is ideal but is rarely available in the emergency department. A first-morning void can be obtained at home when follow-up urine cultures are necessary. Diagnosis of UTI is based on a urine culture indicating a colony count of more than 100,000 organisms/ml. Growth of several different organisms is an indication that the specimen was contaminated, in which case the culture should be repeated.

Uncentrifuged urine should be gram stained and examined with high-power fields to determine the presence of significant bacteria. Routine urinalysis may reveal red blood cells, white blood cells, protein, and bacteria.

Management. The goal of treatment is directed toward eradication of the infecting microorganism and prevention of recurrence. Antibiotic treatment is initiated before cultures are available if the patient is symptomatic and urinalysis and gram stain are suggestive of UTI.

Newborns with UTI should be hospitalized for intravenous antibiotics. A combination of intravenous gentamicen and ampicillin are usually administered. Older infants and children with UTI are treated with ampicillin, 100 mg/kg/day, given orally in four divided doses, or sulfisoxazole (Gantrisin), 100 to 200 mg/kg/day given in four divided oral doses on an outpatient basis.

Parents need to be instructed in the proper amount and administration of medication, increased fluid intake, and use of sitz baths to relieve discomfort. Parents should be advised to return to the emergency department or to see their physician if the child is unable to retain the medication due to persistent vomiting or if oliguria, high fever, lethargy, or signs of dehydration are present. Irregardless of how the child is progressing clinically, another culture should be obtained and should be found negative after 24 to 48

hours of antibiotic therapy. If the repeat culture is positive, a different antibiotic should be prescribed according to the sensitivity report. The child will need to be recultured after another 24 to 48 hours. Because recurrence is common, the child will need to be followed carefully upon completion of the antibiotic therapy. Parents should also be taught proper perineal care, such as "front to back" wiping, to prevent subsequent UTIs.

Acute Glomerulonephritis

Acute glomerulonephritis [AGN], an immune complex disease, is the most common noninfectious renal disease in childhood. Poststreptococcal glomerulonephritis is the most common form of glomerulonephritis in children. Most cases are related to a previous infection with nephritogenic strains of group A beta-hemolytic streptococci. There is a latent period of 10 to 14 days between the streptococcal infection and the onset of clinical manifestations.

Acute glomerulonephritis occurs most frequently in children aged 3 to 12 years of age, with a peak incidence at 7 years of age. Males are affected more often than females.

Etiology and Pathophysiology. In the northern sections of the United States the initial streptococcal infections usually involve pharyngitis and upper respiratory infection, whereas impetigo, infected insect bites, and scabies are the leading causes in the southern states. Children with acute glomerulonephritis usually recover completely, and recurrence is unusual.

The renal involvement is thought to result from an antigen-antibody response, which is stimulated by the initial streptococcal infection, followed by an immune-complex reaction. These immune complexes become trapped in the glomerular capillary loop.[9]

The kidneys are normal to moderately enlarged during the initial phase. Microscopic examination reveals a diffuse proliferative exudative process. The glomerular capillary loops become obliterated by edema, and the filtration rate is reduced. This results in a reduced capacity to form filtrate from plasma flow. This decreased plasma filtration results in excessive retention of sodium and water, followed by expanded plasma and interstitial fluid volumes that may result in circulatory congestion and edema.[10]

History. There may be a history of pharyngitis in the preceding week or two; skin infection, such as impetigo; headache; hematuria; dysuria; edema; and weight gain. With increasing degrees of renal failure there may be a history of nausea, vomiting, and abdominal pain.[11]

Assessment. The child's airway, breathing, and circulation (ABCs) should be carefully assessed and supported. The child may be found to have edema, hypertension, and, in severe cases, signs of congestive heart failure. The edema may be noted primarily in the face in the morning but then spreads to the extremities and abdomen during the day. Congestive heart failure results from fluid retention that leads to vascular overload. The child may appear pale, lethargic, and irritable.

In severe cases the patient may have seizure activity secondary to hypertension or cerebral ischemia or have oliguria or anuria, the result of acute renal failure.

Laboratory Data. Urinalysis results will usually include a high specific gravity, protein, red blood cells, white blood cells, epithelial cells and casts, but no bacteria. A complete blood count, serum ASO and streptozyme titers, serum complement levels C3 and C4, serum creatinine, blood urea nitrogen (BUN), urine culture, and chest radiographs should be obtained. A positive throat culture is useful in establishing the diagnosis. In most cases, however, the throat culture is negative. Throat cultures should be obtained from all household members and other close contacts.

An electrocardiogram (ECG) may reveal elevation or depression of the ST segment, prolonged QRS and ST segments, lengthening of the PR interval, and flattened or inverted T waves. The chest radiograph may show cardiac enlargement, pulmonary congestion, and plural effusion during the acute phase.

Management. Management of acute glomerulonephritis is generally supportive. If hypertension is present, hydralazine (Apresoline) 0.15 mg/kg intramuscularly is usually effective in lowering blood pressure within 15 to 60 minutes.[12] This dose may be doubled or tripled if necessary and may be repeated every 3 to 6 hours as needed.[13] Reduction in the vascular circulatory volume is also necessary to lower blood pressure. This can be achieved through administration of a diuretic such as furosemide (Lasix), 1 mg/kg intravenously. Decreased sodium intake will limit the reaccumulation of fluid and the recurrence of hypertension. Fluid intake (oral and intravenous) should be restricted. Intake and output should be carefully measured and recorded. Electrolyte balance should be carefully maintained.

If acute renal failure with marked oliguria is present, severe restriction of sodium, potassium, protein, and fluid intake is necessary. Occasionally peritoneal dialysis or hemodialysis will be necessary. All patients with acute glomerulonephritis should be admitted to a pediatric intensive care unit for close observation.

Psychosocial Support and Parent Education. The child and parents are often anxious and will need much reassurance while in the emergency department. All procedures should be carefully explained. Both the child and parents will need to be prepared for the child's admission to the hospital.

Acute Renal Failure

Acute renal failure (ARF) occurs when there is an abrupt loss of renal excretory function due to impaired blood flow. The kidneys are unable to regulate the volume and composition of urine. ARF is uncommon in children, but mortality is high in this age group. Prognosis depends on the etiology and prompt identification and treatment. ARF is categorized by changes in creatinine clearance.

Etiology and Pathophysiology. Causes of ARF include renal trauma, shock, toxic agents, and dehydration. Causes of ARF are usually classified as prerenal, renal, and postrenal. Prerenal causes are the most common cause of ARF in children and are related to reduction of renal perfusion to a normal kidney. Dehydration secondary to gastroenteritis, shock, surgery, trauma, burns, diabetic ketoacidosis, congestive heart failure, and sepsis are other common causes. Postrenal causes, uncommon in children over one year of age, include upper urinary tract obstruction or bladder neck obstruction. Renal causes include diseases such as glomerulonephritis or nephrotoxic agents that damage the glomeruli, tubules, or renal vasculature.

ARF is characterized by a severe reduction in glomerular filtration rate, elevated serum urea nitrogen level, decreased tubular reabsorption of sodium from the proximal tubule, with increased concentration of sodium in the distal tubule. Glomerular filtration is reduced, which prevents urinary losses of sodium.

History. The infant or child in renal failure may present with a history of oliguria (less than 0.5 cc/kg/hour), symptoms related to acute glomerulonephritis, a history of ex-posure to nephrotoxic substances such as carbon tetrachloride or heavy metals or ingestion of prescribed medications such as sulfonamides, neomycin, or kanamycin. In most cases the child initially has signs and symptoms of a precipitating disorder, such as shock, burns, near drowning, acute glomerulonephritis, or dehydration. In such cases the possibility of developing ARF should be anticipated and carefully monitored.

Assessment. The ABCs should be continually assessed. Signs of volume overload, such as edema, rales, and cardiac gallop, may be present. Vital signs should be carefully monitored. There may be hypertension, seizures, lethargy, coma, and fever.

Laboratory Data. Urine electrolytes and urinalysis with specific gravity should be obtained. A complete blood count, serum electrolytes, BUN, creatinine, and arterial blood gases should also be obtained. Table 20–5 outlines the abnormal laboratory values associated with ARF.

Management. Treatment of ARF is directed toward the etiology, management of any complications, and supportive therapy. If dehydration exists and has caused inadequate perfusion, volume replacement by intravenous therapy is essential. A Foley catheter should be inserted immediately upon diagnosis to collect urine for analysis and a highly accurate measurement of output. Urine output should be measured on an hourly basis. If oliguria exists in the presence of adequate hydration, a rapid-acting diuretic may be administered while the patient is still in the emergency department.

Hyperkalemia, if present, will need to be corrected immediately if concentrations are in excess of 7.0 mEq/L. Careful cardiac monitoring will be necessary due to the risk of arrhythmias associated with hyperkalemia. A prolonged QRS complex, de-

TABLE 20-5. ABNORMAL LABORATORY VALUES ASSOCIATED WITH ARF

Determination	Findings in ARF	Normal Values
Potassium	Hyperkalemia	Newborn 5.0–7.7 mEq/L Infant 4.1–5.3 mEq/L Child 3.5–4.7 mEq/L
Sodium	Hyponatremia	Newborn 139–162 mEq/L Infant 139–146 mEq/L Child 138–145 mEq/L
Calcium	Hypocalcemia	Newborn 3.7–7.0 mEq/L Infant 5.2–6.0 mEq/L Child 5.0–5.7 mEq/L
Creatinine serum	Elevated	0.3–1.1 mg/dl
BUN	Elevated	Newborn/Infant 5–15/dl Child 10–20 mg/dl
Arterial blood gases	Metabolic acidosis	PO_2 Newborn 60–70 mm Hg Child 80–90 mm Hg PCO_2 35–45 mm Hg pH 7.35–7.45

pressed ST segment, high-peaked T waves, bradycardia, or heart block may occur with hyperkalemia. The effects of hyperkalemia may need to be corrected with one of the following temporary measures:

- calcium gluconate, 0.5 ml/kg intravenously over 2 to 4 minutes;
- glucose 25 percent and insulin 0.1 unit/kg intravenously, which causes glucose and potassium to move into the cells; or
- administration of polystyrene sodium sulfonate (Kayexalate) 1 g/kg orally or rectally to bind potassium and to remove it from the body.

Nursing care for the infant or child with ARF includes precise measurement of intake and output and careful monitoring of all vital signs. Hypertension may occur in ARF due to overexpansion of extracellular fluid volume. An antihypertensive such as hydralazine may be ordered. Fluids and sodium are restricted in patients with hypertension. Children with ARF require dialysis when there is severe fluid overload that does not respond to diuretic therapy. The patient must be contin-

ually observed for any signs of congestive heart failure. The child's neurologic status should be closely monitored for changes in mental status or any seizure activity.

Psychosocial Support and Parent Education. Both child and parents will need a tremendous amount of support. All diagnostic procedures and treatments should be carefully explained. The parents need to be kept continually informed of the child's condition. The child will require admission to a pediatric intensive care unit for close monitoring.

NOTES

1. J.E. Paradise. Vaginal bleeding. In G. Fleisher, and S., Ludwig (Eds.), *Textbook of Pediatric Emergency Medicine.* Baltimore: Williams & Wilkins, 1983, p. 255.
2. Ibid., p. 258.
3. Ibid.
4. K.C. Edelin. Vulvovaginitis in children. In R.M. Reece (Ed.), *Manual of Emergency Pediatrics* (3rd ed.). Philadelphia: W.B. Saunders, 1984, pp. 576–577.
5. J.W. Chamberlain. Balanitis. In R.M. Reece

(Ed.), *Manual of Emergency Pediatrics* (3rd ed.). Philadelphia: W.B. Saunders, 1984, p. 547.

6. N.R. Feins. Paraphimosis. In R.M. Reece (Ed.), *Manual of Emergency Pediatrics* (3rd ed.). Philadelphia: W.B. Saunders, 1984, p. 213.

7. Kogan, S.T., Levitt, S.B., & Smey, P. Genitourinary emergencies. In E. Crain, & J. Gershel (Eds.), *A Clinical Manual of Emergency Pediatrics*. Norwalk, Conn.: Appleton-Century-Crofts, 1986, p. 220.

8. H.M. Snyder. Urologic emergencies. In G. Fleisher, & S. Ludwig (Eds.), *Textbook of Pediatric Emergency Medicine*. Baltimore: Williams & Wilkins, 1983, p. 925.

9. L.F. Whaley, & D.L. Wong. Acute glomerulonephritis. In *Nursing Care of Infants and Children* (2nd ed.). St. Louis: Mosby, 1983, pp. 1123–1124.

10. Ibid.

11. H. Trachtman. Renal emergencies. In E.F. Crain, & J.C. Gershel (Eds.), *A Clinical Manual of Emergency Pediatrics*. Norwalk, Conn.: Appleton-Century-Crofts, 1986, p. 465.

12. R.P. Gottlieb. Acute glomerulonephritis. In R.M. Reece (Ed.), *Manual of Emergency Pediatrics* (3rd ed.). Philadelphia: W.B. Saunders, 1984, p. 596.

13. Ibid.

BIBLIOGRAPHY

Ginsburg, C.M., & McCracken, G.H. Urinary tract infections in young infants. *Pediatrics* April 1982, pp. 409–412.

Hoover, D.L. Genitourinary trauma. *Topics in Emergency Medicine* October 1982, pp. 55–60.

Kaplan, G.W. Recurring urinary infections: Current dilemmas, observations, reflections. *Pediatric Consultation* 4(1980):1–8.

Kidd, P.S. Trauma of the genitourinary system. *Journal of Emergency Nursing* September/October 1982, pp. 232–238.

Knasel, A.L. Venereal disease in children. In *Sexual Abuse of Children: Selected Readings*. Washington, D.C.: U.S. Department of Health and Human Services, 1980, pp. 17–20.

Lanros, N.E. Genitourinary emergencies. In *Assessment and Intervention in Emergency Nursing* (2nd ed.). Bowie, Md.: Robert Brady, 1983, pp. 331–334.

Link, D.A. Acute renal failure. In Cohen, S.A. (Ed.), *Pediatric Emergency Management*. Bowie, Md.: Robert Brady, 1982, pp. 268–271.

McAninch, J. Traumatic injuries to the urethra. *Journal of Trauma* 21(1981):291–297.

McCoy, J.A. Preliminary diagnosis of urinary tract infection in symptomatic children. *Nurse Practitioner* January 1982.

Norman, M.E. Renal and electrolyte emergencies. In Fleisher, G.R., & Ludwig, S. (Eds.), *Textbook of Pediatric Emergency Medicine*. Baltimore: Williams & Wilkins, 1983, pp. 415–459.

Paradise, J.E. Pediatric and adolescent gynecology. In Fleisher, G.R., & Ludwig, S. (Eds.), *Textbook of Pediatric Emergency Medicine*. Baltimore: Williams & Wilkins, 1983, pp. 603–631.

Reece, R.M. (Ed.). Genitourinary and gynecological disorders. In *Manual of Emergency Pediatrics* (2nd ed.). Philadelphia: W.B. Saunders, 1978, pp. 449–497.

Schwartz, W. Dysuria. In Fleisher, G.R., & Ludwig, S. (Eds.), *Textbook of Pediatric Emergency Medicine*. Baltimore: Williams & Wilkins, 1983, pp. 136–138.

Selden, R.V., et al. Managing urinary tract infections in children. *Pediatric Annals* 10(1981):12–24.

Siegel, S.R., et al. Urinary infections in infants and preschool children. *American Journal of Diseases in Children* April 1980, pp. 371–372.

Snyder, H.M. Urologic emergencies. In Fleisher, G.R., & Ludwig, S. (Eds.), *Textbook of Pediatric Emergency Medicine*. Baltimore: Williams & Wilkins, 1983, pp. 921–929.

Stann, J.H. Urinary tract infections in children. *Pediatric Nursing* 5(1979):49–52.

Stoeppel, A., & Oakes, A. Care of the child with a disorder of the renal system. In Oakes, A. (Ed.), *Critical Care Nursing of Children and Adolescents*. Philadelphia: W.B. Saunders, 1981, pp. 201–219.

Thomas, C.T. Childhood urinary tract infection. *Pediatric Nursing* April 1982, pp. 114–119.

Whaley, L.F., & Wong, D.L. Acute glomerulonephritis. In *Nursing Care of Infants and Children* (2nd ed.). St. Louis: Mosby, 1983, pp. 1123–1129.

**EMERGENCY DEPARTMENT CARE GUIDE FOR THE CHILD
WITH A GENITOURINARY PROBLEM**

Nursing Diagnosis	Interventions	Evaluation
Alteration in renal tissue perfusion related to infection	Administer diuretic as ordered Restrict fluid intake Obtain laboratory specimens Carefully monitor serum electrolytes Administer antibiotics as ordered Continually monitor vital signs	Urinary output is adequate (>1 ml/kg/hour) Serum electrolytes are within normal range Vital signs are stable
Fluid volume excess related to renal disease	Administer diuretic as ordered Restrict fluid intake Carefully measure and record fluid intake and output Carefully monitor blood pressure	Urinary output increases Blood pressure remains stable
Alteration in pattern of urinary elimination related to dysuria or urinary tract infection	Administer antibiotics as ordered Encourage child to void even though it is uncomfortable Obtain urine culture, urinalysis, and specific gravity Administer pyridium for dysuria	Urinary output increases
Hyperthermia related to infection of genitourinary tract system	Administer antipyretic Provide tepid sponge bath to infant or young child Administer initial dose of antibiotic as soon as possible	Body temperature returns to normal
Knowledge deficit related to child's illness or injury	Carefully explain all procedures and treatments to child and parents Inform parents of the discharge care of their child, including medication administration and fever control If child is to be admitted, explain admission procedures to child and parents	Child and parents indicate an understanding of procedures and treatments Parents demonstrate knowledge of medication administration and fever control

Nursing Diagnosis	Interventions	Evaluation
Fear related to painful procedures and emergency department environment	Carefully explain all procedures to child Allow parents to remain with child at all times Encourage parents to remain overnight in hospital if child is admitted	

21 | Orthopaedic Emergencies

Kathleen Rourke
Anne Phelan
Martha C. Miller

In considering the anatomic, physiologic, and psychosocial differences of children, it becomes readily apparent that children are not just small adults. While children can sustain musculoskeletal injuries very similar to those seen in adults, there are problems that are primarily seen in children, and some specific considerations in assessment, treatment, and follow-up must be kept in mind.

ANATOMIC AND PHYSIOLOGIC CONSIDERATIONS

The part of a child's skeleton that is most different from adults and that is of greatest concern and importance is the growth cartilage. This growth cartilage, often referred to as the growth plate or epiphyseal plate, is a radiolucent cartilagenous disc located between the epiphysis and the metaphysis at both the proximal and distal ends of long bones. This is the area that is primarily responsible for the longitudinal growth of bone in children.[1]

The outer covering, or periosteum, of a child's bone is thicker and stronger than that of an adult. It is these characteristics that give a child's bone its flexibility, or plasticity. Because the periosteum is more resistant to tearing, children's fractures are often undisplaced and incomplete, that is, the outer covering or "cortex" of the bone

remains intact. These fractures are commonly referred to as greenstick fractures.[2]

The porous nature of a child's bone also influences the type of fractures seen in children. The compact bone found in adults is most likely to fail in tension, while the porous nature of a child's bone commonly causes failure in compression as well as tension. Fractures that occur near the metaphysis of the bone, the area of greatest porosity, are commonly referred to as buckle or torus fractures. Buckle fractures are seen more often in the young child than in the older child who is near the end of the growth period. It is interesting to note that bone in an elderly person is also very porous, and older people are also likely to sustain compression fractures as well as those fractures caused by failure in tension.

The specific nature of the periosteal covering of a child's bone also makes it capable of producing great amounts of callus, or new bone, in a very short period of time. This gives children an advantage in fracture healing, but gives the clinician less time to manipulate and correct problem deformities that may recur after a fracture has been initially reduced. Fracture healing in children is also remarkable for the fact that children are capable of a process called remodeling. This term refers to the fact that certain fracture deformities are corrected over time, after the bone has

418

healed. The capability of a child's bone to remodel seems to be related to the process of continual growth and can be seen in some instances of adult fractures, but to a very limited degree. It is important to remember that only a limited amount of correction can be obtained through this process. Varus and valgus deformities, deformities secondary to malrotation, or severe deformities of angulation do not correct with remodeling and must be corrected by reduction. Remodeling is most likely to occur in children with open epiphyses and in fractures close to the epiphyseal plate.[3]

ASSESSMENT AND TREATMENT CONSIDERATIONS

The initial assessment of any child who has sustained some form of trauma demands immediate attention to and assessment of the basic ABCs: airway, breathing and circulation. Injuries to the musculoskeletal system generally are not life-threatening, and have last priority except where excessive bleeding is involved or where neurovascular deficits are present. Establishing and maintaining a patent airway always has first precedence.

Children are easily frightened and demand careful explanation of and participation, where possible, in all aspects of asessment and treatment. When assessing a specific injury, ask the child where it hurts rather than attempt to initially examine the injury yourself. The best way to assess the use or movement of an extremity is to observe the child or to ask the child to move or use it rather than attempt to move the extremity yourself. Often you can coax a child to reach for an object or perform common movements, such as clapping the hands or waving good-bye. It is important to remember that you will often have only one chance to gain a

child's trust or cooperation. This is a situation where first impressions really count.

When a fracture is suspected, the extremity should be splinted prior to obtaining x-rays, and when possible x-rays should be taken by positioning the machine and not the extremity. Children will usually splint or immobilize an injured extremity themselves and are most likely to cooperate when they are in control of how the extremity is handled.

A very important aspect of examining a child with a suspected musculoskeletal injury is the assessment of neurovascular status. This examination is performed to detect any existing neurovascular impairment or deficit so that measures may be quickly instituted to correct the condition, thus preventing permanent deformity and disability. Circulation and innervation should be assessed, with major emphasis on the distal aspect of the extremity.

In addition to performing a neurovascular examination as part of the initial assessment of an injured child, the assessment should be ongoing and repeated at regular intervals to detect any changes that may occur. Assessment is particularly important before and after casting, splinting, the application of traction, the reduction of a fracture or dislocation, and after surgery.

The components of the circulatory assessment include evaluation of color, capillary filling, pulses, temperature, and edema. The examination for innervation includes assessment of both motor and sensory components of the nerves involved.[4]

Because this type of examination can be very difficult to perform on a child, parental participation is particularly valuable. Children may respond to parents rather than to hospital staff. Children, for a variety of reasons, will often refuse to move an injured extremity, but it is important to persist and to be patient until you have established whether the child cannot or will not perform the requested motion. Information about pain and sensation may be difficult to elicit from adults, and obtaining accurate information about these parameters is even more difficult when assessing members of the pediatric population.

Children have difficulty relating to the various words that emergency department staff may use. Most children do not know what "numb" means. Other descriptions, such as feeling "fuzzy," "funny," "different," or "asleep" are better understood by a child.[5]

The use of stories, dolls, puppets, or drawings may be very helpful in obtaining accurate information from a child. In general, for children under 7 years of age nonverbal data is much more reliable than what can be obtained verbally.[6] The child's behavior and facial expressions should be noted throughout the evaluation. Carefully observe the child for signs of grimacing and for evidence of muscle spasms. Other physiologic signs of pain include dilated pupils, pallor or flushing of the skin, nausea, vomiting, increased pulse and respirations, diaphoresis, and changes in blood pressure.

Injuries that involve a joint are often difficult or impossible to evaluate on x-ray. This is particularly true in the very young child. If there is any question of the presence of an abnormality, comparison views of the opposite extremity are indicated and are mandatory when trying to evaluate an elbow injury in a young child. As with adults, there can be more than one injury in an extremity, and x-rays should include the areas proximal and distal to the obvious site of injury. If all clinical signs point toward a significant injury and x-ray data is unclear, it is best to err on the side of overtreatment, with the consideration being to treat the child and not the x-ray.

Because children's fractures heal very quickly, follow-up should be early and frequent when there is specific cause for concern. Parents need to thoroughly understand the importance of follow-up and must be informed of the possible consequences of a delay in reevaluation.

PSYCHOSOCIAL CONSIDERATIONS

The child and the parents of a child with a musculoskeletal injury need to be treated in a gentle, caring, and informative manner. The nature of the injury, the specific intervention, and the expected outcome need to be explained in as much detail as possible. Where outcomes are uncertain or problems can be anticipated, details should be repeated several times, and possibly written, to avoid confusion or misunderstanding.

When possible children should participate in their treatment to gain their trust and cooperation and to make them feel more in control. Most orthopaedic injuries sustained by children do not require hospitalization, but when it is necessary this information should be presented calmly and reassuringly.

There is little that one can do to alleviate the terror that a cast saw has for a young child, but once again a calm and reassuring manner is extremely important. It is helpful if you demonstrate that the cast saw will not cut the child's skin by first using it on your skin. Children will also be less frightened if the noise of the cast saw is described as a "buzzing" noise and the vibration is described as "tickling." Dolls and puppets can be used to demonstrate a variety of hospital procedures, including bandaging, splinting, and casting. Older children may enjoy looking at their x-rays and receiving copies to take home, especially if a fracture is highly evident and easily seen. Making finger casts is often a good introduction to what a cast feels like, and these can be turned into finger puppets with the quick application of a "happy face" using magic marker. The presence of a friendly skeleton is often a fun way to teach children about where and what bones have been injured.

EPIPHYSEAL INJURIES

Injuries to the epiphyses in children are usually traumatic, although damage can be caused by disease processes such as osteomyelitis. Epiphyseal injuries need to be carefully evaluated, with the primary concern being the potential for the injury to cause a disturbance in growth. When the growth plate is damaged, longitudinal growth may completely cease or be retarded, resulting in a shortened extremity. Progressive angular deformities may occur when an injury causes growth to be asymmetical.[7]

Although the mechanisms of injury can be similar in children and adults, the results may be dramatically different. The trauma that frequently causes a dislocation in an adult is more likely to cause an epiphyseal separation in a child. Because ligaments in children partially attach to epiphyses and are stronger than growth cartilage, a valgus stress injury to a child's knee usually results in an injury to the distal femoral epiphysis, while the same injury in an adult is likely to cause a tear of the medial collateral ligament.

Epiphyseal injuries can be the result of shearing, splitting, avulsion, or compression-type forces. These forces determine the seriousness of the injury and the prognosis for uncomplicated recovery. Growth plate injuries are most commonly classified according to the Salter-Harris system (Fig. 21-1).[8]

Type I injuries are caused by a shearing or avulsion force that separates the epi-

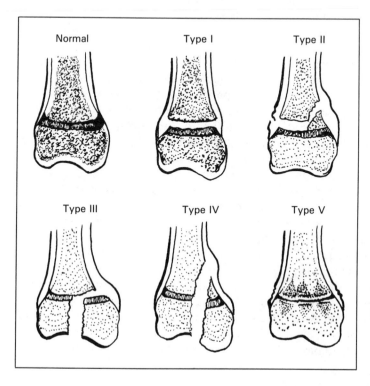

Figure 21-1. The Salter-Harris classification system used in epiphyseal injuries. *(From R.R. Simon, & S.J. Koenigsknecht. Emergency Orthopedics: The Extremities (2nd ed.). Norwalk, Conn.: Appleton & Lange, 1987, p. 19.)*

physis from the metaphysis. This often occurs without any x-ray evidence of a fracture. Because the separation is usually spontaneously reduced, the injury is not clearly visible on x-ray and may only be correctly diagnosed by tenderness to palpation directly over the growth plate rather than over ligaments. While x-ray examination will not show the cartilage, soft tissue swelling over the epiphysis is usually present and is also apparent on clinical examination.

Type II injuries, which seem to be the most common injuries, involve a separation of the epiphysis from the metaphysis, accompanied by an avulsion of a portion of the metaphysis. If properly diagnosed and treated, type I and type II injuries rarely result in growth disturbance and generally have an excellent prognosis.

Type III injuries are intra-articular and are most often seen at the lateral condyle of the distal humerus. They are caused by a splitting force that results in a fracture that extends through the growth plate into the metaphysis. Despite accurate reduction, angular deformities may develop; these injuries have a variable prognosis and are often best treated with operative fixation.

Type IV injuries are also intra-articular and not only extend from the joint surface through the epiphysis and across the epiphyseal plate but also include a portion of the metaphysis. These injuries frequently require open reduction and internal fixation.

Type V injuries are rare, usually occur in the knee or ankle, and are caused by axial compression that results in a crushing of the epiphyseal plate. These injuries often look benign, are easily overlooked, and carry a very poor prognosis even when identified and properly treated. Any injury that interferes with the blood supply to the epiphyseal plate is likely to have a poor result. This is particularly true in the areas of radial and femoral heads where the blood supply is normally somewhat limited.

An epiphyseal injury must be suspected in any child with a history of signs and symptoms of trauma near the ends of a long bone, the most common areas being the distal radius and the distal tibia.[9] Children are usually unwilling to use an injured joint when the upper extremity is involved and are unwilling to bear weight or may walk with a limp when a lower extremity is injured. Physical examination is remarkable for localized swelling and point tenderness over the growth plate. With severe injuries there may be obvious deformities of the joint. Oblique and comparison x-ray views are mandatory if there is any difficulty in defining the presence or extent of a fracture. When reduction is required the procedure should be done as soon as possible and as gently as possible. Forceful reductions may cause further injury to the epiphyseal plate and may result in premature closure of the plate and cessation of growth. The goal of reduction is to achieve anatomic congruity of the fragments and to decrease the possibility of discrepancy and distortion of growth.

In general the type of injury dictates the ultimate prognosis. Problems of growth disturbance are most common in types III through V but occur with any of these injuries.[10] The young child is more likely to suffer growth disturbances than the older child who is near the end of his or her growth period. The majority of growth plate injuries heal well and carry minimal risk for growth disturbance. Treatment should involve both the child and the parents. Careful communication is necessary if problems are anticipated. Follow-up should be consistent and should include observation of the child for the duration of his or her growing years.

FRACTURES OF THE UPPER EXTREMITIES

Figure 21–2 illustrates the various fractures of the upper extremity that can result from the force in a fall on the outstretched hand.

Clavicle Fractures

Fractures of the body of the clavicle (Fig. 21–3) are fairly common in childhood. These fractures usually result from a fall or blow to the shoulder or from a fall on the outstretched hand. The clavicle may also be fractured as a result of the passage of the shoulder through the birth canal.[11] The prognosis for uncomplicated healing of the fractured clavicle is good, and any residual deformity is usually completely resolved within 1 year.[12]

The child with a fractured clavicle will usually present with a history of pain and inability to move the arm or shoulder on the affected side. A careful history of the event surrounding the injury should be elicited. In the case of a witnessed accident or fall of a small child or with a child old enough to verbalize the mechanism of injury, the history will usually be consistent with direct impact on the shoulder or the extended arm.

Assessment. The deformity may be visible or palpable. Palpation should be performed beginning at the medial aspect of both clavicles. Using only the fingertips, gently palpate laterally, moving along both sides simultaneously for comparison.

Management. As soon as the diagnosis of a fractured clavicle is suspected, the emergency department nurse should immobilize the affected shoulder while supporting the arm on that side. This may be accomplished through the use of a simple sling with the arm flexed at 90 degrees. Immobilization and support may be further en-

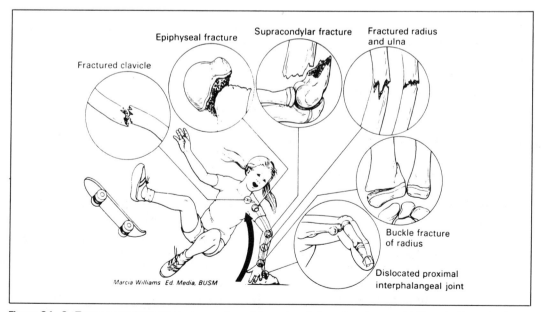

Epiphyseal fracture

Supracondylar fracture

Fractured radius and ulna

Fractured clavicle

Marcia Williams Ed. Media, BUSM

Buckle fracture of radius

Dislocated proximal interphalangeal joint

Figure 21–2. Trauma resulting from progression of force in a fall on the outstretched hand. *(From D. Segal. Pediatric orthopedic emergencies. Pediatric Clinics of North America 26, no. 4, November 1979.)*

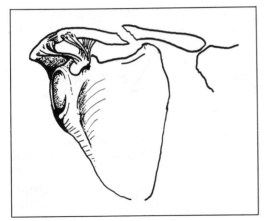

Figure 21-3. Displaced middle third fracture of the clavicle. *(From R.R. Simon, & S.J. Koenigsknecht. Emergency Orthopedics: The Extremities (2nd ed.). Norwalk, Conn.: Appleton & Lange, 1987, p. 174.)*

hanced by the use of an Ace wrap around the chest and arm.

Documentation by the emergency department nurse should include a history of the mechanism of injury and a description of any local physical findings. The documented assessment of neurovascular status must include any signs of axillary artery or brachial plexus compression, the presence or absence of distal pulses and their intensity, any temperature or color variation between the arm on the affected side and its unaffected counterpart, and any specific degree and direction of limited motion or refusal to move. The presence of any bruising in the area of the clavicle or shoulder must also be documented.[13]

Once the clavicle radiographs have confirmed the presence of a fracture, the emergency department nurse may be needed to assist the orthopaedist in the placement of the figure-of-eight clavicle splint or harness, or in the placement of swathing over the sling. When manual manipulation or reduction is not necessary, the immobilization procedure is not painful, and premedication is not necessary. If manual reduction is necessary the child should be given an analgesic prior to reduction. Care should be taken to pad the axilla to prevent chafing. Fractures of the distal third of the clavicle should be treated in the same manner as an acromioclavicular separation.[14]

Parent Education. Parents should be advised that immobilization will be necessary for 2 to 3 weeks. Parents should be informed that any deformity caused by displacement or by developing callus will disappear within 1 year. Progress will be monitored through follow-up visits with the orthopaedist.[15]

SHOULDER INJURIES

Acromioclavicular Separations

Acromioclavicular (AC) separations are more common in older children and are usually the result of a fall or blow with direct impact on the shoulder itself. The child will usually have pain and swelling over the AC joint.

Assessment. In instances in which the child is not able to move the shoulder at all, the most noted limitation of motion will be the inability to perform the abduction-adduction function. The most severe separations may be palpable due to the upward displacement of the distal end of the clavicle.[16] When the emergency department nurse suspects such an injury, shoulder films with views of both the affected and unaffected sides should be obtained, as comparison is often necessary to distinguish the minor separations.

Documentation of nursing assessment in the emergency department must include a description of the mechanism of injury, a description of any observable or palpable deformity, the presence or absence and intensity of distal pulses, and any evidence or lack of evidence of neuro-vascular compromise.

Management. The emergency department nurse should immediately provide support and immobilization of the shoulder through the application of a sling. Swathing with an Ace bandage may enhance comfort, and ice may be applied to any swelling.

Treatment of the minor (less than 1 cm of upward displacement of the clavicle) is similar to that of the fractured clavicle. The orthopaedist may utilize a sling and swath, shoulder immobilizer, or figure-of-eight strap to support the shoulder girdle in proper alignment and to promote healing. With the more severe cases of AC separation (greater than 1 cm of upward displacement of the distal clavicle), the orthopaedist must become involved in the management of this child as soon as possible, as surgery may be necessary for optimum reduction and healing.[17]

Parent Education. Discharge teaching should include instructions for the removal and reapplication of immobilization devices to assist in bathing. The importance of follow-up at recommended intervals with the orthopaedist cannot be overemphasized to assure uncomplicated healing and the return of normal function. The parents should be advised that reported feelings of numbness, tingling, or altered sensations of the fingers or hand should be taken seriously and evaluated right away.

Anterior Shoulder Dislocation

Anterior displacement of the humeral head is the most common type of shoulder dislocation in childhood. This type of injury is usually the result of a fall on the extended arm while it is abducted from the trunk and externally rotated.

Assessment. Physical assessment findings will usually indicate that the humeral head is palpable anteriorly and that the deltoid musculature is flat. In addition, the emergency department nurse should document any findings of decreased sensation over the shoulder or deltoid area indicative of an axillary nerve compomise or any positive or negative findings of vascular compromise.[18]

Management. Support of the shoulder by the application of a sling with the affected arm in internal rotation is desirable prior to obtaining films. Reduction of anterior shoulder dislocations is necessary and usually requires premedication of the child. Diazepam is used to achieve muscle relaxation in a dose of 0.1 to 0.2 mg/kg. Meperidine is the preferred drug used for analgesia in a dose of 1 to 2 mg/kg intramuscularly or intravenously (maximum dose of 50 mg). Reduction is usually complete 20 to 30 minutes after the application of weights (1 lb per 7 kg of body weight). Weights are applied with the child lying flat on his or her abdomen with the injured arm and shoulder hanging off the bed. Reduction may also be achieved by the manipulation of the humeral head and scapula by the orthopaedist. Postreduction films may show a fracture not noted previously. This may occur as a complication of the reduction process, which then must be managed clinically, as they often require surgery.[19]

Parent Education. Those children not requiring surgical intervention are usually sent home once sufficiently recovered from the analgesia and postreduction physical assessment reveals no neurovascular compromise. Parents should be instructed on the removal and replacement of immobilization (sling and swath or shoulder immobilizer) with emphasis on maintenance of the arm in the internal rotation, adducted position. Four weeks of immobilization are usually required for healing. Follow-up with the orthopaedist is essential, especially because this injury has an approximate 70 percent recurrence rate in children and may require surgery. As with all injuries of the upper extremities, parents should be advised to take seriously any complaints of paresthesias (numbness, tingling) or temperature or color changes in the hand on the affected side and to return for assessment as soon as these symptoms develop.[20]

Fractures of the Scapula

Scapular fractures are rare in childhood and are usually the result of severe blunt trauma. This child may well have several associated injuries. Swelling and any tenderness directly over the scapula are indications for the inclusion of scapular views along with other films that may be necessary. When uncomplicated, fractures of the scapula may be managed with a sling and swath and then followed by the orthopaedist.[21]

Pulled Shoulder

The torn shoulder capsule is frequently seen in toddlers and young children who have been pulled suddenly or lifted by the arm or hand.

Assessment. This child usually presents with refusal to move or to use the affected arm, and a painful response will be initiated on any attempt at passive range of motion of the shoulder. Shoulder films will be negative for fractures and dislocation.

Management. Immobilization with a sling for 7 to 10 days is necessary to allow healing of the capsule. In addition to advising the parents of the more serious possibilities for injury resulting from such traction on the arm, the parents should be shown

how to quickly lift a child without potential for injury. The emergency department nurse should demonstrate the lift by stooping, wrapping the adult arm around the chest under both axilla, and lifting the child onto a hip. Parents should also be advised that if pain persists past one week, they should bring the child back to the orthopaedist for repeat evaluation and films to rule out the possibility of a fracture or separation of the proximal humeral epiphysis that was undetectable at the time of the original visit.[22]

Fractures of the Proximal Humeral Epiphysis

The most common occurrence in older children and adolescents with shoulder injuries is a Salter II epiphyseal fracture—separation of the proximal humerus. This injury may be caused by direct blunt trauma but is more frequently the result of a fall backwards landing on the extended arm.[23]

Assessment. On physical assessment the emergency department nurse should document the presence of pain, local swelling, and bruising, as well as limitations of motion and any indication of possible neurovascular compromise distally. There may be an absence of palpable bony deformity, as anterior angulation or displacement is usually minimal.

Management. Clinical management of the minor proximal epiphyseal injury with separation less than 1 cm and angulation of less than 20 to 40 percent and no malrotation is usually accomplished with the application of a shoulder immobilizer or sling and swath. Injuries with a greater degree of angulation usually necessitate a closed reduction. In fractures involving three pieces of the proximal humeral head, surgery is usually indicated.[24]

Parent Education. As with other shoulder injuries, parents should be instructed on the removal and reapplication of the immobilization device, the importance of follow-up with the orthopaedist, and the importance of having reported sensations of numbness or tingling in the hand or arm evaluated rapidly.

Humeral Fractures

Fractures of the humeral shaft are seen less frequently in children than in adults. The mechanism of injury in infants may be birth injury or the inflicted physical injury in child abuse. In the toddler and young child, battered child syndrome should be a strong suspicion, as the spiral fracture of the body of the humerus is usually the direct result of a twist.[25] In older children the possibility of abuse continues to exist, but the fracture may also be the result of a fall on the extended arm. Transverse fractures of the humeral shaft are usually the result of a direct blow.[26]

Assessment. Fractures of the humeral shaft are rarely displaced due to the thickness of the periosteal sleeve around the humerus (Fig. 21–4). Bony deformity may therefore not be an obvious presenting sign. There may be swelling and ecchymosis locally, as well as the inability to move the arm. The emergency department nurse should immediately immobilize the upper arm with a suitable splint to reduce pain caused by bone grating on movement. The child must also be assessed for the possibility of neurovascular compromise. Documentation should include presence or absence and intensity of distal pulses, color or temperature variations from the opposite limb, and motion and sensation distal to injury site. Films should include shoulder and elbow to rule out associated injuries.

Management. In a humeral shaft fracture not involving severe angulation or displacement, alignment can easily be maintained by the application of a long arm plaster splint (sugar tong) from wrist to axilla with the elbow flexed at 90 degrees. The splinted arm is then supported in a sling and may be swathed. After application of the splint and sling the emergency department nurse should again document the neurovascular status distal to the injury site.[27]

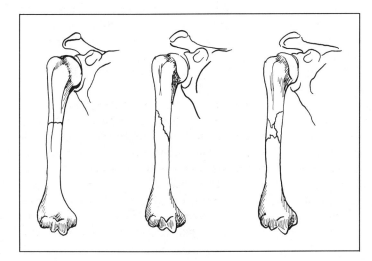

Figure 21–4. Nondisplaced or minimally displaced humeral shaft fractures. *(From R.R. Simon, & S.J. Koenigsknecht. Emergency Orthopedics: The Extremities (2nd ed.). Norwalk, Conn.: Appleton & Lange, 1987, p. 146.)*

Parent Education. Parents should be instructed to keep plaster dry, as it may change shape or break down if wet. They should also be alert to complaints of pain, pressure sensations, or feelings of numbness or tingling by the child, as these may be indications that further swelling has occurred, and revision of the splint may be necessary. Close follow-up with the orthopaedist is desirable, and the splint will usually need to remain in place for 4 to 6 weeks.

INJURIES TO THE ELBOW

Supracondylar Fractures of the Humerus

The supracondylar humeral fracture is the most common type of elbow fracture. It usually occurs between the ages of 3 and 12 years with peak incidence at 5 to 8 years of age. This fracture is usually the result of a fall on the outstretched arm with some elbow flexion and pronated forearm.[28] Supracondylar fractures of the humerus constitute an emergent condition requiring prompt and effective intervention.

Assessment. The child will usually arrive with the history of injury, pain, and very little ability to move the elbow. Neurovascular condition of the injury site and distal portions of the arm must be assessed and documented carefully and frequently. Bleeding, hematoma, and swelling are likely to occur due to the displacement of the distal fragment posteriorly on the proximal fragment and the resultant stretch of the brachial artery and vein. Compartment syndrome may occur as a result of the vascular damage in combination with swelling in the fascial compartments of the forearm. The degree of actual deformity is dependent on the degree of displacement.[29]

Management. When there is minimal displacement, conservative immobilization with a splint is often sufficient. As soon as the diagnosis of significant displacement is confirmed by radiographic examination, the reduction must be planned. Closed manipulation reduction is usually performed under general anesthesia to assure complete relaxation of the musculature. Since closed manipulation reduction is often difficult, open reduction with stabilization by Kirchner wires is sometimes preferred.[30]

In cases of supracondylar fractures, the child is usually admitted for at least the first 24 hours so that careful and frequent observations of neurovascular status can be made. Pain, poor perfusion, pallor, cyanosis, and decreased sensation are the most significant assessment parameters as well as the intensity of the radial pulse. At any indication of impending Volkmann's contracture or compartment syndrome, emergency surgical intervention to explore the vasculature is often necessary.[31]

Fractures of the Capitellum

Capitellum (lateral condyle) fractures are usually Salter IV injuries that transect the epiphysis. These injuries are usually seen in 3- to 15-year-olds who give the history of a fall on the extended arm. This injury represents a serious potential for further complications because malunion is likely to occur from minimal displacement if the fracture site is not properly stabilized.[32]

Assessment. Because these children may not have significant deformity, the history of the fall, the presence of pain, and swelling over the lateral aspect of the distal humerus become the most important clinical cues of the possibility of a fractured capitellum. Films of the injured elbow as well as of the other side will be helpful for comparison to assure accurate diagnosis. Assessment parameters for the emergency department nurse include neurovascular status distal to the injury as well as the ability to pronate-supinate the forearm.

Management. The potential late complications of this injury include joint stiffness, severe cubitus valgus, and traction palsy of the ulnar nerve, which can produce paralysis years later. Due to the gravity of these potential complications, management of the capitellum fracture in its early stages is very important. When there is no displacement, conservative treatment with a splint is acceptable. The importance of close follow-up with the orthopaedist, however, cannot be overemphasized, as a slight migration of the fragment may lead to the problems discussed above. Children who have even minimal displacement usually undergo open reduction under general anesthesia to assure proper stabilization and fixation. These children always require hospital admission.[33]

Fractures of the Medial Humeral Epicondyle

These injuries are rarely seen in children, but when they occur they have the same potential complications discussed in association with the lateral condyle, due to the proximity of the ulnar nerve.

Management. Displacement of less than 1 cm is usually managed with splinting and follow-up. Open surgical reduction is usually only necessary with displacement greater than 1 cm or demonstrated compression of the ulnar nerve. These fractures produce marked swelling and bleeding that may extend to the forearm. Due to the possibility of compartment syndrome, children with medial epicondylar fractures are usually admitted for frequent and careful observation of their neurovascular status.[34]

Posterior Elbow Dislocation

Posterior elbow dislocation (Fig. 21-5) represents the second most common type of dislocation seen in children. It is usually caused by a fall on the hyperextended arm.

Assessment. These children will show marked deformity, swelling, and joint effusion. There may be associated fractures, usually supracondylar. Neurovascular status must be assessed carefully, as compromise is not infrequent.

Management. Prior to reduction the child should be medicated with diazepam (0.1 to 0.2 mg/kg) for muscle relaxation or merperidine (1 to 2 mg/kg) for pain. The child is placed lying flat on his or her abdomen with the arm hanging over the side of the bed. Gentle traction is exerted on the forearm to relocate the elbow. Neurovascular assessment is also essential in the immediate postreduction phase, as is a second motor function examination. Postreduction films should be obtained to assure proper alignment and to check for associated fractures. The elbow is then flexed at 90 degrees, and a splint is placed. Radial pulse should be checked after flexion to assure vascular integrity. The parents should be advised that the splint will remain in place for 2 to 3 weeks, and follow-up is essential with the orthopaedist.[35]

Radial Head Dislocation or Subluxation

The "nursemaid's elbow" is most commonly seen in the young child and is usually the result of a sudden pull on the pronated forearm.

Assessment. The child will usually arrive with the affected arm held in pronation and will refuse to move it. Attempts at supination yield a pain response. Elbow

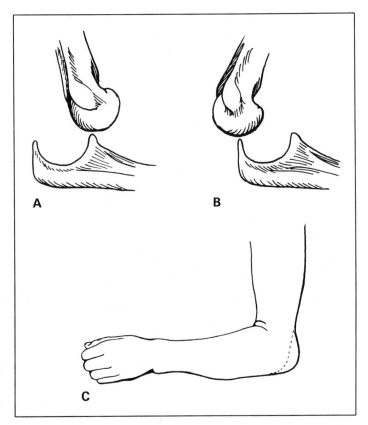

Figure 21–5. Posterior **(A)** and anterior **(B)** dislocations of the elbow. Note the posterior protuberance of the olecranon in a posterior dislocation **(C)**. *(From R.R. Simon, & S.J. Koenigsknecht. Emergency Orthopedics: The Extremities (2nd ed.). Norwalk, Conn.: Appleton & Lange, 1987, p. 320.)*

films will usually be negative, as the supinated position required for the films usually reduces the dislocation.[36]

Management. Relief is usually immediate upon reduction of the dislocation by the physician. Immobilization with a sling is only necessary for comfort.

Parent Education. Parents should be instructed on the negative effects of pulling or lifting a child by the hand or forearm. They should also be advised to return with the child if he or she has any further refusal to move his or her arm.

Radial Neck Fractures

When the proximal radial head has separated from the shaft of the radius at more than 30 degrees of angulation, open reduction may be necessary (Fig. 21–6). Proper realignment is necessary to assure normal bone growth and the pronation-supination function of the forearm.[37]

FRACTURES OF THE FOREARM

Forearm fractures account for up to 20 percent of all childhood fractures. These children will usually give the history of a fall landing on the palm of the hand or a direct blow to the forearm, swelling, and obvious deformity. Since there is often an associated injury, forearm films should always include views of the elbow and wrist. Splinting will often reduce pain for the child caused by bone grating on motion.[38]

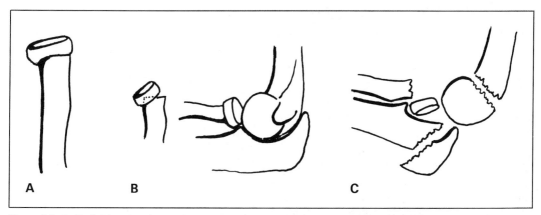

Figure 21-6. Radial head and neck fractures (epiphyseal fractures in children). **A.** Nonangulated (15 degrees angulation). **B.** Angulated (greater than 15 degrees angulation). **C.** Displaced radial head. *(From R.R. Simon, & S.J. Koenigsknecht. Emergency Orthopedics: The Extremities (2nd ed.). Norwalk, Conn.: Appleton & Lange, 1987, p. 102.)*

Types of Fractures

Monteggia's fracture produces an overriding fracture of the shaft of a single bone (usually the ulna) with associated dislocation of the radial head. The radial head involvement is a critical clinical feature that may be missed if the elbow is not included in the films.[39]

Torus (buckle) fractures are common in children and usually have no displacement or clear fracture line. They are frequently seen as a disruption of the smooth cortex, usually at the distal end, and may involve both bones.

A greenstick fracture is a linear fracture involving the diaphysis of either long bone. The fracture line does not transect the shaft of the bone but runs laterally along one side of the cortex.

Colles' fractures transect the distal radius, with dorsal angulation occurring simultaneously with a Salter II epiphyseal fracture of the ulnar styloid.

The antithesis of the Colles' fracture is a Smith's fracture in which volar angulation occurs. This is usually caused by a blow to the forearm while it is held in pronation.

Barton's fracture consists of a marginal fracture of either the dorsal or volar surface of the radius with corresponding dislocation of the carpal bones and hand.

Galeazzi's fracture is a common fracture of the forearm occuring at the junction of the middle and distal third of the radial shaft. Radioulnar subluxation may accompany this fracture.[40]

Management. Ongoing documented assessment of the neurovascular status distal to the fracture site is essential, as compromise is a possible complication of most fractures of the forearm. Reduction becomes necessary if angulation exceeds 15 degrees. Open reduction with internal fixation is usually necessary if both the radius and ulna are fractured. Due to the possibility of further swelling, fractures of the forearm are usually immobilized with wrapped anterior and posterior splints or a bivalved cast. Casting is usually maintained for 4 to 6 weeks.[41]

Parents will need instructions in cast care and application of the sling. Parents will also need instruction in administration of an analgesic, such as acetaminophen, for pain in the first 48 to 72 hours.

Hand Injuries

Hand injuries are a common occurrence in childhood, and their accurate assessment and management are very important due to the possibilities of later functional impairment. The history of the mechanism of injury is important to elicit, as it provides the initial direction of the physical assessment. If the history is inconsistent with the physical findings, the possibility of child abuse must be considered and investigated.

Assessment. The presence and location of hand swelling and tenderness are the best clinical cues for focusing the physical assessment. As is true with most pediatric problems, the emergency department nurse should begin the assessment with the least painful features and proceed quickly and systematically. Observe the hand at rest for obvious location of swelling, deformities, or discolorations. If the fingers override on flexion, a malrotation injury should be suspected. Assess the fingertips and nail beds for cyanosis and capillary filling.

The presence of sweating on the palmar aspect of the hand is indicative of intact sympathetic functioning of the digital nerve. Sensation distal to the injury must be assessed as a parameter of function of these three major nerves: radial nerve (web space), median nerve (tip of index finger), and ulnar nerve (tip of little finger). The motor ability of each finger should be assessed by supporting the joints immediately below and by asking the child to alternately flex and extend the distal interphalangeal, phalangeal interphalangeal, and metacarpal interphalangeal of each affected finger.[42]

Types of Injuries

Navicular Fractures. The carpal bones are largely composed of cartilage and rarely become fractured in childhood. Navicular fractures (scaphoid bone), however, are likely to occur in older children as the result of a fall on the dorsiflexed hand. These children typically have tenderness over the navicular and weakened grip strength. Even though the initial films may not show irregularities of the navicular, the clinical findings alone are sufficient to warrant immobilization of the wrist and thumb until films are repeated 10 days later. Approximately 50 percent of the time no fracture will be seen on the follow-up films, and immobilization may be discontinued. If the fracture line does become evident on the follow-up films, however, parents should be advised that immobilization and follow-up must continue for an additional 6 weeks to prevent nonunion and the resultant avascular necrosis.[43]

Metacarpal Fractures. Metacarpal bone fractures are likely to occur from a direct blow to the hand. These children will arrive with swelling, joint tenderness, deformity, and displacement. A boxer's fracture is a fracture of the metacarpal head of the little finger. The rarer Bennett's fracture occurs at the metacarpal base of the thumb. Immobilization of these fractures consists of splinting from distal phalanges to mid-forearm with wrist extended and metacarpal phalangeal joint flexed. Parents should be advised that immobilization will continue for 3 to 4 weeks.[44]

Finger Fractures. Finger fractures are a common occurrence in childhood. Perhaps the most common injury is the crush of the distal phalanx, resulting from entrapment of the child's finger in a door or machinery. When concurrent lacerations occur, copious irrigation, some suturing, and sterile dressings may be required, but as a general rule these injuries heal well in children. Fractures or exposure of the distal tuft occurring in association with amputation of the distal fingertip may require some skin grafting and nail repair, but these also heal well.

Mallet finger deformities are frequently the result of epiphyseal separation of the phalanges. These are usually managed by splinting the finger in hyperextension.

Fractures of the shaft of the phalanx usually result in some angulation requiring reduction and careful splinting to prevent malalignment.

Fractures of the proximal phalanx may be difficult to reduce requiring surgery and open fixation when a spiral fracture is present or when the head is irreversibly displaced.[45]

FRACTURES OF THE LOWER EXTREMITIES

Pelvic Fractures

The most important aspect of pelvic fractures is the possibility of damage to the viscera or major vessels. The bony damage is of secondary importance.[46] Classification of pelvic fractures is varied; however, the following types may be used as a general guide: (1) avulsion fractures, (2) fractures of the pelvic ring, and (3) fractures involving the acetabulum.[47]

Crush fractures of the pelvis seldom occur in childhood because of the elasticity of the bony ring with its interposed cartilage buffers. A more common injury consists of a separation or compression injury to the pelvis. These injuries are many times the result of overzealous activity in sports. Fractures involving the acetabulum are also rare in children.

Patients with simple stable fractures of the pelvis have a good prognosis for uncomplicated healing. Crush injuries of the pelvis occur, in the majority of cases, as a result of high-energy accidents and usually involve multiple trauma. A rapid and thorough assessment is essential for the successful treatment of these patients.

Mild Displacement Injuries

Assessment. Children with mild displacement injuries experience weakness and pain with activity. Close attention to the history, especially to any involvement in sports, will usually provide the source of the injury. There is usually no difficulty in the diagnosis of severe crush injuries; the child complains of pain in the pelvic region, and bruising and swelling in the perineum is often present. If, however, severe multiple injuries have occurred, evaluation of the amount of trauma to the associated systems will take precedence.[48]

Management. Less severe pelvic injuries, namely those that do not involve the weight-bearing columns, can be treated simply by a period of bedrest for 2 to 4 weeks and guarded ambulation until symptoms subside. If the fracture is unstable, the child may be placed in a spica cast or pelvic sling. The emergency department nurse should immobilize the child until the diagnosis is confirmed. Support and an explanation of the future treatment and rehabilitation process should also be provided to the family.

Severe Crush Injuries

In the case of severe crush injuries, it is the damage to the contents of the pelvis that is of primary importance. Evaluation and treatment of these patients should begin at the accident site with gentle handling, proper splinting, and careful transport.[49]

These cases often involve multiple trauma. An adequate airway must be established and ventilation supported if required. The treatment of injuries to any organs will begin with early fluid and blood replacement. If there has been major soft tissue damage associated with the fracture, the general principles of open fracture and wound care must be applied. Radiologic examination will usually be postponed until the child's condition is stable.

Assessment. The nurse must assess the patient carefully. The initial hospital examination requires complete exposure of the patient and the recording of all injuries, whether obvious or suspected. The emergency department nurse should take particular care with the documentation of this assessment. The emergency department nurse may need to assist the orthopaedist with a fixation device if so prescribed. Surgical intervention may be necessary to repair other involved organs or severe pelvic fractures. If surgery is required the emergency department nurse should prepare the patient, explain the procedure to the parents, and provide emotional support.

Parent Education. The importance of following all instructions regarding ambulation and weight bearing must be stressed to the parents and child. Parents should be cautioned that the child may feel like ambulating before the healing process has been effective. Long-term follow-up will be necessary to observe for any residual deformity.

Hip and Femoral Fractures

The management of fractures of the femur presents problems not found with other long bones of the skeleton. The femur is a primary weight-bearing bone and is enveloped by some of the most powerful muscles of the body. About 70 percent of all fractures of the shaft of the femur in children occur in the middle third, 18 percent in the proximal third, and the remaining 12 percent in the distal end.[50] Most children's fractures are transverse, oblique, or spiral in direction. Simple fractures of the femur occur most often during childhood games. The modern machine age has also contributed to the number of complex injuries. Hip fractures in children are very uncommon as compared to hip fractures in adults.

Most children with simple fractures of the femur have a satisfactory outcome with any reasonable form of treatment. The problem fractures of the femur include severely comminuted fractures with extensive soft tissue trauma or bone loss. A significant functional deformity may follow severe trauma (Fig. 21-7).[51]

Assessment. Deformity, swelling, and tenderness are present on physical examination; however, radiographic examination will confirm the diagnosis. The emergency department nurse plays a most important role in implementing neurovascular assessment of the injured limb. The color, warmth, and sensation of the limb must be checked at regular intervals. The evaluation of the extremity must include palpation for distal pulses and mobility of the toes.

Management. Immobilization of the injured limb will precede any treatment. Close observation of the limb must begin at that point to avoid future complications such as nerve palsy. Once the diagnosis has been confirmed, the most common form of treatment includes closed reduction of the fracture followed by traction or casting. Operative stabilization of severe fractures includes external pin fixation, intramedullary pins or rods, or plates. Although internal fixation is justified in special situations, the routine use is inappropriate. The foot must be supported

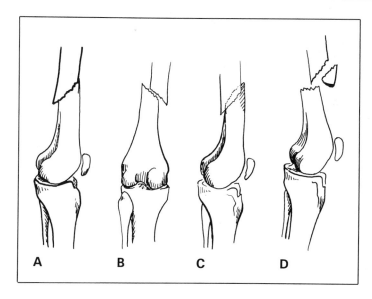

Figure 21–7. Femoral shaft fractures. **A, B,** and **C.** Displaced fractures. **A.** Minimal displacement. **B.** Moderate displacement. **C.** Displacement with overriding of fragments (lateral view). **D.** Comminuted fracture. *(From R.R. Simon, & S.J. Koenigsknecht. Emergency Orthopedics: The Extremities (2nd ed.). Norwalk, Conn.: Appleton & Lange, 1987, p. 224.)*

to prevent an equinus deformity and care taken to avoid skin damage from the pressure of any support.

Parent Education. The parents should be advised of the immobilization period needed in the treatment of the child's fracture. This time will vary according to the severity of the fracture. Both the parents and the child (if old enough to understand) should be taught basic neurovascular assessment. The parents should be concerned if the child complains of continued pain, loss of sensation, or refusal to move the toes. Such symptoms should be reported immediately to the orthopaedist. The long-term rehabilitation plan, including physical therapy requirements, should be clearly outlined to the family.

Knee Injuries

The importance of these injuries lies not only in the fact that the lower extremity is used for mobilization, transportation, and weight bearing but that the child differs from the adult because of the tremendous growth potential about the knee. The area about the knee determines approximately

65 percent of the longitudinal growth of the lower extremity. An injury could cause an inhibition in the growth plates of the knee resulting in significant leg length discrepancy.[52] Careful treatment and follow-up is crucial due to the very real threat of deformity from abnormal growth following an injury.

Injuries of the knee may be grouped as follows: (1) fracture separation of the lower femoral epiphysis, (2) injuries of the patella, (3) fractures of the tibial spine, and (4) fracture of the upper tibial epiphysis.[53]

Sports injuries account for the majority of cases seen, with automobile accidents also contributing a large number. A smaller number occur in newborns at the time of delivery.

Assessment. The patient is usually unable to walk or to bear weight on the injured limb immediately after sustaining an injury. The pain is often quite severe. Effusion of the knee and soft tissue swelling develop rapidly, and a deformity may be evident if the separation is displaced. If the injury has caused an impingement on the popliteal artery, the pulses may be diminished or absent and the foot may be cold and pale.

The emergency department nurse must assist in a careful assessment of patients with knee injuries. Diagnosis of knee fractures is sometimes difficult, and the nurse's observations are essential. Documentation should include the patient's activity previous to the injury and all physical findings. The neurovascular status of the affected limb must be evaluated carefully. Impingment of a nerve or vessel could occur not only from the injury itself but also from support or immobilization devices.

Management. Once the diagnosis has been confirmed by the radiographic findings, treatment will vary according to the severity of the injury. The majority of knee injuries in children are treated with gentle manipulation or closed reduction followed by cast or brace application. Open reduction is performed only if closed reduction fails to produce realignment or if a fragment requires internal fixation. Care is taken to avoid disturbing the growth plates if possible.[54] The emergency department nurse may assist the orthopaedist in the manipulation of the knee or in the application of a cast or brace.

The child may be medicated if the pain has been severe, and standard procedure for a medicated patient should be followed.

Parent Education. Explanations to the child and family are especially important due to the possible residual deformity following a knee injury in the young patient. The nurse should make certain that the family understands the long-range treatment and rehabilitation plan. The patient may be discharged from the hospital in a cast or brace. The basic circulatory checks (warmth, sensation, and color of the foot and leg) should be explained to the par-

ents. Written instructions should be given to the family on the application and care of a knee brace or routine cast care, if applicable.

Fractures of the Tibia and Fibula

These injuries can be divided into two groups: (1) fractures of the upper tibial metaphysis and (2) fractures of the shafts of the tibia and fibula (Fig. 21–8).[55]

The complications and treatment of injuries involving the upper tibial metaphysis were discussed in the preceding "Knee Injuries" section. Fractures of the tibial shaft are the most common injuries of the lower limb. Complete fractures occur more often than greenstick fractures (where the bone is partially bent and partially broken). These fractures may occur

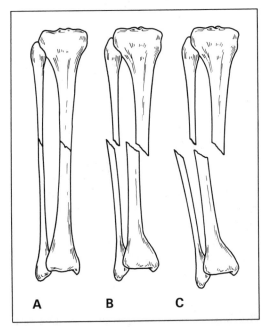

Figure 21–8. Tibial and fibular shaft fractures. **A.** Zero to 50 degrees displacement. **B.** Greater than 50 degrees displacement but with bony contact. **C.** Complete displacement. *(From R.R. Simon, & S.J. Koenigsknecht. Emergency Orthopedics: The Extremities (2nd ed.). Norwalk, Conn.: Appleton & Lange, 1987, p. 249.)*

as the result of an indirect force, such as a twisting motion, or as a result of direct violence. Although fractures of the tibia and fibula heal readily, complications such as leg length discrepancy are not uncommon due to the interrupted growth pattern. Corrective surgery may be necessary at some point following healing to prevent a deformity that could lead to joint degeneration.

Assessment. The signs and symptoms of shaft fractures differ according to the force involved in the injury. There may be no history of trauma or sign of injury. An incomplete or greenstick fracture may not prevent the child from walking; however, there will be complaint of pain and a limp. The child should be questioned carefully to find out the exact location of pain. Any activity prior to the injury should also be noted to try to determine the force involved. Neurovascular checks should include documentation of warmth, color, and sensation of the foot and a comparison of pulses on the affected limb to the uninjured leg. Diagnosis may only be made after careful evaluation of anteroposterior and lateral radiographs of the limb.

Management. Regardless of whether the injury is obvious or suspected, the limb should be immobilized. Unless the fracture is complicated or massive tissue damage has occurred, these fractures are treated with closed reduction and immobilization in a long leg cast for 5 to 8 weeks. The emergency department nurse may need to assist in the cast application.

Parent Education. Instructions should be given to the child and family concerning the care of casts. Basic neurovascular checks should also be taught. The child should be given a basic understanding of the injury and the long-term treatment and rehabilitation. The importance of following the physician's orders for activity resumptions and continued follow-up visits must be reinforced by the nurse.

Ankle Injuries

The pattern of ankle fractures in children differs from that of adults because the majority involve the lower tibial epiphyseal plate. A common cause for ankle fracture is a fall while the foot is fixed. Crush injuries of the ankle occur less but may involve multiple trauma. The seriousness of these injuries lies in the possibility of displacement of a part of the epiphyseal plate. Consequently there is bound to be some interference with bone growth and a chance of ankle deformity. If no displacement of the plate has occurred, then the effect upon bone growth is minimal. The prognosis for ankle fractures must be cautious until the child has been observed for several years.[56]

Assessment. Close observation with detailed documentation of the injured area is essential. Neurovascular signs should be noted along with any obvious trauma, such as swelling or bruising.

Management. Immobilization of the ankle is necessary for transport. Closed reduction with casting is the treatment of choice, although open reduction and internal fixation may be needed to reduce the displacement.

Parent Education. The possibility of a residual deformity should be explained to the parents so that they will cooperate in maintaining the lengthy follow-up of their child. Routine cast care, neurovascular checks, and ambulation instructions should be outlined clearly.

Foot Injuries

The child's foot is so flexible that a force applied to it is usually transmitted higher up to produce the fracture. Almost all fractures of the foot are due to direct trauma in which the associated injuries would take precedence.[57] The most notable feature of foot injuries is that almost all of the fractures of the foot heal well with a minimum of treatment.

Assessment. Pain, soft tissue swelling, and discoloration will usually be present; however, radiographs are needed to confirm the diagnosis.

Management. The emergency department nurse should note the nature of the injury. Treatment of any severe tissue damage will take precedence. If there is no evidence of trauma, the foot will be elevated and ice applied until a diagnosis is confirmed. The majority of fractures will be treated with a toe splint, a flexible bandage for support, or a cast. Seldom is surgical intervention necessary. The nurse will need to assist in the application of a support device and observe for good alignment.

Parent Education. Although the severity of a fracture in the foot may appear less severe than an injury involving one of the long bones, the patient still needs support and teaching. Instruction in cast care, neurovascular evaluation, and follow-up care should not be neglected.

NOTES

1. N.E. Hilt, & W.E. Schmitt. *Pediatric Orthopedic Nursing.* St. Louis: Mosby, 1975, p. 12.
2. J.C. Adams. *Outline of Fractures* (5th ed.). London: E&S Livingstone, 1968, p. 7.
3. Hilt, & Schmitt, *Pediatric Orthopedic Nursing,* p. 16.
4. F.L. McCullough, & L.M. Evans. Assessment of neurovascular status in children. *Orthopaedic Nursing* 4, no. 4(July/Aug 1985):21.
5. McCullough, & Evans, Assessment of neurovascular status, p. 23.
6. Ibid., p. 24.
7. W.H. Oh, C. Craig, & H.H. Banks. Epiphyseal injuries. *Pediatric Clinics of North America* 21, no. 2(May 1974):409.
8. Ibid., p. 409.
9. Ibid., p. 418.
10. Ibid., p. 411.
11. W.J.W. Sharrard. *Paediatric Orthopaedics and Fractures.* Oxford, England: Blackwell Scientific, 1971, p. 932.
12. A.H. Crawford, & A.S. Cionni. Management of pediatric orthopedic injuries by the emergency medicine specialist. *Topics in Emergency Medicine* October 1982, p. 69.
13. Sharrard, *Paediatric Orthopaedics,* p. 934.
14. D. Mayeda. Orthopedic injuries. In R.M. Barkin, & P. Rosen (Eds.), *Emergency Pediatrics.* St. Louis: Mosby, 1984, p. 409.
15. Crawford, & Cionni, Management, p. 69.
16. Mayeda, Orthopedic injuries, p. 409.
17. Ibid., p. 410.
18. Sharrard, *Paediatric Orthopaedics,* p. 491.
19. Mayeda, Orthopedic injuries, pp. 410–411.
20. Ibid., p. 411.
21. Ibid., p. 412.
22. Sharrard, *Paediatric Orthopaedics,* p. 943.
23. H.H. Sherk. Musculoskeletal injuries. In Fleisher, G., & Ludwig, S. (Eds), *Textbook of Pediatric Emergency Medicine.* Baltimore: Williams & Wilkins, 1983, p. 957.
24. Mayeda, Orthopedic injuries, p. 412.
25. Sherk, Musculoskeletal injuries, p. 958.
26. Mayeda, Orthopedic injuries, p. 413.
27. Ibid.
28. Ibid.
29. Sherk, Musculoskeletal injuries, p. 959.
30. Ibid.
31. Skolnick, et al. Supracondylar fractures of the humerus in children. *Orthopedics* 3, no. 5(May 1980), p. 405.
32. Sherk, Musculoskeletal injuries, p. 961.
33. Skolnick, Supracondylar fractures, p. 404.
34. Sherk, Musculoskeletal injuries, p. 964.
35. Mayeda, Orthopedic injuries, p. 414.
36. Ibid., p. 415.
37. Sharrard, *Paediatric Orthopaedics,* p. 974.

38. Sherk, Musculoskeletal injuries, p. 966.
39. Sharrard, *Paediatric Orthopaedics*, p. 978.
40. Mayeda, Orthopedic injuries, p. 416.
41. Ibid., pp. 416–417.
42. Ibid., p. 418.
43. Sherk, Musculoskeletal injuries, p. 972.
44. Mayeda, Orthopedic injuries, p. 420.
45. Sherk, Musculoskeletal injuries, pp. 974–975.
46. A.G. Pollen. *Fractures and Dislocations in Children*. Baltimore: Williams & Wilkins, 1973, p. 141.
47. J.C. Hohl. Symposium on fractures and other injuries in children. *Orthopedic Clinics of North America* 7, no. 3(1976):616.
48. L.F. Peltier. The fractured pelvis. *Medical Times* 104, no. 1(1976):78.
49. Ibid., p. 77.
50. W.D. Blount. *Fractures in Children*. Baltimore: Williams & Wilkins, 1954.
51. C.A. Rockwood, K.E. Wilkens, & R.E. King (Eds.), *Fractures in Children*. Philadelphia: Lippincott, 1984.
52. Hohl, Symposium on fractures, p. 880.
53. Pollen, *Fractures and Dislocations*, p. 170.
54. Rockwood, *Fractures in Children*, p. 903.
55. Pollen, *Fractures and Dislocations*, p. 179.
56. Ibid., pp. 220–207.
57. Hohl, Symposium on fractures, p. 677.

BIBLIOGRAPHY

Pediatric Orthopaedic Emergencies

Bernstein, S., King, J., & Sanderson, R. Fractures of the medial epicondyle of the humerus. *Contemporary Orthopaedics* 3, no. 7(July 1981):637–641.

Crawford, A.H., & Cionni, A.S. Management of pediatric orthopedic injuries by the emergency medicine specialist. *Topics in Emergency Medicine* October 1982, pp. 61–73.

DeLee, J., Wilkins, K., Rogers, L., & Rockwood, C. Fractures—separation of the distal humeral epiphysis. *Journal of Bone and Joint Surgery* 62, no. 8(December 1980):46–51.

Denton, J.R., & Goldsmith, H.S., (Eds.). *Orthopedics*, vol. 2. Philadelphia: Harper and Row, 1984.

Fahmy, N.R.M. Unusual monteggia lesions in children. *Injury: The British Journal of Accident Surgery* 12, no. 5(1981):399–404.

Harrington, I.J. & Tountas, A.A. Replacement of the radial heads in the treatment of unstable elbow fractures. *Injury: The British Journal of Accident Surgery* 12, no. 5(1981).

Hilt, N.E., & Schmitt W.E. *Pediatric Orthopedic Nursing*. St. Louis: Mosby, 1975.

Hilt, N.E., & Cogburn, S. *Manual of Orthopaedics*. St. Louis: Mosby, 1980.

Holda, M., & LaMont, R. Epiphyseal separation of the distal end of the humerus with medial displacement. *Journal of Bone and Joint Surgery* 62, no. 8(December 1980):52–57.

Lee, B., Esterhai, J., & Dias, M. Fractures of the distal radial epiphysis. *Clinical Orthopaedics and Related Research* 185(May 1984):90–96.

Lucas, G., & Sachtjen, K. An analysis of hand function in patients with Colles' fracture treated by rush rod fixation. *Clinical Orthopaedics and Related Research* 155(March-April 1981):172–179.

Macy, N.J. Orthopedic emergencies. In Crain, E.F., & Gershel, J.C. (Eds.), *A Clinical Manual of Emergency Pediatrics*. Norwalk, Conn.: Appleton-Century-Crofts, 1986, pp. 415–428.

Mayeda, D. Orthopedic injuries. In Barkin, R. (Ed.), *Emergency Pediatrics*. St. Louis: Mosby, 1984.

McCullough, F.L., & Evans, L.M. Assessment of neurovascular status in children. *Orthopaedic Nursing* 4, no. 4(July/August 1985):19.

McMinn, D.J.W. Mallet finger fractures. *Injury: The British Journal of Accident Surgery.* 12, no. 6(1981):477–479.

Morrissey, R., & Wilkins, K. Deformity following distal humeral fracture in childhood. *Journal of Bone and Joint Surgery* 66-A, no. 4(April 1984):557–561.

Rockwood, C.A. Jr., Wilkins, K.E., & King, R.E. *Fractures in Children*. Philadelphia: Lippincott, 1984.

Segal, D. Pediatric orthopedic emergencies. *Pediatric Clinics of North America* 26, no. 4(November 1979):793–801.

Sharrad, W.J.W. *Paediatric Orthopaedics and Fractures*. Oxford, England: Blackwell Scientific, 1971.

Sherk, H.H. Musculoskeletal injuries. In

Fleisher, G., & Ludwig, S. (Eds.), *Textbook of Pediatric Emergency Medicine*. Baltimore: Williams & Wilkins, 1983.

Siffert, R.S. Injuries to the growth plate and the epiphysis. In *Instructional Course Lectures*, *American Academy of Orthopaedics Surgeons*, vol. 29. St. Louis: Mosby, 1980.

Skolnick, et al. Supracondylar fractures of the humerus in children. *Orthopedics* 3, no. 5(May 1980):395–405.

EMERGENCY DEPARTMENT CARE GUIDE FOR THE CHILD WITH AN ORTHOPAEDIC EMERGENCY

Nursing Diagnosis	Interventions	Evaluation
Alteration in comfort: pain related to musculoskeletal injury	Assess child's level of pain Administer analgesic as indicated Apply ice to decrease swelling to injured site Immobilize and elevate injured extremity	Child describes a decrease in pain Child's injured extremity is immobilized
Fear related to injury and emergency treatments	Carefully explain all procedures and treatments to child Allow parents to remain with child at all times	Child remains calm and cooperative Parents remain with child
Impaired physical mobility related to injured extremity	Explain purpose of immobilization of extremity to child Teach child and parents care of immobilized extremity	Child and parents demonstrate understanding of importance of immobilization of injured extremity
Knowledge deficit related to musculoskeletal injury	Explain all emergency department procedures to child and parents Teach child and parents care of injured extremity Teach parents importance of follow-up appointment with orthopaedist Instruct parents in cast care and sensory checks	Child and parents demonstrate understanding of emergency treatment Child and parents demonstrate understanding of discharge care

22 | Infectious Disease Emergencies

Susan J. Kelley

Sepsis

Sepsis, or septicemia, refers to a profound, life-threatening bacterial infection of the blood stream. Neonates, especially those born prematurely, are highly susceptible to sepsis. Neonatal sepsis refers to the clinical syndrome of systemic illness associated with bacteremia during the first 4 weeks of life. All neonates evaluated in the emergency department with rectal temperature of 101F or above should be considered to be septic until proven otherwise.

The incidence of sepsis in the United States is estimated to be anywhere between 1 to 8 cases per 1000 live births.[1] The frequency of infection is almost twice as great in male infants as in females. The associated mortality rate among male infants is also higher than with females. The overall mortality rate is in the 15 to 50 percent range, depending on the infecting organism. The high-risk infant has a four-times-greater chance of developing sepsis than the healthy newborn.

Etiology and Pathophysiology.

In the neonatal period the pathogens most frequently responsible for sepsis are *Escherichia coli* and group B streptococcus. In infants and children over 1 month of age the organisms under suspicion are the same as those that produce meningitis in this age group. These organisms include *Hemophilus influenzae, Streptococcus pneumoniae,* and *Neisseria meningitidis.*

Maternal risk factors for neonatal sepsis include endometritis, bacteremia, vaginal infection, premature rupture of the membranes, or a traumatic delivery. Infant risk factors include premature birth, low birth weight, fetal distress, and an Apgar score at 1 minute of 5 or less. Neonates in the nursery are at risk for self-infection and cross-contamination from other infants, hospital personnel, and inanimate objects. Bacterial infections can occur through the umbilical stump, skin, mucous membranes of the eyes, nose, pharynx, and ears, as well as through the respiratory, gastrointestinal, nervous, and urinary systems.

History.

The neonate, or infant under 6 weeks of age, may have a general history of "not doing well." A careful history may reveal poor feeding, vomiting, diarrhea, abdominal distension, respiratory distress, apnea, lethargy, irritability, and seizures. The history obtained in the infant or child older than 1 month of age may include fever, petechial-purpuric rash, lethargy, irritability, vomiting, diarrhea, and poor feeding. A history of a localized infection, such as a respiratory tract infection, may be given. A careful history of any chronic or terminal illness, such as sickle cell disease, leukemia, or acquired immune deficiency syndrome (AIDS), should alert clinicians to a child at increased risk of sepsis.

Diagnostic Procedures. Laboratory studies should include a complete blood count with differential, at least one blood culture, serum electrolytes with glucose, platelet counts, prothrombin time (PT), partial thromboplastin time (PPT), and arterial blood gas values. A urine culture should be obtained through a suprapubic bladder tap in infants and by a clean-voided specimen in the older child. A lumbar puncture should be performed and cerebrospinal fluid analyzed to rule out meningitis. Approximately 20 to 30 percent of neonates with septicemia will also have bacterial meningitis. The nasopharynx, ear canals, and any skin lesions should be cultured in hopes of yielding the infective organism. In neonates the umbilical stump should be cultured. If indicated a chest x-ray should be obtained to rule out the presence of pneumonia.

Assessment. An initial nursing assessment should include evaluation of airway, breathing and circulation (ABCs). The infant or child should next be evaluated for indicators of septic shock. Symptoms of septic shock include tachycardia, hypotension, tachypnea, decreased level of consciousness, poor peripheral circulation, and decreased urinary output. Vital signs and temperature must be continually assessed. Tachycardia occurs early in the course of sepsis, often exceeding 200 beats per minute in infants under 3 months, 175 beats per minute between 4 months and 2 years, and 150 beats per minute in children over 2 years.[2] It is important to note that infants under 3 months of age who are septic are often afebrile. Septic infants under 1 month of age are often hypothermic. Fluid intake and output must be carefully recorded. Respiratory status should be

carefully assessed. The skin is often cold and should be carefully examined for presence of petechiae, purpura, jaundice, pallor, cyanosis, or mottling. Central nervous system involvement should be assessed with special attention to the child's level of consciousness, level of activity, irritability, seizure activity, and bulging fontanels. The infant or child should also be assessed for jaundice and hepatomegaly.

Management. Table 22–1 summarizes the nursing management priorities for the septic patient. Early recognition and treatment of sepsis and septic shock is essential to increase the chances for survival and to decrease long-term sequelae. Oxygen should be administered at 100 percent. An intravenous route must be established, and a volume expander, such as normal saline with 5 percent dextrose, should be administered at 20 ml/kg/hour. The unstable patient requires central venous, arterial, and urinary catheters.[3] If present, metabolic acidosis should be corrected with sodium bicarbonate, 1 to 2 mEq/kg/dose.

Antibiotic therapy is instituted immediately upon diagnosis or high suspicion of sepsis. For the neonate, a penicillin such as ampicillin (100 mg/kg/day) and an aminoglycoside such as gentamicin (5.0 to 7.5 mg/kg/day) are administered intravenously even before culture results are available. In the older infant and child sepsis is usually treated with ampicillin (200 to

TABLE 22–1. PRIORITIES IN THE NURSING CARE FOR THE INFANT OR CHILD WITH SEPSIS

Support airway, breathing, and circulation (ABCs)
Evaluate for signs of septic shock: hypotension, tachycardia, poor peripheral circulation
Prompt administration of intravenous fluids and antibiotics
Careful measurement of intake and output
Adminster blood products as needed
Provide emotional support to child and parents

400 mg/kg/day to a maximum daily dose of 8 to 12 grams) and chloramphenicol (100 mg/kg/day to a maximum daily dose of 4 grams). Neonates and older infants who are septic often become hypoglycemic; therefore a 25 percent solution of glucose 1 g/kg may be administered.

Blood components are given as indicted by results of the initial hematologic studies. If the hemoglobin is less than 10 g/dl, packed red blood cells are administered at 10 ml/kg. Thrombocytopenia is corrected with platelet concentrates at 0.2 units/kg. Decreased clotting factors are replaced with fresh frozen plasma at 10 ml/kg. A corticosteroid, such as methylprednisolone, 120 mg/kg/day divided into four doses, may be given during the first 24 hours.[4]

The patient with sepsis or septic shock warrants close monitoring in the emergency department. The infant or child with sepsis is always admitted to the hospital for intravenous antibiotic therapy and close monitoring.

Psychosocial Support and Parent Education. The septic infant or child has usually become quite ill suddenly, which is very frightening to parents. Parents may experience feelings of guilt for not observing changes in their child sooner or for not seeking medical attention earlier. Parents need to be reassured that they took the appropriate measures by bringing the child to the emergency department. Because parents are usually separated from their child during the diagnostic procedures, they should be continually informed of their child's status. Parents are particularly frightened by lumbar punctures. Although the risk of a complication arising from a lumbar puncture is minimal, many parents fear their child may become paralyzed by the procedure. This procedure should therefore be carefully explained in a sensitive manner. Once the diagnostic proce-

dures are completed, the parents should be allowed to remain with their child.

Parents often become upset when they are informed that their child is going to be admitted to the hospital. One or both parents should be encouraged to remain at the hospital overnight, if hospital policy permits. Separation from parents is particularly stressful for an ill infant or child and should be avoided whenever possible.

Acute Rheumatic Fever

Rheumatic fever (RF) is an inflammatory process that may affect the heart, joints, central nervous system, and subcutaneous tissue. The major sequelae to RF is heart damage in the form of scarring of the mitral valve, referred to as rheumatic heart disease. Rheumatic heart disease is the most common cause of acquired heart disease in children. It rarely occurs before age 3 in children born in the United States. It has, however, been known to occur earlier than this in children from the Caribbean and Far East.[5]

Etiology and Pathophysiology. There is usually a preceding group A beta-hemolytic streptococcal infection 2 to 3 weeks prior to onset of symptoms. In some cases, however, there may be a longer period between the acute streptococcal infection and onset of RF. Most often the preceding streptococcal infection is pharyngitis. Prevention or prompt treatment of group A beta-hemolytic streptococcal infections will prevent rheumatic heart disease. Changes in the heart include swelling, fragmentation, and alterations in the connective tissue of the heart. The structures most often affected are the mitral and aortic valves. These valves may become swollen and edematous. The pulmonic and tricuspid valves are rarely affected in children.

History. A history of a recent upper respiratory tract infection, especially pharyngitis, should be sought. The onset of symptoms, length of illness, presence of fever, and medications taken, if any, should be elicited. Any joint pain should be noted.

Assessment. Careful evaluation of the ABCs is important. Clinical presentation of the child with acute rheumatic heart disease may include fever, tachycardia, and carditis. The diagnosis of carditis is based on the presence of one or more of the following findings: abnormal murmurs, pericardial friction rub, cardiomegaly, and congestive heart failure.[6] Changes in the conductivity of the heart as seen on electrocardiogram include prolonged PR interval and nonspecific ST or T wave changes.

Joints should be carefully examined for motion, tenderness, swelling, warmth, and redness. Joint involvement in RF tends to localize in the larger joints of the extremities. The most frequently affected joints are the knees and ankles, followed by the wrists, elbows, and hips. The hands, feet, shoulders, and small joints are least frequently involved. If the only joints involved are the temporomandibular or vertebral joints, a cause for the arthritis other than RF should be sought.[7]

The skin should be carefully examined for subcutaneous nodules and erythema marginatum. Subcutaneous nodules are found over extensor surfaces of joints. These nodules are firm, nontender, and movable. Erythema marginatum is normally found on the trunk and extremities. Chorea is an unusual finding in RF. It is characterized by involuntary and purposeless movements of the extremities and facial grimacing. Emotional lability may be present.

When there is evidence of preceding streptococcal infection, the diagnosis of RF is usually based on the presence of two major or of one major and two minor manifestations from the revised Jones Criteria for RF (Table 22–2).

TABLE 22–2. REVISED JONES CRITERIA RHEUMATIC FEVER MANIFESTATIONS

Major Manifestations	Minor Manifestations
Carditis	Fever
Polyarthritis	Arthralgia
Erythema marginatum	Elevated erythrocyte
Subcutaneous nodules	sedimentation rate
Chorea	ECG changes, prolonged P to R interval
	History of previous rheumatic fever

Laboratory Data. Complete blood count with differential will indicate leukocytosis and anemia. Sedimentation rate (ESR) and C-reactive protein levels will be elevated. An increased or rising antistreptolysin-O (ASO) titer is the most commonly used serologic test to detect previous group A streptococcal infection. The multiple antibody test (Streptozyme) can also provide serologic confirmation of recent streptococcal infection.

Throat cultures (two) should be obtained before penicillin therapy is started. Blood cultures should also be obtained to rule out subacute bacterial endocarditis.

Electrocardiogram will indicate prolonged PR interval and nonspecific ST or T wave changes. A chest film should be obtained to assess the heart size, to verify the presence of carditis, and to gauge the severity of the carditis.

Management. The emergency treatment of rheumatic heart disease involves eradication of the hemolytic streptococci, control of congestive heart failure, prevention of permanent cardiac damage, and prevention of recurrences of the disease. Penicillin is the drug of choice for combatting the underlying infection. Erythromycin or sulfonamides are used for those allergic to penicillin. If cardiac failure is severe, steroids such as prednisone may be administered to reduce the inflammatory process. Digoxin and diuretics may be used to treat congestive heart failure. Strict bed rest and isolation for all patients suspected of RF should begin in the emergency department.

Upon stabilization in the emergency department the patient should be admitted to a pediatric intensive care unit or inpatient unit, depending on the patient's condition. The child and parent will need emotional support and information regarding the disease and treatment. Prevention of recurrent attacks is crucial. Prophylaxis may continue for 10 to 15 years after the initial diagnosis. Some patients with RF are treated for a lifetime.

CENTRAL NERVOUS SYSTEM INFECTIOUS DISEASES

The two most important central nervous system infections in the pediatric population are meningitis and encephalitis. Since children with Reye's syndrome often come to the emergency department with clinical manifestations similar to meningitis and encephalitis and since Reye's syndrome involves the central nervous system, it will be discussed in this section.

Meningitis, encephalitis, and Reye's syndrome are of special challenge to the emergency department nurse. Each of these diseases needs early identification and intervention to prevent serious sequelae and death. Although these central nervous system infections and postinfectious disease syndromes are critical illnesses, their initial presentations may resemble those of many minor pediatric illnesses and complaints. Infants and children with a central nervous system infection often have such common pediatric complaints as fever, irritability, lethargy, vomiting, or headache. The emergency department nurse must therefore be knowledgeable in identifying and differentiating between the minor pediatric illnesses and the serious CNS diseases of meningitis, encephalitis, and Reye's syndrome. These

life-threatening pediatric diseases are amenable to therapy if they are diagnosed early in the emergency department.

Meningitis

Meningitis, a potentially fatal infectious disease, is an inflammation of the meninges. It is caused by bacterial or viral infection of the meninges. The meninges, the three membranes investing the spinal cord and brain, include (1) the dura mater (external); (2) the arachnoid (middle); and (3) the pia mater (internal).

Meningitis is one of the most serious of the infectious diseases and occurs frequently in the pediatric population. It is estimated that annually there are 30,000 cases of bacterial meningitis and over 3000 deaths attributable to meningitis. Estimated risk to a child of developing bacterial meningitis by 5 years of age is between 1 in 400 and 1 in 2000. It carries a mortality rate of 1 to 5 percent in infants and young children. In neonates it carries a mortality rate between 20 and 50 percent.[8] If treated early the prognosis is generally good. Early clinical recognition and treatment is therefore essential to decrease morbidity and mortality. Long-term effects of meningitis include delayed psychomotor development, seizure disorders, hydrocephalus, speech defects, visual and hearing impairments, mental retardation, and behavior changes.

Etiology. Bacterial meningitis can be caused by a variety of bacterial agents. *H. influenzae* (type B), *S. pneumoniae*, and *N. meningitidis* (meningococcus) organisms are responsible for bacterial meningitis in 95 percent of children over 2 months of age. *H. influenzae* is the predominant causative organism in children 3 months to 3 years of age.[9] In the neonate group B streptococci and *E. coli* are the most frequent causative organisms. The most common causative organisms in viral (aseptic) meningitis are coxsackie B., echovirus, rubella virus, mumps virus, and herpes simplex.

Factors that predispose children to meningitis include preexisting central nervous system anomalies, neurosurgical procedures, sickle cell disease, immunoglobulin deficiencies, immunosuppressant drug therapy, severe head trauma, or primary infections elsewhere in the body. Maternal factors that increase the risk of meningitis in the neonate include premature rupture of the membranes, maternal infection during the last week of pregnancy, or prolonged labor.

Pathophysiology. The central nervous system offers minimal resistance to infection. Organisms that are weakly pathogenic elsewhere become serious infective agents when they invade the central nervous system.

Bacterial meningitis is transmitted by droplet infection, with an incubation period of 1 to 7 days. The organisms reside in the nasopharynx, and the infection then spreads to the vascular system. The blood supply of the meninges lies adjacent to the venous system of the nasopharynx, mastoid process, and middle ear. This area provides an excellent environment for bacterial colonization because of the slower rate of venous circulation.[10] Next, the invading organism gains entry into the cerebrospinal fluid and then spreads throughout the subarachnoid space. The infective process causes the brain to become hyperemic, edematous, and covered with a layer of purulent exudate. Sequelae may include hydrocephalus, subdural effusions, venous thrombosis, and temporary or permanent damage to the cranial nerves.[11]

History. A careful history should be obtained in all cases of suspected meningitis. The history obtained should include any recent febrile episodes; the child's recent level of activity, with special attention given to any history of irritability or lethargy; decrease in appetite; total fluid intake during the last 24 hours; vomiting; diarrhea; seizures; or signs of respiratory distress. There may be a history of a recent otitis media or upper respiratory infection.

The clinical presentation of meningitis varies with the age of the patient. Diagnosis of meningitis in the neonate or infant is difficult. Often the only clinical sign in infants is irritability. Irritability associated with meningitis often cannot be alleviated by any measure, not even maternal comforting. With any infant whose mother describes irritability or other change in behavior, the nurse must maintain a high index of suspicion for meningitis. Fever may or may not be present. Bulging of the fontanels is a late sign. Table 22–3 summarizes the clinical signs and symptoms of meningitis in infants.

In children over the age of 2, the symptoms become more specific for central nervous system involvement. These patients may present with classic meningeal symptoms of headache, nuchal rigidity, vomiting, and fever. Table 22–4 summarizes the clinical presentation of meningitis in children over 1 year of age. In either age group meningitis may be abrupt in onset or more insidious, often with a history of respiratory infection.

Assessment. As in all critically ill patients, the first priority is assessment and

TABLE 22–3. CLINICAL PRESENTATION OF MENINGITIS IN INFANTS

Irritability	Petechiae below the
High-pitched cry	nipple line
Fever	Purpura
Bulging anterior	Seizure activity
fontanel	Apnea
Poor feeding	Nuchal rigidity
Vomiting	General appearance of
Lethargy	"sick infant"
Altered sleep pattern	

TABLE 22–4. CLINICAL PRESENTATION OF MENINGITIS IN CHILDREN

Headache	Altered level of con-
Vomiting	sciousness
Fever	Petechiae
Nuchal rigidity	Purpura
Positive Kernig's sign	Photophobia
Positive Brudzinski's	Seizure activity
sign	Coma

support of the ABCs. Apneic episodes are common in infants with meningitis. Breath sounds should be assessed for sign of pneumonia, which may accompany meningitis. Any respiratory distress should be noted. Cardiac monitoring should be used. Vital signs should be carefully monitored.

The infant with meningitis is often hypothermic. The older infant or child may be febrile. The child's temperature should be carefully monitored. The patient's neurologic status should be continually assessed for signs of increased intracranial pressure. This includes assessment of the child's level of consciousness, irritability, pupillary responses, cranial nerve assessment, equality of movement, and strength of extremities. The fontanels in infants should be assessed for bulging.

The patient should be continually assessed for septic shock. Septic shock is often associated with meningococcemia. Vital signs should be monitored every 15 minutes or more frequently if the patient is unstable. The signs of septic shock include fever, tachycardia, hypotension, decreased capillary filling, tachypnea or apnea, decreased level of consciousness, and decreased urinary output.

Laboratory Data

Lumbar Puncture. A lumbar puncture (LP) should be performed immediately on all patients in whom meningitis is sus-

pected (Fig. 22–1). The LP should include measurement of opening and closing pressures, cerebrospinal fluid cell and differential count, gram stain to identify the particular bacterial organism, and cerebrospinal fluid glucose, protein, and culture. While holding the child or infant for the LP the nurse must continually assess the child's respiratory status. An infant or child who has eaten prior to the LP is at risk for aspiration.

Venipuncture. Serum electrolytes with glucose should be obtained. Decreased serum sodium and serum osmolarity may indicate syndrome of inappropriate antidiuretic hormone (SIADH). The majority of children with bacterial meningitis show evidence of SIADH. Careful monitoring of fluid and electrolytes is therefore imperative.

A serum glucose level should be obtained prior to the LP, as the stress of the LP may artificially raise the serum glucose level. The serum glucose level is compared to the cerebrospinal fluid glucose level. In bacterial meningitis the cerebrospinal fluid glucose level will be reduced or will be one half the serum glucose level. Infants are prone to becoming hypoglycemic when critically ill, which can lead to seizures and respiratory arrest.

A complete blood count with differential will help to differentiate between bacterial and viral meningitis. A platelet count should also be obtained.

One or more blood cultures should be obtained because of the high incidence of associated septicemia. The blood culture will yield the infecting organism in 50 percent of cases of bacterial meningitis.

Urine Specimens. The urine electrolytes should include potassium, sodium, and urine osmolarity. These values will assist in the diagnosis of SIADH. A urine culture and urinalysis should be obtained, be-

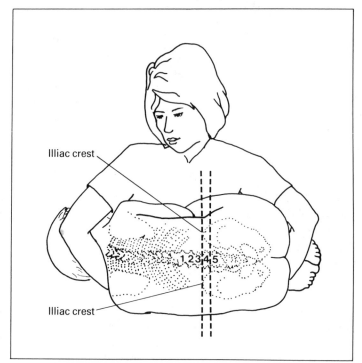

Figure 22-1. Position for lumbar puncture. The desired sites are the interspaces between L-3 and L-4, or L-4 and L-5.

cause there may be a concurrent urinary tract infection. The specific gravity of the urine is important in monitoring fluid and electrolyte balance.

Other Cultures. A throat culture may yield the infecting organism. Cultures of purpuric lesions, abscesses, or middle ear infections should also be obtained.

Radiographs. A chest x-ray should be obtained if pneumonia is suspected.

Management. Meningitis is a true emergency that requires immediate detection and institution of therapy to prevent death and to avoid permanent neurologic impairment. Refer to Table 22-5 for a summary of nursing intervention priorities in the child with meningitis. The child's ABCs must be continually assessed and supported. Humidified oxygen should be administered to all infants and children

who are pale, cyanotic, or show signs of shock. Intubation and assisted ventilation are necessary in some cases. Intravenous access should be ensured.

If the signs of septic shock previously described are present, shock may be corrected with rapid infusion of packed red blood cells or intravenous solutions.

If bacterial meningitis is identified or suspected, rapid administration of the appropriate antibiotic(s) is essential. Antibiotics are usually administered until cul-

TABLE 22-5. PRIORITIES IN THE NURSING MANAGEMENT OF THE CHILD WITH MENINGITIS

Support airway, breathing, and circulation (ABCs)
Evaluate and treat shock
Institute antibiotic therapy
Monitor and prevent increased intracranial pressure
Monitor fluid therapy and electrolyte balance
Prevent spread of infection in emergency department
Provide emotional support to child and parents

tures are available. Refer to Table 22–6 for the appropriate antibiotic therapy. Antibiotics should be given immediately upon completion of the lumbar puncture.

Increased intracranial pressure and cerebral edema may occur with meningitis. All measures should be taken to prevent, monitor, and treat cerebral edema and increased intracranial pressure (ICP). There should be continual assessment of the patient's neurologic status. Intravenous and oral fluid intake must be restricted to two thirds maintenance level in order to decrease the volume of fluid in the brain. Carefully monitor fluid and electrolyte balance. If necessary hyperventilate the patient to control Pco₂ levels to between 25 and 30 mm Hg. Elevate the head of the bed to 30 degrees, and maintain the head in a midline, neutral position to prevent obstruction of cranial venous return.

If intracranial pressure is acutely elevated, one or more osmotic diuretics may be administered in the following dosages: mannitol (20 percent solution), 0.5 to 1.0 g/kg/dose every 4 to 6 hours intravenously; or furosemide (Lasix), 1 mg/kg/dose every 4 to 6 hours. The use of steroids such as dexamethasone in the treatment of meningitis remains controversial.[12] Temperature regulation is important, since hyperthermia compounds cerebral edema. Antipyretics should be administered orally if the patient is alert and rectally if the patient is unable to take medications by mouth. Acetaminophen, 15 mg/kg (maximum dose 650 mg), is administered every 4 hours for temperatures over 101F. Tepid sponging or cooling blankets may also be required. Rubbing alcohol should never be used, since the alcohol may be absorbed through the skin and has been associated

TABLE 22–6. ANTIBIOTIC DOSAGE IN BACTERIAL MENINGITIS

Age or Organism	Drug	Dosage	Route of Administration
Infants < 7 days old (organism unknown)	Ampicillin and	100 mg/kg/day, divided doses given every 12 hr	IV, IM
	gentamicin	6 mg/kg/day, divided doses given every 12 hr	IV, IM
Infants > 7 days old (organism unknown)	Ampicillin and	300 mg/kg/day, divided doses given every 8 hr	IV, IM
	gentamicin	7.5 mg/kg/day, divided doses given every 8 hr	IV, IM
Infants > 2 months (organism unknown)	Chloramphenicol and	100 mg/kg/day, divided doses given every 6 hr	IV
	ampicillin	300 mg/kg/day, divided doses given every 4 hr	IV, IM
H. influenzae	Chloramphenicol and ampicillin	Same as above for unknown organism	
Pneumococcus	Penicillin G	250,000 U/kg/day divided doses given every 4 hr	IV
Meningococcus	Penicillin G	250,000 U/kg/day, divided doses given every 4 hr	IV

Abbreviations; IV = intravenously; IM = intramuscularly.

with acute toxicity and even death in some instances.

All necessary precautions should be taken in the emergency department to protect one's self and others from possible exposure to meningitis. All suspected cases should be isolated upon arrival to the emergency department. Precautions also include the wearing of masks, gowns, and gloves when having direct contact with the patient.

Patients with meningitis are admitted for close observation, intravenous antibiotic therapy, and supportive measures.

Prophylaxis for Contacts. The children at greatest risk for developing *H. influenzae* meningitis are siblings under 6 years of age and children attending the same day care center. Adult and child household members and classmates at day care should receive rifampin prophylaxis. Infants less than 1 month are treated with rifampin, 10 mg/kg every 24 hours for 4 days. Infants and children between 1 month and 12 years are treated with rifampin, 20 mg/kg every 24 hours for 4 days. Children over 12 and adults are treated with rifampin, 600 mg every 24 hours for 4 days.[13]

Prophylaxis is recommended for all close contacts of a child with meningococcal meningitis. Infants less than 1 month should be given rifampin, 5 mg/kg every 12 hours for 2 days. Infants and children 1 month to 12 years should receive rifampin, 10 mg/kg every 12 hours for 2 days. Children over 12 years and adult contacts should receive rifampin, 600 mg every 12 hours for 2 days.[14]

Routine prophylaxis of hospital personnel who have come into contact with the patient with meningitis is usually not necessary. Circumstances in which prophylaxis is indicated for health professionals include direct contact with the patient's saliva through mouth-to-mouth resuscitation or prolonged close contact with the patient prior to the institution of antibiotic therapy. Those at risk of infection should receive rifampin prophylaxis with rifampin, 600 mg daily for 2 or 4 days, as described above depending on the infective organism.[15]

Currently prophylactic agents will not reliably abort incipient meningitis. Close observation of those with exposure is therefore extremely important. With the first sign of fever, sore throat, otitis media, rash, or other sign of infection, contacts should be evaluated promptly.[16]

Viral (Aseptic) Meningitis. Viral, or aseptic meningitis, is generally much milder in clinical presentation than bacterial meningitis. Usually it is self-limiting, without specific therapy. The presenting symptoms are similar to those seen in bacterial meningitis and include nuchal rigidity, headache, malaise, photophobia, seizures, abdominal pain, sore throat, and generalized muscle aches. The onset of symptoms may be abrupt or insidious. Increased intracranial pressure is infrequent in cases of viral meningitis. The assessment and management of viral meningitis is similar to bacterial meningitis, except that antibiotic therapy is of no value in the treatment of viral meningitis. Antibiotic therapy may be administered and isolation enforced, however, until a definitive diagnosis is made and the possibility of bacterial meningitis is eliminated. All patients with viral meningitis should be admitted for close monitoring.

Psychosocial Support and Parent Education. The term meningitis still provokes thoughts of death or permanent disability in the minds and emotions of most lay persons. It is therefore important to provide emotional support and accurate information to the child and parents. The child and parents will need careful explanations of all procedures and treatments. Lumbar punctures are particularly frightening to the patient as well as the parents. Fears need to be allayed with information and reassurance. Many parents mistakenly assume that in a lumbar puncture the spinal needle goes through the spinal cord and thus can potentially cause paralysis. The parents therefore need to be informed that the needle does not enter the spinal cord itself but rather is placed between two lumbar vertebrae below where the spinal cord ends. Parents will also need to be prepared for the child's admission to the hospital.

Encephalitis

Encephalitis is an inflammatory process of the brain that produces altered function of the central nervous system. The encephalitis process is usually created by the direct invasion of a virus into the central nervous system or postinfectious involvement of the central nervous system after a viral disease.[17]

Etiology and Pathophysiology. Encephalitis due to direct invasion is often caused by the arboviruses (arthropod-borne viruses) acquired through an arthropod vector. The vector reservoir for these arboviruses is the mosquito. In the United States the four arboviruses that are the major causes of encephalitis are (1) the eastern equine encephalomyelitis (EEE) found primarily in eastern and north central United States; (2) St. Louis encephalitis (SLE), found in most sections of the United States, with the exception of the Northeast; (3) Western equine encephalomyelitis (WEE), found primarily in the western United States and Canada and scattered areas further east; and (4) California viruses (CE), found throughout the United States.[18]

Measles, mumps, varicella, rubella, enteroviruses, and herpes simplex may cause encephalitis as a complication of the disease process. In rare cases encephalitis may occur as a complication of a routine vaccination for smallpox, poliomyelitis, diphtheria, pertussis, or influenza. In recent years, however, more than 60 percent of encephalitis cases reported to the Centers for Disease Control have been of indeterminate cause.[19]

Encephalitis is associated with greater morbidity and mortality than bacterial or viral meningitis. Recovery may take days, weeks, or months. Death may result. Residual effects of encephalitis may include developmental delays, brain damage, seizure disorders, hydrocephalus, hemiparesis, hemiplegia, loss of hearing, and focal or sensory deficits. Herpes simplex type I encephalitis carries the worst prognosis, causing death or serious neurologic sequelae in over 70 percent of patients.

History. The onset of the disease may be dramatic or insidious. There may be a history of headache, fever, nuchal rigidity, decreased level of consciousness, seizure activity, ataxia, photophobia, diplopia, nausea, vomiting, or facial twitching. Table 22–7 summarizes the clinical indicators of encephalitis.

Assessment. The patient's ABCs should be carefully assessed and supported. A neurologic assessment should be performed including a cranial nerve assessment, level of consciousness, pupillary responses, and extraocular eye movements. The fontanels in infants should be assessed for tenseness or bulging. Vital signs should be carefully monitored.

TABLE 22–7. CLINICAL INDICATORS OF ENCEPHALITIS

Alterations in level of consciousness/mental status	Headache
	Fever
Neurologic deficits	Vomiting
Seizure activity	Nuchal rigidity

Laboratory Data

Lumbar Puncture. A lumbar puncture is performed to differentiate between encephalitis, meningitis, Reye's syndrome, and an intracranial bleed. The cerebrospinal fluid is often within normal limits, with normal to moderately elevated pressure and a normal glucose level. Five to a few hundred cells with a predominance of lymphocytes and leukocytes may be found. A viral study of the cerebrospinal fluid is necessary for identification of the causative organism. Viruses of herpes, mumps, measles, and enteroviruses may be detected in the cerebrospinal fluid. Arboviruses are rarely detected in the cerebrospinal fluid or blood.

Cultures. Viral cultures of the blood, pharynx, and stool may yield the infecting organism. Bacterial cultures should also be obtained of the blood, urine, and pharynx to rule out bacterial meningitis.

Venipuncture. A complete blood count with differential will help distinguish between bacterial meningitis and viral encephalitis. In cases of encephalitis, the blood count will usually show a mild polymorphonuclear or mononuclear leukocytosis. Serum electrolytes should be obtained to rule out SIADH, which may accompany encephalitis.

Urine. Urine electrolytes and osmolarity should be obtained to rule out SIADH. A urinalysis and culture should also be obtained.

Management. The patient's ABCs should be continually assessed and supported. If present, acidosis should be corrected. Increased intracranial pressure should be carefully monitored and treated by hyperventilation if necessary. The head of the patient's bed should be elevated to 30 degrees, with the head in a midline position to prevent obstruction of cerebral venous return. Fluid intake should be carefully monitored and limited to two thirds maintenance. Electrolytes should be carefully monitored. Osmotic diuretics or steroids may be administered. Urine output should be carefully monitored. If critically ill, a urinary catheter should be inserted for accurate urinary output measurement.

If the patient is febrile, antipyretics should be administered, since hyperthermia compounds cerebral edema by increasing metabolism, which in turn causes an increase in cerebral blood flow. A cooling blanket may be necessary if the child's fever fails to respond to antipyretics. Antibiotics are not administered, since they are of no value in viral infections. If the patient is thought to have herpes simplex type I encephalitis, however, antiviral therapy with adenine arabinoside may be administered pending the results of a brain biopsy. Since patients with encephalitis are prone to seizures, precautions should be taken. Anticonvulsants will be necessary if the patient begins seizing in the emergency department. Refer to the chapter on seizure disorders for the management of seizure activity in the emergency department.

Psychosocial Support and Parent Education. The child with encephalitis has often become ill suddenly and may deteriorate rapidly. Parents are frightened by the sudden serious condition of their child and need reassurance that all that is possible is being done. All procedures and treatments should be carefully explained to the child and parents.

The parents should be encouraged to remain at the child's bedside as much as possible while in the emergency department. They will also need to be prepared for the hospitalization of their child and should be encouraged to remain with the child once admitted to the hospital.

Reye's Syndrome

Reye's syndrome is a pediatric disease characterized by encephalopathy and fatty degeneration of the liver. The first description of this entity was reported in 1963 by Australian pathologist H.D.K. Reye. Since then this distinct malady has been classified as Reye's syndrome and has been identified with increasing frequency.

Reye's syndrome is characterized by fever, profoundly impaired consciousness, and liver dysfunction. The peak incidence occurs at 6 to 11 years of age. Cases involving patients 2 months to 21 years of age, however, have been documented. Characteristically Reye's syndrome occurs in late winter or early spring. Distribution is worldwide, with no preference for either sex.

Etiology and Pathophysiology. The etiology of Reye's syndrome is still uncertain. Viral infections have been implicated. The viruses associated include influenza types A and B, varicella, coxsackie, adenovirus, echovirus, rubeola, and herpes simplex. Influenza in an epidemic pattern and varicella in a sporadic pattern are most notable.[20] Research continues to link chemical toxins such as pesticides and fertilizers to Reye's syndrome, since a higher incidence of these cases are reported in suburban and rural areas.[21] Other studies reported to the Centers for Disease Control suggest a relationship between salicylates and antiemetic drugs taken during a viral illness.[22] The American Academy of Pediatrics recommends that aspirin products not be given to infants or children with symptoms of viral illnesses, especially when a child has chicken pox.

The pathophysiology of Reye's syndrome includes disruption of the liver mitochondria or urea cycle, resulting in a buildup of fatty deposits in the liver due to inadequate lipid metabolism, which leads to metabolic encephalopathy.[23] Electron microscopy reveals abnormally large and swollen mitochondria in the liver and brain cells. Hyperammonemia is caused by a reduction in the enzymes that convert ammonia to urea. Brain dysfunction and death are the end result of swollen and damaged cells.[24]

History. Early detection and intervention will affect the course of the disease. Reye's syndrome should be suspected in any infant, child, or adolescent who has an altered mental status and who recently appeared to have recovered from an upper respiratory infection or other viral illness such as varicella (chicken pox). The history obtained from parents may include intractable vomiting and central nervous system dysfunction, which may be manifested by seizures, alterations in breathing patterns, including apnea, and decreased level of consciousness. In infants there may be a history of high-pitched, abnormal crying.

The course of the illness has two phases. In the first phase the child has a viral illness for 5 to 7 days with apparent recovery. In the second phase the child develops recurrent vomiting, followed by a progressive disturbance in level of consciousness that can range from very mild lethargy to coma.

Clinical Staging. Staging criteria have been developed by Lovejoy et al.[25] that are correlated with the patient's level of consciousness, cardiorespiratory status, and reflexes. These stages are described in Table 22–8. The patient is evaluated upon diagnosis, and a numerical grade of severity assigned. The stage at time of diagnosis

TABLE 22-8. LOVEJOY'S CLINICAL STAGING OF REYE'S SYNDROME

Stage I	Vomiting, lethargy, drowsiness, liver dysfunction
Stage II	Disorientation, delirium, combative-ness, aggressiveness, hyperventila-tion, hyperactive reflexes, liver dysfunction
Stage III	Obtunded, comatose, hyperventila-tion, decorticate posturing, liver dysfunction
Stage IV	Deepening coma, decerebrate rigidity, large and fixed pupils, divergent eye movements, loss of corneal re-flexes, minimal liver dysfunction
Stage V	Seizures, respiratory arrest, flaccidity, loss of deep tendon reflexes

dictates the therapeutic interventions as well as the anticipated prognosis.

Assessment. The patient's ABCs should be continually assessed. Acute respiratory failure and cardiac arrhythmias may occur. A cardiac monitor should therefore be used continually while the patient is in the emergency department. Vital signs should be monitored every 15 minutes.

The patient's neurologic status should be continually assessed for changes in level of consciousness, disorientation, com-bativeness, posturing, ridigity, and seizure activity.

Signs of increased intracranial pres-sure should be carefully monitored. Changes in respiratory rate and depth are early indictors of increasing intracranial pressure. Hyperventilation may indicate the body's attempt to normalize intra-cranial pressure because hypocarbia pro-duces cerebral vasoconstriction, which de-creases intravascular volume. Tachycardia and hypotension may indicate hypovo-lemia.[26]

Laboratory Data

Venipuncture. Serum ammonia is ele-vated (150 to 750 $\mu g/dl$) in early stages of the disease and often returns to normal within 48 to 72 hours. Elevation of ammo-nia levels is the product of initial virus-toxin interaction. Elevation is thought to be correlated with the severity of the dis-ease.

Liver function test results, including serum glutamic-oxaloacetic transaminase (SGOT), serum glutamic-pyruvic transam-inase (SGPT), and lactic dehydrogenase (LDH), are elevated. PT and PTT are twice the upper limit of normal range. Blood urea nitrogen and creatinine levels may show mild to moderate elevation.

Serum glucose levels may indicate hypoglycemia. Serum glucose levels may fall to below 50 mg/dl with reduced insulin levels and diminished glucagon response.

Arterial blood gases may reflect a blend of respiratory alkalosis with meta-bolic acidosis.

A lumbar puncture is performed to rule out meningitis or encephalitis. In Reye's syndrome the cerebrospinal fluid is essentially normal, although the pressure may be elevated.

A liver biopsy is the definitive diag-nostic study for Reye's syndrome and is usually performed in the pediatric inten-sive care unit. The biopsy reveals a charac-teristic cell morphology.

Management. The priorities in the man-agement of the patient with Reye's syn-drome are summarized in Table 22-9. The ABCs should be continually assessed and supported. Children at the coma stage (stage III and above) are electively intu-bated and placed on a respirator as a means of preventing cerebral ischemia. An arterial line may be inserted to monitor blood pressure and for direct access for

TABLE 22-9. PRIORITIES IN THE NURSING MANAGEMENT OF REYE'S SYNDROME

Early identification	Electrolyte balance
Support of airway, breathing, and circulation (ABCs)	Temperature control
	Close monitoring of vital signs
Control of increased intracranial pressure	Admission to pediatric intensive care unit
Seizure control	Emotional support to child and parents
Fluid restriction	

blood gas studies. A central venous pressure line may be inserted to monitor right ventricular pressure. Arterial PO_2 levels of 100 to 150 torr should provide adequate oxygen for brain cell metabolism despite decreased cerebral perfusion. The $PaCO_2$ is maintained between 20 to 30 mm Hg. This will decrease cerebral blood volume and reduce intracranial pressure.[27]

Fluid and electrolyte balance must be carefully maintained. Restrict fluids to 50 to 75 percent of daily maintenance. Record intake and urine output with specific gravity hourly. A Foley catheter should be inserted for accurate urinary output. A minimum urine output of 0.5 ml/kg/hour is necessary to ensure kidney function. Monitor serum electrolytes carefully.

Children with Reye's syndrome are prone to developing hypoglycemia. Infants are particularly intolerant of hypoglycemia and may have a seizure or respiratory arrest. Untreated hypoglycemia will lead to increased production of ammonia and fatty acidemia. An attempt is made to maintain a serum glucose level of 200 to 300 mg/dl with hypertonic glucose IV solutions. The solution chosen will depend on the child's glucose and electrolyte levels in the range of 10 to 20 percent dextrose in 50 to 75 percent NaCl. Potassium may be added to the intravenous solution if the need is indicated by electrolyte values and kidney function is assured.[28]

Closely monitor for and prevent increased intracranial pressure. Elevate the head of the bed to 30 degrees, and maintain the child's head in a midline, neutral position to prevent obstruction of cranial venous return. Body temperature should be maintained between 36.5C and 37C, because hyperthermia compounds cerebral edema by increasing cerebral metabolism, which in turn demands an increase in cerebral blood flow.[29]

An intracranial pressure monitoring device will be inserted when the patient arrives in the intensive care unit. ICP should be controlled at levels less than 20 torr. Decadron may be administered at regular intervals to lessen the effects of cerebral edema. Mannitol or glycol may be administered to elevate blood osmolality, which in turn causes fluid to move out of edematous tissue.

Vitamin K, 1 to 5 mg, may be administered to correct clotting abnormalities, which are the result of hepatic and cellular dysfunction and decreased production of clotting factors.

Psychosocial Support and Parent Education. The patient and parents need a great deal of emotional support. They are usually quite frightened by the suddenness and severity of the illness. Children in the early stages are often disoriented and confused and will therefore need simple, clear explanations that they can comprehend and calm reassurance from the emergency department nurse. All procedures and laboratory data should be carefully explained to the parents. The parents should be continually updated on their child's condition while in the emergency department and should be prepared for the child's admission to an intensive care unit. All suspected cases of Reye's syndrome should be admitted to a pediatric intensive care unit for close observation and supportive care.

Families and professionals can obtain information on Reye's syndrome from the National Reye's Syndrome Foundation, 8293 Homestead Road, Benzonia, MI 49616.

NOTES

1. B. Dashefsky. Sepsis. In R.M. Reece (Ed.), *Manual of Emergency Pediatrics* (3rd ed.). Philadelphia: W.B. Saunders, 1984, p. 289.
2. G. Fleisher. Sepsis. In G. Fleisher, & S. Ludwig (Eds.), *Textbook of Pediatric Emergency Medicine,* Baltimore: Williams & Wilkins, 1983, p. 359.
3. Ibid., p. 360.
4. Ibid.
5. H.L. Chernoff, & M.B. Kreidberg. Rheumatic fever. In R.M. Reece (Ed.), *Manual of Emergency Pediatrics* (3rd ed.). Philadelphia: W.B. Saunders, 1984, p. 506.
6. Ibid., p. 507.
7. Ibid., p. 506.
8. E.Y. Oppenheimer, & N.P. Rosman. Meningitis. In R.M. Reece (Ed.), *Manual of Emergency Pediatrics* (3rd ed.). Philadelphia: W.B. Saunders, 1984, p. 189.
9. L.F. Whaley, & D.L. Wong. *Nursing Care of Infants and Children* (2nd ed.). St. Louis: Mosby, 1983, p. 1415.
10. K.M. Anderson. Meningitis. In G.M. Scipien (Ed.), *Comprehensive Pediatric Nursing* (2nd ed.). New York: McGraw Hill, 1979, p. 568.
11. Whaley, & Wong, *Nursing Care of Infants and Children,* p. 1416.
12. R.M. Barkin, & P. Rosen (Eds.). *Emergency Pediatrics.* St. Louis: Mosby, 1984, p. 595.
13. E.Y. Oppenheimer, & N.P. Rosman. Meningitis. In R.M. Reece (Ed.), *Manual of Emergency Pediatrics* (3rd ed.). Philadelphia: W.B. Saunders, p. 197.
14. Ibid.
15. G.D. Overturf. Meningitis. *Topics in Emergency Medicine* 3(1982):24.
16. R.J. Coffey. Pediatric neurological emergencies. *Topics in Emergency Medicine* 3(1982):77–78.
17. L.F. Whaley, & D.L. Wong. Encephalitis. In *Nursing Care of Infants and Children* (2nd ed.). St. Louis: Mosby, 1983, p. 1420.
18. Ibid.
19. C. Trump. Encephalitis. In R.M. Reece (Ed.), *Manual of Emergency Pediatrics* (3rd ed.). Philadelphia: W.B. Saunders, 1983, p. 132.
20. F.P. Riordan. Reye's syndrome. *Critical Care Quarterly* 3(June 1980):10.
21. R.S. Dunne, & R.C. Perez. Reye's syndrome: A challenge not limited to critical care nurses. *Issues in Comprehensive Pediatric Nursing* 5(July-August 1981):254.
22. *Morbidity and Mortality Weekly Report* 7(1980):532–533.
23. Dunne, & Perez, Reye's syndrome, p. 254.
24. Whaley, & Wong, *Nursing Care of Infants and Children,* p. 1421.
25. F.H. Lovejoy, A.L. Smith, & M.J. Bressman, et al. Chemical staging in Reye's syndrome. *American Journal of Diseases in Children* 128(1974):36–41.
26. M.E. Martelli. Reye's syndrome: An update. *Journal of Emergency Nursing* 10 (1984):290.
27. Ibid., p. 291.
28. Ibid., p. 290.
29. Ibid.

BIBLIOGRAPHY

Sepsis

Crone, R.K. Acute circulatory failure in children. *Pediatric Clinics of North America* 27(1980):525.

Dashefsky, B. Sepsis. In Reece, R.M. (Ed.), *Manual of Emergency Pediatrics* (3rd ed.). Philadelphia: W.B. Saunders, 1984, pp. 288–298.

Fleisher, G. Sepsis. In Fleisher, G., & Ludwig, S. (Eds.), *Textbook of Pediatric Emergency Medicine.* Baltimore: Williams & Wilkins, 1983, pp. 358–360.

Grodin, M., & Crone, R. Shock in the pediatric patient. *Pediatric Clinics of North America* 26(1979):821.

Lamb, L.S. You think you know septic shock. *Nursing '82* 12(1982):34–43.

Morse, T.S. Shock in infants and children. In Pierog, J.E., & Pierog, L.J. (Eds.), *Pediatric Critical Illness: Assessment and Care*. Rockville, Md.: Aspen Systems, 1983, pp. 181–186.

Whaley, L.F., & Wong, D.L. Sepsis. In *Nursing Care of Infants and Children* (2nd ed.). St. Louis Mosby, 1983, pp. 322–324.

Yabek, S.M. Management of septic shock. *Pediatric Review* 2(1980):83–87.

Acute Rheumatic Fever

Chernoff, H.L., & Kreidberg, M.B. Rheumatic fever. In Reece, R.M. (Ed.), *Manual of Emergency Pediatrics* (3rd ed). Philadelphia: W.B. Saunders, 1984, pp. 506–508.

Gewitz, M.H., & Vetter, V.L. Acute rheumatic fever. In Fleisher, G., & Ludwig, S. (Eds.), *Textbook of Pediatric Emergency Medicine*. Baltimore: Williams & Wilkins, 1983.

Huntington, J. Rheumatic fever and rheumatic heart disease. In Oakes, A.R. (Ed.), *Critical Care Nursing of Children and Adolescents*. Philadelphia: W.B. Saunders, 1981, pp. 135–36.

Pasternack, S.B., & Lybarger, P. Acute rheumatic fever. In Scipien, G.M. (Ed.), *Comprehensive Pediatric Nursing* (2nd ed.). New York: McGraw-Hill, 1979, pp. 671–674.

Whaley, L.F., Wong, D.L. Rheumatic fever. In *Nursing Care of Infants and Children* (2nd ed.). St. Louis: Mosby, 1983, pp. 1330–1335.

Meningitis

Anderson, K.M. Meningitis. In Scipien, G.M. (Ed.), *Comprehensive Pediatric Nursing*. New York: McGraw Hill, 1979, pp. 568–570.

Barkin, R.M., & Rosen, P. (Eds.). *Emergency Pediatrics*. St. Louis: Mosby, 1984.

Coffey, R.J. Pediatric neurological emergencies. *Topics in Emergency Medicine* July 1982, pp. 67–78.

Edwards, M.S., & Baker, C.J. Complications and sequelae of meningococcal infections in children. *Journal of Pediatrics* 99(1981):540–545.

Fleisher, G.R., & Ludwig, S. (Eds.). Infectious disease emergencies. *Textbook of Pediatric Emergency Medicine*. Baltimore: Williams & Wilkins, 1983, pp. 356–414.

Green, G.H. Management of the child with fever and infection. *Topics in Emergency Medicine* April 1981, pp. 19–42.

Jacob, J., & Kaplan, R.A. Bacterial meningitis. *American Journal of Diseases in Children* 131(1977):46–56.

Krugman, S., & Katz, L.L. *Infectious Diseases of Children* (7th ed.). St. Louis: Mosby, 1981.

Langner, B.E., & Schott, J.H. Nursing implications of central nervous system infections in children. *Issues in Comprehensive Pediatric Nursing* 2(1979):38–53.

McCracken, G.H. Neonatal septicemia and meningitis. *Hospital Practice* 11(1979):89–97.

Oppenheimer, E.Y., & Rosman, N.P. Meningitis. In Reece, R.M. (Ed.), *Manual of Emergency Pediatrics* (3rd ed.). Philadelphia: W.B. Saunders, 1984, pp. 189–198.

Overturf, S.D. Meningitis. *Topics in Emergency Medicine* April 1982, pp. 16–25.

Whaley, L.F., & Wong, D.L. *Nursing Care of Infants and Children* (2nd ed.). St. Louis: Mosby, 1983.

Encephalitis

Heiber, J.P. Encephalitis/meningitis. In Levin, D.L. (Ed.), *A Practical Guide to Pediatric Intensive Care*. St. Louis: Mosby, 1979.

Oakes, A.R. (Ed.). *Critical Care Nursing of Children and Adolescents*. Philadelphia: W.B. Saunders, 1981.

Packer, R.J., & Berman, P.H. Encephalopathy. In Fleisher, G., & Ludwig, S. (Eds.), *Textbook of Pediatric Emergency Medicine*. Baltimore: Williams & Wilkins, 1983, pp. 339–341.

Trump, C. Encephalitis. In Reece, R.M. (Ed.), *Manual of Emergency Pediatrics* (3rd ed.). Philadelphia. W.B. Saunders, 1984, pp. 132–135.

Whaley, L.F. & Wong, D.L. Encephalitis. In *Nursing Care of Infants and Children* (2nd ed.). St. Louis: Mosby, 1983.

Reye's Syndrome

Belkengren, R.P., & Sapala, S. Reye's syndrome: Clinical guidelines for practitioners in ambulatory care. *Pediatric Nursing* 7(1981):26–28.

Boutras, A.R., et al. Reye's syndrome: A predictable curable disease. *Pediatric Clinics of North America* 27(1980):539–552.

Budd, R., & Hobbell, E. Reye's syndrome. *Critical Care Nursing* 3(1983):94–97.

Dalgas, P. Reye's syndrome update. *Maternal Child Nursing Journal* 8(1983):345–349.

Dunne, R.S., & Perez, R.C. Reye's syndrome: A challenge not limited to critical care nurses. *Issues in Comprehensive Pediatric Nursing* 5 (July-August 1981):253–263.

Kolata, G.B. Reye's syndrome: A medical history. *Science* 207(1980):1453–1454.

Martelli, M.E. Reye's syndrome: An update. *Journal of Emergency Nursing* 10(1984):287–293.

Martelli, M.E. Teaching parents about Reye's syndrome. *American Journal of Nursing* 82(1982):260–263.

Miller, J., & Arensenault, L. Reye's syndrome.

Journal of Neurosurgical Nursing 15(1983):154–164.

Lovejoy, F.H., Smith, A.L., Wood, J.N., et al. Clinical staging in Reye's syndrome. *American Journal of Diseases in Children* 128(1974): 36–41.

Riordan, T.P. Reye's syndrome. *Critical Care Quarterly* 3(June 1980):9–25.

Shaywitz, B.A., et al. Monitoring and management of intracranial pressure in Reye's syndrome. *Pediatrics* 66(1980):198–202.

Trauner, D.A. Treatment of Reye's syndrome. *Journal of National Reye's Syndrome Foundation* 1(1980):85–89.

Whaley, L.F., & Wong, D.L. *Nursing Care of Infants and Children* (2nd ed.). St. Louis: Mosby, 1983.

EMERGENCY DEPARTMENT CARE GUIDE FOR THE CHILD WITH AN INFECTIOUS DISEASE

Nursing Diagnosis	Interventions	Evaluation
Hyperthermia related to infectious process	Identify source of fever Administer antipyretics as ordered Give tepid sponge bath to reduce fever Obtain necessary laboratory specimens Administer antibiotics as ordered	Child's body temperature returns to normal Source of fever and infection is identified Antibiotics are administered as soon as possible
Fluid volume deficit related to increased metabolic needs and decreased intake	Assess child's hydration status Administer intravenous fluids Carefully monitor fluid intake and output Monitor serum electrolytes	Child's skin turgor and mucus membranes indicate adequate hydration Serum electrolytes are within normal range
Alteration in patterns of urinary elimination: decreased urinary output	Measure urinary output Obtain urine-specific gravity	Urinary output remains adequate (> 1 ml/kg/hr)
Potential for infection of hospital staff, family members, and other patients in the emergency department	Isolate child with infectious disease from other patients in emergency department Utilize infectious disease precautions as indicated, such as masks, gowns, and secretion and excrement precautions	Other patients in emergency department remain free from exposure to infectious pathogens Emergency department staff utilize effective precautions

Nursing Diagnosis	**Interventions**	**Evaluation**
Knowledge deficit related to care of child with infectious disease	Carefully explain all procedures and treatments to parents Instruct parents in administration of antibiotics Teach parents methods of fever control Inform parents to return to emergency department or to telephone physician if child's condition worsens	Parents demonstate an understanding of all treatments and procedures Parents demonstrate an understanding of child's care at home

Instructions to Parents

INSTRUCTIONS TO PARENTS OF A CHILD WITH FEVER

When your child has a fever you can do several things to decrease the fever and to make your child more comfortable. Always remember that a fever is a sign that your child is ill. You should contact your doctor if your child's fever is high (greater than 102 degrees Fahrenheit) or persists for several days, if your child is under 6 months of age, or if your child appears ill to you.

To decrease your child's fever you should:

1. Remove any heavy clothing while indoors. Light clothing will allow heat to escape through the skin. Avoid wrapping the child in heavy blankets.
2. Give your child plenty of fluids. Drinking fluids is more important than eating when a child is ill. If your child also has vomiting or diarrhea, avoid fluids that are heavy, such as milk.
3. If your child's temperature is over 101 degrees Fahrenheit, you may give acetaminophen (Tylenol) in the following dosages:

Age	Dose of Tylenol
Under 6 months of age	Consult your physician
6 to 11 months	80 mg (½ tsp of elixir, 160/5 ml; or 0.8 ml dropperful)

Age	Dose of Tylenol
1 to 2 years	120 mg (¾ tsp of elixir, 160/5 ml; or 1.2 ml dropperful; or 1½ chewable tablets, 80 mg each)
2 to 3 years	160 mg (1 tsp of elixir, 160 mg/5 ml; or 1.6 ml dropperful; or 2 chewable tablets, 80 mg each)
4 to 5 years	240 mg (1½ tsp of elixir, 160/5 ml; or 2.4 ml dropperful; or 3 chewable tablets, 80 mg each)
6 to 8 years	320 mg (2 tsp of elixir, 160/5 ml; or 4 chewable tablets, 80 mg each)
9 to 10 years	400 mg (2½ tsp of elixir, 160/5 ml; or 5 chewable tablets, 80 mg each)
11 to 12 years	480 mg (3 tsp of elixir, 160/5 ml; or 6 chewable tablets, 80 mg each; or 1½ adult tablets, 325 mgs each)

4. If your child's temperature remains high, you may give your child a bath or sponge bath with lukewarm water for

10 to 15 minutes. Never use cold water or rubbing alcohol. Placing alcohol on your child's skin or in the bath water is dangerous, because the alcohol may be absorbed through the skin.

DISCHARGE INSTRUCTIONS FOR HEAD TRAUMA

Your child has suffered a head injury that may cause problems. The first 12 to 24 hours is the most crucial period. The first night following the injury or during his or her usual nap time you should be able to awaken your child easily every 2 to 3 hours. Please closely observe your child for the following warning signals. If any of these warning signals occur, *call your doctor* or the *emergency department*.

Warning Signals
1. Unusual sleepiness or excessive drowsiness
2. Repeated vomiting (more than once or twice)
3. Any problems with seeing (blurred vision), hearing, speaking, walking, or having trouble using his arms or legs
4. One pupil larger or different than the other
5. Severe headache occurs
6. Irregular or labored breathing
7. Convulsion or seizure (If a seizure occurs place your child on one side where he cannot fall. *Call an ambulance immediately.*)

Other instructions: _____

_____

Emergency department telephone number:

_____

Doctor's name: _____

Nurse's name: _____

Prepared by Nancy Sullivan Flint.

INSTRUCTIONS TO PARENTS OF A CHILD WITH CROUP

Your child has a virus that causes swelling of the voice box and other parts of the airway. This is called croup, and the swelling causes that harsh, barking cough. Because croup is a virus, there is no specific medicine for it. But there are some important things you can do at home to make your child's breathing easier and to help him or her rest.

1. Give lots of cold fluids, such as ice water, cold sodas, fruit juices, sherbet, Popsicles, or Jello.
2. Make a mist tent: using a cool mist vaporizer, point the mist at the child's crib. Add only water to the vaporizer. Attach a sheet across the top of the crib and let it hang down to cover the side opposite the vaporizer. This cool, damp air soothes the throat and keeps mucus loose. Use this day and night.
3. Use fever control if your child's temperature goes above 101 degrees Fahrenheit rectally.

Watch for other signs that mean the croup is getting worse:

1. Breathing becomes faster, noisier, or both.

2. A paleness or bluish color appears around the mouth, nose, eyes, or ears.
3. Coughing becomes more frequent, and the child is not able to rest well.
4. Your child will not take liquids or is drooling much more than usual.

Prepared by Anne Phelan.

5. The dents above the breast bone, below the breast bone, or in between the ribs become deeper.

If any of these things should happen, you should call your doctor or bring your child back to the emergency department. Save this paper, because your child may catch this virus again.

INSTRUCTIONS TO PARENTS OF A CHILD WITH PNEUMONIA

Your child has been found to have pneumonia. This means that a small part of one of the lungs has become congested with mucus. Many times medicines such as antibiotics are prescribed. If your doctor has given you a prescription, please make sure you understood how to use the medicine so that it will work most effectively.

There are other important things for you to do to help your child feel comfortable and to get better faster.

1. Give lots of fluids. Sick children often do not feel like eating solid foods and milk products may also be heavy on their stomachs. Fluids like fruit juices, soup broths, water, sodas, Jello, and Popsicles help to thin out and move the mucus out of the lung.
2. Use a cool mist vaporizer. Add only water to the vaporizer, and point it toward the head of the child's bed.
3. Do chest physical therapy. Position the child on his or her stomach with the shoulders a little lower than the waist. Make a cup with the palms of your hand and clap the child's back in the direction of the shoulder blades. Make sure your child's nurse has shown you this as well as different positions for drain-

ing different sections of the lung. With small children it is sometimes helpful to call this a coughing game to cough up and spit out the mucus. This should be done about every 4 hours while the child is awake.
4. Use fever control if your child's temperature goes over 101 degrees Fahrenheit, rectally or orally.

There are also some signs to watch for that mean the child's breathing is getting more difficult:

1. Breathing becomes faster, noisier, or both.
2. You notice a bluish or greyish color around the nose or mouth.
3. You can see dents above or below the breast bone or in between the ribs when the child breathes in.
4. The fever remains above 103 degrees Fahrenheit rectally, even after fever control.
5. The child won't drink fluids or starts to choke on liquids.
6. Vomiting occurs so often that the child cannot keep the medicine down.

If one or more of these things start to happen, you should call your doctor or bring your child back to the emergency department.

Prepared by Ann Phelan.

INSTRUCTIONS TO THE PARENTS OF A CHILD WITH A COLD

Your child has an upper respiratory tract infection, or cold. The cold is caused by a virus and must run its course. There is no specific medicine to cure a cold, but there are several things you can do to make your child more comfortable:

1. Fever control. Follow the instructions on the fever control sheet. Tylenol will also help the aches and pains.
2. Rest. Encourage quiet activities and frequent naps.
3. Fluids. Extra liquids help to thin out the mucus, keep fever down, and replace lost water.

Prepared by Anne Phelan.

4. A cool mist vaporizer may help to keep the mucus loose.
5. Babies need salt water nose drops and bulb suctioning to pull out mucus from the nose.
6. Cough syrups should usually not be used with children because the cough is the body's way of loosening mucus in the lungs.

   Call your doctor if the fever is high (over 102 degrees Fahrenheit rectally) and will not decrease with fever control, if the cough interferes with rest or drinking fluids, or if the child seems to get worse instead of better.

INSTRUCTIONS TO PARENTS OF A CHILD WITH ASTHMA

Your child has a breathing problem called asthma. This usually happens in children who have allergies or when there has been asthma in other family members. During an asthma attack the small breathing tubes in the lungs are squeezed tight, and extra mucus is made. This causes the child to have fast or noisy breathing. Older children may seem nervous and may be able to tell you that they can't breathe right. Asthma attacks can be caused by many different things; for example, exposure to something the child is allergic to, a cold or pneumonia, or an emotional upset. In children the most frequent cause is an allergy. If your child is over 4 years old, he or she should be tested to see what things he or she is allergic to.

You will most likely be given a prescription for a liquid, pills, or inhaler for your child to take at home. Please be sure

that the nurse or doctor has explained when and how to give the medicines. One of the important things to remember about asthma medicines is that they only stay in the blood stream for a certain length of time. If too much time passes before the medicine is given again, the wheezing can return.

Give your child plenty of fluids to drink. Milk and other thick liquids should be avoided. Clear liquids are best until the asthma attack has subsided.

Your should call your doctor or return to the emergency department if:

1. Your child begins to have wheezing when he or she has taken the asthma medicine.
2. Your child has persistent vomiting and is unable to keep the medicine down.

3. Your child is breathing fast or is using extra muscles to breathe (dents between ribs or above or below breast bone.)

4. Your child's lips or skin turn blue or gray.

Prepared by Ann Phelan.

INSTRUCTIONS FOR PARENTS OF A CHILD WITH BRONCHIOLITIS

Your child has a virus called bronchiolitis. This is why the baby's breathing is noisy (wheezing) and difficult. Since this is a virus, there is no special medicine that will make your child better. Bronchiolitis usually clears up very quickly about 3 days after the breathing trouble began. Even though there is no quick "cure," there are some important things you can do to help the baby breathe easier.

1. Give the baby lots of liquids. When children are sick they often do not feel like eating and milk may also be heavy for them. Offer your baby lots of juices, water, soup broth, flat sodas, or Jello water. Young babies should drink some Pedialyte or Lytren, a special mineral water.

2. Use a cool mist vaporizer. Add only water, and point it directly at the baby's crib. For extra relief you may turn on the warm water of the shower and let the bathroom fill with steam, then sit in the room with the child.

3. Have the baby lie on his or her stomach when sleeping. This helps push out the extra trapped air. No pillows are needed.

4. Keep the baby's nose clear. You can clean the nostrils with a cotton swab or use a suction bulb to pull out the mucus.

5. Use fever control if the baby's temperature reaches 101 degrees Fahrenheit or higher rectally.

There are also some things to watch for that mean the baby is having more trouble breathing:

1. Breathing is faster or noisier.
2. Small dents appear above, below, or in between the ribs when the baby breathes in.
3. There is a paleness or bluish-grey color around the nose and mouth.
4. The baby seems unable to relax or to sleep well.
5. The baby refuses or chokes on liquids.

If any of these things start to happen, call the doctor who saw your baby for this illness or bring your baby back to the emergency department.

Prepared by Anne Phelan.

INSTRUCTIONS TO PARENTS REGARDING ACCIDENTAL POISONINGS

Accidental poisoning is one of the leading causes of death in infants and small children. Many things that are used in the home can injure or even kill a child if they are swallowed.

These common household substances

are poisonous and should be kept locked away:

- Ammonia, bleach, detergents
- Drain and oven cleaners
- Furniture polish
- Soaps, shampoos
- Paints, paint thinner, turpentine
- Pesticides or rat poisons
- Cosmetics (including nail polish, removers, perfumes, permanent wave solutions)
- Alcoholic beverages
- Moth balls
- Medicines of all kinds, including over-the-counter drugs, vitamins, cough syrups

Poisoning can be prevented. Here are some things that you can do to protect your child:

1. Store all nonfood items in their original containers. Store them high in a locked cabinet or medicine chest, separated from food.
2. When your child must take medicine, never call it "candy."
3. Buy brands of products that have safety caps. Even if they have safety caps, lock them away in a safe place.
4. Be careful when visiting friends or family that your child does not have access to any of their medicines or household products.

Keep a bottle of Ipecac syrup in the house. It is the safest way to make a person vomit. It is also a poison, however, and should be used only when the poison control center or a medical person tells you to give it to your child.

Should a poisoning occur, take the following actions:

1. Try to determine what substance was swallowed.
2. *Immediately* call the Poison Control Center or your doctor for advice.
3. Save the poison container and a sample of the vomit, if any. During vomiting, turn head to the side.

Vomiting should not be induced if:

1. A corrosive such as lye or a strong acid has been swallowed; or
2. The child is drowsy, unconscious, or convulsing.

A child who has swallowed a poison is likely to attempt the same thing again within a year. Practice poison prevention.

Prepared by Elena Hopkins-Lotz.

Normal Pediatric Laboratory Values

HEMATOLOGY

Age	2 wk	1 mo	3 mo	6 mo	1 yr	2–6 yr	7–12 yr	Adult female	Adult male
Hemoglobin gm/dl	13–20	14–16	9.5–14.5	10.5–14	10.5–14	10.5–14	11.0–16.0	12.0–16.0	14.0–18.0
Hematocrit %	42–66	53	31–41	33–42	33–42	33–40	33–40	37–47	42–52
White Blood Cells per mm^3	5000–20,000	6000–18,000	6000–17,000	6000–16,000	6000–15,000	7000–13,000	5000–13,500	5000–10,000	5000–10,000
Polymorphonuclear Leukocytes %	40	30	30	45	45	45	55	55	55
Lymphocytes %	48	63	63	48	48	48	38	35	35
Eosinophils %	3	2	2	2	2	2	2	3	3
Monocytes %	9	5	5	5	5	5	5	7	7
Platelet Count	150,000–200,000	250,000	300,000	300,000	300,000	300,000	300,000	300,000	300,000

SERUM AND BLOOD CHEMISTRY

Test	Normal Values	Test	Normal Values
Albumin	3.8–5.0 g/dl	Glucose	Infants: 60–80 mg/dl
Alkaline phosphatase	Infants: 8–12 BU		Children: 90–125 mg/dl
	Children: 4–10 BU	Lead	< 20 μg/100 ml WB
Amylase	<150 units	Phosphorus	3.5–4.5 mg/dl
Bilirubin	Direct <0.4 mg/dl	Potassium (K)	3.5–4.5 mEq/L
	Total <1.0 mg/dl	Protein (total)	6–8 g/dl
BUN	Birth to 2 years: 5–15 mg/dl	Prothrombin time	12–15 seconds (depends on control)
	> 2 years: 10–20 mg/dl	SGOT	8–36 OD units
Calcium	9–11 mg/dl	SGPT	6–35 OD units
Chloride (serum)	95–110 mEq/L	Sodium	135–148 mEq/L
Cholesterol	150–250 mg/dl	Uric acid	3–5 mg/dl
Creatinine serum	1 to 5 years: 0.3–0.5 mg/dl 5 to 10 years: 0.5–0.8 mg/dl		

BLOOD GASES

Arterial	Venous
P_{O_2} Newborns 60 to 70 mm Hg Older children and adults 80 to 90 mm Hg P_{CO_2} 35 to 45 mm Hg pH 7.35 to 7.45	P_{O_2} 10 to 25 mm Hg P_{CO_2} 41 to 51 mm Hg pH 7.32 to 7.42

URINALYSIS

Test	Age	Normal Values	Test	Age	Normal Values
Microscopic			pH	Newborn/neonate	5–7
White blood cells	All ages	0–4/high-power field		Infants and children	4.8–7.8
Red blood cells	All ages	Rare/high-power field	Specific gravity	Newborn/infant	1.001–1.020
Casts	All ages	Rare/high-power field		Children	1.002–1.030
Osmolality	Premature and newborn	100–600 mosm/L			
	Infants and children	50–1400 mosm/L			

Recommended
Immunization Schedules

RECOMMENDED SCHEDULE FOR ACTIVE IMMUNIZATION
OF NORMAL INFANTS AND CHILDREN

Recommended Age	Immunization(s)	Comments
2 mo	DTP[a], OPV[b]	Can be initiated as early as 2 wk of age in areas of high endemicity or during epidemics
4 mo	DTP, OPV	2-mo interval desired for OPV to avoid interference from previous dose
6 mo	DTP (OPV)	OPV is optional (may be given in areas with increased risk of poliovirus exposure)
15 mo	Measles, mumps, rubella (MMR)[c]	MMR preferred to individual vaccines; tuberculin testing may be done
18 mo	DTP[d,e], OPV[e]	
24 mo	HBPV[f]	
4–6 yr[g]	DTP, OPV	At or before school entry
14–16 yr	Td[h]	Repeat every 10 yr throughout life

[a]DTP—Diphtheria and tenanus toxoids with pertussis vaccine.

[b]OPV—Oral, poliovirus vaccine contains attenuated poliovirus types 1, 2, and 3.

[c]MMR—Live measles, mumps, and rubella viruses in a combined vaccine.

[d]Should be given 6 to 12 months after the third dose.

[e]May be given simultaneously with MMR at 15 months of age.

[f]*Haemophilus* b polysaccharide vaccine.

[g]Up to the seventh birthday.

[h]Td—Adult tenanus toxoid (full dose) and diphtheria toxoid (reduced dose) in combination.

For all products used, consult manufacturer's package insert for instructions for storage, handling and administration. Biologics prepared by different manufacturers may vary, and those of the same manufacturer may change from time to time. The physician should therefore be aware of the contents of the package insert.

Reproduced with permission from the Report of the Committee on Infectious Diseases (20th ed.). Elk Grove Village, Ill.: American Academy of Pediatrics, 1986.

RECOMMENDED IMMUNIZATIONS SCHEDULES FOR CHILDREN NOT IMMUNIZED IN THE FIRST YEAR OF LIFE

Recommended Time	Immunization(s)	Comments
Children Less Than 7 Years Old		
First visit	DTP[a], OPV[b], MMR[c]	MMR if child ≥ 15 mo old; tuberculin testing may be done
Interval after first visit		
1 mo	HBPV[d]	For children 24–60 mo
2 mo	DTP, OPV	
4 mo	DTP (OPV)	OPV is optional (may be given in areas with increased risk of poliovirus exposure)
10–16 mo	DTP, OPV	OPV is not given if third dose was given earlier
Age 4–6 yr (at or before school entry)	DTP, OPV	DTP is not necessary if the fourth dose was given after the fourth birthday; OPV is not necessary if recommended OPV dose at 10–16 mo following first visit was given after the fourth birthday
Age 14–16 yr	Td[e]	Repeat every 10 yr throughout life
Children 7 Years Old and Older		
First visit	Td, OPV, MMR	
Interval after first visit		
2 mo	Td, OPV	
8–14 mo	Td, OPV	
Age 14–16 yr	Td	Repeat every 10 yr throughout life

[a]DTP—Diphtheria and tetanus toxoids with pertussis vaccine.

[b]OPV—Oral, poliovirus vaccine contains attenuated poliovirus types 1, 2, and 3.

[c]MMR—Live measles, mumps, and rubella viruses in a combined vaccine.

[d]*Haemophilus* b polysaccharide vaccine. Can be given, if necessary, simultaneously with DPT (at separate sites). The initial three doses of DTP can be given at 1- to 2-month intervals; so, for the child in whom immunization is initiated at 24 months old or older, one visit could be eliminated by giving DTP, OPV, MMR at the first visit; DTP and HBPV at the second visit (1 month later); and DTP and OPV at the third visit (2 months after the first visit). Subsequent DTP and OPV 10 to 16 months after the first visit are still indicated.

[e]Td—Adult tetanus toxoid (full dose) and diphtheria toxoid (reduced dose) in combination.

Reproduced with permission from the Report of the Committee on Infectious Diseases (20th ed.). Elk Grove Village, Ill.: American Academy of Pediatrics. 1986.

Anthropometric Charts

Anthropometric (growth) charts are important tools for determining if a child's height, weight, and head circumference are within the normal range for the child's age. Growth measurements are related to both genetic and environmental factors. Information on the parents' stature and weight is important when assessing a child's growth because heredity will play an important role in the child's growth pattern. Environmental factors that will influence a child's growth include psychosocial problems and feeding disorders and undernutrition. Some chronic illnesses also will interfere with normal growth and development.

For children 36 months old and younger, the child's length, weight, and head circumference are obtained and each plotted according to age on the chart of the correct gender. For children over 3 years of age, height and weight are plotted. The percentiles obtained for each measurement should be documented in the child's medical record.

Changes over time in percentile ranks are important clinical indicators. Height and weight measurements below the 10th percentile may be related to undernutrition and the child should be referred to his or her primary care provider for evaluation. Children with weights below the third percentile are often admitted to the hospital for evaluation. A head circumference that is found to be in a significantly higher or lower percentile than other measurements may indicate a neurological disorder and warrants an evaluation. Nonorganic failure-to-thrive is characterized by measurements in which weight is at a lower percentile rank than length and length is at a lower percentile rank than head circumference.

GIRLS: BIRTH TO 36 MONTHS PHYSICAL GROWTH NCHS PERCENTILES

NAME_____ RECORD #_____

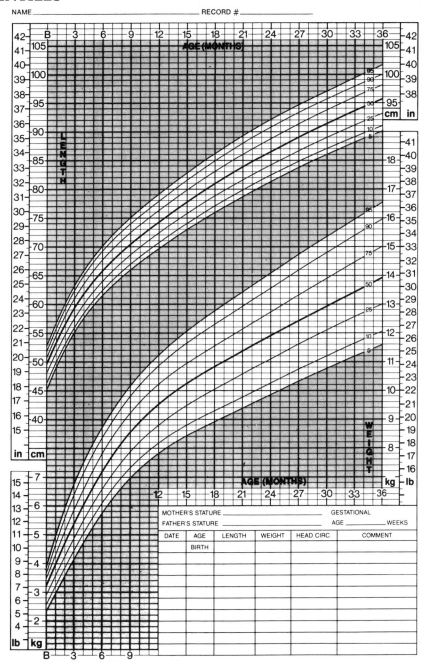

Adapted from P.V.V. Hammill, T.A. Drizd, C.L. Johnson, et al.: Physical growth: National Center for Health Statistics percentiles. American Journal of Clinical Nutrition 32(1979):607–609. Data from the Fels Longitudinal Study, Wright State University School of Medicine, Yellow Springs, Ohio. Courtesy of Ross Laboratories.

BOYS: BIRTH TO 36 MONTHS PHYSICAL GROWTH NCHS PERCENTILES

NAME_____ RECORD #_____

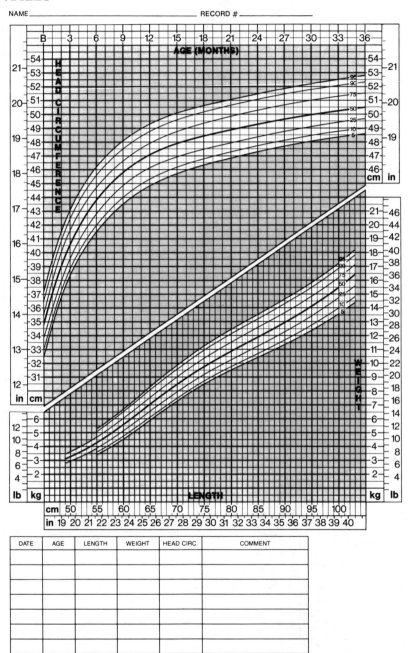

DATE	AGE	LENGTH	WEIGHT	HEAD CIRC.	COMMENT

Adapted from P.V.V. Hamill, T.A. Drizd, C.L. Johnson, et al.: Physical growth: National Center for Health Statistics percentiles. American Journal of Clinical Nutrition 32(1979):607–609. Data from the Fels Longitudinal Study, Wright State University School of Medicine, Yellow Springs, Ohio. Courtesy of Ross Laboratories.

GIRLS: BIRTH TO 36 MONTHS PHYSICAL GROWTH NCHS PERCENTILES

NAME _____ RECORD # _____

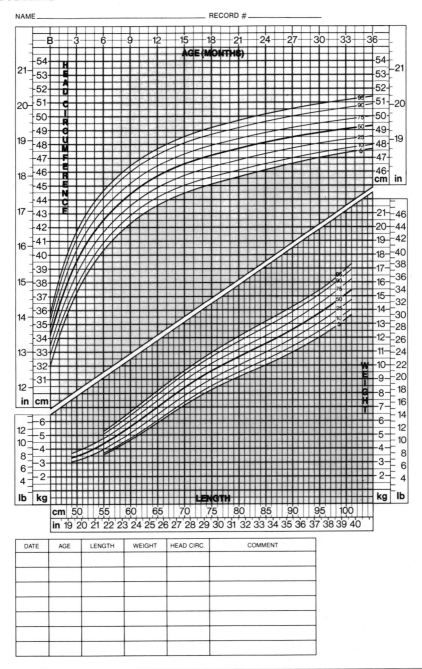

DATE	AGE	LENGTH	WEIGHT	HEAD CIRC.	COMMENT

Adpted from P.V.V. Hamill, T.A. Drizd, C.L. Johnson, et al.: Physical growth: National Center for Health Statistics percentiles. American Journal of Clinical Nutrition 32(1979):607–609. Data from the Fels Longitudinal Study, Wright State University School of Medicine, Yellow Springs, Ohio. Courtesy of Ross Laboratories.

BOYS: BIRTH TO 36 MONTHS PHYSICAL GROWTH NCHS PERCENTILES

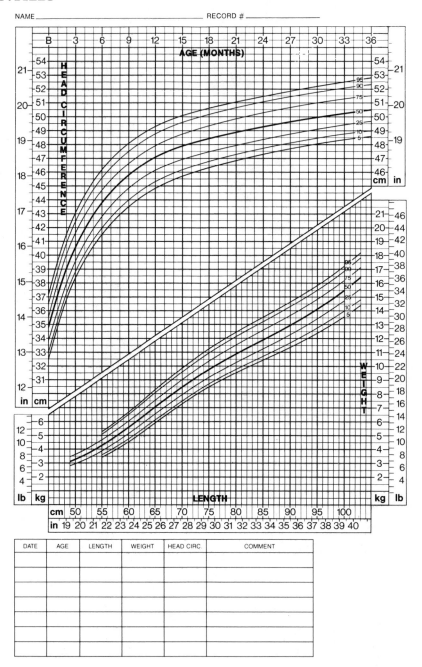

NAME_____   RECORD #_____

DATE	AGE	LENGTH	WEIGHT	HEAD CIRC	COMMENT

Adapted from P.V.V. Hamill, T.A. Drizd, C.L. Johnson, et al.: Physical growth: National Center for Health Statistics percentiles. American Journal of Clinical Nutrition 32(1979):607–609. Data from the Fels Longitudinal Study, Wright State University School of Medicine, Yellow Springs, Ohio. Courtesy of Ross Laboratories.

GIRLS: 2 TO 18 YEARS PHYSICAL GROWTH NCHS PERCENTILES

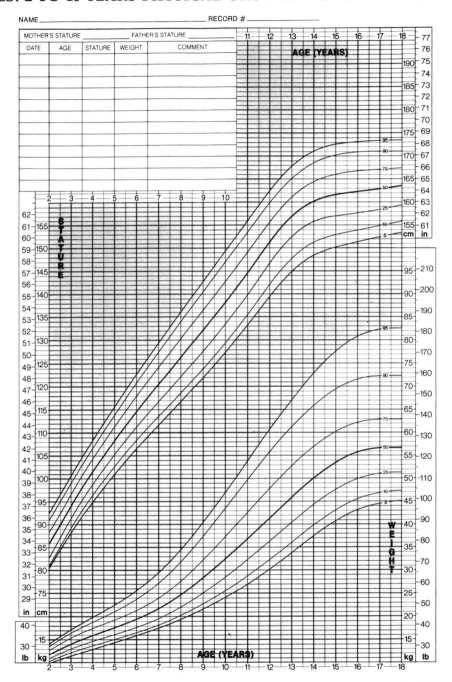

Adapted from P.V.V. Hamill, T.A. Drizd, C.L. Johnson, et al.: Physical growth: National Center for Health Statistics percentiles. American Journal of Clinical Nutrition 32(1979):607–609. Data from the National Center for Health Statistics (NCHS), Hyattsville, Md. Courtesy of Ross Laboratories.

BOYS: 2 TO 18 YEARS PHYSICAL GROWTH NCHS PERCENTILES

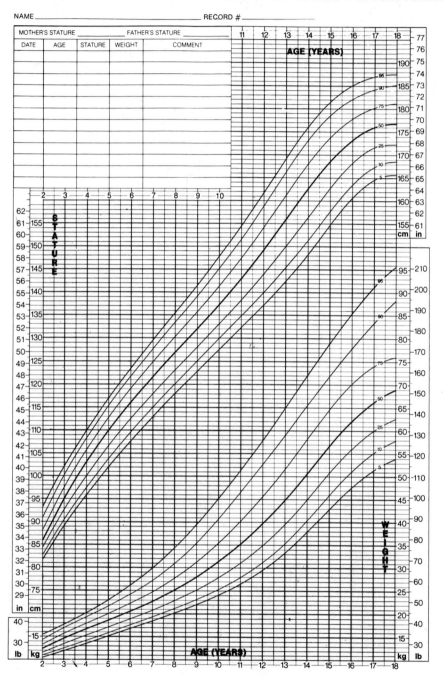

Adapted from P.V.V. Hamill, T.A. Drizd, C.L. Johnson, et al.: Physical growth: National Center for Health Statistics percentiles. American Journal of Clinical Nutrition 32(1979):607–609. Data from the National Center for Health Statistics (NCHS), Hyattsville, Md. Courtesy of Ross Laboratories.

GIRLS: PREBUBESCENT PHYSICAL GROWTH NCHS PERCENTILES

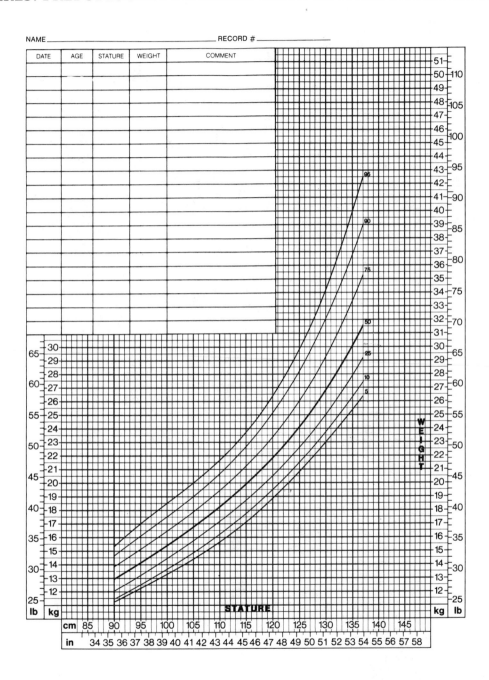

Adapted from P.V.V. Hamill, T.A. Drizd, C.L. Johnson, et al.: Physical growth: National Center for Health Statistics percentiles. American Journal of Clinical Nutrition 32(1979):607–609. Data from the National Center for Health Statistics (NCHS), Hyattsville, Md. Courtesy of Ross Laboratories.

BOYS: PREBUBESCENT PHYSICAL GROWTH NCHS PERCENTILES

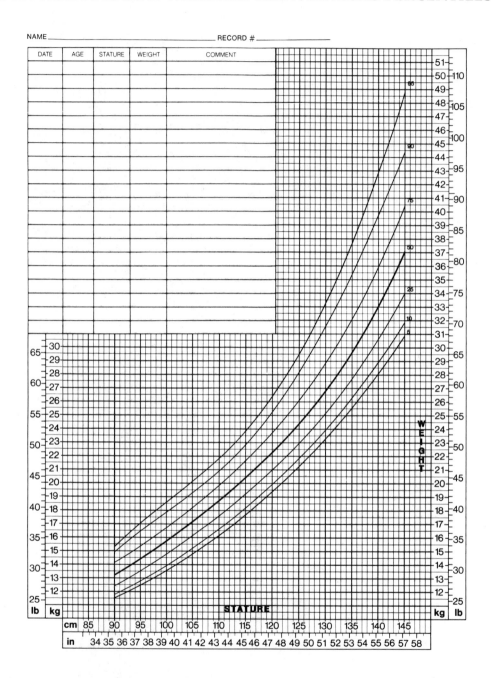

Adapted from P.V.V. Hamill, T.A. Drizd, C.L. Johnson, et al.: Physical growth: National Center for Health Statistics percentiles. American Journal of Clinical Nutrition 32(1979):607–609. Data from the National Center for Health Statistics (NCHS), Hyattsville, Md. Courtesy of Ross Laboratories.

Index

Page numbers followed by *f* refer to illustrations.
Page numbers followed by *t* refer to tables.

Page numbers followed by *f* refer to illustrations.
Page numbers followed by *t* refer to tables.

Page numbers followed by *f* refer to illustrations.
Page numbers followed by *t* refer to tables.

Page numbers followed by *f* refer to illustrations.
Page numbers followed by *t* refer to tables.

Page numbers followed by *f* refer to illustrations.
Page numbers followed by *t* refer to tables.

Page numbers followed by *f* refer to illustrations.
Page numbers followed by *t* refer to tables.

Page numbers followed by *f* refer to illustrations.
Page numbers followed by *t* refer to tables.

Page numbers followed by *f* refer to illustrations.
Page numbers followed by *t* refer to tables.

Page numbers followed by f refer to illustrations.
Page numbers followed by t refer to tables.